Affective Neuroscience

SERIES IN AFFECTIVE SCIENCE

Series Editors
Richard J. Davidson
Paul Ekman
Klaus Scherer

The Nature of Emotion: Fundamental Questions
Edited by Paul Ekman and Richard J. Davidson

Boo! Culture, Experience, and the Startle Reflex
by Ronald Simons

Emotions in Psychopathology: Theory and Research
Edited by William F. Flack, Jr. and James D. Laird

What the Face Reveals: Basic and Applied Studies of Spontaneous Expression Using the Facial Action Coding System (FACS)
Edited by Paul Ekman and Erika Rosenberg

Shame: Interpersonal Behavior, Psychopathology, and Culture
Edited by Paul Gilbert and Bernice Andrews

Affective Neuroscience: The Foundations of Human and Animal Emotions
by Jaak Panksepp

Extreme Fear, Shyness, and Social Phobia: Origins, Biological Mechanisms, and Clinical Outcomes
Edited by Louis A. Schmidt and Jay Schulkin

Cognitive Neuroscience of Emotion
Edited by Richard D. Lane and Lynn Nadel

The Neuropsychology of Emotion
Edited by Joan C. Borod

Anxiety, Depression, and Emotion
Edited by Richard J. Davidson

Persons, Situations, and Emotions: An Ecological Approach
Edited by Hermann Brandstätter and Andrzej Eliasz

Emotion, Social Relationships, and Health
Edited by Carol D. Ryff and Burton Singer

Appraisal Processes in Emotion: Theory, Methods, Research
Edited by Klaus R. Scherer, Angela Schorr, and Tom Johnstone

Music and Emotion: Theory and Research
Edited by Patrik N. Juslin and John A. Sloboda

Nonverbal Behavior in Clinical Settings
Edited by Pierre Philippot, Robert S. Feldman, and Erik J. Coats

Memory and Emotion
Edited by Daniel Reisberg and Paula Hertel

Psychology of Gratitude
Edited by Robert A. Emmons and Michael E. McCullough

Thinking about Feeling: Contemporary Philosophers on Emotions
Edited by Robert C. Solomon

Bodily Sensibility: Intelligent Action
by Jay Schulkin

Who Needs Emotions? The Brain Meets the Robot
Edited by Jean-Marc Fellous and Michael A. Arbib

Affective Neuroscience

The Foundations of Human and Animal Emotions

JAAK PANKSEPP

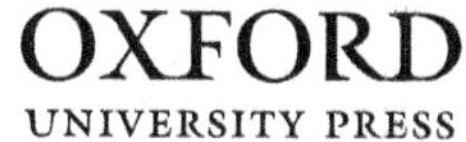
OXFORD
UNIVERSITY PRESS

OXFORD
UNIVERSITY PRESS

Oxford New York
Auckland Bangkok Buenos Aires Cape Town Chennai
Dar es Salaam Delhi Hong Kong Istanbul Karachi Kolkata
Kuala Lumpur Madrid Melbourne Mexico City Mumbai Nairobi
São Paulo Singapore Taipei Tokyo Toronto

Published by Oxford University Press, Inc.
198 Madison Avenue, New York, New York 10016

www.oup.com

First issued as an Oxford University Press paperback, 2005

Library of Congress Cataloging-in-Publication Data
Panksepp, Jaak.
Affective neuroscience : the foundations of human and animal emotions / Jaak Panksepp.
p. cm. — (Series in affective science)
Includes bibliographical references and indexes.
ISBN-13 978-0-19-517805-0 (pbk.)

1. Emotions. 2. Emotions and cognition. 3. Emotions—Social aspects. 4. Psychobiology. 5. Psychology, Comparative. I. Title. II. Series.
BF531.P35 1998
156′.24—dc21 98-15955

Printed in the United States of America
on acid-free paper

I dedicate this book to my lost child, Tiina, and my friend Anesa, who supported me when I was in need.

When the world came down upon me
and the sky closed like a door,
sounds filled my ears from far away.
I lay down on the floor.
And no one near could find me,
and nothing near was mine.
I sank into the floorboards
from the voices, soft and kind.
Until one thought got through to me,
one image filled my mind:
a pencil and a paper lying
close to hand, nearby.
Somehow I took them up and traced
one word and then the next,
until they linked together in a chain
that first perplexed the darkness
in my eyes, then,
rowing on my paper barque,
I soon was far away
and saw the water trail I'd left
rise up into a chain—
a ladder reaching high above
to light and sound and friends.
And that's how I climbed out
of the grief that has no end.

Anesa Miller,
A Road Beyond Loss, 1995

Preface

The Aims of This Book

This book was written with the student firmly in mind, but it is not a traditional textbook. It is an attempt to clarify the interrelations between brain and mind as expressed in the fundamental emotional processes that all mammals share. I will explore how our knowledge of the animal brain can help clarify the affective nature of the human mind and how our ability to appreciate the basic emotions of the human mind helps us understand the functional organization of the mammalian brain. This borderland of knowledge between the many disciplines that study the animal brain and the human mind—the various subareas of neuroscience and behavioral biology and the many schools of psychology and philosophy—should be rich in intellectual commerce. Unfortunately, this is not so. At present, these disciplines are only slowly being introduced to each other, like Europe and the Far East a millennium ago, and xenophobia prevails. Just as the trade routes between those distant cultures were opened slowly by explorers and adventurers, interchange between the disciplines that view human nature from above (i.e., the viewpoint of our recently evolved rational and cultural mind) and those that view it from below (the ancient networks of our brains) remains tortuous and unsatisfactory. This book offers one view of how the needed trade routes may be constructed in the area of emotions and motivations.

A motive of the old explorers was adventure under the guise of economics—the search for new vistas and knowledge in behalf of what is useful. The motives that underlie the writing of this book are the same. The aim is to enrich our knowledge about the brain/mind interface, but the more primal motive is the adventure of exploring uncharted spaces. At times, the conceptual paths of the brain/mind charts presented here will be like the routes on ancient maps that never really depicted the immensity of the journey. At present, ignorance is more abundant than knowledge in this field, often forcing me to oversimplify in order to formulate any coherent ideas and explanations at all. It will be a while before we have a true and lasting science of emotions as opposed to the fragmentary knowledge that now exists. But instead of just summarizing a patchwork of existing theories that are endemic in the field, I will aspire to provide a cohesive map to guide future navigations. We are still in the early stages of analyzing the psychobiology of emotions, and many additional generations of careful work will be needed before we have precise maps.

This book is dedicated to a new synthetic psychology of the future that will be more catholic than the present variants—one that will be built jointly on evolutionary, neuroscientific, behavioristic, affective, and cognitive foundations. I will attempt to take nature on its own terms by coming to grips with those intrinsic, ancient processes of the brain/mind that mediate between environmental events and the natural classes of action tendencies that animals spontaneously generate in the real world. The basic premise here is that the brain is a "symbolic organ" that reflects an evolutionary epistemology encoded in our genes. The mammalian brain not only represents the outside world in symbolic codes based on the properties of its sensory-perceptual systems but also has intrinsic operating systems that govern ingrained psychobehavioral tendencies for coping with those ever-present challenges that our ancestors confronted in their evolution. Many of these operating systems arouse emotional states, which are probably internally felt by other animals in ways not that different from humans. While modern neuroscience has achieved great success in deciphering the anatomical and physiological substrates of many sensory and motor processes at the neuronal level, it has made only a modest beginning in deciphering the functional characteristics of that "great intermediate net" that intervenes between inputs and outputs. Here, I advocate the position that many intervening neuropsychological processes, such as the basic emotions, can now be understood in neuroanatomical, neurophysiological, and neurochemical terms. But that level of understanding does require more theorizing and utilization of indirect evidence than is common in the field.

This new, integrative form of psychobiology is still in its early stages. Its development has been permitted only by the recent growth of neuroscience. The best evidence concerning emotional mechanisms has emerged largely from brain research on kindred animals such as birds, rats, guinea pigs, dogs, cats, and monkeys. Some comes from work on creatures even "lower" in the evolutionary "bush," and an ever-increasing amount is also now coming from studies of humans treated with various psychoactive drugs and hormones, as well as those with brain damage. We must use many sources of knowledge to reveal the nature of emotionality—what it really means to feel anger, fear, lust, joy, loneliness, happiness, and the various other desires and vexations of the human "heart."

In my more optimistic moments, I hope that the lines of evidence summarized here could serve as a foundation for a "new psychology" that recognizes that the discipline must be grounded on solid neuroscience foundations. Although psychology can continue to deal with the loftiest human aspirations, it also must become rooted in the evolutionary realities of the brain if it is to become a true science. But that metamorphosis will be a difficult one, since most of what psychologists do is not clearly linked to brain issues. Since few psychologists are doing brain research, it is hard to convince them that their thinking should be premised on a deep respect for and understanding of the organ of the mind. Substantive neurobiological offerings are still not part of the traditionally mandated curricular requirement of many psychology programs. All too often the neural facts are offered in such a dry manner that students shy away from immersion in such materials. My aim here has been to provide a treatment with a bit more literary merit than may be typical for a book of this type. I have aimed to maintain a friendly, readable style, in the hope of attracting the attention of many readers who truly wish to appreciate the underlying complexities of the human mind and to understand how our highest aspirations often remain tethered to the values elaborated by ancient parts of our animal brain.

I did choose to cast the present coverage in textbook format, with enough chapters for a typical semester, divided into convenient thirds. Although this type of course is not yet a traditional offering in psychology, I hope it will gradually emerge as one for advanced undergraduates and graduate students studying the psychology of emotions and motivations, as well as neuroscience and behavioral biology students who wish to have an appreciation of functional processes shared by all mammals. Also, the work will cover issues that should be essential for related disciplines such as neurophilosophy and biological psychiatry. In sum, I have tried to write a book for those interested in psychology who wish to know more about brain matters and for those interested in neurosciences who wish to know more about psychological matters. I have tried to write in such a way that little neuroscience or psychological background is necessary to follow the story lines. At times, the going may be difficult, especially when it comes to the essential background issues presented in Chapters 4–6 on neuroanatomy, neurophysiology, and neurochemistry. However, I trust that even the novice will find them reasonably interesting.

I have also sought to keep the lay reader in mind by including enough general material to make the more detailed materials worthy of continued attention. Many people are interested in gaining a new and better understanding of the evolutionary sources of the human mind, which must largely be obtained from brain research. Unfortunately, there are few places to go to obtain a substantive, yet interesting, coverage of emotional issues. Accordingly, in this book I have taken a conceptual approach as much as an empirical approach. This is also reflected in the referencing style, where I have tried to put ideas and carefully selected facts in the foreground and to leave personalities who have done the hard investigative work, as well as the myriad research details, in the background. I have used endnotes in preference to the traditional name-date approach. I mention names only when we encounter the work of investigators of considerable historical importance. However, the author index should allow effective retrieval of those whose work has been covered. Obviously, there exists much more raw material to be cited than I have chosen to cover. For instance, I recently received two reviews on two of the topics covered here, hypothalamic control of feeding and aggression, and each cited more than 1,000 original pieces of research. It would have been possible to cite thousands of references for every chapter of the book, but my aim, more than anything, was to generate a readable text. Thus, my strategy in referencing materials was to focus equally on review articles and research reports, with a view to maximizing the possibility that students could access related materials reasonably efficiently.

I have also tried to sustain a fairly natural style through the explicit recognition that we humans are storytelling creatures. Our cultural evolution (and perhaps even our cerebral evolution; see Appendix A) has been guided by aeons of sitting around campfires, sharing our deepest perspectives about the worlds in which we live. The best teaching must try to rekindle this spirit around the intellectual campfire of the modern classroom. Thus, one of my main goals is to encourage a renewed interest in the types of experimental inquiries that can take us toward a substantive understanding of how emotions are organized in the brain. Unfortunately, in the present scientific climate (where we often reward knowing more and more about less and less), there is remarkably little integrative work by active investigators in the field and remarkably little work on the psychobiology of emotions. Brain scientists are typically unwilling to use mentalistic words in discussing their empirical findings, and psychologists, because of their lack of training in the neurosciences, are typically unable to link their psychological concepts to brain functions. The present effort is based on the assumption that our ability to pursue such linkages, first verbally and then empirically, is essential for future scientific progress in understanding emotions. Accordingly, I have used the unusual literary device throughout this book of labeling major emotional systems in folk-psychological terms, using capitalized letters to highlight that I am focusing on certain necessary albeit not sufficient neural substrates for distinct types of emotional processes.

Our stories and our semantic habits have profound consequences for how we proceed in empirical inquiries, and as I will repeat, perhaps ad nauseum, there is really no other way to obtain biological knowledge about emotional matters except through arduous brain research (usually in other species), guided by meaningful psychological concepts. Thus, this book is written especially for those students who wish to bridge psychological and neurological issues in scientifically sound ways. For them, I have attempted to mill the abundant factual peppercorns into tempting conceptual spices. I have tried to make this difficult journey into the brain as stimulating as possible without doing injustice to the facts, even though I had to neglect many important lines of evidence to prevent the book from becoming too cumbersome. In any event, I hope that there are a number of students of philosophy, psychology, and the neurosciences who will find my efforts sufficiently refreshing and provocative that they will eventually set out on their own empirical journeys in search of answers to the many scientific questions that remain to be asked.

An Overview

This book is divided into three parts: (1) Background issues are discussed in Chapters 1–6, (2) the primitive emotions and motivations are covered in Chapters 7–11, and (3) the social emotions form the topic of Chapters 12–16.

In Part I, Chapters 1–3 will elaborate key concepts related to the functional systems in the brain and taxonomic issues. Chapters 4–6 offer an essential background for understanding the substantive individual topics covered in Parts II and III. Chapter 4 provides a relatively user-friendly summary of neuroanatomy, Chapter 5 touches upon relevant aspects of neurophysiology, and Chapter 6 addresses key neurochemical issues. These sections may be tough going for readers who have little knowledge of the brain, but I have tried to make them sufficiently concise and interesting that, after several readings, even a novice may gain a sense of mastery of the material. I have also tried to write so that experienced readers will enjoy them as thumbnail sketches of the enormous fields they are. Other basic background issues, such as the details of sensory and motor processes, will not be covered here, since they are peripheral to our major goal. I have also generally avoided peripheral autonomic and psychophysiological issues, which are typically well handled in many other basic physiological psychology and neuroscience texts.

In Part II of this book, I will discuss topics that are typically covered in most physiological psychology texts, but my approach will be atypical—it will focus not simply on basic behaviors but also on the probable affective consequences of these behaviors for the organism. In Chapter 7, I will discuss how sleep is organized in the brain and especially how dreaming may relate to the brain organization of emotionality. In Chapter 8, I will provide a new view of how so-called reward or reinforcement systems (i.e., those that animals like to "self-stimulate") participate in the organization of natural behaviors and mental life. The assertion will be that in both animals and humans, these brain systems control foraging, seeking, and positive expectancies rather than what is traditionally called pleasure. Chapter 9 will focus on how the body maintains certain constancies, such as of energy and water, through the auspices of pleasure and aversion mechanisms of the brain. I will discuss how such affective processes help inform animals of the homeostatic status of various bodily functions. Finally, Chapter 10 will focus on the nature of anger in the brain, and Chapter 11 will cover what we know about the brain mechanisms of fear.

Part III offers perspectives on the more subtle social emotions. I will discuss distinct topics in terms of the emotional cascade within the reproductive-developmental phase of the life cycle, starting with sexuality in Chapter 12, followed by nurturance and maternal behavior in Chapter 13, the sources of separation distress, grief, and social bonding in Chapter 14, the basic nature of playfulness in Chapter 15, and the most difficult topic of all, the nature of the self and higher mental processes in Chapter 16. With each successive chapter, we enter topics about which less and less is known, and all conclusions are accordingly more tenuous. Three key issues that did not fit well in the main text are placed in Appendixes A, B, and C: the first on human evolution, the second on the vagaries of human languages, as used in science (especially psychology), and finally a brief discussion of dualism in the brain and behavioral sciences.

In each chapter, I pay special attention to how our present knowledge may impact our understanding of emotional disorders. Throughout, animal and human issues will be blended. This attempt at simplification is a strategy that assumes that an understanding of the similarities will take us toward important scientific insights that can have a positive impact on human welfare more rapidly than a focus on the all-pervasive differences among species.

Acknowledgments

I have tried to steer a middle course between the various polar views that presently characterize different schools of psychology. My attempt at a synthesis is bound to receive some criticism from colleagues who have strong antireductionist biases, for many still do not feel comfortable trying to explain complex psychological phenomena in neurological terms. My approach may also go against the grain of a long-standing tradition in behavioral neuroscience, which mandates that we should not talk about processes that we cannot see with our eyes. Several good friends and scientific colleagues warned me of the dangers in such an enterprise, but ultimately they all encouraged me to proceed. They did this with even greater urgency as, during the middle of the present efforts, I underwent the most painful time of my life: My precious daughter, Tiina Alexandra, died along with three friends, on a dismal Good Friday evening in 1991 when a drunken driver, evading arrest, careened into their car. After that event, my spirit was demoralized, and I could not face the labors of this book for several years. Through the magic of friends and modern psychiatric drugs, my spirits were partially restored. In the fall of 1993, I restarted the project and eventually devoted renewed energies to these labors in loving memory of my daughter. My Tiina was an emotionally rich child who did not hesitate to share her true feelings with others. I recall a conversation I had with Tiina concerning human emotions almost two decades ago, when I was first attempting to summarize the issues that are the foundation of this book, "Toward a General Psychobiological Theory of Emotions,"

Behavioral and Brain Sciences 5 (1982): 407–467). I recorded the following conversation in that article:

> To shed more light on the issue, I turned from my desk to my six-year-old daughter playing at my feet.
>
> "Tiina, can you tell me something? [She looks up agreeably.] How many emotions are there?"
>
> "What's an emotion?" she queries.
>
> "Mm . . . it's the way we feel. How many different ways can we feel?"
>
> She places a finger to her lips and looks briefly puzzled, and then rattles off, "Happy, mad, sad. . . . Is that right, Daddy?"
>
> "I'm not sure—you tell me. Are there any more?"
>
> "Mm, yes, yes, scared! Is that right?"
>
> "You tell me."
>
> "Mm . . . mm . . . mm . . . frowned? Are there any more?" [She is beginning to look exasperated.]
>
> "Hey, that's really good. Can you show me all those in faces?"
>
> As I say "happy," she smiles and jumps up and down clapping her hands; as I say "mad," she frowns, clenches her jaw, and more or less growls at me; as I say "sad," she pantomimes the mask of tragedy; as I say "scared," she retracts her torso, balloons her eyes, and shows a frightened mouth; as I say "frowned," she looks puzzled, scratches her head a little, and finally crunches her face in a way that communicates little to me. (p. 455)

Thanks, Tiina, wherever your spirit may be!

Many others along the way have helped me better understand the nature of emotions and the nature of the scientific enterprise that must be pursued in order to understand the deep, neurological nature of human emotionality. Foremost among those have been the writings of Paul MacLean and students, too numerous to mention, who have joined me in classes and laboratories to explore the nature of emotions. Irreplaceable advice, assistance, and perspective taking have been provided by several close colleagues at Bowling Green State University—especially Pete Badia, Vern Bingman, Bob Conner, Kevin Pang, and John Paul Scott—as well as visiting scholars and friends who came to BGSU to work and talk with me about emotional issues, especially Bruce Abbott, Manfred Clynes, Dwight Nance, and John Jalowiec, who provided insightful input on an entire early version of this manuscript. Lonnie Rosenberg did most of the very fine artwork in this book; the rest was done by myself and several graduate students. I have been fortunate to have had many outstanding investigators who have shared an interest in my work, most especially the editors of Oxford University Press's Series in Affective Science—Richie Davidson, Paul Ekman, and Klaus Scherer. They, along with other colleagues of the core faculty of the ongoing National Institute of Mental Health Postdoctoral Training Program on Emotion Research, are foremost among the scholars who are presently revitalizing emotion research around the world.

Several times I have used drafts of this book for teaching purposes at BGSU and the University of Salzburg, Austria. I wish to thank my hosts in Austria—Guenther Bernatzky and Gustav Bernroider of the Institute of Zoology, Wolfgang Klimesch of the Institute of Psychology, and Patrick Lensing of School Psychology of Upper Austria—for helping create an excellent environment for trying out new ideas. I also thank Joan Bossert and the other good people at Oxford University Press, who were patient and encouraging in my protracted struggle to get this project completed.

However, without a muse and a kindred spirit, all this would not have happened. Dr. Anesa Miller, my wife, supported me well in the many roles that were needed to sustain these efforts—providing emotional support, critical feedback, and her special worldview, poetry, and music as needed. She read most of this book several times and provided endless suggestions on how to make a better, more understandable manuscript. She helped sharpen my thinking and brought clarity to many jumbled words. The readability of this work was enhanced enormously by her remarkable linguistic skills and her sense of beauty, meaning, and personal integrity. Much of this help was provided during a period when her own creative fires were also burning intensely. The book of poetry she wrote to commemorate the tragic passages of our lives—*A Road Beyond Loss* (1995, published by the Memorial Foundation for Lost Children, Bowling Green, Ohio)—is an incomparable expression of the emotions we all experience in times of grief. I thank you, Anesa, for your special help, and I value you for the remarkable person that you are.

To the extent that semantic ambiguities and opacity of thought still abide on these pages, I sincerely apologize, for I have labored earnestly to get at the truth and to convey it more clearly than is possible in this difficult area of human knowledge.

Bowling Green, Ohio J. P.
September 1996

Illustration and Production Credits

The illustrations for this text were constructed with the help of several students and a professional artist, Lonnie Rosenberg, who prepared from my rough sketches and photographs figures 2.7, 3.6, 3.7, 4.8, 4.9, 4.11, 5.3, 8.6, 10.2, 10.5, 10.6, 10.9, 11.2, 12.1, 13.3, 14.9, 14.10, 15.2, 15.6, and B.1. Help with some of the other figures graciously came from Marni Bekkedal (figures 12.2, 12.3, and 12.4), Charles Borkowski (figures 1.2, 1.4, 2.5, 2.6, and 8.3), Meliha Duncan (figures 3.1, 3.2, and 6.3), Barbara Herman (Figure 14.4), and Brian Knutsen (Figure 14.1). The photographs used in Figure 5.4 were generously provided by Dr. Gordon Harris and those in Figure 15.7 by Dr. Steve Siviy. The remaining illustrations, some from previously published works, were done by the author.

The sources for all figures that were redrawn from published data are aknowledged in the figure legends. Ideas for some of the anatomical plates were drawn and modified from other published works, but I will not attempt to trace the confluence of sources; however, I would like to thank all of the original investigators, authors, and illustrators for their high-quality work. Some of the remaining items that are derived directly from the original artwork that I prepared for some of my previously published works were utilized with the publisher's permission, as needed. Certain publishers (e.g., Academic Press) no longer require authors to obtain permission to reuse their own illustrations in subsequent works, and I thank them for having adopted this rational policy. I thank several other publishers for providing permission to reuse some of my previously published illustrations. They are as follows:

Figures 6.6, 7.3, 8.2, 8.3, 9.1, and 10.1 (for full reference, see chap. 3, n. 25) were slightly modified from the work cited in the legends. These adaptations are used with permission, courtesy of Marcel Dekker, Inc.

Figures 3.4 and 3.5 (for full reference, see chap. 3, n. 26) are slightly modified versions of figures that appeared in the work cited in those figure legends. They are adapted, with permission, courtesy of Cambridge University Press.

I would also like to acknowledge the help of Nakia Gordon for preparing the author index for this volume; Anesa Miller, for helping me proof the text; and Will Moore of Oxford University Press, who superbly handled many of the technical details on the publisher's side. Many thanks to everyone that lent a hand on this project.

Contents

Affective Neuroscience

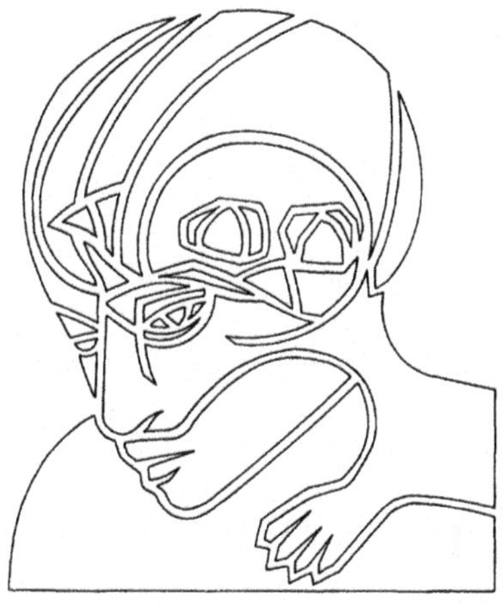

PART I

Conceptual Background

A Suggested Paradigm for the Study of Emotions

To understand the basic emotional operating systems of the brain, we have to begin relating incomplete sets of neurological facts to poorly understood psychological phenomena that emerge from many interacting brain activities. I will first lay out an overall strategy (Chapter 1), then argue why we should accept the existence of various intrinsic psychobehavioral systems in the brain (Chapter 2), and then try to identify the major emotional systems that exist as the genetic birthright of each individual (Chapter 3). At the outset, we must also dwell on many brain facts, including ones neuroanatomical (Chapter 4), neurophysiological (Chapter 5), and neurochemical (Chapter 6), and then, through successive approximations, examine the functional characteristics of the major emotional systems of the brain (the rest of the book).

The use of carefully chosen animal models in exploring the underlying brain processes is essential for making substantive progress. Even with recent advances in functional brain imaging and clinical psychopharmacology, the human brain cannot be ethically studied in sufficient detail to allow the level of analysis needed to understand how emotional systems actually operate. Although emotional circuits, as many other brain systems, exhibit considerable plasticity during the life span of organisms, the initial issue is identification of the genetically dictated emotional operating systems that actually exist in the brain. Such systems allow newborn animals to begin responding coherently to the environments in which they find themselves. There is little doubt that all of the systems I discuss in this book actually exist in both animal and human brains—those for dreaming, anticipation, the pleasures of eating as well as the consumption of other resources, anger, fear, love and lust, maternal acceptance, grief, play, and joy and even those that represent "the self" as a coherent entity within the brain. The doubts that we must have concern their precise nature in the brain.

Because of the provisional nature of our current knowledge, the present synthesis entails necessary simplifications. My main concern, as I undertake these descriptions of brain emotional systems, is that I am trying to impose too much linear order upon ultracomplex processes that are essentially "chaotic" (in the mathematical sense of nonlinear dynamics). I look forward to a day when the topics discussed herein can be encompassed within the conceptual schemes of sophisticated dynamic approaches. The basic emotional systems may act as "strange attractors" within widespread neural networks that exert a certain type of "neurogravitational force" on many ongoing activities of the brain, from physiological to cognitive. Unfortunately, at present we can utilize such dynamic concepts only in vague metaphoric ways.

Although the various forms of emotional arousal do many things in the brain, one of the most important and most neglected topics in neuroscience is the attempt to understand how emotional feelings are generated. An attempt to grapple with this issue is one of the main goals of this text. Although most of the critical evidence remains to be collected, I will try to deal with this difficult problem in a forthright manner. I will accept the likelihood that other animals do have internal feelings we commonly label as emotions, even though the cognitive consequences of those states probably vary widely from species to species. This empirically defensible assumption will allow me to utilize information derived from simpler brains to highlight the fundamental sources of affective experiences in humans. This is not to deny that much of cognitive as well as emotional processing in the brain transpires at a subconscious level but to assert that basic, internally experienced affective states do have an important function in determining how the brain generates behavior and that other animals probably have internally experienced feelings.

In asserting the above, I should emphasize that the complexity of the human brain, especially at its highest neocortical reaches, puts all other brains "to shame." The human brain can generate many thoughts, ideas, and complex feelings that other animals are not capable of generating. Conversely, other animals have many special abilities that we do not have: Rats have a richer olfactory life, and eagles have keener eyes. Dolphins may have thoughts that we can barely fathom. But the vast differences in cognitive abilities among species should not pose a major difficulty for the present analysis, for the focus here will be mainly on those ancient subcortical operating systems that are, to the best of our knowledge, homologous in all mammals. Although detailed differences in these systems exist across species, they are not sufficiently large to hinder our ability to discern general patterns.

In short, many of the ancient, evolutionarily derived brain systems all mammals share still serve as the foundations for the deeply experienced affective proclivities of the human mind. Such ancient brain functions evolved long before the emergence of the human neocortex with its vast cognitive skills. Among living species, there is certainly more evolutionary divergence in higher cortical abilities than in subcortical ones. Hence cognitive subtleties that can emerge from the shared primitive systems interacting with more recently evolved brain areas will receive little attention here. An analysis of those issues will require the types of conceptualizations presently being generated by *evolutionary psychologists*. The species differences in those higher functions are bound to be more striking than the differences in the nature of the basic emotional systems that will be the focus of discussion here. However, to the extent that the subcortical functions are shared, we can create a general foundation for all of psychology, including evolutionary psychology, by focusing on the shared emotional and motivational processes of the mammalian brain. These systems regrettably have been neglected by mainstream psychology.

Why has it taken us so long to recognize the general organizational principles for mind and behavior that are found within the primitive genetically dictated areas of the brain that all mammals share? It is partly because the actions of those ancient brain systems are very difficult to see clearly within our own behavior patterns, especially through the complex cognitive prisms of the human cortex that generate subtle behavioral strategies and layers of learning and culture that are uniquely human. It is partly because until recently we simply did not know enough about the brain to have any confidence in such generalizations. However, it is also because for a long time, 20th century psychology insisted that we should seek to explain everything in human and animal behavior via environmental events that assail organisms in their real-life interactions with the world rather than via the evolutionary skills that are constructed in their brains as genetic birthrights.

The Relationship between "Affective Neuroscience" and Related Disciplines

In the following chapters, I will try to come to terms with the ancient psychobiological processes that emerge from ancient brain activities. This simply cannot be done using a single disciplinary approach. It is essential to synthesize behavioral, psychological, and neurological perspectives. Many disciplines are contributing facts that are useful for achieving the needed synthesis, but there is presently no umbrella discipline to bridge the findings of animal behaviorists, the psychological basis of the human mind, and the nature of neural systems within the mammalian brain. Many come close, but none takes all three levels of analysis seriously. The discipline of *ethology* has dealt effectively with many of the relevant instinctual behavior patterns, but until quite recently it had not delved deeply into the brain mechanisms or neuropsychological processes that generate those behaviors. *Behaviorism* has dealt credibly with the modification and channeling of behavior patterns as a function of learning, but it has not dealt effectively with the nature of the innate sources of behavioral variation that are susceptible to modification via the reinforcement contingencies of the environment. The various *cognitive sciences* are beginning to address the complexities of the human mind, but until recently they chose to ignore the evolutionary antecedents, such as the neural systems for the passions, upon which our vast cortical potentials are built and to which those potentials may still be subservient. It is also refreshing to see that growing numbers of investigators are advocating greater focus on animal cognitions and consciousness, although few have chosen to grapple with the nature of emotional experience and emotional processes at a primary-process neurobiological level. *Sociobiology* and, more recently, *evolutionary psychology* have woven fascinating and often exasperating stories concerning the distal (ancient, evolutionary) sources of human and animal behaviors, but they have yet to deal effectively with the proximal neural causes of those behavior patterns. *Clinical psychology* and *psychiatry* attempt to deal at a practical level with the underlying disturbances in brain mechanisms, but neither has an adequate neuroconceptual foundation of the sources of emotionality upon which systematic understanding can be constructed.

In other words, something is lacking. I would suggest that a missing piece that can bring all these disciplines together is a neurological understanding of the basic emotional operating systems of the mammalian brain and the various conscious and unconscious internal states they generate. This new perspective, which I have chosen to call *affective neuroscience*, may be of some assistance to the growing movement in philosophy to bring neurological issues to bear on the grand old questions concerning the nature of the human mind. I look forward to the day when *neurophilosophy* (as heralded in a book by that name written by Pat Churchland in 1985) will become an experimental discipline that may shed new light on the highest capacities of the human brain—yielding new and scientific ways to talk about the human mind. Parts of this book may serve as a foundation for such future efforts.

Despite its claim to a new view among the psychological sciences, *affective neuroscience* is deeply rooted within *physiological psychology*, *behavioral biol-*

ogy, and the modernized label for all of these disciplines: *behavioral neuroscience*. The present coverage will rely heavily on data collected by individuals in these fields, but it will put a new twist on the evidence. It reinterprets many of the brain-behavior findings to try to account for the central neuropsychic states of organisms. It also accepts the premise that most animals—certainly all mammals—are "active agents" in their environments and that they have at least rudimentary representations of subjectivity and a sense of self. With such assumptions, we can create a more realistic and richer science by recognizing the number of basic processes we share with our kindred animals.

Progress in affective neuroscience will be critically dependent on the development and use of compelling experimental models. Obviously, to do this we must exploit other animals. This leads me to briefly confront, at the very outset, the troublesome issue of ethics in animal research. Because of such issues, animal brain research has diminished markedly in university departments of psychology throughout the United States. While the animal rights movement applauds such change, some of us feel that it compromises the future development of substantive knowledge about the deep sources of human nature that can help promote both human and animal welfare. It can also reduce zoophobia in the human sciences.

On the Decline of Animal Research in Academic Psychology

For various reasons, the amount of animal brain research, as a percentage of research being done in psychology departments of American universities, has diminished markedly over the last few decades. This has occurred for several reasons: because of the difficulty of such research, because more and more psychologists do not appreciate the relevance of this type of research for understanding human problems, and because of a new wave of ethical considerations and regulations promoted by individuals who have grave concerns about the propriety of doing experimental work on captive animals. It is this last issue that has become a vexing concern for biologists, neuroscientists, and many others who wish to study animals, either out of pure curiosity or from a desire to understand aspects of the human mind and body that cannot be understood in any other way.

Although the ethics of using animals in research has been debated with increasing fervor, it is certain that our knowledge of the human brain and body would be primitive were it not for such work. Without animal research, many children would still be dying of juvenile diabetes and numerous other diseases. However, it would be foolish to deny that much of this research has, indeed, caused distress in animals. For that reason, some biologically oriented investigators may not want to deal forthrightly with the nature of animal emotions and subjectivity. However, I believe that most brain scientists support the humane treatment of their animal subjects, even as they make the necessary ethical compromises to obtain new knowledge. Most investigators regard their subjects as fellow animals who deserve their full respect and care.

Since this book seeks to deal with the reality of emotions in the animal and human brain, it is important to clarify my personal position on the propriety of animal brain research at the outset. I will do this in the form of an "Afterthought"—a stylistic medium I will use throughout this book. "Afterthought" is not meant to imply that the material is not important. It is used to give focused attention to key issues, especially historical or conceptual ones, that do not fit well in the main text.

Indeed, the "Afterthoughts" will often highlight the most critical issues, such as the following concern that all sensitive people must have about biological research on live animals.

AFTERTHOUGHT: A Brief Discussion of the Ethics of Animal Research

I summarized my side of the debate over animal research at a conference entitled "Knowledge through Animals" at the University of Salzburg (September 23, 1992). Let me share the abstract of that presentation, which was entitled "Animals and Science: Sacrifices for Knowledge." It is a viewpoint that permeates this book and summarizes my personal research values.

> The debate over the use of live animals in behavioral and biomedical research cannot be resolved by logic. It is an emotional issue which ultimately revolves around the question of whether other animals affectively experience the world and themselves in a way similar to humans—as subjectively feeling, sentient creatures. The topic of subjectivity is one that modern neuroscience has avoided. It is generally agreed that there are no direct, objective ways to measure the subjectivity of other animals, nor indeed of other humans. Only their words and actions give us clues about their inner experiences. But if we consider actions to be valid indicators of internal states in humans, we should also be ready to grant internally experienced feelings to other animals. Indeed, it is possible that the very nature of the brain cannot be fathomed until neuroscience comes to terms with this potential function of the nervous system—the generation of internal representations, some of which are affectively experienced states which establish value structures for animals. A balanced evaluation of the evidence, as well as a reasonable evolutionary account of the nature of the mammalian brain, support the conclusion that other animals also have what may be termed "emotional feelings." Accordingly, our research enterprises with animals should recognize this fact, and aspire to new levels of sensitivity that have not always characterized animal research practices of the past. The practice of animal research has to be a trade-off between our desire to generate new and useful knowledge for the betterment of the human condition, and our wish not to impose stressors on other creatures which we would not impose on ourselves. Those who pursue animal research need to clearly recognize these trade-offs, and address them forthrightly. Indeed, a clearer recognition of these issues may have benefits for certain areas of investigation, such as behavioral brain research, by promoting more realistic conceptions of the nature of brain mechanisms that have long been empirically neglected (e.g., the emotions). It may also promote heightened respect for the many creatures we must study if we are to ever understand the deeply biological nature of human values.

Although animal research will surely not reveal why humans have strong emotions regarding issues such as abortion, rape, and the many civil injustices that still characterize our society and our world, it can provide a substantive answer to questions such as what it means to be angry, scared, playful, happy, and sad. If we understand these important brain processes at a deep neurobiological level (an end result that can be achieved only with animal brain research), we will better understand the fundamentally affective nature of the human mind. Thereby, we will also be in a better position to help animals and humans who are in emotional distress. The aim of this book is to nurture the growth of such knowledge.

1

Affective Neuroscience

History and Major Concepts

Literary intellectuals at one pole—at the other scientists. . . . Between the two a gulf of mutual incomprehension—sometimes (particularly among the young) hostility and dislike, but most of all lack of understanding. They have a curious distorted image of each other. Their attitudes are so different that, even on the level of emotion, they can't find much common ground.

C. P. Snow, *Two Cultures and the Scientific Revolution* (1959)

The "emotions" are excellent examples of the fictional causes to which we commonly attribute behavior.

B. F. Skinner, *Science and Human Behavior* (1953)

CENTRAL THEME

Our emotional feelings reflect our ability to subjectively experience certain states of the nervous system. Although conscious feeling states are universally accepted as major distinguishing characteristics of human emotions, in animal research the issue of whether other organisms feel emotions is little more than a conceptual embarrassment. Such states remain difficult—some claim *impossible*—to study empirically. Since we cannot directly measure the internal experiences of others, whether animal or human, the study of emotional states must be indirect and based on empirically guided theoretical inferences. Because of such difficulties, there are presently no direct metrics by which we can unambiguously quantify changes in emotional states in any living creature. All objective bodily measures, from facial expressions to autonomic changes, are only vague approximations of the underlying neural dynamics—like ghostly tracks in the bubble chamber detectors of particle physics. Indeed, all integrative psychological processes arise from the interplay of brain circuits that can be monitored, at present, only dimly and indirectly. Obviously, a careful study of behavioral actions is the most direct way to monitor emotions. However, many investigators who study behavior have argued that emotions, especially animal emotions, are illusory concepts outside the realm of scientific inquiry. As I will seek to demonstrate, that viewpoint is incorrect. Although much of behavioral control is elaborated by unconscious brain processes, both animals and humans do have similar affective feelings that are important contributors to their future behavioral tendencies. Unfortunately, the nature of human and animal emotions cannot be understood without brain research. Fortunately, a psychoneurological analysis of animal emotions (via a careful study of how animal brains control certain behaviors) makes it possible to conceptualize the basic underlying nature of human emotions with some precision, thereby providing new insights into the functional organization of all mammalian brains. A strategy to achieve such a cross-species synthesis will be outlined here. It is based largely on the existence of many psychoneural homologies—the fact that the intrinsic nature of basic emotional systems has been remarkably well conserved during the course of mammalian evolution. Although there is a great deal of diversity in the detailed expressions of these systems across species, the conserved features allow us to finally understand some of the fundamental sources of human nature by studying the animal brain.

Do Psychologists Need to Understand Emotions to Understand Behavior? Do Neuroscientists Need to Understand Emotions to Understand the Brain?

Imagine an archetypal interaction: A cat is cornered by a dog. The cat hisses, its body tensely arched, hairs on end, ears pulled back. If the dog gets too close, the cat lashes out, claws unsheathed. If we could see the cat's heart, it would be pounding "a mile a minute." The dog barks loudly, bounding forward and backward, but coming only so close, as not to get slashed by the cat. What is motivating their behavior? "Fear" and "anger" might be a satisfactory answer in everyday terms. A slightly more sophisticated explanation might be that the dog's initial attack was produced by the anticipation of a good chase, but the cat's affective defenses successfully thwarted the dog's intentions and provoked frustration. That really aroused the dog's ire and got emotional volleys of anger and fear bouncing back and forth.

Although such everyday instinctual, emotional, and mentalistic descriptions were used widely by psychologists in the early years of the 20th century, they soon came to be regarded as unsatisfactory scientific explanations of behavior. What does it mean to be angry or scared, to have anticipations, frustrations, and intentions? Investigators began to realize that it adds little to our scientific understanding to try to explain something observable—namely, behavior—in terms of feelings and thoughts that could not be directly observed. To this day, such mental states are still not generally accepted as credible *scientific* explanations of animal actions, even though they remain widely used as everyday "explanations" for the many impulsive things that animals and humans do.

During the height of the "behaviorist era" in psychology, many investigators questioned whether emotions and thoughts really influence human behavior. That extreme level of skepticism was so unrealistic, and at such variance with everyday experience, that it was abandoned in most branches of psychology with the gradual victory of the "cognitive revolution" that enthralled psychology a few decades ago. However, such a metamorphosis did not come to pass in animal research, and now a great intellectual chasm divides those who pursue the study of human psychology from those who pursue the most basic form of the discipline, the analysis of how the brain controls animal behavior. Because of the lack of consensus on fundamental issues, psychology became splintered into a multitude of subareas, with no generally accepted foundation. Nonetheless, an increasing number of brain scientists are beginning to believe that neuromental processes do contribute to the control of animal behavior, and this emerging view, especially to the extent that it can generate new predictions, has the potential to heal and solidify psychology as a unified discipline. *Affective neuroscience* can be a cornerstone of such a foundation.

The great intellectual achievement that is allowing us to realistically reconsider this long-forbidden alternative to the study of the animal and human mind is the recent "neuroscience revolution." Newfound information about the brain, with the many anatomical, neurochemical, and neurophysiological *homologies* that exist across all mammalian species, has the potential to render such neuromental processes as emotional feelings measurable, manipulable, and hence scientifically real (see Appendix A). But this is no easy task—either empirically, conceptually, or politically, for that matter. Because of the many vested interests in established intellectual traditions, a habitual tendency remains among behaviorally oriented psychologists (including most animal behaviorists and behavioral neuroscientists) to dismiss such endeavors as scientifically unrealistic. However, their skepticism is misplaced and counterproductive if internally experienced emotional processes do, in fact, exist in the brains of other mammals.

Obviously, final resolution of such issues will require a great deal more thought, discussion, and research. Nonetheless, we can already be confident that all mammals share many basic affective processes, since many homologous neural systems mediate similar emotional functions in both animals and humans. This fact is strategically important for the substantive growth of future knowledge concerning the human condition: Our most realistic hope to adequately understand the sources of our own basic emotions is through the deployment of animal models that allow us to study the underlying neural intricacies in reasonable detail. However, this project cannot get off the ground unless it is done in conjunction with a credible analysis of the fundamental emotional feelings that all humans experience. Thus, my answers to both of the questions that head this section are affirmative. Furthermore, I believe that it is only through a detailed study of animal emotions and their brain substrates that a satisfactory foundation for understanding human emotions can emerge.

Why Has the Neural Understanding of Emotions Been Delayed?

Earlier in this century, psychologists did not have the abundance of neuroscientific knowledge that we now possess. In its absence, rigorous scientists had to look elsewhere for the causes of behavior. Starting with John Watson's[1] 1924 manifesto *Psychology from the Standpoint of a Behaviorist*, and followed in 1938 by B. F. Skinner's[2] *The Behavior of Organisms*, most experimentalists looked to the diversity of environmental events and relationships in order to find the factors that control organismic actions. Those views captivated mainstream American psychology for many years. The analysis of intermediary psychological and neural states, the so-called inner causes of behavior, were deemed irrelevant, and many academic psychologists discouraged and even forbade discussion of these presumably pseudoscientific issues. This eventually led to dissatisfaction within academic psychology, partly due to the scorn of scholars in other fields. Gradually, starting about a quarter century ago, conceptual constraints were relaxed as the discipline of psychology, except for my own field of behavioral neuroscience, underwent a cognitive revolution that accepted the complexity of the human mind but, regrettably, was not well grounded in evolutionary principles.[3] More recently, an emerging backlash against certain forms of cognitivism has generated a new and growing conceptual view, commonly known as *evolutionary psychology*. This view readily accepts that many complex adaptive strategies have been built into the human brain and that many of them may serve functions that are not readily apparent to our conscious mind.[4] To an outsider, it may seem remarkable that these new disciplines have not more fully embraced a study of the brain. Partly this is because human brain research is remarkably difficult to conduct, both practically and ethically. No doubt, it is also due to the fact that most investigators interested in the brain mechanisms of animal behavior remain strongly committed to behaviorist traditions, which, on the basis of first principles, reject the possibility that inner psychological states help control animal behaviors.

Still, a metamorphosis is slowly unfolding within the brain sciences. Experimental psychologists who are interested in human behavior but work on animal models are beginning to recognize the many conceptual opportunities that our newly acquired brain and evolutionary knowledge provide. We can now conceptualize basic psychological processes in neurological terms that appeared terminally stuck in unproductive semantic realms only a few years ago. Neuroscientific riches are now so vast that all subfields of psychology must begin to integrate a new and strange landscape into their thinking if they want to stay on the forefront of scientific inquiry. This new knowledge will have great power to affect human welfare, as well as human self-conceptions. It is finally possible to credibly infer the natural order of the "inner causes" of behavior, including the emotional processes that activate many of the coherent psychobehavioral tendencies animals and humans exhibit spontaneously without much prior learning. These natural brain processes help create the deeply felt value structures that govern much of our behavior, whether learned or unlearned. This new mode of thought is the intellectual force behind *affective neuroscience*.

In the traditional behaviorist view, it was not essential to understand such natural "instinctual" tendencies of animals. Psychologists' province was largely restricted to examining the laws of learning. The intrinsic limitations of the behaviorist approach became fatally apparent when it was found that the "laws of behavior" varied substantially, at least in fine detail, from one species to another.[5] In other words, the general principles of learning were muddied by the vast evolutionary/instinctual variability that existed across species.

To their initial chagrin and eventual delight, more and more investigators began to note that animals trained according to behaviorist principles would often "regress" to exhibiting their own natural behavioral tendencies when experimental demands became too severe. For instance, raccoons that had been trained to put coins in piggy banks to obtain food (for advertisement purposes) would often fail to smoothly execute their outward demonstrations of learned "thriftiness," instead reverting to rubbing the coins together and manipulating them in their hands as if they were food itself. Apparently, the instinctual, evolutionary baggage of each animal intruded into the well-ordered behaviorist view that only reinforcement contingencies could dictate what organisms do in the world. These observations were enshrined in the now famous article, "The Misbehavior of Organisms,"[6] which led to the widespread recognition that there are biological constraints on learning.[7]

Although the empirical wealth provided by the behaviorist paradigm was vast and continues to grow (see the "Afterthought" of this chapter), so was the barrier it created to understanding the psychological and behavioral tendencies that evolution had created within the brains of animals. This, of course, was not the first time scientists had built powerful and useful methodologies and conceptual systems on faulty assumptions, nor will it be the last. Just as each growing child must initiate creative activities for developmental progress to occur, new ideas need to be entertained in psychology, along with the hope that the inevitable mistakes will be corrected by the collection of more evidence.

A great challenge for psychology at present is to identify and unravel the nature of the intrinsic operating systems of the mammalian brain—to distinguish coherently functioning psychobehavioral "organ systems" among the intricate webs of anatomical, chemical, and electrical interactions of neurons. Why has progress at this level of analysis been so slow in coming? Partially because there has been a widespread aversion to approaches that sought to localize functions in the brain after the embarrassing era of *phrenological* thinking in the 19th century (i.e., the notion that one could read psychological characteristics by measurement of cranial topography). Rejection of those simple forms of neurologizing about complex psychological matters led to a general failure of the discipline to incorporate the new findings from neuroscience into its mainstream ideas. Psychology, the discipline that should be most concerned with revealing the intrinsic functional nature of the human brain/mind, stalled on the road to finding a neural infrastructure for its fundamental concepts.

To put some of the recent historical sources for that failure in stark relief, I will share a short segment of a lengthy letter I once sent to B. F. Skinner, widely considered to have been the most influential psychologist of the 20th century (although it now seems that the writings of Charles Darwin and his modern followers may come to fill that bill). My aim in writing this frank letter (the full text was eventually published elsewhere)[8] was to coax Skinner to consider once more, in his twilight years, some critical issues concerning the role of neuroscience and internal emotional states in a coherent understanding of behavioral processes.

During the years just before his death, Skinner had written a series of sententious articles with such titles as "Whatever Happened to Psychology as the Science of Behavior?,"[9] in which he vigorously defended the basic correctness of his own view of psychology and debunked branches of the discipline, especially clinical, cognitive, and humanistic psychologies, that no longer followed the behaviorist paradigm. In my letter, I sought to reemphasize that psychology is inherently interdisciplinary and should always try to blend information from many sources.

At the beginning of my letter of September 7, 1987, I stated:

> It is clear from your paper that you admire evolutionary concepts and even wish to conceptualize behaviorism along the lines of evolutionary principles of "variation" and "selection." Although behaviorism has provided a reasonable analysis of the "selection" processes that go into the molding and construction of many adaptive behaviors, you continue to ignore the preexisting behavioral "variation" factors of the behavioral equation. The evidence indicates that initial behavioral "variation" (prior to the changes induced by reinforcement contingencies) is not simply the result of a "random behavior generator" but emerges from a diversity of coherently operating brain systems which can generate psychologically meaningful classes of adaptive behavioral tendencies. . . . How shall we identify, categorize and study these essential psychoneural functions of the brain, if not by speaking of inner causes? If psychology ignores such intrinsic functions of the brain, we will, by necessity, continue to have a very fragmented science.

At the end of that letter, I concluded:

> Although I have long admired the intellectual, methodological and technological achievement of the "behaviorism" which you helped create, I have also long been perplexed by your apparent unwillingness to nurture the natural growth of your own brainchild. . . . Psychology, as a scientific discipline, must be constituted by its very nature from an uncomfortable recipe: one-third brain science, one-third behavioral science (including ethological approaches), and one-third experiential science (which will have to include the best that even cognitive psychology, humanistic psychology, psychotherapy, and the other sub-disciplines of psychology have to offer). It makes me sad that such a realistic hybrid approach has yet to fully materialize. Most psychologists continue to be poorly trained in one of our foundation disciplines—the brain sciences. The "black-box" tenets of behaviorism have encouraged that. Let us be a coherent discipline and take nature on her own terms rather than the terms stipulated by restrictive and limited schools of thought! I think it would be a major contribution if you were to throw your intelligence and considerable reputation behind the development of a hybrid science of psychology which has a true internal integrity.

A few weeks later, in October 1987, Professor Skinner replied:

> A behavioral account has two unavoidable gaps—between stimulus and response, and between reinforcement and a resulting change in behavior. Those gaps can be filled only with the instruments and techniques of neurology. A science of behavior need not wait until neurology has done so. A complete account is no doubt highly desirable but the neurology is not what the behavior really is; the two sciences deal with separate subject matters. A third discipline may very well wish to deal with how the two can be brought together, but that is not my field.

In this succinct and telling reply, Skinner accepts the obvious conclusion that the two vast gaps in behavioral knowledge will have to be filled with information from the neurosciences. While acknowledging that the chasm between environmental change and behavioral response needs to be studied, he continued to maintain that such pursuits are not the business of psychologists. That was, of course, a remarkably hollow view of psychological science at the end of the 20th century. Here I continue to take up Skinner's challenge to contribute to a new approach. I will develop the position that a hybrid discipline focusing on the neurobiological nature of brain operating systems (especially those that mediate motivational and emotional tendencies) is needed as a foundation for a mature and scientifically prosperous discipline of psychology. A guiding assumption of this approach is that a common language, incorporating behavioral, cognitive, and neuroscientific perspectives, must be found for discussing the fundamental psychoneurological processes that all mammals share. Accordingly, I will argue that some of the old emotional words used in everyday folk psychology can still serve our purposes well, since they approximate the realities that exist, as genetic birthrights, within mammalian brains.

In my estimation, the most important reason for cultivating this new view is that it may be the only scientific way to come to terms with our human and animal natures. A key question in this endeavor will be: Do other mammals also have internal affective experiences and if they do, do such experiences control their behaviors? On the basis of a great deal of evidence summarized in this text, I will argue for the affirmative view. If that is correct, we have no strategic option but to confront, head-on, the troublesome issue of how affective consciousness is organized within the mammalian brain.

Words and Environmental Events Cannot Explain Basic Behaviors; Brain Processes Can

Ultimately, an understanding of all our mental activities must begin with our willingness to use words that approximate the nature of the underlying brain processes. Our thinking is enriched if we use the right words—those that reflect essential realities—and it is impoverished if we select the wrong ones. However, words are not equivalent to physical reality; they are only symbols that aid our understanding and communication (see Appendix B). This book is premised on the belief that the common emotional words we learned as children—being angry, scared, sad, and happy—can serve the purpose better than many psychologists are inclined to believe. These emotions are often evident in the behaviors animals spontaneously exhibit throughout their life span. We must remember that the words we select are not causes for behavior; they only begin to specify the types of brain processes we must fathom in order to comprehend behavior. One reason psychologists became hesitant to use traditional emotional terms was because they could not adequately define most of them. Without brain knowledge, such terms could be defined by behavioral criteria, but the ensuing verbal circles did not really help us predict new behaviors. With the advent of the neuroscience revolution, we can now hone definitions to a finer edge than was ever possible before.

For some—even modern psychologists—it may still come as a bit of a surprise that words alone, which can arouse such intense feelings among people, are not powerful enough to scientifically specify the nature of those feelings. Many generations of psychologists who tried to discuss internal processes with folk psychological words found it impossible to agree on essential matters, such as what are we really talking about when we assert that someone did something because they felt this way or that way? It took psychologists some time to realize that the only things they could agree upon scientifically were visually evident empirical observations, such as the latency, speed, frequency, and quality of behavioral actions. For a long time, this made behavioral psychology a highly productive but conceptually conservative and intellectually sterile field (at least to those not initiated into its intricacies).

After modest study of the underlying issues, one can understand why scientists must be conservative with their concepts. In order to make real scientific progress, as opposed to merely generating creative ideas, we must seek rigorous definitions for the concepts we use. All key concepts should be defined in clear and consistent ways, and they must be deployed experimentally (operationally) in ways that help us predict new behavioral acts. Until the recent achievements of modern neuroscience, our desire to explain human and animal behaviors in a scientific manner using emotional terms could not succeed. Now it can—because of advances in brain research. If thoughts and feelings do, in fact, control human and animal behaviors, scientific progress will depend critically on our ability to specify what we mean by thoughts and feelings, at least in part, on a neural level. Of course, a full and accurate definition depends on the fullness and accuracy of our knowledge, and in the midst of our current ignorance we must start with approximations.

I would submit that it is correct to assume that primary-process affective feelings in humans (i.e., "raw feels") arise from distinct patterns of neural activity that we share with other animals, and that these feelings have an important role in controlling behavior, especially conditionally. In the following chapters I will begin to focus on the murky outlines of those genetically ingrained emotional circuits that provide an affective infrastructure to the animal and human mind. The necessary operational and conceptual reference points for my definitions for the various emotions will be discrete types of instinctual behaviors that can be conditioned and the neural systems from which they arise. To facilitate communication, the emotion-mediating neural systems that have now been identified within the mammalian brain will be labeled with common affective terms, and a general definition for emotional circuitry will also be provided in due course (see Chapter 3). The foremost question, but one that will have to be answered by future research, is where and how, among the various circuit interactions, does the actual experience of emotional feelings arise? I will try to provide a provisional answer to that sticky problem in the final chapter of this text.

In sum, the original sticking point that hindered progress in the field was this: Without a concurrent neural analysis, emotional concepts cannot be used *noncircularly* in scientific discourse. We cannot say that animals attack because they are angry and then turn around and say that we know animals are angry because they exhibit attack. We cannot say that humans flee from danger because they are afraid and then say we know that humans are afraid if they exhibit flight. Such circular word juggling does not allow us to make new and powerful predictions about behavior. However, thanks to the neuroscience revolution, we can begin to specify the potential brain mechanisms that are essential substrates for such basic emotions. When we do that, we begin to exit from the endless rounds of circular explanations. A modern sticking point will be the following: Why is a focus simply on the biological mechanisms of the brain an insufficient basis for discussing and dissecting such issues? I suspect that is because the complexity of the systems that evolved to generate emotional feelings (see Chapter 16) are such that a comprehensive understanding will necessitate the use of several integrated conceptual approaches to make sense of complex phenomena such as emotions, in the same way that "wave" and "particle" perspectives are essential to make sense of certain physical phenomena.

A Summation of the Aims of Affective Neuroscience

The existential reality of our deepest moods and emotions cannot be adequately explained with mere words, even though the environmental reasons they are evoked can be so clarified. The most difficult part of the analysis—the clarification of the *proximal causes* which generate the actual feeling states and behavioral acts—can only arise from an integrative neuroscience approach. It is the same for all basic psychological concepts. How could we ever define the experience of redness with words? We can study the environmental manifestations of redness and describe the external physical properties of electromagnetic radiation that trigger our experience of redness, but we cannot define the experience itself. Redness, like all other subjective experiences, is an evolutionary potential of the nervous system, one that was "designed" to allow us to appreciate the ripeness of fruits, the readiness of sexuality, and perhaps even the terror and passion of blood being spilled. The subjective nature of redness can only be explained by neuroanatomical, neurochemical, and neurophysiological studies done in conjunction with appropriate behavioral and psychological observations.

Emotional feelings must ultimately be understood in similar ways. As I will describe, that intellectual journey has finally started in earnest. Until recently, investigators had few options but to remain at the periphery—studying the various environmental events that trigger and soothe our feelings, the accompanying facial expressions, bodily postures, and behavioral acts, and changes in various peripheral organs and chemistries of the body.[10] We could also study the many subtleties of emotional expressions in human languages and cultures. Important as those issues are, they will receive relatively little attention here, for they are not directly relevant to the problem at hand, and they have been well covered elsewhere.[11] Here I will focus on those neural processes that undergird our emotional experiences and actions—essential mechanisms for the generation of the basic emotional forces that we still share with other mammals. Careful theorizing on the basis of accumulated data will allow us to understand the sources of many emotional tendencies in neuroscientific terms. Will we ever see into the subjectivity of other minds? Obviously, all approaches will have to be indirect, but if we do not try, we may never truly fathom the organizational nature of the mammalian brain.

The Major Premises of Affective Neuroscience

A central, and no doubt controversial, tenet of affective neuroscience is that emotional processes, including subjectively experienced feelings, do, in fact, play a key role in the causal chain of events that control the actions of both humans and animals. They provide various types of natural internal values upon which many complex behavioral choices in humans are based. However, such internal feelings are not simply mental events; rather, they arise from neurobiological events. In other words, emotional states arise from material events (at the neural level) that mediate and modulate the deep instinctual nature of many human and animal action tendencies, especially those that, through simple learning mechanisms such as classical conditioning, come so readily to be directed at future challenges. One reason such instinctual states may include an internally experienced feeling tone is that higher organisms possess neurally based self-representation systems. I would suggest that subjectively experienced feelings arise, ultimately, from the interactions of various emotional systems with the fundamental brain substrates of "the self," but, as already mentioned, an in-depth discussion of that troublesome issue will be postponed until Chapter 16.

It is here assumed that basic emotional states provide efficient ways to mediate categorical types of learned behavioral changes. In other words, emotional feelings not only sustain certain unconditioned behavioral tendencies but also help guide new behaviors by providing simple value-coding mechanisms that provide self-referential salience, thereby allowing organisms to categorize world events efficiently so as to control future behaviors. At present, the simplest way to access the natural taxonomy of these systems is through (1) major categories of human affective experience across individuals and cultures, (2) a concurrent study of the natural categories of animal emotive behaviors, and (3) a thorough analysis of the brain circuits from which such tendencies arise. At each of these levels, we are beginning to learn how to sort out the various distinct processes. Homologies at the neural level give us solid assurance of common evolutionary origins and designs.

Once we can specify distinct brain systems that generate emotional behaviors, we can also generate biologically defensible (as opposed to simply intuitive and behaviorally based) taxonomies of emotions. Obviously, if we are to remain data-based, our initial taxonomies must be quite conservative and for the time being open-ended. At the simplest level, world events can produce *approach* or *withdrawal*, but careful analysis of the evidence now suggests that both of these broad categories contain a variety of separable, albeit interactive, processes that must be distinguished to reveal a proper taxonomy of affective processes within the brain. The main criterion here for an emotional system will be whether a coherent emotional response pattern can be activated by localized electrical or chemical stimulation along specific brain circuits, and whether such arousal has affective consequences as measured by consistent approach or avoidance responses. Such constraints prevent the analysis from getting more complex than the existing neuroscience evidence. For that reason, I will have to avoid many of the emotional complexities that seem apparent from the perspective of modern evolutionary psychology.[12] Although I find those modes of thought to be on the right track, most cannot yet be linked to neural analyses in anything more than highly speculative ways.

At the empirical level, we can presently defend the existence of various neural systems that lead to the limited set of discrete emotional tendencies described in this book. I will argue that a series of basic emotional processes arises from distinct neurobiological systems and that everyday emotional concepts such as anger, fear, joy, and loneliness are not merely the arbitrary taxonomic inventions of noncritical thinkers. These brain systems appear to have several common characteristics. As discussed fully in Chapter 3, they reflect coherent integrative processes of the nervous system. The core function of emotional systems is to coordinate many types of behavioral and physiological processes in the brain and body. In addition, arousals of these brain systems are accompanied by subjectively experienced feeling states that may provide efficient ways to guide and sustain behavior patterns, as well as to mediate certain types of learning.

Further, it seems reasonable to assume that when such neural activities continue at low levels for extended periods of time, they generate moods and, ultimately, such personality dimensions as the differential tendency to be happy, irritable, fearful, or melancholy. These systems help create a substantial portion of what is traditionally considered universal "human nature." Obviously, a complete study of emotional systems is also essential for understanding the many psychiatric disturbances that assail humans—the schizophrenias, autisms, manias, depressions, anxieties, panics, obsessive-compulsive disorders, post-traumatic stress disorders, neuroses, and other vexations of the human spirit.

At present, the grand new brain-imaging procedures for measuring human brain geographies (the functional MRIs and PET scans; see Chapter 5) are revealing the cerebral topographies of psychiatric disorders,[13] but we will not be able to understand the underlying neurodynamics of emotional systems without a great deal of concurrent animal brain research. Here, I will seek both to lay out the *general* neural principles that create the major emotions in the brains of all mammalian species and to outline a strategy of how we can effectively come to know more. Pervasive differences in behavioral details among species will be de-emphasized. Rather, I will focus on communalities at the neural level that arise from the impressive degree of genetic relatedness between ourselves and other mammals (see Appendix A).

As a simplifying maneuver, I will assume that recent evolutionary diversification has more vigorously elaborated surface details of behavior and cognitive abilities than it has altered the deep functional architecture of the ancient brain systems that help make us the emotional creatures that we are. Thus, fear is still fear, whether in a cat or a frightened human. Rage is still rage, whether in a dog or an angry human. Sexual lust and maternal acceptance are very similar in both humans and many other mammals. Presumably, the major evolutionary differences within the subcortical operating systems are matters more of emphasis than of kind. For example, rabbits may have more fear circuitry, while cats have more anger circuitry. Other differences may also be striking—the precise bodily appearance of emotional patterns, the variety in the details of sensory and motor apparatuses, as well as specific psychobehavioral strategies. But at deeper levels, very similar emotional systems guide many of the spontaneous behavioral tendencies of all mammals.

So let us imagine another archetypal interaction not much different from the one that opened this chapter: You are cornered in a dark, dead-end street by a crazed mugger wielding a stiletto. He desperately needs money to satisfy the artificial craving aroused in his brain by periodic drug use. Societal laws have made the satisfaction of his craving a criminal business. The most important motivation in his mind is to obtain the resources needed to alleviate the primal psychic strain and pain that are now surging through his hyperemotional brain. His worries have now become yours. He has challenged your right to your possessions. Your body is filled with tension, your heart pounds, you feel cold, weak, and trembly, but you are almost reflexively putting on a valiant, but perhaps foolish, effort to keep him at bay by shouting, flailing your arms, and throwing handfuls of pebbles at him. He is shouting that he will really get you for that. He is now angry, and it's not just your wallet or purse that he wants; he wants your life. By a stroke of luck, passing police officers notice the commotion in the alley, and they save you. The police take the criminal away, but he struggles, kicks, and fiercely shouts that he will really get you the next time. You are filled with a lingering dread and horror. For several nights your dreams are filled with symbolic variations of the incident. Months later you are still prone to recount how you felt, how you had never been more scared in your life, how relieved you were to see the police arrive, how you now support more stringent drug laws. Whenever you think about that final threat, you again become infused with feelings of anxiety and avoid going out alone, especially at night. Only a fool would deny that the memory of your emotional experiences continues to control your behavior for some time to come. Although other animals will not have thoughts comparable to ours, there are good reasons to believe that our deep feeling of dread emerges to a substantial extent from the same brain systems that create fearful states for other animals. Still, an understanding of such simple emotional behaviors cannot be separated from the environmental and social contexts in which they occur.

On the Nature-Nurture Controversy: As Always, a Fifty–fifty Proposition

Many social scientists want to understand the causes behind the mugger's act of aggression. As yet, there is no single satisfactory answer. We do know that men are more likely than women to perpetrate aggressive, antisocial acts. Such behavior is also more common in culturally and economically disadvantaged individuals who have little to lose.[14] It is especially likely to occur among those who have become dependent on illegal drugs.[15] In addition, we know that there are genetic personality predispositions for aggression and drug addiction.[16] However, if we fail to consider that aggressive and fearful urges emanate from distinct brain systems, we cannot adequately describe what happened in that archetypal situation.

Because of our failure to fully acknowledge the functional role of circuits constructed in our brains during the long course of evolution, we occasionally still have needlessly polarized controversies over the role of nature and nurture in the genesis of psychological processes. But nature and nurture provide different things in our final toolbox of skills—nature gives us the ability to feel and behave in certain ways, and learning allows us to effectively use those systems to navigate the complexities of the world. These tendencies are especially well mixed in those individualistic styles of thinking, feeling, and behaving that we call personality.

The best recent estimates of heritability of human personality, using identical twins reared apart, suggest that about half of observed variation must be attributed to nature, while half must be attributed to nurture. In fact, heritability is around 50% for all the major temperamental variables that are measured in modern personality theory.[17] Of course, the degree of influence for each specific trait is more lopsided—some appear to have stronger genetic loadings, and others have greater socioenvironmental ones. Moreover, every estimate of environmental and genetic influence varies depending on the specific cultural context in which the measures are taken. It must also be emphasized that no behaviors are ever inherited in a formal sense; the only things that can be inherited are the potentials of bodily tissues. DNA only encodes information for the construction of protein chains, which can combine with each other and with environmentally derived molecules in a variety of temporal and spatial ways. When we sometimes say in shorthand that "this or that behavior is inherited," what we should actually be saying is that certain psychobehavioral *tendencies* can be represented within the intrinsic brain and body constructions that organisms inherit. No specific thoughts or behaviors are directly inherited, but dispositions to feel, think, and act in various ways and in various situations certainly are. Although these tendencies do not necessarily dictate our destinies, they powerfully promote certain possibilities and diminish others.

While nature provides a variety of intrinsic potentials in the brain, nurture provides opportunities for these potentials to be manifested in a diversity of ways in real life. Thus, while basic emotional circuits are among the tools provided by nature, their ability to permanently change the life course and personalities of organisms depends on the nurturance or lack of nurturance that the world provides. In more precise scientific terms, everything we see is *epigenetic*, a mixture of nature and nurture. If you plant two identical tomato seeds in two different environments, you will have two plants of strikingly different size and overall shape, but they will still be discernibly tomato plants. There is no longer any question that brain tissues create the potential for having certain types of experiences, but there is also no doubt that the experiences, especially early ones, can change the fine details of the brain forever.

Endless functional examples fill the textbooks of psychology and history, but there are structural examples as well. One of my favorites is that monkeys trained to use a certain finger to solve a behavioral task gradually exhibit larger areas of cortical representation for that finger.[18] This may also help explain how an aspiring pianist gradually becomes a skilled artist, and it has been shown that right-handed guitarists have richer cortical representations of that hand within their left hemispheres.[19] But such plasticity does not tell us why, across different individuals and species, the representations of fingers are found in essentially the same relative locations within their brains—a brain area that in humans is situated just beneath the temples near the tips of the ears. The rest of the body is also represented systematically (and upside down, with one's rear pointing up and the head down, as if one were getting a spanking) on nearby tissue of the precentral and postcentral gyri. The cortical areas for bodily representations are encoded, in some presently unknown way, within the same genes of all mammals. However, a little farther down from the hand and arm area of motor and sensory cortex, we have the speech cortex, which is uniquely enlarged in humans but whose sophisticated multimodal functions still emerge from the ancestral ability of that multimodal (i.e., associative) brain tissue to interrelate many different sensations and perceptions, and hence to symbolize complex ideas. Human speech cortex dramatically highlights the plasticity of the brain—the cerebral tissues of young children are especially malleable, and many different areas of the brain can elaborate communicative functions if other, preferential areas are damaged (see Appendix B and Figure B.1).

Disregarding the complexities of underlying molecular mechanisms for the time being (which are presently being worked out at a fever pitch), the plasticity in the brain that arises from experience is *conceptually* not all that different from the types of changes we see in our bodies as a function of use. Exercise makes our muscles stronger, and with disuse they become smaller.

"Use it or lose it," as the saying goes. Still, we do not generate totally new muscles through exercise. Similarly, experience is more influential in changing the quantitative expressions of neural systems rather than their essential nature. Presumably, the same principles hold for the brain's emotional systems. On top of genetically determined vigor of the neural substrates, emotional systems can surely be strengthened by use and weakened by disuse. Unfortunately, only modest data are available on such important topics at the present time.

For the discipline of affective neuroscience, the most important issue in emotion research for the foreseeable future will be the accurate specification of the underlying brain circuits, in anatomical, neurochemical, and neurophysiological terms. An additional and even more difficult task is to unravel how emotional feelings emerge from the neurodynamics of many interacting brain sytems. The nature of emotional representations cannot be decoded without reference to all of these levels of analysis. However, the second goal can succeed only when there has been a credible resolution of the first, so here I will largely aspire to do that—to provide a provisional anatomical and neurochemical overview of some of the brain systems that are essential participants in the genesis of the basic emotional behaviors. Regrettably, because of space constraints, my discussion of experiential issues will be limited to those rare occasions where some especially compelling data are available.

One related apology: At times it may seem that I am talking about brain emotional systems as if they could operate independently of interactions with real-life events. I do not wish to give that impression, although to some extent the reality of emotions in the brain is independent of the environment: We can evoke strong emotions in animals and humans by electrically stimulating subcortical sites within the brain.[20] These ancient systems respond to world events, but because of their genetically ingrained nature, they can generate free-floating affective states of their own. This is reflected in the potential for spontaneous neural firing within these systems. However, the expressions of all emotional functions will normally be dictated by their effectiveness or lack thereof in dealing with real-life events.

Homologies and Analogies

At this point, it is important to focus a bit on the concepts of *homology* and *analogy*, especially as they apply to brain mechanisms. *Homology* is a term used in anatomy to indicate genetic relatedness of bodily structures. For instance, human arms and bat wings are *homologous* because they both arise from the genetic information that controls forelimb development. Although the functions have diverged markedly, one can still get a great deal of insight about the use of human forelimbs by analyzing the arm movements of any other mammalian species.[21] On the other hand, the wings of birds and bees are *analogous*—serving a similar function—even though they do not share a common genetic inheritance. In a strict sense, these are morphological terms used to discuss body structures, and they should not be used to discuss such issues as brain functions.[22] However, the neuroanatomical and neurochemical similarities in the underlying behavioral control processes are presently sufficient to lend great credence to the likelihood that pervasive homologies are present in these types of basic psychoneural functions in all mammals. Occasional problems will arise in certain cross-species comparisons, not only because of variety in the supporting sensory and motor mechanisms but also because of *exaptations,* whereby evolution has modified homologous parts for very different ends in different species (e.g., the gill arch supports of fish eventually evolved into the middle ear bones of mammals, and surprisingly, terrestrial lungs were apparently converted to flotation controlling swim bladders in fish).[23]

Also, many hidden potentials remain masked within the DNA of each species, ready to be functionally enshrined (i.e., as informational potentialities within DNA become biological realities) when critical environmental changes occur. Such occurrences can make argument by homology difficult and risky indeed. But we have few alternatives, if we aspire to do more than merely describe the seemingly endless diversity of species. At the present time, our scientific aim can be more profitably focused on the shared foundations rather than the many surface differences and particularities of each species.

Interestingly, at the present time scientists are discouraged from inferring the existence of cross-species processes in the brain by prevailing research funding policies. Obviously, a strong argument of homology cannot be made until a great deal of relevant neurological data has been collected in a variety of species, and at the present time the collection of such data has to be done in a different guise than argument by homology. To argue for the likelihood that homologous processes exist is to seriously diminish the possibility of obtaining research support from peer-reviewed funding sources. In any event, because of some deep-seated philosophical and evolutionary perspectives, I have chosen to pursue this debatable course of thought and action for the past quarter of a century, and I will continue that journey in this text. I believe it is the strategy that can lead most effectively to an understanding of the neural foundation of human and animal emotions. Because both neuroscientists and psychologists are loathe to conceptualize such issues, vast areas of brain integrative processes remain open for insightful investigation. For instance, neuroscientists have almost completely neglected the study of integrative brain processes such as those that generate anger, loneliness, and playfulness. At the same time there is now abundant research on the topic of brain substrates of fearfulness, even though few of the active investigators are willing to assume their animal subjects actually experience fear in a way that resembles human fear.

A Case in Point: Innate Fears and the Play of Rats

Let me share a concrete example to highlight some of the preceding issues. If one puts two young rats, that have been individually housed, together in a single cage, they immediately exhibit a flurry of chasing, pouncing, and wrestling that may appear quite aggressive. When I once demonstrated this very robust phenomenon to a senior behavioral scientist visiting our lab, he asked me, "How did you train the animals to fight that way?" With some amusement, I said, "I didn't train them. *Evolution* did. . . . And, by the way, they are not fighting. They are playing." As will be discussed more fully in Chapter 15, the young of most mammalian species exhibit vigorous forms of social play that share a category resemblance, even though many of the specific actions do vary substantially among species. At present, it does seem likely, at least to me, that a basic form of roughhousing play emerges from *homologous* neural circuits in the brains of all mammals, but because of interactions with many other systems, play is expressed outwardly in measurably different ways. However, the detailing of differences is less likely to give us major insights into human nature than a probing of the similarities.

The biological sources of play behavior have now been studied systematically under well-controlled laboratory conditions (see Chapter 15). To the best of our knowledge, a basic urge to play exists among the young of most mammalian species, with very similar controls. In all species that have been studied, playfulness is inhibited by motivations such as hunger and negative emotions, including loneliness, anger, and fear. These effects probably indicate that very similar neural influences modulate the circuits that instigate play across different species.

Let us briefly focus on the innate effect of fear (Figure 1.1) on several measures of play in rats, including the number of (1) "dorsal contacts" or play solicitations, which is the way animals pounce on each other to instigate play motivation in their partners, and (2) pins, which reflect how animals fare in their wrestling bouts. Although there are many other behaviors that could be measured, these are excellent general indicators of the amount of play. In this experiment, young rats were first allowed five-minute play periods on four successive days, and then on the fifth, half were exposed to a small tuft of cat hair on the floor of their "playroom." During that session, play was completely inhibited. The animals moved furtively, cautiously sniffing the fur and other parts of their environment. They seemed to sense that something was seriously amiss. In other words, they seemed to have an innate knowledge that they should be cautious when such predatory smells are about.

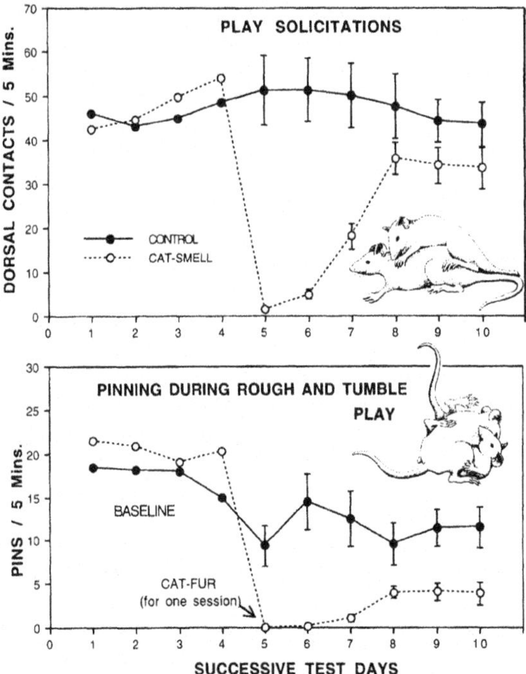

Figure 1.1. Following four baseline days of play, cat smell was introduced into the play chamber for a single test day (i.e., during a standard five-minute observation session). Although the chamber was clean on all subsequent days, play solicitations (i.e., dorsal contacts) were markedly reduced for three days, while pinning was reduced for all five subsequent test days. For a description of these play behaviors, see Chapter 15. The control group (solid lines) was not exposed to any cat fur. Data are means and ±SEMs. (According to unpublished data, Panksepp, 1994.)

Evolution must have put this innate stimulus for wariness into their brains, for these animals had been born in the lab and had never had anything to do with cats prior to the first test. This effect can also be produced with the fur of other predators such as ferrets but not the smell of mice, chickens, or certain breeds of dog. Since I was personally spending a great deal of time studying play in laboratory rats, it was essential for me to determine whether the odor of my Norwegian elkhound, which might be lingering on my hands and clothes, would affect the play of my animals. To my relief, covering the entire floor of the play chamber with Ginny's fur did not disrupt the play of young rats in the least, which suggests that the ancestors of such domestic dogs did not normally prey upon rats in the wild.

However, the powerful effect of cat odor should make us wonder how many behaviorists in the past, being cat fanciers, have inadvertently carried the smells of their predatory pets into the laboratory. Such undetected variables could have led to dramatic changes in the behavior of their rodent subjects. Indeed, I know of several labs where cats and rats have been kept in nearby quarters, and in our experience it is difficult to replicate certain phenomena from those labs unless the cat-smell variable is reintroduced into the testing situation. For a while we also had a few cats in the lab, and we now know that low doses of morphine very powerfully increase play in the presence of cat smell, but the effect is comparatively weak in the absence of anxiety-provoking stimuli.

The inhibition of behavior provoked by cat odor is remarkably powerful and long-lasting. As summarized in Figure 1.1, following a single exposure to cat odor, animals continued to exhibit inhibition of play for up to five successive days. Our interpretation of this effect is that some unconditioned attribute of cat smell can innately arouse a fear system in the rat brain, and this emotional state becomes rapidly associated with the contextual cues of the chamber. On subsequent occasions, one does not need the unconditioned fear stimulus—the feline smell—to evoke anxiety. The contextual cues of the chamber suffice. This, in essence, is *classical* or *Pavlovian conditioning*. The flow of associations is outlined more formally in Figure 1.2, and as we will see, classical conditioning is still one of the most powerful and effective ways to study emotional learning in the laboratory.

In the present context, it is important to emphasize that unlike many other unconditional fear stimuli, such as foot shock, the power of the cat-smell stimulus to provoke fear is probably restricted to species that are normally preyed upon by cats. Cat smell is a species-typical rather than a species-general fear stimulus, while pain is an example of the latter. This demonstrates that there will be enormous species variability in the natural stimuli that can access emotional systems, even though the nature of the underlying fear systems remains, to the best of our knowledge, remarkably similar across all mammalian species.Thus, rats have an innate connection from the olfactory apparatus to emotional circuitry that can disrupt ongoing behavior patterns, but it would be maladaptive for cats to have such a sensory-perceptual input into their own fear system. Since emotional systems have widespread consequences in the brain, virtually all other behaviors are typically affected by emotional arousal. Had our young rats been tested in a feeding situation, they would have exhibited inhibition of feeding, and so on.

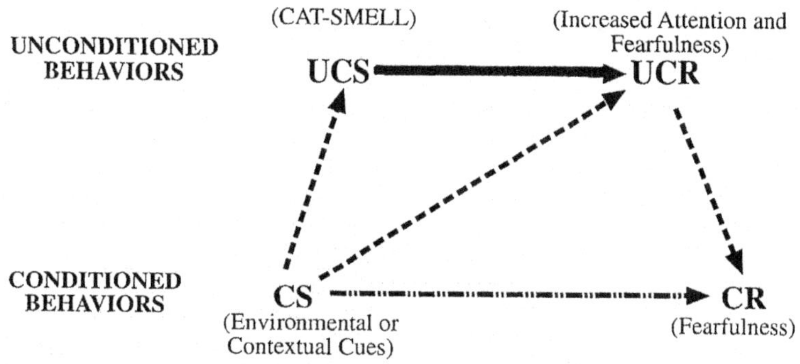

Figure 1.2. Schematic summary of classical conditioning, using the specific example studied in Figure 1.1. The natural response to the unconditional stimulus (UCS) of cat odor is for rats to exhibit the instinctual unconditioned response (UCR) of elevated attention and cautious/fearful behavior patterns. When this pairing simply occurred in the regular test environment, the environmental or "contextual" cues served as a conditional stimulus (CS) that could arouse the conditioned response (CR) of fear, which was incompatible with continuation of playfulness in this situation. In classical conditioning of this type, it is not certain whether the CS produces the CR directly or indirectly via activation of UCS or UCR processes in the brain. Although the most likely connection is directly to the UCR system, direct learned connections could also be made to UCS representations in the brain, while direct connections to the CR seem less likely since the CR, at least in this specific situation, may simply be a conceptual entity that consists of nothing more than arousal of the unconditioned fear processes in the brain, which in this specific case may consist of arousal of the specific FEAR systems such as those described in Chapter 11 (see Figure 11.1).

The Monists' View of "Mind": Psychology Is Neurodynamics

Although some investigators still choose to believe that human emotions are unique and acquired through social learning, here we will proceed with the data-based premise that the ultimate sources of human feelings are biological, and that these foundations are essential for all of the many acquired complexities that characterize the detailed expressions of human emotions in the real world. In short, the present view will be a reductionistic one where we shall seek the sources of emotionality within the evolutionarily shared neurodynamics of the older parts of the mammalian brain. The traditional distinction between bodily and psychological processes becomes blurred as we come to increasingly appreciate that mental abilities are bodily functions of the brain.

Conversely, I would hasten to reemphasize, some of the most important brain questions require a psychological analysis. Psychological and brain analyses must remain two-way streets. For instance, to understand the nature of the brain, we must understand emotions, but to understand the diversity of real-life emotions, we must understand the intrinsic operating systems of the brain. To help clarify such complex interactions, I will focus on the machine that has changed human lives most during the second half of the 20th century—the digital computer.

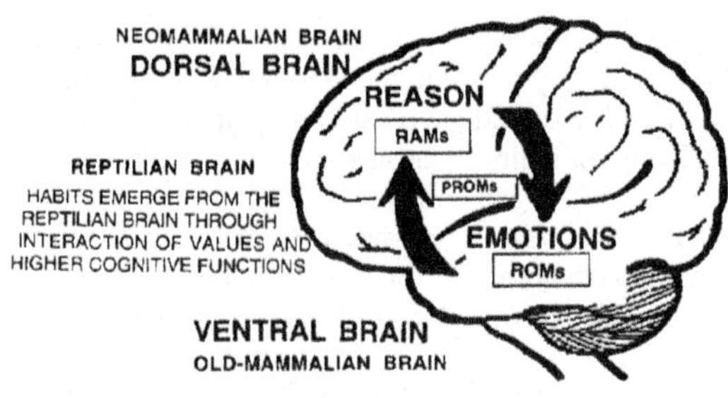

Figure 1.3. Conceptual schematic of ROM- and RAM-type processes in the brain. The basic emotional value-systems are conceived to be genetically ingrained operating systems that are heavily concentrated in ventral parts of the "old-mammalian" brain, which include hypothalamic-limbic circuits, while the flexibility of learning is mediated more by RAM-type processes in dorsal "neomammalian" parts of the brain, which are elaborated more by thalamic-neocortical systems. The interactions of these processes can yield programmable read-only memories (PROMs), which emerge ultimately from the convergence of the above two layers of brain organization onto the "reptilian" brain yielding the habit structures of organisms, many of which may be mediated by classical conditioning principles such as those summarized in Figure 1.2.

To use a simplified computer analogy, we need to understand the operating systems in read-only memories (ROMs) of the brain-biocomputer before we can really fathom how the intricacies of brain software (or complex modes of learning and cognition) are elaborated in the random-access memory (RAM) types of neural processors within the brain. Obviously, all software functions of modern digital computers would be useless without the competencies built into operating systems, and likewise the programmable parts of the mammalian brain would remain mute without the intrinsic forces of the ancient and genetically dictated operating systems. In general, ROM functions are more ancient and reside in lower, subcortical regions of the brain, while RAM functions are more recent and are concentrated in the neocortex (Figure 1.3). Here we will conceptualize some of the ROM functions as basic emotional operating systems, while the RAM functions more closely resemble cognitive abilities. In other words, the subcortical ROM structures and functions of the mammalian brain resemble the "hidden units" of neural-net computers, and their proper conceptualization is the aim of this text. Although the manner in which information processing occurs in the RAM-like space of the brain is a very important neuropsychological problem that is being tackled by many disciplines ranging from *cognitive neuroscience* to *artificial intelligence*, those higher issues will tend to be ignored in the present coverage.

The mental complexities that can emerge from the software/programmed functions of the neocortex, especially speech areas, have encouraged some thinkers to advocate dualist views in which brain functions and mind functions are considered distinct entities (see Appendix C). Most investigators now accept that they are not, even though the highly interrelated intrinsic "hardware" functions of the brain and the acquired "software" functions surely do need to be distinguished.

To proceed further with this simplifying analogy, all mammals appear to have very similar ROM functions, while humans obviously have far more RAM-like neuro-computational space than other mammals (i.e., they have more neocortex and other brain areas that can elaborate learned software functions of the brain). However, because of the similarities in genetically dictated ROM functions in all mammals, we can use animal models effectively to analyze the basic, subcortical nature of the human condition. Activities in these operating systems constitute what in common parlance are called the emotions, passions, or hungers—issues that have been sadly neglected during the massively tangled growth of 20th century neuroscience and psychology.[24] The aim of affective neuroscience is to understand the neural nature of these basic operating systems,[25] which only by loose analogy resemble the ROM functions of digital computers. Of course, by clarifying such issues, we do not begin to approximate a complete description of human experience. It is only a scientific foundation that allows us to understand some of the major anchor points (i.e., intrinsic values) that continue to tether all of our complex psychological functions.

The reason psychology, as a discipline, has been so successful while generally disregarding the study of these ROM functions of the brain is similar to the reason we can be so successful in using our personal computers without knowing much about how they really work. These machines do our bidding as if by magic, so it is easy to take their essential nature for granted. The same dynamic applies to basic neuropsychological processes—we can readily generate successful end results without understanding much about the inner workings. Fortunately, we now know enough about the brain and body to seek a deep understanding of such matters.

Toward a Synthesis of Divergent Views

The integration of neurological, behavioral, and mental concepts is the next great frontier of psychology. This emerging synthesis was poignantly highlighted by the late Heinz Pagels in his final book, *The Dreams of Reason: The Computer and the Rise of the Sciences of Complexity.*[26] In considering the dilemma of human understanding, Pagels suggests that we need to seriously consider the fundamental correctness of the traditional materialist worldview, which has long been distasteful to humanistically oriented scholars:

> Most natural scientists hold a view that maintains that the entire vast universe, from its beginning in time to its ultimate end, from its smallest quantum particles to the largest galaxies, is subject to rule—the natural laws—comprehensible by a human mind. Everything in the universe orders itself in accord with such rules and nothing else. Life on earth is viewed as a complex chemical reaction that promoted evolution, speciation, and the eventual emergence of humanity, replete with our institutions of laws, religion, and culture. I believe that this reductionalist-materialist view of nature is basically correct.

He then suggests that we need to seriously consider that the traditional humanist worldview, which is rather closer to traditional psychology than the materialist worldview, is also correct:

> Other people, with equal intellectual commitment, maintain the view that the very idea of nature is but an idea held in our minds and that all of our thinking about material reality is necessarily transcendent to that reality. Further, according to this view, the cultural matrix of art, law, religion, philosophy, and science forms an invisible universe of meaning, and the true ground of being is to be found in this order of mind. I also believe that this transcendental view, which affirms the epistemic priority of mind over nature, is correct.

Pagels recognized the possibility of a synthesis, and my aim here is to aspire toward such a goal, which the discipline of psychology desperately needs.

These two views of reality—the natural and the transcendental—are in evident and deep conflict. The mind, it seems, is transcendent to nature. Yet according to the natural sciences that transcendental realm must be materially supported and as such is subject to natural law. Resolving this conflict is, and will remain, a primary intellectual challenge to our civilization for the next several centuries.

Modern psychology must now seek to simultaneously deal with the issue of how environmentally acquired representations of our present world interact with the evolutionarily provided neural representations of worlds past that still exist within the genetically dictated connections and neurodynamics of our brains. Obviously, all cognitive and emotional facts that we use as specific living skills are learned, while many of the underlying cognitive and emotional potentials of the brain are our birthright. For instance, our brains are designed to have a sense of causality between certain temporally related events and also to classify and categorize objects and events in certain ways. Here, we will be more concerned with the fundamental sources of the genetically ingrained affective potentials of our brains—the innate values that are elaborated by our inherited emotional operating systems—rather than the vast diversity of learning these systems can support. Indeed, our understanding of learning and memory mechanisms, a main focus of modern behavioral neuroscience,[27] will be broadened and deepened by an understanding of the basic emotional circuits that they serve.

In sum, we can finally be quite certain that all mammals share many basic psychoneural processes because of the long evolutionary journey they have shared. Neural homologies abound in the lower reaches of the mammalian brain. Even though our unique higher cortical abilities, especially when filtered through contemporary thoughts, may encourage us to pretend that we lack instincts—that we have no basic emotions—such opinions are not consistent with the available facts. Those illusions are created by our strangely human need to aspire to be more than we are—to feel closer to the angels than to other animals. But when our basic emotions are fully expressed, we have no doubt that powerful animal forces survive beneath our cultural veneer. It is this ancient animal heritage that makes us the intense, feeling creatures that we are.

As we come to understand the neural basis of animal emotions, we will be clarifying the primal sources of human emotions. Of course, because of our richer cortical potentials and the resulting evolution of human cultures, the ancient emotional systems have a much vaster cognitive universe with which to interact. Evolution may have created a greater diversity of specific cognitive potentials across species than affective potentials, even though there are also bound to be many general principles that govern the seemingly distinct cognitive styles of different species. For instance, within the spatial maps of the hippocampus,[28] the "well-grounded" navigational thoughts of groundhogs may be organized around similar neural principles as the soaring spatial thoughts of falcons. In any event, the empirically based premise of the present work is that at the basic affective level, neural similarities will abound.

AFTERTHOUGHT: The Accomplishments of Behaviorism in a Historical Context

From an overall historical vantage, the thesis of *mentalism*, which governed psychology around the turn of the century, was challenged by the antithesis of *behaviorism* in America and *ethology* (the study of the natural behaviors of organisms) in Europe. In its early stages, behaviorism was a solid and useful addition to American psychology because it brought with it a desperately needed empirical and conceptual rigor. No longer were mere verbal concepts and unseen attributes of mind a sufficient basis for explaining behavior. Rather, behavior was seen to arise from objective occurrences and contingencies in the environment. Lawful relations were finally established between specific environmental events and patterns of behavior emitted by organisms. Mentalistic concepts such as feelings and thoughts were erased from the official lexicon of psychology. At the time these changes occurred, they were healthy ones: An earlier psychology had reached the sorry state where ill-defined verbal conceptions (especially labels for various instincts) were too widely used as explanations of behavior.

Behaviorists generated a remarkable series of major accomplishments—among the most important being the general laws of learning. Because of their careful empirical work, we now have a rich description of how organisms behave in token economies that simulate capitalistic systems (Figure 1.4), and these findings have implications for areas as diverse as drug abuse.[29] Useful general principles have been uncovered by studying the detailed patterns of lever pressing of hungry rats and pecking of hungry pigeons working for their daily food on various schedules of reinforcement. Animals doing "piece-work" (i.e., working on fixed-ratio schedules, requiring a certain number of responses to get each reward) perform very rapidly and take some

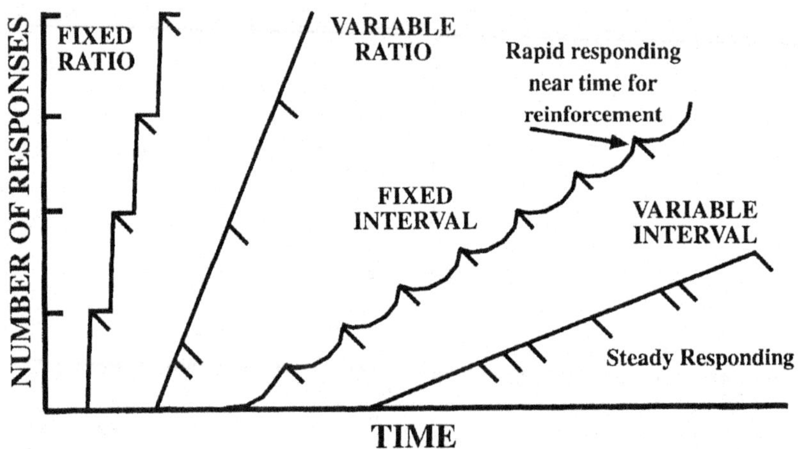

Figure 1.4. Schematic depiction of some of the laws of operant behavior. Representative types of response patterns (arbitrary scales) of animals working on traditional partial reinforcement schedules of reward. Animals on fixed-ratio (FR) schedules work at high constant rates and exhibit short postreinforcement pauses after acquiring each reward. On variable-ratio (VR) schedules, animals respond at fast constant rates that are somewhat slower than rates on FR schedules. On fixed-interval (FI) schedules, animals exhibit slowly accelerating modes of responding, with the most rapid rates exhibited just prior to each reward (which reflects an "expectancy type" of gradually intensifying pattern of behavioral arousal). On variable-interval (VI) schedules, responding is very steady but generally much slower than any of the other schedules of reinforcement. Obviously, gambling places such as Las Vegas prefer to keep their clients working on VR schedules of reinforcement.

time off after each reinforcement, yielding the "post-reinforcement pause." When required to work for set wages for a certain amount of time at work (i.e., a fixed-interval schedule, where one merely has to wait a certain amount of time before a single response will bring a reward), they tend to work slowly during the first part of the interval, gradually increasing behavioral output as "paytime" arrives (yielding a scalloped curve). When placed on variable-ratio and variable-interval schedules, where things are unpredictable (as in Las Vegas), animals work at constant steady rates, but the rates are substantially faster with variable-ratio schedules (just the way profiteers in Las Vegas want us to behave when playing one-armed bandits). Both humans and animals work in about the same way on such schedules. Unfortunately, behaviorism provided no cogent mechanistic explanation of why and how the brain generates such consistent learned behavior patterns. That would have required brain research, of the type that is summarized in Chapter 8.

Once the fundamental environment-behavior relations were worked out, behaviorism should have encouraged ever stronger connections to surrounding levels of analysis—biological principles below and psychological principles above the behavioral ones that had been established. This would have been the natural evolution of the field. Unfortunately, rather than changing with the times, the tenets of behaviorism became dogma, the intellectual wagons were drawn together into ever tightening circles, and an intellectual battle was waged with the rest of the field that desired to seek broader and deeper knowledge about problems of mutual interest. This failure to accept the obvious led to the intellectual rebellion that we now know as the cognitive revolution.

One regret we must have is that, as a result of such battles for intellectual dominance, many of the important empirical contributions that rigorous behavioral analysis provided now have less impact than they deserve in the current curriculum of mainstream psychology. For instance, at present it is generally agreed that one of the best ways to teach autistic children specific new ways to behave in the world is single-trial behavioral approaches where one systematically rewards and punishes (mildly!) specific behaviors. Ivar Lovaas, who popularized this approach, has claimed that almost half of autistic children can be mainstreamed in the school system with intensive, 40-hour-a-week implementation of such discrete-trial learning procedures.[30] The reason this approach has had to struggle for recognition (which is presently coming rapidly, at least from parents of autistic children) is because it was seen as dehumanizing, since the "whole person" was not the target of therapy. While behaviorism is by no means dead, and it rightfully continues to flourish in fields as diverse as pharmacology and economics,[31] it can no longer be deemed an adequate paradigm for unraveling many of the remaining mysteries of the brain and mind.

Suggested Readings

Barkow, J., Cosmides, L., & Tooby, J. (eds.) (1990). *The adapted mind: Evolutionary psychology and the generation of culture*. New York: Oxford Univ. Press.

Bunge, M. (1990). What kind of discipline is psychology: Autonomous or dependent, humanistic or scientific, biological or sociological? *New Ideas in Psychology* 8:121–137.

Byrne, R., & Whiten, A. (eds.) (1988). *Machiavellian intelligence*. Oxford: Oxford Univ. Press.

Churchland, P. (1985). *Neurophilosophy*. Cambridge, Mass.: MIT Press.

Clynes, M., & Panksepp, J. (eds.) (1988). *Emotions and psychopathology*. New York: Plenum Press.

Griffin, D. R. (1984). *Animal thinking*. Cambridge, Mass.: Harvard Univ. Press.

Lewis, M., & Haviland, J. M. (eds.) (1993). *Handbook of emotions*. New York: Guilford Press.

MacLean, P. D. (1990). *The triune brain in evolution*. New York: Plenum Press.

Plutchik, R. (1980). *Emotion: A psychoevolutionary synthesis*. New York: Harper and Row.

Wilson, E. O. (1975). *Sociobiology: The new synthesis*. Cambridge, Mass.: Harvard Univ. Press.

2

Emotional Operating Systems and Subjectivity

Methodological Problems and a Conceptual Framework for the Neurobiological Analysis of Affect

That the experience-hypothesis, as ordinarily understood, is inadequate to account for emotional phenomena, will be sufficiently manifest. If possible, it is even more at fault in respect to the emotions than in respect to the cognitions. The doctrine maintained by some philosophers, that all desires, all the sentiments, are generated by the experiences of the individual, is so glaringly at variance with hosts of facts, that I cannot but wonder how anyone should ever have entertained it.

Herbert Spencer, *Principles of Psychology* (1855)

CENTRAL THEME

Ultimately the emotional systems of the brain create mixtures of innate and learned action tendencies in humans, as well as in the other creatures we must study in order to fully understand the neural substrates of affective processes. As we now know, there are no credible, routine ways to unambiguously separate the influences of nature and nurture in the control of behavior that will apply across different environments. To understand the aspects of behavior that derive their organizational essence mainly from nature, we must first identify how instinctual behaviors emerge from the intrinsic potentials of the nervous system. For instance, animals do not learn *to search their environment* for items needed for survival, although they surely need to learn exactly when and how precisely to search. In other words, the "seeking potential" is built into the brain, but each animal must learn to direct its behaviors toward the opportunities that are available in the environment. In addition, animals do not need to learn to experience and express fear, anger, pain, pleasure, and joy, nor to play in simple rough-and-tumble ways, even though all of these processes come to modify and be modified by learning. Evidence suggests that evolution has imprinted many spontaneous psychobehavioral potentials within the inherited neurodynamics of the mammalian brain; these systems help generate internally experienced emotional feelings. Indeed, affective experience appears to be closely linked to brain programs that generate emotional behaviors, as well as the incoming sensory experiences that result from emotive behaviors. The function of subjectively experienced feeling states may be to sustain ongoing behavior patterns and to augment simple and effective learning strategies. Accordingly, in order to understand the neural nature of emotional feelings in humans, we must first seek to decode how brain circuits control the basic, genetically encoded emotional behavioral tendencies we share with other mammals. Then we must try to determine how subjective experience emerges from or is linked to those brain systems. Progress on these issues has been meager. In general, both psychology and modern neuroscience have failed to give sufficient credence to the fact that organisms are born with a variety of innate affective tendencies that emerge from the ancient organizational structure of the mammalian brain.

An Example of an Instinctual System in Action

Consider an archetypal situation: A cricket has outgrown its old cuticle and must successfully molt in order to proceed into the world in its new exoskeleton. The behaviors that achieve this transformation were not left to chance by evolution but are programmed into the cricket's neurobehavioral repertoire. As described by Truman:

> The initial behaviors involve anchoring the old cuticle [i.e., shell] to a substrate and swallowing air. This causes the body to swell and aids in rupturing the old cuticle. The ecdysis [i.e., molting] movements then involve a complex series of motor patterns, the major one consisting of rhythmic bouts of peristaltic contractions that move the abdomen up and propel the old cuticle backwards along the body. Coordinated with these abdominal movements are specific motor subroutines that extract each appendage (legs, antennae) from its sheath of old cuticle. There are additional behavioral subroutines that are not displayed during a normal ecdysis. If certain aspects of the behavior go awry, such as when an appendage becomes stuck, these behaviors are then called into play.[1]

This behavioral program is activated by a specific hormone. Other hormone-driven behavioral routines allow caterpillars to become moths or butterflies and human children to become adults.

Without inherited behavioral potentials, no creature could survive. Do the "lower" creatures feel delight and pleasure once their fixed patterns of behavior have yielded the appropriate results? Probably not, especially if the behavior is "hardwired," exhibiting little response flexibility, but we may never know this for certain because their behaviors and nervous systems are so fundamentally different from ours. Although it was long deemed impossible, we should now be able to answer such questions empirically for our close relatives, the other mammals, whose nervous systems and hormonal controls are homologous to ours. For instance, the analysis of subcortical brain circuits and hormonal influences on animal and human behavior has revealed many powerful cross-species generalizations.[2] An especially provocative example is the ability of the same gonadal steroids to promote energized psychosexual arousal in both animals and humans, and the discovery that such effects arise from similar circuits of the brain (see Chapter 12). There are many other examples, ranging from the nature of the pituitary adrenal stress response (see Chapter 6) to the neurochemistries that control social feelings (see Chapter 14). By studying such homologous processes in other mammals, we can establish a solid foundation for understanding the sources of human emotions and motivations.

However, we must always keep in mind that evolution generates variety. Thus, even though we can derive useful general principles concerning human emotions from studying animal brains, there are bound to be many differences in detail. This didactic point can be highlighted by focusing on the many uses of the tail across mammalian species. In monkeys, the tail can serve as a useful appendage for unique forms of locomotion. Whales and porpoises use their tails for swimming. Cows, horses, and many other ungulates use the tail as a flyswatter to dispel insects from their anal zones. Many species also use their tails, presumably unconsciously, to convey social signals. This tendency has been markedly amplified in canine species, where the position of animals' tails and their tendency to wag can tell us much about the animals' emotional states and social relationships. And then we have the great apes, who have no tails at all, except during fetal stages of development. Ultimately, along came humans, who are prone to tell many tall tales, one of the most popular being that we are completely different from all the other species. Of course, when we do encounter structural and functional diversity across species, even within homologous brain circuits that control basic emotions, we will have to deal with them forthrightly. However, at the present time, we are still in the early stages of such work—trying to identify the major emotional pathways that exist in the mammalian brain—and I will not focus on the many fine and troublesome details that characterize the variety of nature.[3]

Thesis: All Mammals Possess Intrinsic Psychobehavioral Control Systems

All mammals, indeed all organisms, come into the world with a variety of abilities that do not require previous learning, but which provide immediate opportunities for learning to occur. The influence of these systems varies as a function of the life span in each species (Figure 2.1). Analysis of the emotion systems that control behavior is complicated by the fact that the intrinsic arousability of underlying brain systems may change in many ways as organisms age. Still, the present premise will be that emotional abilities initially emerge from "instinctual" operating systems of the brain, which allow animals to begin gathering food, information, and other resources needed to sustain life. As such emotive systems mature and interact with higher brain areas, where they undergo both rerepresentation and refinement, organisms learn to make effective behavioral choices. Emotional tendencies such as those related to fear, anger, and separation distress emerge at early developmental stages, allowing young animals to cope with archetypal emergency situations that could compromise their survival. Gradually, through their effects on other parts of the brain, these systems allow animals to have more subtle social feelings and to anticipate important events and deal with them in increasingly complex ways. Others, such as sexual lust and maternal devotion, emerge later to promote reproductive success. Additional social processes, such as play and the seeking of dominance, start to control behavior with differential intensities during later phases of life and help promote the establishment of

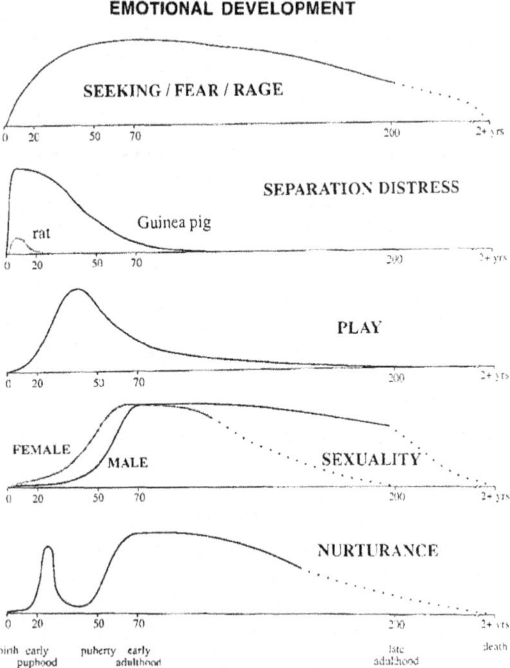

Figure 2.1. Schematic representation of the approximate developmental age course of changes in the expression of various emotional processes in the laboratory rat (with one additional species depicted for separation distress to highlight striking species differences that exist in some emotional systems). The developmental progressions of RAGE and FEAR systems are less well studied, but they are probably relatively constant across the life span, similar to the trajectory of the SEEKING system. As is evident, sexuality and nurturance tend to parallel each other, suggesting common controls. The youthful peak in nurturance may indicate a period that corresponds to the phase when young animals exhibit an intense interest in other young animals. It is noteworthy that dominance tendencies also parallel sexual urges.

stable social structures and the propagation of the most fortunate and the most able.

It is an understatement to say that at present we do not know how, precisely, affective states are generated within the brain. Primary-process affective consciousness (i.e., raw feels) may have evolved because such internal states allowed animals to make better behavioral choices. For instance, the ability of learned associations to activate internally experienced affective schema could have provided a simple coding device to promote generalized adaptive responses that could be molded by further learning.

Here I will argue, on the basis of a great deal of empirical data, that the distinct emotional "command" systems (as outlined in the next chapter and detailed in Chapters 7–15) activate various types of affective feelings. These may be quite specific for individual emotional systems or they may be nonspecific, as reflected in generalized feelings of pleasure and aversion that are shared by several emotional systems. In either case, affective feelings help animals to better identify events in the world that are either biologically useful or harmful and to generate adaptive responses to many life-challenging circumstances.[4]

In addition to responding to emergency situations, mild arousal of these brain systems presumably helps generate characteristic moods and coaxes animals to perform their everyday activities in characteristic ways. Even when there is no clear environmental reason for emotional arousal, these systems may continue to prompt organisms to undertake new activities (as in the case of exploration or play), all the while providing internal values (i.e., positive and negative feelings) for life choices.

Because of learning and the rapid development of behavioral habits, one can never capture innate emotional dynamics in their pure form, except perhaps when they are aroused artificially by direct stimulation of brain areas where those operating systems are most concentrated. I will refer to such experiments in subsequent chapters as one of the main lines of evidence to support the existence and provisional localization of emotional operating systems. It is now well established that one can reliably evoke several distinct emotional patterns in all mammals during electrical stimulation of homologous subcortical regions. Typically, animals either like or dislike the stimulation, as can be inferred from such behavioral criteria as conditioned approach and avoidance. If the electrodes are not placed in the right locations, no emotional behaviors are observed. For instance, most of the neocortex is free of such effects. Even though cortical processes such as thoughts and perceptions (i.e., appraisals) can obviously instigate various emotions, to the best of our knowledge, the affective essence of emotionality is subcortically and precognitively organized. This last issue has been a bone of contention for emotion researchers for some time,[5] but in the present context, precognitive is taken to mean that these systems have an internal organization so that they could, in principle, generate emotional feelings with no direct input from either unconditioned or learned environmental inputs. For instance, a ill-placed tumor could generate a chronic state of emotional arousal, even though the underlying neural system is designed to be normally governed by external inputs.

Although cognitive and affective processes can be independently conceptualized, it comes as no surprise that emotions powerfully modify cortical appraisal and memory processes and vice versa.[6] The innate emotional systems interact with higher brain systems so extensively that in the normal animal there is probably no emotional state that is free of cognitive ramifications.[7] It is more likely that in humans there may be some thoughts that are free of affect. Clearly, there is much more variety among mammals in cortical functions than in subcortical ones. However, if those cortical functions were evolutionarily built upon the preexisting subcortical foundations, providing ever-increasing behavioral sophistication and flexibility, we must obviously understand the latter in order to make sense of the functions of the former.

The most primal affective-cognitive interaction in humans, and presumably other animals as well, is encapsulated in the phrases "I want" and "I don't want." These assertions are reflected in basic tendencies to approach and avoid various real-life phenomena. However, there are several distinct ways to like and dislike events, and a proper classification scheme will yield a more complex taxonomy of emotions than the simple behavioral dimension of approach and avoidance. For instance, it seems unlikely that the dislike of bitter foods and the dislike of physical pain emerge from one and the same avoidance system. It is equally unlikely that the desire for food and the urge to play emerge from the same brain systems. As outlined in the next chapter, evolution has constructed a variety of emotional systems in the ancient recesses of the mammalian brain. To the best of our knowledge, these systems still exist in human beings as well.

When these affective systems are overtaxed or operate outside the normal range, we call the end results *psychiatric disorders*. Underactivity of certain systems may cause depression and variants of personality disorders. Overactivity can contribute to mania, paranoid schizophrenia, and anxiety, obsessive-compulsive, and post-traumatic stress disorders (PTSDs). Other problems such as autism and childhood schizophrenia appear to emerge from "wiring" problems in brain circuits. Because of the social importance of these human problems, a substantive understanding of the ancient neurobiological value systems and the manner in which they can become overtaxed is of great scientific and societal concern.

The extent to which the emotional operating systems exhibit neuronal plasticity—changes in the efficiency of synaptic connections and dendritic arborization as a function of experience—is becoming an increasingly important avenue of empirical inquiry. Practically every brain system changes with use and disuse. For instance, the "archetypal situations" described in the previous chapter are the types of experiences that lead to PTSD, and it is presently widely believed that persistent neural traces of emotional traumas reflect the development of long-term sensitization in areas of the brain such as the amygdala, which are known to mediate fearfulness. Indeed, newly emerging disorders such as *multiple chemical sensitivities*, which may have contributed to that mysterious recent outbreak known as the *Gulf War syndrome*, may be due to a change in the sensitivity of emotional circuits that can be induced, especially in temperamentally predisposed individuals, by exposure to environmental toxins.[8] Although our knowledge about the chronic changes that can occur in emotional circuits remains rudimentary, it is likely that all emotional systems exhibit forms of plasticity, which eventually will help us understand much about the underlying neuronal nature of psychiatric disorders.

The Challenge of Studying Intrinsic Brain Operating Systems

I will use the general term *brain organ system*, and more specifically *emotional operating system*, to designate the complex neural interactions that generate such inborn psychobehavioral tendencies. Although each instinctual psychobehavioral process requires the concurrent arousal of numerous brain activities (Figure 2.2), our scientific work is greatly simplified by the fact that there are "command processes" at the core of each emotional operating system, as indicated by the ability of localized brain stimulation to activate coherent emotional behavior patterns.[9] We can turn on rage, fear, separation distress, and generalized seeking patterns of behavior. Such central coordinating influences can provoke widespread cooperative activities by many brain systems, generating a variety of integrated psychobehavioral and physiological/hormonal response tendencies. These systems can generate internally experienced emotional feelings and promote behavioral flexibility via new learning. Similar *command systems* have also been found in many invertebrates.[10] For instance, crayfish and lobsters exhibit a stereotyped flight response. Although we may never know with any sense of assurance whether these creatures have what we might call "affective consciousness," it is noteworthy that their seemingly fixed behavioral responses are really not that fixed. Even their emotional responses can be modulated by fairly subtle social contextual variables, such as their positions in status hierarchies.[11]

Each emotional system is hierarchically arranged throughout much of the brain, interacting with more evolved cognitive structures in the higher reaches, and specific physiological and motor outputs at lower levels. As depicted schematically in Figure 2.2, the emotional systems are centrally placed to coordinate many higher and lower brain activities, and each emotional system also interacts with many other nearby emotional systems. Because of the ascending interactions with higher brain areas, there is no emotion without a thought, and many thoughts can evoke emotions. Because of the lower interactions, there is no emotion without a physiological or behavioral consequence, and many of the resulting bodily changes can also regulate the tone of emotional systems in a feedback manner.

As can be readily appreciated from Figure 2.2, taxonomies of emotions are bound to differ depending on an investigator's preferred level of analysis. For instance, subtle social emotions like shame, guilt, and embarrassment may emerge from separation-distress

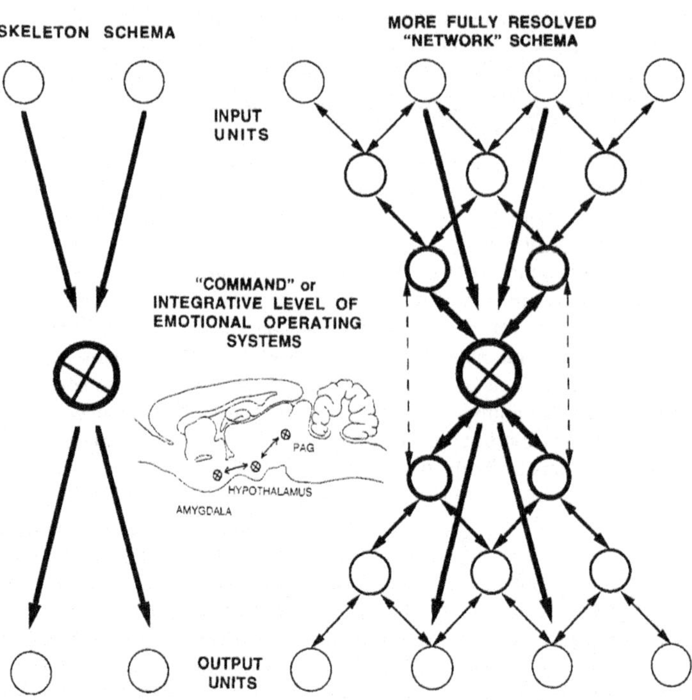

Figure 2.2. Two schematic representations of an emotional operating system. In simplest terms (*left*), emotional "command" systems integrate unconditional inputs and generate instinctual behavior output patterns. In more resolved conceptualizations (*right*), there are many hierarchical levels of control within both input and output components, with multiple feedbacks across levels and also strong interactions between different emotional systems (not shown). Within this conceptualization, central executive components (indicated by "comparator" circles with Xs and highlighted a bit more realistically on the saggital depiction of an emotional system such as the one for RAGE; see Figure 10.4) can synchronize the whole system into a coherent form of emotional responsivity. The central integration of each specific emotional response appears to be coordinated by specific neuropeptide circuits.

systems (see Chapter 14) interacting with higher brain functions. In any event, at the present time, the lower command level provide the best organizational principles for neuroscientific inquiries. We can now be confident that a limited number of executive structures for emotionality were created in our brains by our genetic heritage, but we cannot yet be certain how many exist and how widespread they are in the nervous system. However, we can be confident about the approximate locations of some half a dozen systems, and we can approximate their ramifications in the brain using various neuroscience techniques. An analysis of the core structures of the major emotional command systems will be the main focus of this text.

Many of the emotional command influences are mediated by specific neuropeptides, of which several hundred have already been characterized (see Chapter 6). Several discrete emotions can now be manipulated via the stimulation and blockade of individual neurochemistries. Since these neurochemistries can be easily visualized using neuroanatomical techniques, such as *immunocytochemistry*, our ability to tease coherent systems out of the massive webwork of the brain has become possible in the last few decades. This allows fairly impressive specification of the neuroanatomical trajectories of the executive influences of certain emotional systems. Likewise, the ability of new genetic techniques to highlight those neurons that are activated during certain psychobehavioral experiences (e.g., visualization of transiently activated gene products such as *Fos* protein expression in neurons; see Chapter 4) allows us, in conjunction with other tools, to estimate how widespread are the brain influences of specific forms of emotional arousal. In general, because of the inexorable spread of neural activities within the brain, they are much wider than the executive circuits that will be discussed here. Still, we should always remember that such new techniques only visualize the activities of brain tissues. How shall we ever see the neurodynamics of a thought process or a feeling state objectively? Probably through a combination of neurochemical, neurophysiological, and behavioral techniques (Chapters 5 and 6), blended with theoretical inference.

Currently our most open psychological window into the emotional mind is the use of modern introspective techniques in humans, such as diary and other verbal reports,[12] but empirical developments in this area have been slow because of the conceptual biases of previous times. At the turn of the century, introspectionism was found to have fatal flaws, and it continues to be evident that humans often do not adequately understand the causes of their own behaviors. Thus, we must remain cautious of introspective approaches for providing much in the way of causal knowledge. Most of emotional processing, as of every other psychobehavioral process, is done at an unconscious level. However, introspection can help identify many of the distinct emotional categories and other basic brain functions that need to be elucidated by science.

To study emotions in animals, we have to remain sensitive to their natural needs and values, and develop more subtle measures of their natural tendencies in many different situations. As we saw in the previous chapter, we cannot reasonably study the playfulness of young rats in the presence of predator odors. Likewise, we cannot study the courting, reproductive, dominance, and migratory urges of birds unless the lighting is right (e.g., the lengthening daylight hours of spring, which allow their reproductive systems to mature each year). If we do not pay attention to a host of variables that reflect the adaptive evolutionary dimensions of the animals we study, we will not obtain credible answers concerning their natural emotional tendencies. Thus, some of our best insights may come from observation of animals in the wild. As an example, let me share a striking description of Darwin's finches courting in the Galápagos Islands:

> Mating season begins with all the black cocks on the island singing in the rain. Each male broadcasts from his singing post, and while he sings he scans his territory. If a female alights near one of the display nests that he has built, he darts from his singing post and flies to her. If she is one of his own kind, he sings and shakes his wings at her, makes them quiver tremulously. Then he flies to the nearest nest. (Any nest will do, even the nest of a rival if the rival is out.) He goes in and out, in and out of the nest, looking back at the female over his shoulder. Sometimes he picks up a bit of grass in his beak and puts it down again, rapidly, over and over, as if he were trying to catch her eye.[13]

Do these birds have emotional experiences during these activities, or are their movements consciousness-independent *fixed-action patterns*? Do they have internal feelings, or are they robots with vacuous minds like our personal computers? At present, no one knows for sure, but laboratory tests are now available to evaluate such important brain issues (i.e., conditioned place preference and aversion measures).

How Can We Study Internal Processes That We Cannot See in Animals?

How are we to address the issue of feelings when we deal with creatures that do not communicate with us directly? The traditional academic "solution" to the problem of neurosubjectivity in animal brain research has been to ignore it—to study behavior and simply disregard the troublesome probability that a focus on the affective and cognitive experiences may be essential for a clear and accurate picture of how the brain operates. Thus, students of energy and fluid regulation have typically been encouraged to study the neural correlates of food and water intake and to forget that subjective motivational terms such as hunger and thirst exist. Students of reproduction are advised to study the courting and copulatory movements of animals, and to disregard the possibility that animal brains might be filled with specific forms of erotic arousal. Because the richness and visual objectivity of behavioral change allows us to focus our empirical attention, the neurobiology of internal states continues to be neglected.

In any event, neuroscientists and psychologists have finally started to deal effectively with unseen entities, in the same way particle physicists started to envision a universe of complexity within atoms about a century ago. Even though physicists still cannot "see" clearly inside atoms, their theoretically inferred knowledge has changed the world. The same will happen with brain research on emotions and motivations. Progress at this level requires the continual application of the time-honored but fallacious form of scientific logic known as "affirmation of consequents" (Figure 2.3). Although the logical flaw of this most common mode of scientific reasoning—induction—is obvious,[14] there is no alternative way to extract general principles from observed facts. Thus, the study of experienced feelings remains a difficult, some say "insoluble," challenge for the analysis of animal behavior, but it does become a workable problem when we add the dimension of cross-species brain research. By using spontaneous behaviors and various preference tests as our initial indicator variable for internal processes, and the subsequent evaluation of the neuroscience conclusions in humans, one can infer how both animal and human feelings are organized. Interpretive flaws in such research can be corrected through the falsification of predictions, successive approximations toward better theories, and the weight of converging evidence.

In humans, the study of subjectivity is a bit easier to pursue. We can ask people to speak to us or to indicate on some other output device when they are having various emotional experiences. Simultaneously we can measure many of the brain and body changes to which new technologies provide access.[15] Of course, the mere act of responding in this way may change the processes being observed, especially in inexperienced subjects. In humans we can now observe some of the internal dynamics of the brain, even though a standardized measure of emotionality that operates in a real-time window is not yet available. Functional *magnetic resonance imaging* (fMRI) is beginning to approximate the ideal, but, as summarized in Chapters 4 and 16, serious interpretive problems remain. For instance, fMRI can estimate brain activities by measuring regional blood flow or oxygenation changes throughout the brain, but emotions may have undiscovered and unpredictable effects on brain blood parameters that are not simply reflective of neural activities. For instance, it is possible that certain emotions such as fear are characterized by reductions of blood flow to many brain areas as a secondary consequence of emotional intensity rather than as a result of local metabolic needs to fuel neuronal activity. Although the problem of validation in such experiments is almost as enormous as in animal research, the combination of animal and human approaches

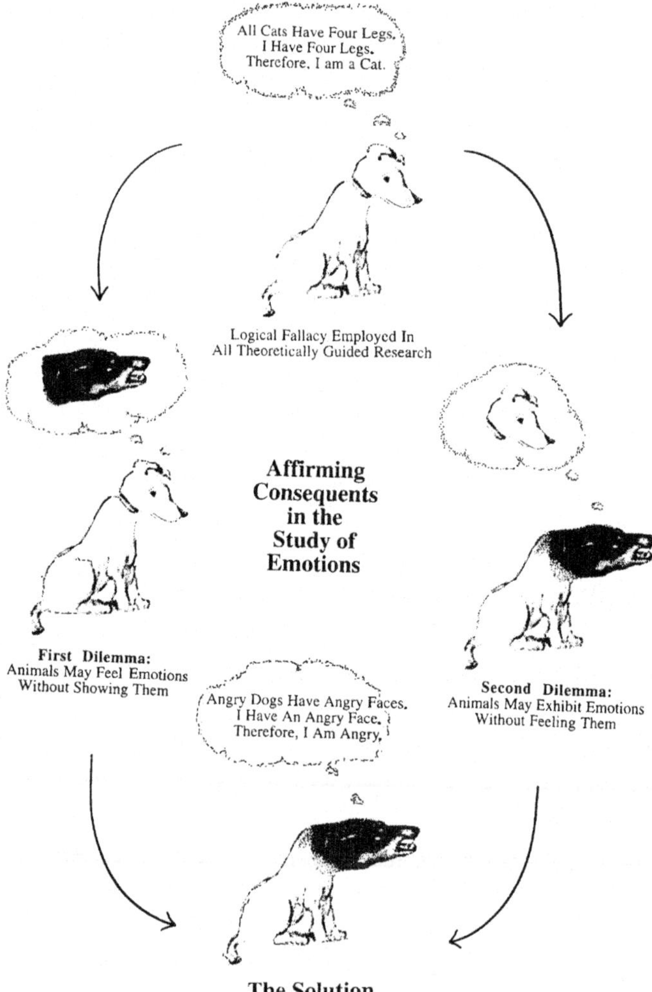

Figure 2.3. All theoretically guided research proceeds via "affirmation of consequents," which is, of course, a logical fallacy since every individual observation can potentially be explained by a variety of theories. The two major types of flaws (or dilemmas) that this type of reasoning poses for emotion research are depicted, but to make progress on the more subtle functions of the nervous system, there is no alternative but to accept such weaknesses and to proceed with the realization that any mistakes can be corrected by the procedures of disconfirmation. Namely, if hypothesized experimental predictions do not hold, they negate the general principles from which they were derived. Conversely, through the use of converging manipulations that confirm predictions, and through the resultant "weight of evidence," we can have considerable confidence in theoretical ideas. (Adapted from Panksepp, 1991; see n. 41.)

presently allows us to converge on concepts in ways that were unimaginable just a few years ago.

Thus, the nature of central affective states must be theoretically inferred from a variety of brain measurements and manipulations, which are related to new predictions of behavioral changes in animals. The resulting conclusions, in turn, must be validated against the verbal reports of human subjects (Figure 2.4). Through such triangulation procedures involving brain manipulations, behavioral changes in animals, and, where possible, reported mental changes in humans, the scientific conundrum of subjectivity can finally be credibly addressed (Figure 2.3). Obviously, one critical but underappreciated key to this strategy is behavioral brain research in other animals. To really understand the basic human emotions, we cannot simply stay at the human level. Conversely, to understand animal emotions, we probably cannot simply stay at the animal-behavior level. An integrated interdisciplinary approach, with an active attempt to link levels of analysis, is essential for understanding the shared nature of human and animal emotions.

Contrasting the Study of Cognitions and Emotions in Animals

Obviously, studies of the intrinsic functions of the brain, such as the nature of the various emotions, are among the most difficult to pursue in neuropsychology. Related topics, like the nature of the self, the will, and thinking processes, also remain neglected by neuroscientists. Only recently has human psychology returned its attention to these questions under the banner of *cognitive neuroscience*.[16] Many animal behaviorists have also started to study the nature of animal cognitions.[17] The renewed effort to understand cognitive representations, imagery, and thought is notoriously difficult, but it is decidedly easier than the study of emotions. Cognitive representations can often be treated as logical propositions that can be precisely linked to explicit referents in the external world, which allows investigators to initiate credible empirical studies.

For instance, it has now been demonstrated that pigeons can generate internal representations of moving visual stimuli, and can use these representations to solve problems when the visual stimuli are temporarily out of sight. This was achieved by using a video image of a rotating, constant-velocity clock hand as the cue, and requiring test animals to respond to the internally imaged speed of the clock hand during periods when the video display was briefly turned off. Pigeons that were able to accurately keep the temporal progression of such an image in mind could obtain food by responding appropriately in a timely manner. Pigeons acquired such tasks remarkably well, and a host of control manipulations indicated that the pigeons were in fact responding to sustained internal representations of the visual displays within their brains.[18] The success of such experiments has been based upon experimenters' ability to cleverly manipulate environmental contingencies in strictly controlled ways.

Subjective emotional feelings, on the other hand, do not follow the rules of propositional logic, and external reference points—the natural stimuli that evoke emotions—are not as clear-cut except in a few examples such as the smell of predators described in Chapter 1. Even if such trigger stimuli (or "sign stimuli" in ethological terminology) can be identified, the objects of our feelings (e.g., the people we love or the foods we enjoy) rarely have intrinsic logical qualities (like the constant speed of the aforementioned clock hand) that allow us to conceptually anchor the nature of an animal's internal representations to world events.

With affective feelings, other important, but as yet unstudied, internal representations may be the anchor points for felt experience. For instance, the reference process for specific emotional states may be the arousal of specific neurochemical circuits and anatomical areas of the brain. Furthermore, the actual generation of affective feelings may arise from the interaction of those circuits with yet other brain systems such as those that generate the internal preconscious process of "I-ness" or self-identity as discussed in Chapter 16.

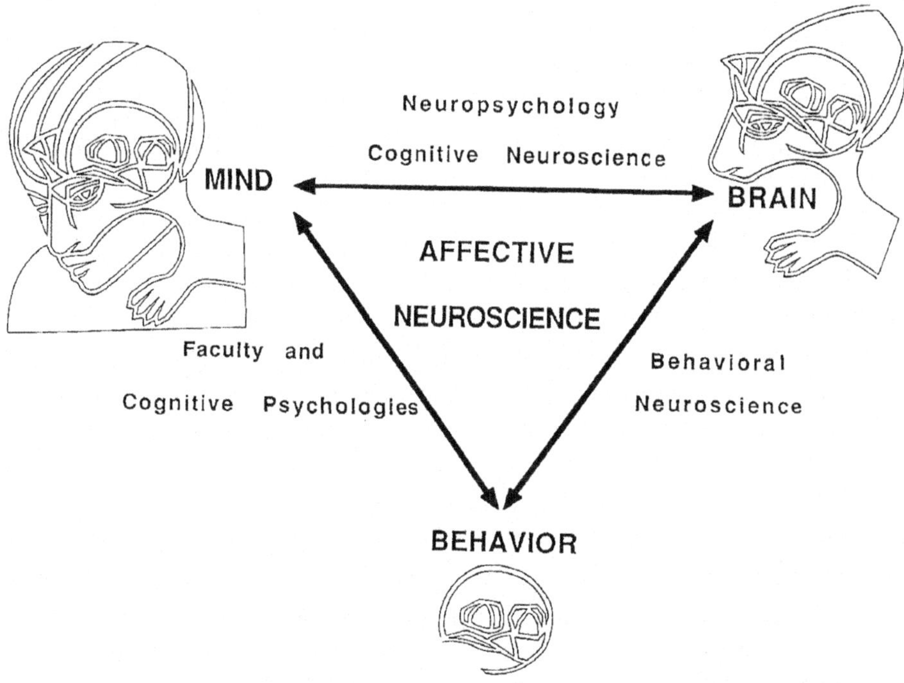

Figure 2.4. Progress in understanding the biological nature of affective processes can only proceed through the integration of psychological, behavioral, and neuroscientific approaches. At present, there is no discipline that utilizes all of these approaches in a balanced manner. The various disciplines that bridge two of the three components are indicated. Affective neuroscience aspires to bridge all three, and the dissection of the logo used for this book helps symbolize the complexities we face: We need to come to terms with ancient reptilian brain functions, old mammalian brain functions, as well as the crowning glory of the human cortex.

Although there have been several previous heroic efforts to link emotions to bodily events (e.g., the James-Lange theory of emotions described in the "Afterthought" of Chapter 3), at present the major reference processes appear to be largely within the evolved functions of the brain rather than in peripheral physiological changes. Thus, we experience feelings of thirst not primarily because of having a dry mouth but because certain neural circuits automatically and unconsciously inform us that our body does not have enough water or that the concentration of salts has become too high within our cells. The notion that emotions are simply the result of our higher cognitive appreciation of certain forms of bodily commotion has been largely negated by the observation of essentially normal emotional responsivity in people who have suffered massive spinal cord injuries.[19]

The actual neural mechanisms that create emotional feelings is the central question of affective neuroscience. My assumption is that neural interactions elaborate a variety of distinct periconscious affective states that have little intrinsic cognitive resolution except various feelings of "goodness" and "badness." I use the term *periconscious* to suggest that higher forms of consciousness had to emerge evolutionarily from specific types of preconscious neural processes, and that the primitive affective systems that will be described in this text may have been the major gateways for the development of cognitively resolved awareness of values that appear to exist in the world.

As a result of mental maturation, those periconscious affective systems eventually inform our higher cognitive apparatus how world events relate to our intrinsic needs—thereby gradually establishing our higher value systems. For instance, one can produce the appearance of anger in an infant simply by restraining its movement.[20] However, only through maturation can such primitive experiences of anger be symbolically generalized to world events: that some specific person or institution is attempting to symbolically constrain our freedom of action or trying to take something valuable away from us, even something as subtle as our peace of mind. Obviously, those higher interpretations that eventually come to surround our emotional states (let us call them "attributions," as is so common)[21] can only emerge from higher brain functions.

According to current evolutionary thinking, the cognitive apparatus of higher brain areas has ingrained tendencies to dwell upon such affective challenges with various forms of retribution—which arise from a sense of justice and/or desire for revenge.[22] Although an analysis of cognitive consequences is of great societal and social-psychological importance (and can yield a more complex taxonomy of emotions than the one pursued here), those levels of analysis will not give us any clear answer to the primal nature of the powerful neuropsychic "energies" that we share with other creatures—the neural processes that constitute the primitive emotional forces that we call anger, fear, desire, and distress. To my knowledge, the type of affective neuroscience strategy outlined here is the only way we can scientifically understand the neural foundations of the emotions that may be essential substrates for the genesis of the more complex, hybrid forms of human feelings. Because of the sheer magnitude of the task before us, my attention will be restricted largely to those neurobehavioral topics that will help us clarify the foundation issues.

The Possible Functions of Subjective Emotional Experiences

Besides the obvious difficulties in measurement, the main dilemma that has reduced the willingness of investigators to utilize affective concepts in neuroscience has been our difficulty in envisioning how internally felt subjective states could have any mechanistic influence in the causal chain of neural events intervening between environmental stimuli and responses. It has traditionally been assumed that feelings and other mental processes are immaterial and hence cannot act as material causes for anything else. Also, it has been difficult to see why internally experienced emotional states would be needed for immediate behavioral control. Neural explanations without any psychological qualities should suffice to explain most instinctual behaviors. Hence, some have been tempted to suggest that if emotional feelings do exist, they are simply epiphenomena, mechanistically passive by-products of the neural activities that actually control behavior.

Of course, as the computer revolution has taught us by the simple fact that software functions can control hardware functions, there are many nondualistic ways around this dilemma: we can readily assume (1) that feeling states are not immaterial but rather true reflections of specific types of neural circuit interactions, and (2) that subjective feelings have other functions than the mere governance of unconditional behavioral outputs (i.e., more than the mere generation of instinctual behaviors). For example, internal feelings may directly mediate learning by coding behavioral strategies for future use, or perhaps they do this indirectly by interacting with "self-representational" systems within the brain. Indeed, such an assumption is a central tenet of the present thesis.

To put this troublesome issue into a more formal perspective, let us note four major ways in which emotional feelings might be represented within the normal flow of information from instigating events to behavioral and other bodily responses (Figure 2.5). In the first version, which might be called the *traditional folk-psychological view*, the interpretation of instigating events establishes a feeling state that generates bodily changes ranging from behavior to various types of visceral arousal. The apparent flaw with this simpleminded

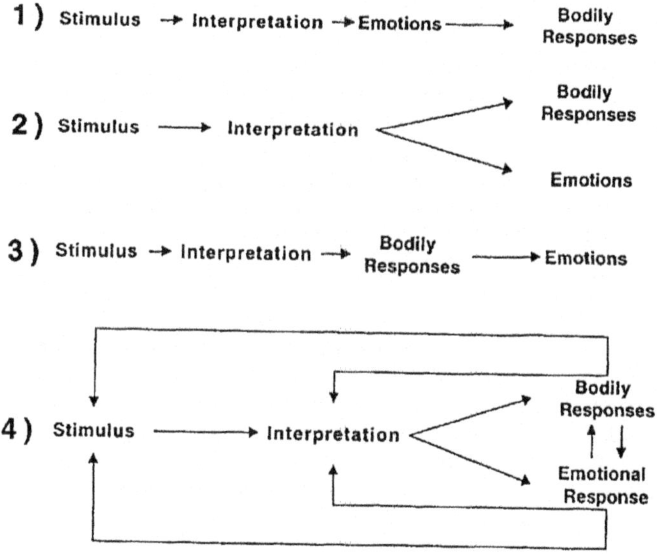

Figure 2.5. Four possible ways of viewing the role of affective consciousness in the generation of adaptive behaviors in emotional situations: (1) the "commonsense" view that emotions cause bodily responses; (2) the possibility that the two are independently but concurrently organized; (3) the counterintuitive James-Lange type of view that emotions arise by the way we bodily respond in emotional situations; and (4) a more realistic view, which suggests that all levels of information processing in the generation of emotional responses interact with each other. Although all of these schemes suggest that stimulus "interpretation" is important for emotions, it is also possible to evoke emotions directly by artificially activating certain brain circuits.

view is that a great deal of evidence suggests emotional responses are much too rapid for feelings to have been aroused. For instance, it takes less than a hundredth of a second for a fear-potentiated startle reflex to be initiated,[23] and it is often claimed that nociceptive information gets into the relevant flexor reflex circuits more rapidly than it takes for the conscious experience of pain to emerge.[24] The use of such facts to argue against the existence of consciousness in emotional behaviors fails to recognize that the generation of an affective response may be as important for guiding future behaviors as for immediate ones. Thus, fearful contextual stimuli associated with pain may induce a central state of fear that only gradually leads an animal to freeze and to apparently get "uptight."[25]

Some investigators have advocated the second variant (Figure 2.5), which suggests that emotional affective responses may be epiphenomena, occurring in parallel with emotional responses but having little role in the control of behavior. In line with such a view, many investigators are still willing to simply assume that affective consciousness is present only in humans.[26] These simpleminded views also fail to fully consider that the ancient neural mechanisms of affective responsivity may sustain central nervous system readiness for future response selection that animals exhibit as a result of conditioning. Although it is likely that humans have a more sophisticated appreciation of their own affective consciousness than other animals, it presently seems most reasonable to assume that the "raw feels" of emotions are a shared mammalian experience that does have functional consequences for an animal's behavior.

Because of the difficulty of dealing scientifically with questions of consciousness, early investigators, such as William James, suggested a third version in the flow of emotional information in his famous statement that "the bodily changes follow directly the PERCEPTION of the exciting fact and . . . our feeling of the same changes as they occur is the emotion."[27] James postulated that affective feelings emerge as a result of the cognitive interpretation of the many energetic bodily responses that are instigated by various emergency situations. In other words, we feel scared of approaching bears because of our exertions in running away from them. Although this view has enjoyed much popularity in academic psychology, like all the preceding views, it suffers from a failure to recognize the full complexity of the brain substrates. At the time James suggested his counterintuitive but not unreasonable view, we did not know there was a visceral-emotional nervous system in the brain. For instance, a modern version of the James-Lange theory might suggest that emotional feelings reflect higher cerebral readout of the activities of basic emotional circuits in subcortical areas of the brain, but such a view has not been adequately developed in psychology.

In fact, it presently seems most likely that a hybrid version of these several views is closest to the true nature of things. Accordingly, a more complex view is taking hold in emotion research (the fourth model in Figure 2.5), which accepts that emotions operate in a dynamically interactive way at many hierarchical levels within the brain. Two-way communication among levels characterizes the overall organization of an emotional response. In this view, there is a great deal of room for internally experienced affective consciousness to influence behavior in a variety of ways. Since the acceptance of subjective experience in the control of behavior has been one of the main sticking points in the study of animal emotions, the following point probably cannot be overemphasized: Affective consciousness may not be as important in instigating rapid emotional responses as it is in longer-term psychobehavioral strategies. Indeed, in humans the cognitive apparatus can greatly shorten, prolong, or otherwise modify the more "hardwired" emotional tendencies we share with the other animals.

In this view, the "interpretation" or "appraisal" component of the full emotional response is generally deemed to be complex, including many rapid and unconscious neural processes, as well as slow, deliberative responses that characterize the conscious contents of a human mind dwelling on how to deal with emotionally challenging situations.[28] In line with traditional thinking on these matters, I accept the supposition that it is scientifically meaningful to distinguish the various types of cognitive interpretive responses from basic affective ones. Although these two types of neural processing interact massively, the distinction allows us to focus on the primitive affective issues, with more clarity than we might otherwise.

As we will see in subsequent chapters, evidence indicates that internally experienced emotional states are neurologically rather primitive, since they appear to be triggered by the arousal of various subcortical emotive circuits. This suggests that the mechanisms of affective experience and emotional behavior are intimately intertwined in comparatively ancient areas of the mammalian brain, but we are just beginning to figure out exactly where and how. It may be in the higher reaches of emotional systems such as the amygdala, and frontal and cingulate cortices, as many believe; it may be in various regions of the brain stem (as discussed in Chapter 16), or, as is most likely, in distributed hierarchical representations throughout the executive emotional systems that course between higher and lower levels of the brain. My premise here will be that an analysis of these intervening neural systems, which serve a *commanding* role in triggering and coordinating instinctual emotion patterns (as detailed in Chapters 9–15), constitutes our best current strategy for understanding, in some biological detail, how affective feeling states are mechanistically generated within the brain.

In sum, a comprehensive discussion of emotions must pursue a difficult triangulation—considering affective experience, behavioral/bodily changes, and the operation of neural circuits *concurrently*. For research purposes, it may be useful to separate these levels of analysis (Figure 2.4), but for a comprehensive understanding of both the mind and the brain, as well as for more accurate prediction of behavior, the various lines of knowledge need to be blended together into an integrated whole, as they are in the functioning organism.

Conscious and Unconscious Emotions

Since emotional and other instinctual operating systems go back to a dim evolutionary past, we must assume that consciously experienced emotions emerged from preconscious processes. At present, we do not know where to draw the line between such processes. In general, the assumption here will be that the minimal criterion for the existence of consciously experienced affect in animals is the ability to demonstrate classical conditioning of emotional arousal (see Figure 1.2). For instance, I will assume that an animal may have experienced fear only if it exhibits conditioned fearful behaviors to cues that have been previously associated with unconditioned fearful behaviors. Although this is a necessary criterion, it is not a sufficient one. One must also be able to demonstrate that, given a reasonable opportunity, animals will instrumentally learn to avoid stimuli that generate such conditioned states. Also, there is a criterion related to our human ability to self-reflect: The underlying neural systems should be able to modulate the appropriate kinds of internally experienced affective changes in humans. At present, such criteria have been most completely fulfilled for the FEAR system of the brain (see Chapter 11).

However, as has been the tradition in experimental psychology, we should remain wary of using introspective reports of consciousness to reveal the nature of the mechanisms that control behavior. Obviously, a great deal of sensory and motor processing that animals and humans exhibit occurs at an unconscious level, and it is as unwise to ascribe too large a function for consciousness in the control of action tendencies as it is to give it no role in the behavioral choices that animals make. The overriding premise here is that the most fruitful search for a fundamental understanding of affective consciousness will emerge from a study of preconscious neural mechanisms that represent the organism as a coherently acting creature in the world.

How far back such periconscious mechanisms go is anyone's guess, but we can be certain that some type of evolutionary progression took place. The overall view that guides the present coverage is summarized in Figure 2.6. It is important to clearly recognize how little we really know about the emotional consciousness of humans and other animals. The truly important ideas must be cast in ways that can lead to empirical predictions. At present, there are very few ideas that meet such criteria, and for that reason behavioral neuroscience has had little tolerance for talk about such matters. However, even in the absence of definitive knowledge, it is still important to recognize how deceptively wrong our explanatory schemes may be if we do not take the nature of emotional consciousness into consideration when we study the brain mechanisms that control behavior. If basic forms of consciousness emerged in ancestral species that preceded humans on the face of the earth, an understanding of the neural instantiation of those processes, as reflected in all living descendants, is bound to inform us profoundly about the nature of our own conscious abilities. For instance, an understanding of affective consciousness may set the stage

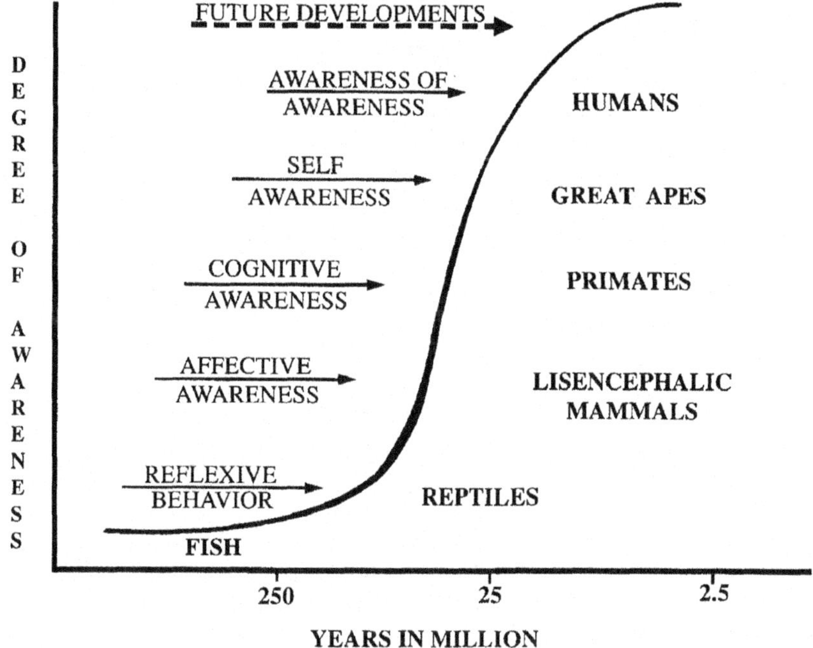

Figure 2.6. An approximation of the emergence of affective consciousness in evolution. The important point is that different levels of consciousness probably emerged during different phases of brain evolution. Chapter 16 will provide a specific view of how neural systems may mediate affective states of consciousness.

for understanding the higher forms, some of which are surely unique to humans. Although a great deal of important information about the causes of animal behavior can be obtained without addressing such matters,[29] I do not think we will be able to solve the riddle of the brain without trying to make such neurodynamic intangibles tangible.

Since we may never be able to specify when affective consciousness emerged in brain evolution with any precision, I will begin my substantive discussion of available research by introducing some of the basic operating systems of the *Aplysia*, a creature that probably operates totally preconsciously. This ancient shell-less mollusk displays a very simple repertoire of instinctual tendencies (Figure 2.7). The study of this creature, commonly called the "sea hare," serves to highlight many of the behavioral procedures and concepts that must be used to study and discuss emotions. We certainly do not know whether such primitive creatures as the *Aplysia* have subjective feelings, and perhaps we never will: Their nervous systems are so different that cross-species generalizations based on neural circuit homologies may be difficult to evaluate empirically. However, despite their apparent emotional and cognitive limitations, these animals are remarkably skilled in taking care of their own simple needs. A major key to understanding them has been through a study of their natural behavioral patterns and the neural generators governing those behavior patterns, especially through the application of simple learning techniques such as classical and operant conditioning tasks—empirical strategies that are similar to those we must use to understand the nature of mammalian emotions.

"Operating Systems" in a Model Creature: *Aplysia californica*

The saltwater sea slug, which goes by the proud scientific name *Aplysia californica*, is a workhorse of the many laboratories that are seeking a precise mechanistic understanding of the neuronal dynamics mediating learning and memory. The advantages of relying on this "model system" have been great.[30] This creature, along with several related invertebrates, has provided a preliminary understanding of nonassociative forms of learning such as *sensitization* (the spontaneous increment in behavior that can occur with repetition of a stimulus), *habituation* (the spontaneous decrement in behavior that can occur with repeated stimulation), and *dishabituation* (the elevated response tendency that occurs when stimulation has been withheld for a period of time).

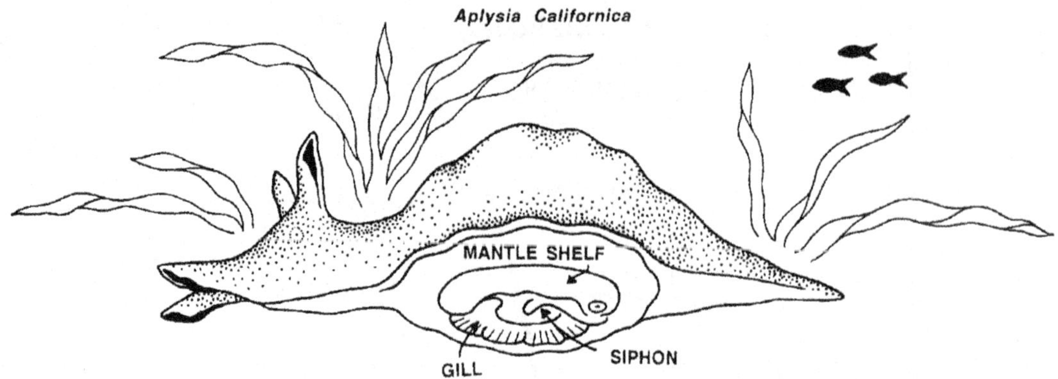

Figure 2.7. The marine snail *Aplysia californica* has a simple nervous system of about 20,000 nerve cells and a set of defensive reflexes that have been used effectively to study the neuronal basis of learning (especially classical conditioning; see Figure 1.2). For instance, touching the siphon or gill leads to a withdrawal of these organs, but this response habituates rapidly. If, however, this type of conditioned stimulus (touch) is paired with electric shock to the tail, the animal develops a conditioned gill-withdrawal response to touch. Although this type of classically conditioned learning has been most extensively studied in this creature, there has been some success in training these animals to also exhibit instrumental learning.

The *Aplysia*'s behavioral repertoire emerges from an experimentally manageable set of gigantic neurons within the abdominal ganglion. Studies of this simple animal have provided a provisional understanding of how enforced learning, or *classical conditioning,* is generated in a nervous system. As summarized in Figure 1.2, classical conditioning occurs when biologically "irrelevant," or so-called conditioned, stimuli develop the ability to elicit *conditional responses* (CRs) through repetitive pairing with various biologically relevant events, or *unconditioned stimuli* that themselves have the intrinsic ability to generate *unconditional responses* (UCRs). For example, electric shock, acting as an unconditional stimulus (UCS), normally produces a UCR of withdrawal in most organisms; when the shock is repeatedly preceded by a tone, functioning as a conditional stimulus (CS), organisms gradually begin to exhibit CRs in the form of anticipatory withdrawal. This form of simple learning has also been demonstrated in the *Aplysia.*[31] The animals will learn to withdraw their feeding siphons as anticipatory responses to neutral stimuli such as mild touch, but only after the touch has repeatedly been paired with a strong electrical stimulation of the body mantle, a stimulus that itself evokes an unconditional siphon withdrawal response.

But investigators wondered if animals would also exhibit instrumental behaviors—whether they would acquire new responses to obtain rewards or avoid punishments. This proved more difficult. Such higher forms of learning provide new levels of complexity in behavioral control that presumably reflect the rudiments of intentional behavior. For a while, the *Aplysia* seemed quite unwilling to do any of the things experimenters hoped they might do in order to obtain rewards. The failures were largely due to the fact that response requirements were not within the natural behavioral repertoire of the *Aplysia.* However, successful *instrumental conditioning* was achieved, and insights into the underlying mechanisms were generated, when it was recognized that the *Aplysia* comes into the world with a spontaneous behavioral repertoire, developed through aeons of evolution, which is capable of being modified by reinforcement contingencies.

Instrumental or operant conditioning occurs when animals begin to emit seemingly "intentional" or "voluntary" responses to obtain certain changes in the environment, such as the avoidance of negative events or the occurrence of positive ones. The trick to generating the fastest and most successful forms of operant conditioning is to rely on response systems that animals use spontaneously in their everyday interactions with the world. Animals are most likely to emit conditional instrumental responses by molding preexisting tendencies within their spontaneous behavioral repertoires. For instance, a rat's FEAR system can produce unconditional freezing and flight, which are quite easy to obtain during simple contextual fear conditioning. Simply giving an animal a foot shock in a test box is sufficient to evoke freezing whenever the animal is returned to that environment. However, if the animal has an avenue of flight, it will rapidly learn to escape the situation. By comparison, it is difficult to train rats to press a lever to avoid foot shock. Such responses are quite unnatural for the animal.

Success in producing instrumental conditioning in the *Aplysia* was achieved by heeding this insight. The *Aplysia* is generally a sluggish and behaviorally inflexible creature that crawls along the seabed, sucking in nutrients such as seaweed and the waste products of other animals. In its journey from rock to rock, it uses an intrinsic behavioral strategy of reaching out and swinging from side to side in search of a new anchor point. In so doing, it exhibits a phototactic preference for darker rather than lighter environments. The swinging response is normally inhibited when the animal is placed on a solid surface, a reaction known as *contact inhibition*, but the behavior can be instigated simply by suspending the animal in water. This behavior is very similar to that of a laboratory rat as it twists to and fro in search of a solid support when suspended by its tail. The *Aplysia*'s swaying movement is clearly aroused by an endogenous behavior generator, since the response will continue for hours without reinforcement. It ceases only when the animal fatigues.

Many labs have now successfully obtained instrumental conditioning by utilizing this instinctual tendency of the *Aplysia*. The clever maneuver used to obtain stable conditioning was to punish the animal with a bright light whenever it swayed to one side of the chamber, while providing darkness whenever it swayed to the other side. As would be expected, the *Aplysia* learned to do most of their swaying toward the side of the chamber where they remained in darkness. This instrumental response could then be observed in the individual muscles that control swaying, as well as in the motor neurons in the abdominal ganglion that control those muscles. Now the "big question" could finally be addressed: Where in the intermediate neural net of the abdominal ganglion does this learned flexibility occur, and how is it mediated in biophysical and neurochemical terms? The evidence suggests that such learning can occur locally within the intimate connections of the motoneuron pool that controls the muscular contractions we visually observe, but the story has yet to be completed.

What is important here is that *Aplysia*, as all other animals, have endogenous behavior generators that make them spontaneously active creatures in their environment. Indeed, intrinsic motor pattern generation may have been the earliest solution for exerting coherent behavioral control. One of the earliest animal behaviors to have evolved was rhythmic undulation in the primordial seas. The possibility for instrumental response modification was initially built upon such spontaneously active neurobehavioral tendencies. A biological understanding of such intrinsic neural processes provides an essential foundation for the construction of a coherent scientific understanding of mammalian emotionality. Each major emotion has intrinsic response patterning mechanisms, and one of the main functions of higher brain evolution has been to provide ever-greater flexible control over such mechanisms.

However, it is important to remember that neither animals nor humans can learn everything simply through the clever manipulation of reinforcement contingencies, as some early behaviorists believed. The range of flexibility is sometimes constrained by the design features of emotional systems. To share one anecdote: In the early years of my career, I made an open challenge to my department's graduate students in psychobiology to train a hungry rat to run down an alleyway backward to obtain food. I assumed that this would be very unlikely, since nature had designed a SEEKING system in the brain (see Chapter 8) so that rats would always forage for food with their nose instead of their butts. Many students, still believing the behaviorist gospel and not believing the evolutionary constraints on learning that were being noted in the literature, thought my challenge might be easy to master. Many tried, but none succeeded. I am not saying it is impossible, but the lesson is obvious. The emotional response systems of animals can be rather inflexible.

The Evolution of "Active Organisms" and Behavioral Flexibility

However, a certain amount of output flexibility is a design characteristic of most brain operating systems (Figure 2.2), including emotional ones, providing several behavioral options that may be the raw material for optimization of learned behavioral strategies. For instance, most insects exhibit such "creativity" when they lose a leg. Normally, cockroaches run in a tripod fashion, keeping two distal legs on one side and the middle leg on the other always planted on the ground, so the animal progresses by rhythmically advancing upon two stable sets of tripods. If this type of locomotion simply reflected the output of a totally "hardwired" internal pattern generator, one would expect the animal to fall over after amputation of the middle legs on both sides. However, when this bit of nastiness is done, a cockroach spontaneously shifts to another strategy, where front and back legs on opposite sides alternate rather than moving together.[32] Although this behavioral readjustment can easily be explained by sensory feedback,[33] by a readjustment in the scaling of "fixed-action patterns," it does highlight the intrinsic creativity that can be found even in simple neural systems.

The existence of intrinsic but behaviorally flexible brain systems has been repeatedly demonstrated by investigators of animal behavior, in simple and elegant experiments. For instance, most young birds do not learn to fly. They will fly at the appropriate age (i.e., maturational stage) even when deprived of the opportunity to exercise such skills prior to their first flight.[34] But they still need to learn where to fly. A similar pattern is seen with rough-and-tumble play: Young rats do not need early experiences with play in order to exhibit outwardly normal ludic interactions as juveniles.[35] But they still need to learn which moves are most effective.

Of course, the expressions of most intrinsic behavior control systems are intermediate: Intrinsic components are rapidly modified by procedural learning. For instance, whereas the courting songs of some avian species appear to be largely innate, other species acquire their characteristic song with the help of learning. They must be exposed to the song of their species when they are young so as to have an appropriate memory template later in life for generating their species-characteristic song. Indeed, the acquired template of some species is so flexible that members will try to imitate the songs of other species if these are all they have heard during critical periods of early development.[36] As always, most behaviors are intermixtures of innate and learned tendencies.

Consider the reaction of cats to one of their natural prey objects, rodents. Their predatory system is based in part on innate tendencies, but these can easily be counteracted by early experiences. Most cats that have been reared only with other cats will hunt and kill mice and rats, but those that have been reared with rats from the time of birth show no such inclination.[37] Does this mean that hunting is a learned response, or is it an instinctual response that can be countered by experience? Probably both to some extent, which highlights the methodological difficulty of studying intrinsic brain systems in sophisticated species living in the real world. As soon as newborn animals interact with the world, their brains are changed forever. In any event, it is a socially important fact that "mere exposure" can make cats friendly with other species. In a similar way, mere exposure to objects and situations probably also increases our comfort level with and preferences for many items and events (see "Afterthought," Chapter 13). This is a very hopeful finding for the future of the human race: We may be able to develop positive bonds to other cultures and other viewpoints, especially if we use television and other modern modes of communication effectively. In short, our natural xenophobia may be counteracted by certain kinds of early education.

We do not know to what extent these long-term behavioral effects reflect changes in how animals and humans consciously process information. All of the preceding phenomena could be mediated at unconscious levels of neural processing. It is only when we begin to see very complex adjustments of behavior sequences in response to systematic challenges that we need to strongly suspect the presence of conscious processes in action.

Let me share one final, and again somewhat nasty, example that demonstrates the adaptive flexibility of conscious behavior in our brethren animals. This is a verbatim description of the exquisite flexibility of maternal care exhibited by a squirrel monkey mother when the arms of her week-old infant were taped behind its back. As the infant screamed on the floor, the mother

> pressed down with her abdomen upon the young, which normally would have facilitated its grasp of her hair. This behavior gave way to visual inspection of the infant, particularly its face, coupled with successive lifting movements using one arm at a time in a manner that positioned the infant ventrally. When the infant still failed to grasp the mother, the predicted maternal behavior occurred: the mother picked up the infant with both arms, cradled it, then walked bipedally away from the experimenter for a distance of 4 ft. and a total of 13 steps.[38]

The overall lesson seems clear: Higher animals are not simply passive reflex machines responding to environmental stimuli in stereotyped ways; rather, they are spontaneously active, spontaneously flexible generators of adaptive behaviors guided by an apparently conscious appreciation of events. But even at the lowest levels, behavioral spontaneity is achieved through the types of flexible neural circuits animals possess, whereby behavioral "master routines" govern a variety of subroutines (Figure 2.2). At some point in brain evolution, behavioral flexibility was achieved by the evolution of conscious dwelling on events and their meaning, as guided by internally experienced emotional feelings. I will argue that these emotional values are a fundamental property of emotional command systems, and that such values are instantiated by "raw feels"—the various forms of affective consciousness that all mammals can experience in the intrinsic neurodynamics of their brains/minds when specific neurochemical systems of the brain become active.

On top of the intrinsic values and the relatively limited flexibilities of the basic emotional systems of the brain, there are layers of learning mechanisms that can yield greater behavioral flexibility and new habits when an animal's circumstances change. Although we now know a great deal about the neural mechanisms that mediate various forms of learning,[39] the basic nature of the *reinforcement processes* that mediate the emotional learning remain largely unknown. At least we now know where to seek answers to such questions—within the neural interactions of the emotive command systems of the brain. Only by understanding such processes can the "unavoidable gaps" between "stimulus and response" and "reinforcement and a resulting change in behavior" (as quoted from the letter from B. F. Skinner in Chapter 1) be filled with substantive knowledge.

A Synopsis of the Foundations of Behavioral Complexity

To rephrase much of the foregoing, the great difficulty in analyzing affective representations arises from the fact that the initial impetus for the construction of such intrinsic brain functions transpired a very long time ago.

Affective experiences are internally generated by neuronal mechanisms that arose to respond to categories of life-challenging events that bombarded our ancestors during the long course of brain evolution. For instance, hunger helps signal energy depletion, not necessarily because immediate energy reserves are dangerously low but because certain forms of energy depletion were encoded as affective anticipatory tendencies within the brain during untold aeons of evolutionary development. In other words, it is more adaptive to anticipate future energy needs than to respond simply to energy emergencies when they arise. Apparently there was no simpler way to do this than for evolution to generate the potential for aversive hunger-type feelings within the mammalian brain. Emotions, especially when they connect up with learning mechanisms, also appear to have this type of anticipatory character. The arousal of feeling states helps channel activities of the cognitive apparatus and thereby facilitates behavioral choices. Thus, it is easy to understand why basic emotional systems evolved to control much of the cognitive apparatus. It is safer and wiser to anticipate possibilities rather than to deal with them once they are squarely in your face.

Because of the emerging complexity of acquired behavioral and cognitive controls in growing organisms, especially advanced ones such as human children, it might be argued that the type of approach pursued here will not really help us understand human behavior. That is most certainly wrong. Although it will not inform us about the details of specific experiences and hence the way each and every outward behavior is controlled, it will provide an understanding of the evolutionary roots that still bind us to our brethren animals, providing a solid foundation for many of our action tendencies and basic value systems.[40]

Because of the massive interaction of emotional systems with the higher cognitive apparatus, it is often tempting to conflate the two into a seamless whole, but as I have argued,[41] a reasonably clear distinction between affective and cognitive processes may exist in the brain, at least in the lower reaches, and an understanding of those areas may allow us to make the type of rapid scientific progress that will eventually highlight essential facets of the higher issues.

Indeed, there are good reasons to believe that the cognitive apparatus would collapse if our underlying emotional value systems were destroyed. This assertion is supported by the fact that in young animals, damage to emotional-limbic areas of the brain is much more devastating than damage to the cognitive-neocortical areas.[42]

We are still on the near shore of understanding on these important topics, but a substantive analysis has finally begun. An appropriate rule guiding this journey may be Descartes's third rule for the scientific pursuit of knowledge: "To think in an orderly fashion when concerned with the search for truth, beginning with the things which were simplest and easiest to understand, and gradually and by degrees reaching toward more complex knowledge, even treating, as though ordered, materials which were not necessarily so."[43]

AFTERTHOUGHT: Behavior Genetics and the Heritability of Psychological Traits

To reemphasize an essential issue: All behavior in mammals, at least from the moment of birth, is a mixture of innate and learned components. As we have seen, recent estimates of heritability for many human behaviors (from cross-fostered, identical-twin studies) generally suggest that approximately 50% of basic human behavioral tendencies, as reflected in a diversity of personality factors, can be attributed to genetic factors, while about 50% can be attributed to learning.[44]

The academic discipline that attempts to evaluate such issues is called *behavior genetics*.[45] For many years, study after study of inbreeding has indicated that virtually any behavioral tendency in animals can be enhanced or diminished as successfully as bodily characteristics. Just as animal husbandry capitalizes on the heritability of physical traits, it is now evident that similar processes contribute to psychological traits in humans and other animals. For instance, different strains of mice differ markedly in their tendencies to exhibit aggressive and fearful behaviors.[46] Although behavioral *tendencies* are as capable of being genetically transmitted as external bodily features, investigators have typically not been able to identify the precise genes and gene products that have been selected when temperamental traits are inherited. However, recently developed animals with single-gene deletions, called "knockout" preparations, have alleviated the need to look for a "needle in a haystack." For instance, elimination of the DNA for a single brain enzyme can have devastating effects on the cognitive/memory abilities of mice.[47] Elimination of the gene for another enzyme produces animals that are violent and hypersexual.[48] And this is only the tip of the iceberg of knowledge that is emerging from genetic analyses. We can anticipate that the menagerie of genetically altered animals will tell us a great deal about the biological underpinnings of many psychobehavioral traits in animals, but there are still some severe methodological problems to be overcome before we can do that with the empirical rigor necessary for definitive conclusions.[49]

Traditionally, the idea that human psychological dispositions can be inherited has not been well received by the intellectual community. Historically, people who advocate such views have been suspected of promoting dubious social policies that threaten to infringe on our fundamental human liberties, a prime example being turn-of-the-century *eugenics,* which championed the "improvement" of the human race by selective breeding or destruction.[50] Nazi and Communist criminals during this century experimented with their own variants of such conceptual monstrosities. We should be aware, however, that the threats posed by biological knowledge can be tempered if we always discriminate between "what is" and "what should be" in discussing the human condition. We can accept the former without ascribing to the "naturalistic fallacy" that biological facts provide any logical mandates for "ought" statements.[51]

It will be intriguing to find out how various emotional characteristics of animals are inherited and the extent to which they can be modified by experience. Although emotional traits can be selectively strengthened or weakened by breeding as well as by cross-rearing in animal experiments,[52] comparatively little has been done with a direct neural end point, such as selection for the strength of specific neurochemical systems or the sensitivity of a specific neuronal system. One of the few relevant pieces of work is the demonstration that animals can be selected for high and low lateral hypothalamic self-stimulation tendencies.[53] Other recent work has shown that neurochemical profiles of the brain can be inherited in both animals and humans.[54]

Such analyses have great potential for advancing our understanding of how the innate operating systems of the mammalian brain control the behavioral proclivities that characterize different temperaments, as well as the emotional disorders and other forms of mental illness that can run in families.[55] Although it is likely that affective proclivities can be inherited, we do not yet understand which genes and what aspect of brain organization are conveying different emotional inclinations. Some appreciation of how things might operate is emerging from ongoing work on various neuropsychiatric disorders in humans.

Recently, there has been great success in revealing the genetic mechanisms of certain disorders such as Huntington's disease, which arises from a specific type of degeneration in ancient brain systems called the *basal ganglia* (see Chapter 4) and is accompanied by an emotional lability and cognitive disintegration that initially resemble schizophrenia. After an initial phase of mental deterioration, the normal flow of motor activities becomes impaired and individuals begin to exhibit uncontrollable and irregular muscle movements, the spontaneous "dance" of the motor apparatus known as *Huntington's chorea*. The source of this disorder has been tracked to a segment on the end of the long arm of chromosome 4, where the normal nucleotide repeat of CAG (cytosine, adenine, guanine), which in normal individuals never exceeds 34 repeats and usually comes in 11 to 24 repeats, has increased to more than 42 and even up to 100 among individuals afflicted with Huntington's.[56] Indeed, many other psychiatric and neurological disorders may also be due to similarly excessive "trinucleotide repeats" within other genes.[57]

The most severe forms of Huntington's disease, with childhood onset, have the largest number of repetitions of the CAG triplet, which codes for glutamate, one of the most powerful and important brain transmitters—one that is an essential component of normal emotional, cognitive, and motor responses (see Chapter 6). Excessive generation of glutamate in the brain seems to explain the symptoms of Huntington's disease, and perhaps even the brain damage that eventually develops. It has long been known that high levels of glutamate can be neurotoxic.[58] In the United States, this finding eventually led to an FDA-mandated elimination of monosodium glutamate (MSG) as a taste enhancer in baby foods. In other words, a "good" molecule that normally allows us to behave and think normally becomes a "bad" molecule in excess, destroying a person's normal ability to live in the world.

As we emphasize such issues, we should remember that all brain organ systems, even straightforward sensory ones such as vision, are susceptible to modification at the biological level as a result of early experiences (including intrauterine ones).[59] From this vantage, it will be most interesting to determine whether powerful emotional experiences early in life are able to modify the underlying neural circuits for the life span of an organism. There are now excellent new genetic and anatomical tracing techniques to analyze such questions at the neural level (see Chapter 4).

Suggested Readings

Ekman, P., & Davidson, R. (eds.) (1994). *Questions about emotions.* New York: Oxford Univ. Press.

Gallistel, C. R. (1980). *The organization of action: A new synthesis.* Hillsdale, N.J.: Lawrence Erlbaum.

Konner, M. (1982). *The tangled wing: Biological constraints over the human spirit.* New York: Holt, Rinehart and Winston.

Oaksford, M., & Brown, G. (eds.) (1994). *Neurodynamics and psychology.* New York: Academic Press.

Plomin, R., De Fries, J. C., & McClearn, G. E. (1990). *Behavioral genetics: A primer* (2d ed.). San Francisco: Freeman.

Schulkin, J. (ed.) (1993). *Hormonally induced changes in mind and brain.* San Diego: Academic Press.

Tinbergen, N. (1951). *The study of instinct.* London: Oxford Univ. Press.

Valenstein, E. S. (1973). *Brain control.* New York: Wiley.

Vernon, P. A. (ed.) (1994). *The neuropsychology of individual differences.* New York: Academic Press.

Wright, R. (1994). *The moral animal.* New York: Random House.

3

The Varieties of Emotional Systems in the Brain

Theories, Taxonomies, and Semantics

Concerning the Number of the Passions, as it hath been variously disputed among Philosophers, so in famous Schools, this Division into Eleven Passions, long since grew of use; to wit, the Sensitive Appetite is distinguished into Concupiscible and Irascible, to the first, are counted commonly six Passions, viz. Pleasure and Grief, Desire and Aversions, Love and Hatred; but to the later five, viz. Anger, Boldness, Fear, Hope and Desperation are wont to be attributed. But this distribution of the Affections is not only incongruous, for that Hope is but ill referred to the Irascible Appetite, and Hatred and Aversion, seem rather to belong to this, than to the Concupiscible: But it is also very insufficient, because some more noted Affections, as Shame, Pity, Emulation, Envy, and many others, are wholly omitted: Wherefore the Ancient Philosophers did determinate the Primary to a certain Number, then they placed under their several Kinds, very many indefinite Species.

Thomas Willis, *Two Discourses Concerning the Soul of Brutes* (1683)

The delusion is extraordinary by which we thus exalt language above nature:—making language the expositor of nature, instead of making nature the expositor of language.

Alexander Brian Johnson, *A Treatise on Language*, as quoted by Frank A. Beach, "The Descent of Instinct" (1955)

CENTRAL THEME

Scholars down through the ages have disagreed about the number and nature of basic emotions. Investigators have not even agreed on the criteria to be used in the classification of emotions. A great deal has been written on such matters, but most of it remains controversial. Until recently, this question could not be approached from a neurological perspective. As we will see in this chapter, now it can. First, I will consider how we might define primary emotional systems, or "affect programs," and then summarize the types of basic emotional circuits that exist in the brain. A limited number of powerful primal emotional circuits—those that appear to elaborate fear, anger, seeking, and sorrow—have now been sufficiently well characterized that they can be addressed cogently through brain research. These universally recognized emotions correspond to the "infantile" feelings that young children exhibit. But this is not a comprehensive list. There are surely others related to sexuality and other more subtle social processes, such as social bonding, separation distress, and play. All emotional taxonomies must remain open-ended until more is known about the brain. I will restrict my discussion here to items for which reasonably coherent evidence exists at the neural level. This does not mean we understand these systems fully, but we do have enough conceptual, neuroanatomical, and neurochemical evidence to make a solid start. In addition, there is probably a much larger number of affective feeling states that arise from the activities of motivational systems, such as those that mediate hunger, thirst, and sexual urges. Still others may reflect "mixtures," permutations or evolutionary outgrowths of primary systems, that can only be studied coherently once the neurophysiologies and neurochemistries of the basic emotional systems are better understood. Although the primal emotional systems probably arise from genetic dictates, they mold and are molded by experience throughout the life span.

On the Power of Emotions in Human Lives

Imagine an archetypal situation: You are hospitalized in the grip of a serious disease or as a victim of grievous bodily harm. It would not be unusual if you felt insecure and anxious about the future, fearing the worst. You may feel irritated and angry over small insensitivities of staff who seem not to appreciate your plight, but you also experience delight in acts of unexpected attention, kindness, and care. In addition to your physical sufferings, you are distressed to be isolated from your social support system and you experience a persistent sense of loss, loneliness, and general apprehension, broken occasionally by empathetic contacts from old friends and the superficial sympathies of more emotionally distant acquaintances. You feel a bit envious of their good health and a bit jealous when your spouse shows up with a good-looking mutual friend of the opposite sex. You may feel a bit of shame over your dependence and inability to control events. After a few days in bed, you are restless because your body aches, but when you do get up for brief periods, you tire quickly. You feel disgusted by the food you are served, but at least the desserts are moderately pleasant on the tongue. When recovery and release are imminent, hope begins to blossom, and you savor the possibilities of life once more. When you leave the hospital, your joy is magnified by simple everyday pleasures—the warmth of the sunshine, a reassuring caress, and the freedom to experience the world as you choose.

Clearly, the range of our affective feelings is enormous. Most people have little difficulty recognizing and discussing them for what they are—highly influential processes in our personal lives that affect not only the quality of our other mental states but also our sense of bodily well-being. Although we take them for granted, they are intrinsically mysterious forces in our lives, because we have not found a clear scientific way to understand them. Those who are unable to fully experience and express emotions are considered *alexithymic*, a psychological condition in which individuals rely excessively on their cognitive-rational processes. In their milder forms, such personality styles may be considered sociopathic, while in their most extreme forms they are sometimes deemed psychopathic.[1]

Although it is self-evident that external events provoke our feelings, emotions actually arise from the activities of ancient brain processes that we have inherited from ancestral species. External stimuli only trigger prepared states of the nervous system. The function of ancient emotional systems is to energize and guide organisms in their interactions with the world, but their power arises from their intrinsic nature in the brain. It is useful to document the sundry environmental events and cognitive appraisals that can arouse our emotions, but such peripheral studies can only indirectly inform our scientific understanding of how the brain generates emotions. Accordingly, most of the vast literature that discusses the role of emotions in everyday life will receive little attention here. I will also not cover many subtle human emotions such as jealousy, shame, and vindictiveness, which are discussed in numerous fine monographs and handbooks that have appeared in recent years, some of which are included in the suggested readings at the end of this chapter. It is generally assumed that many of these complex emotions arise from evolutionary elaborations and interactions of the more basic systems with higher brain functions. Here I will focus on those basic emotions that emerge from homologous subcortical brain activities in all mammals.

An Overview of Brain Organization of Emotionality

The organizational principle that has been most commonly used to summarize the neural infrastructure of emotional processes has been Paul MacLean's concept of the *triune brain* (see Chapter 4 for details). According to the classic version of this view (Figure 3.1), which offers a conceptual cartoon of the major layers of neural development, the functional landscape of the brain is organized in three strata of evolutionary progression. The deepest and most ancient layer is the *reptilian brain*, also known as the *basal ganglia*, or *extrapyramidal motor system*. Here many of our basic motor plans, especially axial or whole-body movements, including primitive behavioral responses related to fear, anger, and sexuality, are elaborated by specific neural circuits. The next layer, known as the *limbic system* or the *visceral brain*, contains newer programs related to the various social emotions, including maternal acceptance and care, social bonding, separation distress, and rough-and-tumble play. Finally, surrounding these ancient subcortical regions, which are quite similarly organized in all mammals, we have the *neomammalian brain* or *neocortex*, which is rudimentary in other vertebrates and exhibits the greatest diversification among mammalian species. The neocortex can come to be influenced by emotions and influences them through various appraisal processes, but it is not a fundamental neural substrate for the generation of affective experience. Although the cortex can be powerfully moved by emotions and the human cortex can rationally attempt to understand and influence them (sustaining and reduc-

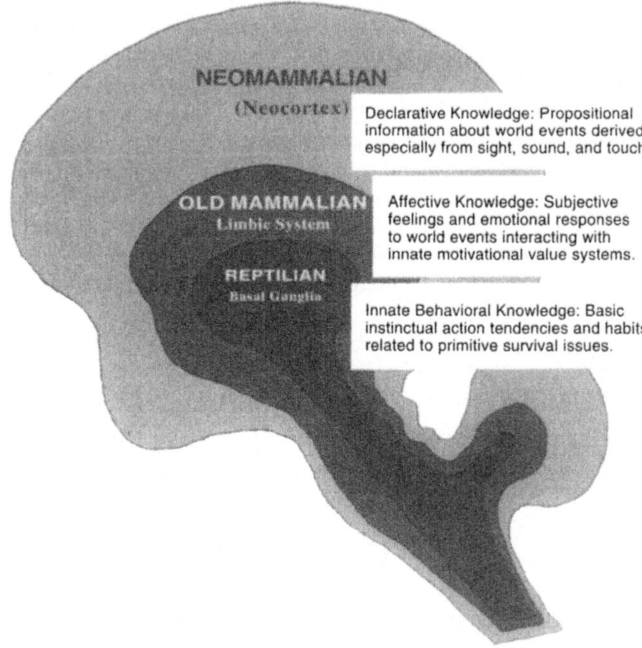
NEOMAMMALIAN
(Neocortex)
Declarative Knowledge: Propositional information about world events derived especially from sight, sound, and touch.
OLD MAMMALIAN
Limbic System
Affective Knowledge: Subjective feelings and emotional responses to world events interacting with innate motivational value systems.
REPTILIAN
Basal Ganglia
Innate Behavioral Knowledge: Basic instinctual action tendencies and habits related to primitive survival issues.

Figure 3.1. Highly schematic representation of MacLean's triune brain concept. The innermost reptilian core of the brain elaborates basic instinctual action plans for primitive emotive processes such as exploration, feeding, aggressive dominance displays, and sexuality. The old-mammalian brain, or the limbic system, adds behavioral and psychological resolution to all of the emotions and specifically mediates the social emotions such as separation distress/social bonding, playfulness, and maternal nurturance. The highly expanded neomammalian cortex generates higher cognitive functions, reasoning, and logical thought. For a more realistic depiction of the same concept, see Figure 4.1. (Adapted from MacLean, 1990; see n. 46.)

ing feelings depending on moment-to-moment appraisals of situations), it apparently cannot generate emotionality without the ancient subcortical functions of the brain. We cannot precipitate emotional feelings by artificially activating the neocortex either electrically or neurochemically, even though, as we will discuss later, emotionality is modified by cortical injury (see Chapters 4 and 16).[2]

Although the triune brain concept is largely a didactic simplification from a neuroanatomical point of view, it is an informative perspective. There appear to have been relatively long periods of stability in vertebrate brain evolution, followed by bursts of expansion. The three evolutionary strata of the mammalian brain reflect these progressions (Figure 3.1): The basic reptilian core is of similar relative size in all mammals (as long as we account for body size). Other vertebrates also have an abundance of this tissue in their small brains. While the limbic system is comparatively small in reptiles, it is large in all mammals and also of similar relative size across different mammalian species. On the other hand, the degree of mushrooming of neocortex varies widely among mammalian species, being modest in rodents and reaching massive proportion in the cetaceans (whales and porpoises) and great apes (the gibbons, orangutans, gorillas, chimpanzees) and attaining its pinnacle in humans. It is the storehouse of our cognitive skills.

In short, the size and complexity of the human neocortical toolbox, even when corrected for body size, are much vaster than in all other mammalian species. By comparison, species differences diminish when we focus on those paleocortical (i.e., ancient limbic cortex) and subcortical systems where the basic emotions are created. Within the cortex, the human brain displays many unique organizational principles, especially among the neural connections that allow us to speak, think, and plan ahead.[3] A similar claim cannot be made about subcortical processes, and the conservation of function in lower areas effectively allows us to triangulate fundamental issues across species, using converging evidence from the brain, behavioral, and mental sciences (see Figure 2.4). Although the remarkable cortical development of the human brain has many affective ramifications, including our ability to conceptualize our emotions in a diversity of artistic forms, to the best of our knowledge, the affective *power* of emotionality arises from subcortical systems that also sway the minds of "lower" animals. Thus, to understand the fundamental nature of emotionality we must decipher the natural order of emotional circuits within the lower reaches of the mammalian brain.

Existing Strategies for the Study of Emotions

Scientists interested in the topic of emotions have yet to agree upon a general research strategy or taxonomy for understanding the basic emotions that can be applied across all mammalian species, and some still reject the notion of "basic emotions" altogether. In experimental psychology, one can presently identify three distinct schools of thought on how we should proceed in our attempts to understand and categorize emotions:

1. *The categorical approach:* Perhaps the most vocal group consists of investigators who posit the existence of a small set of discrete emotions, or "primes," on the basis of either objective analysis of behavioral expressions, human subjective experiences, established brain systems, or a combination of the above.[4] This *categorical approach* assumes that certain affective processes—such as fear, anger, sorrow, and joy—ultimately arise from intrinsic systems of the brain/mind and have a stable and characteristic underlying reality that can be clarified at the biological level. The present analysis is most closely affiliated with this approach, which is contrasted to the next most common approach in Figure 3.2.

2. *The social-constructivist approach:* Others believe that attempts to pigeonhole certain emotions as basic are fundamentally incorrect and even wrong-headed. They have championed several alternative views. Those who are convinced that humans have no instincts and acquire their various affective proclivities

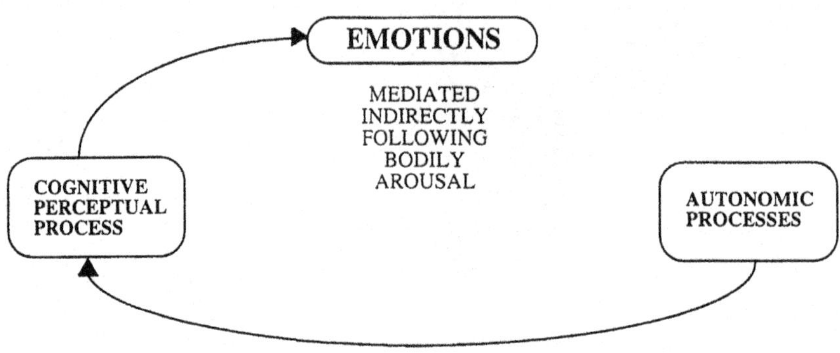

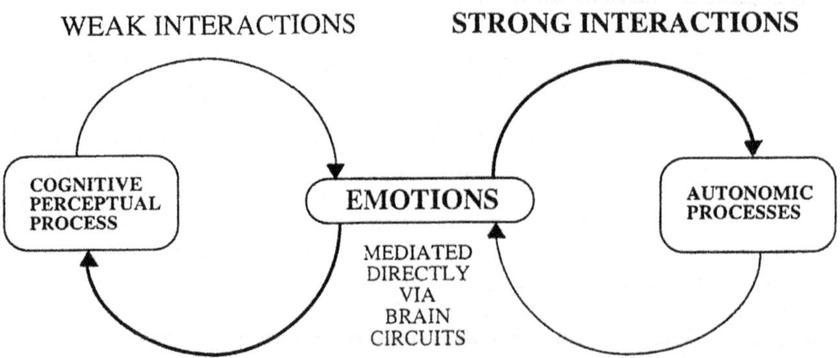

Figure 3.2. Two major current views of how emotions are organized in the brain. The top view represents the essence of the James-Lange perspective (see the "Afterthought" of this chapter), which has guided social-constructivist thinking about emotions to the present day. The bottom view represents a more accurate perspective that is based on existing neuroscience evidence, where centrally situated emotional systems in the brain extensively interact, in strong and weak ways (as highlighted by bolder and lighter lines, respectively), with higher and lower brain functions. A third approach (not shown), the componential one, is really a mixture of the other two. The componential view would be an amalgamation of these views, without the suggestion that there are any coherent emotional systems of the brain. Instead, emotional coordination is achieved by many component responses coming together as a function of learning.

through learning are called *social constructivists*.[5] This approach often focuses its conceptual and experimental inquiries on the way we use words and how we come to label various bodily sensations and patterns of psychic experience. Since all of the words and many cognitive concepts humans apply to affective states must be socially learned, it is assumed that human emotional experience is also constructed by social learning.

Unfortunately, social constructivist frameworks have too commonly disregarded the vast amount of behavioral and physiological evidence for specific emotional response patterns, as well as the wealth of neuroscientific evidence suggesting that there are genetically provided affective infrastructures for different emotions within the brain. The great advantage of constructivist approaches is the full recognition that language is our most important social instrument (see Appendix B). The disadvantage is that this view finds it so easy to overlook the universe of neurobiology that exists independently of our vast, and often deceptive, linguistic abilities.

3. *The componential approach:* There is also a hybrid position advocated by investigators who focus on the appraisal processes that can trigger emotions. These scholars have emphasized that emotions are accompanied by a variety of bodily changes with many cognitive ramifications. This *componential approach* generally asserts that emotions are learned states constructed during early social development from more elemental units of visceral-autonomic experiences that accompany certain behavior patterns. In other words, rather than just being a matter of labeling, as some social-constructivists have argued, the componentialists suggest that biologically given subunits are compiled into full-blown emotional systems via cognitive appraisals and learning.[6] Although this compromise position is applicable to many aspects of emotions, especially the more complex human social emotions, such as shame, guilt, jealousy, embarrassment, and sympathy, a coherent psychobiological research program based on this viewpoint has yet to emerge.

Clearly, every approach has something to offer, and it seems a bit foolish for theoreticians to battle for primacy in this complex area, where provisional ideas and lack of agreement remain abundant. Emotions can be studied at many different hierarchical levels, and at present there is too little cross talk among the levels. The most important issues can only be resolved with more evidence, and the best biological data presently exist at the *categorical* level. Although some psychologists consider the creation of basic taxonomies an unrealistic and even useless enterprise, in fact, all three approaches have a role to play in the analysis of the diversity of emotions manifested in actual human experience. As I have argued, "The categorical, componential and social constructivist approaches need not battle over primacy issues. They work best in different domains of inquiry. The categorical approach can identify basic operating systems that exist in the brain, and the componential and constructivist approaches can provide schemata of how the genetically endowed systems develop their full resolution by interacting with the vast complexity of the real world. It is certain that all of these types of influences contribute to real-life emotional experiences" in humans. However, the psychobiological perspective seems essential for all other levels of analysis. Accordingly, I beseeched, "If we do not fully consider the implications of the neuroscientific evidence (which has largely been obtained through the use of the categorical approach in appropriate animal models), how can the remaining approaches guide us to a rigorous understanding of how emotions are truly constructed in the human brain-mind?"[7]

The constructivist and componential approaches have yet to provide a powerful strategy for addressing neurological questions, so the existing evidence will be discussed here from the categorical perspective. From my utilitarian vantage, the neural organization of the emotional brain is the single most important question in emotion research today. Its importance lies in its vast potential to lay a lasting foundation for our understanding of human nature, providing a way to objectify subjectivity and to promote breakthroughs in our search for new psychiatric tools to alleviate emotional distress. This approach, because of its mechanistic emphasis, eventually may bring new forms of help to those suffering from despair, anxiety, sorrow, mania, and other disturbances of the inner life. The other approaches, because they do not actively seek to understand the brain substrates, are unlikely to yield such benefits. Without inclusion of a brain analysis, the science of emotions cannot provide answers to the grand and fundamental issues of our lives: What does it mean to be angry? How do we come to feel afraid? Where does sorrow come from? What are joy, happiness, frustration, and the many other passions and hungers that constitute the affective mysteries of our lives?

Taxonomies of Emotions

As highlighted at the beginning of this chapter by Thomas Willis's comments on the passions, there have been many taxonomies of emotions down through the ages and all too many sterile controversies.[8] Some scholars, especially those with postmodern deconstructive orientations, believe that psychological processes are intrinsically so complicated by multiple causation that logical analysis through reductionism and manipulation of simple systems (such as those using animal models) will never provide the answers that we need. Diversity of taxonomies and ideas is sustained, and no one's thoughts are excluded. Unfortunately, they cannot all be correct at the biological level.

One response to a proliferation of taxonomies is a movement in the opposite direction—toward a minimalist view of emotions. For instance, it is obvious that emotionality is accompanied by bodily and physiological arousal, and some have claimed that is all there is to emotions. Taking a somewhat more complex view are those who recognize that behavioral arousal can take you away from objects or toward objects, so the next simplified level of analysis accepts only the dichotomous distinction of approach versus avoidance. To this day, many are still attracted by the stark simplicity of such dimensional views,[9] but a careful reading of the available evidence indicates there is greater complexity to emotional matters in the mammalian brain. Although a simple approach-avoidance dichotomy may be defensible for invertebrate species, in which neural homologies are too obscure to illuminate the human condition, this dichotomy is no longer a tenable conceptualization of mammalian emotions. There are simply too many facts, such as the distinct varieties of emotional behaviors that can be evoked by electrical and chemical brain stimulation, that should dissuade us from making very general behavioral gradients the foundation for our thinking about emotional matters.

By arguing that an approach-avoidance dimension is not a sufficient taxonomy for a neuroscientific analysis of emotions, I do not mean to claim that it is not useful in many realms. First, it must be reaffirmed that all emotional systems have dimensional attributes, namely, variations in the intensity of approach-avoidance and affective-arousal gradients that they generate. Also, the measurement of such higher-order constructs as positive and negative affect has yielded useful conceptualizations of personality that have important implications for understanding psychiatric disorders. People high in negative affect seem to be more influenced by emotions such as fear, sadness, anger, and disgust, and tend to be more prone to anxiety and depression. People with high positive affect tend to be outgoing, more playful and sensation-seeking, and more prone to manic disorders.[10] Clearly, though, these broad dimensions subsume many distinct emotional processes under a broad conceptual umbrella, such as might be constructed by generalized affective readout and labeling mechanisms of the neocortex. Although it is easy to understand why higher brain areas might tend to cluster and hence categorize events simply in terms of desirable and undesirable outcomes (i.e., the cortex, perhaps by its linguistic function, can as easily homogenize as discriminate categories), the neurological evidence summarized here indicates that mammals possess highly specific emotional and motivational systems in subcortical regions from which such generalized affective features may be created. However, we should remember that it is still possible that the various discrete emotional systems derive their impact by interacting with a smaller number of positive and negative affect systems (see Chapter 9 for a discussion of such issues).[11]

Here I will seek to restrict our focus to basic emotional systems for which there is a core of agreement among most taxonomists, especially among those who work directly on the brain.[12] Virtually every list ever generated includes *anger*, *sorrow*, *fear*, and *joy*. Although theorists may have different reasons for classifying a given process as basic, the existence of such processes can also be supported by neuroscientific evidence. Simple linguistic analyses also support the primacy of a fairly short list of primary emotions. If one simply asks people to list the four or five basic emotions they experience, one consistently finds agreement on a fairly short list of items. Often "love" is at the top of the list, but if one excludes that option, then at least 60% of people routinely mention some variant of anger, fear, sorrow, and joy, after which there is a sudden drop to less than 20% in the remainder of responses, composed of a long list of items such as "jealousy," "depression," "desire," and "compassion." It is noteworthy that several items such as "surprise" and "disgust," which figure prominently in many taxonomies based on facial analysis, are rarely selected by people as basic emotions in their individual lives.[13]

In recent human research, several prominent emotional taxonomies have been based on the types of facial expressions that people can generate or recognize across different cultures and stages of development. All of these analyses have yielded the four emotions mentioned previously, as well as items such as surprise and disgust, which can also be clearly expressed facially, even though both can be instinctual as well as socially constructed (i.e., sensory versus social disgusts, and fearful versus happy surprise, respectively). However, the use of facial analysis can be easily criticized. I also believe it is a less important criterion than an overall neurobehavioral analysis of action tendencies, but I will not delve into the controversy surrounding the utility of facial analysis. It has been amply aired recently.[14] The essence of the problem is that the face can easily be used as a social display device, which reduces its utility as a monitor of affective states. Here it is important to note that socially constructed and spontaneous facial displays of affect are probably differentially controlled in the brain (i.e., cortically versus subcortically mediated, respectively).[15]

Even though the face can be a fuzzy measure of specific affects in a variety of social situations, the fact that the face spontaneously expresses emotionality is not controversial. The controversy is how it can be used unambiguously as a valid measure of emotionality. In this context, I would note that humans have a much richer affective facial/bodily repertoire than is encompassed in most emotion theories, and individuals who know how to ham it up can easily express disappointment, lustiness, ecstasy, suspicion, shame, regret, sympathy, love, and other emotions, but in doing so they often follow stereotyped culturally based display rules.

Although in humans and some related primates the face is an exquisitely flexible communicative device, that is not the case for most other mammals, which exhibit clear emotional behaviors but less impressive facial dynamics. Although most animals exhibit openmouthed, hissing-growling expressions of rage, and some show an openmouthed play/laughter display, they tend to show little else on their faces.[16] Thus, aside from a few studies in primates, facial analysis provides little evidence for cross-species taxonomic issues. Analysis of body postures, dynamic behavior patterns, autonomic measures, and the study of emotional sounds may provide better data for cross-species comparisons, but these lines of investigation are still comparatively underdeveloped. It is hoped that investigators will eventually develop brain measures that can index the presence of affect more directly.

Since a definitive analysis of the cross-species generalizability of basic emotions must include an analysis of brain systems, it is compelling that the recurring items from the preceding analyses are most clearly supported by data from brain research. Indeed, a brain-systems analysis is finally providing a "gold standard" for all other levels of theorizing. As I will summarize in this text, at present there is good biological evidence for at least seven innate emotional systems ingrained within the mammalian brain. In the vernacular, they include fear, anger, sorrow, anticipatory eagerness, play, sexual lust, and maternal nurturance. There are many more affective feelings, such as hunger, thirst, tiredness, illness, surprise, disgust, and others, but they may need to be conceptualized in terms other than what we will here call basic emotional systems.[17]

Accordingly, before any definitive taxonomy of emotions can be established, we must first have a cogent definition of what it means to be a bona fide emotional process. By failing to do so, investigators have "placed under their several Kinds, very many indefinite Species," as Thomas Willis put it. More recently, I added a similar comment: "The existing lists of basic emotions comprise a menagerie of strange and seemingly incompatible species of dubious evolutionary and epigenetic descent."[18] Why should we not consider the feelings of hunger, thirst, pain, and tiredness to be emotions? They are certainly strong affective feelings. However, they do not fulfill all the neural criteria for an emotional system outlined below. The more traditional and quite cogent conceptual rationale is that it is desirable to exclude peripherally linked regulatory responses such as hunger and thirst from that category and to instead call them motivations (for more on this issue, see Chapter 9). In any event, to establish better taxonomies, we must have better inclusion and exclusion criteria to delimit our topic. If emotions, feelings, and moods come in several natural types, we must aspire to be explicit about the type of classificatory scheme we are trying to construct.

Here I will develop the premise that discrete emotions emerge from a variety of coherently operating brain systems with specific properties. A panoramic view of neural systems will allow us to see the outlines of the major emotional neural "thickets" more clearly. Greater agreement on the use of certain psychological terms will surely be achieved if we anchor them credibly in the objective properties of the brain and body. For these reasons, I will attempt to provide a neurally based definition of emotions, one that specifies *necessary* criteria, even though it falls short on the *sufficiency* dimension, especially when we start to consider the many reflections of emotions in personality and cultural development. Thus, the definitional focus here will be on the general brain characteristics of emotional systems. In addition, we will be able to distinguish systems at anatomical and neurochemical levels, especially with regard to neuropeptide controls. At the same time, it will become quite evident that many distinct emotions also share generalized components such as acetylcholine, norepinephrine, and serotonin systems for the control of attention and general arousal functions. Likewise, glutamate and gamma-aminobutyrie acid (GABA) control all cognitive, emotional, and motivational functions. In the tangled skein of brain systems, emotional specificity has traditionally been difficult to pin down, but as we will see, a great deal of precision is emerging from recent neuroscience studies.

On the Problem of Defining Emotions

As summarized elsewhere,[19] there have been many attempts to define emotions. If we distill them, we might come up with something like this: When powerful waves of affect overwhelm our sense of ourselves in the world, we say that we are experiencing an emotion. When similar feelings are more tidal—weak but persistent—we say we are experiencing a mood. These feelings come in various dynamic forms and are accompanied by many changes in behavior and action readiness, as well as the activities of our visceral organs. Emotions are typically triggered by world events; they arise from experiences that thwart or stimulate our desires, and they establish coherent action plans for the organism that are supported by adaptive physiological changes. These coordinated brain and bodily states fluctuate markedly as a function of time, as a function of minor changes in events, and especially as a function of our changing appraisal of these events. To be overwhelmed by an emotional experience means the intensity is such that other brain mechanisms, such as higher rational processes, are disrupted because of the spontaneous behavioral and affective dictates of the more primitive brain control systems. Although this definition may be adequate for everyday purposes, it does not cover some important aspects of emotional systems, such as how they control personality dimensions, or how emotions really operate to create feelings within the internal psychological landscape of the individuals who experience them.

In any event, the position taken here is that a useful

approach to defining emotions is to focus on their adaptive, central integrative functions as opposed to general input and output characteristics. From this vantage, emotions are the psychoneural processes that are especially influential in controlling the vigor and patterning of actions in the dynamic flow of intense behavioral interchanges between animals, as well as with certain objects during circumstances that are especially important for survival. Each emotion has a characteristic "feeling tone" that is especially important in encoding the intrinsic values of these interactions, depending on whether they are likely to promote or hinder survival (in both the immediate personal and the longer-term reproductive sense). These affective functions are especially important in encoding new information, retrieving information on subsequent occasions, and perhaps also in allowing animals to generalize about new events rapidly and efficiently (i.e., allowing animals to jump to potentially adaptive "snap decisions"). The underlying neural systems may also compute levels of psychological homeostasis or equilibrium by evaluating an organism's adaptation or success in the environment.

In more simple subjective terms, we might say that these systems generate an animal's egocentric sense of well-being with regard to the most important natural dimensions of life. They offer solutions to such survival problems as: How do I obtain goods? How do I keep goods? How do I remain intact? How do I make sure I have social contacts and supports? Such major survival questions, which all mammals face, have been answered during the long course of neural evolution by the emergence of intrinsic emotional tendencies within the brain. Each emotional system interacts with many others at both higher and lower levels of the neuroaxis, and most of the scientific literature on the topic within psychology deals with the indirect psychological, behavioral, and physiological reflections of these interactions. Once we begin to conceptualize the central source processes, we can begin to craft new definitions of emotions on the basis of neural attributes rather than simply on descriptions of external manifestations.

Thus, from the perspective of affective neuroscience, it is essential to have neurally based definitions that can be used equally well in brain research and in the psychological and behavioral studies we conduct on mature humans, infants, and other animals. I have proposed the following: In addition to the basic psychological criterion that emotional systems should be capable of elaborating subjective feeling states that are affectively valenced (a criterion that has so far defied neural specification), there are six other objective neural criteria that provisionally define emotional systems in the brain.[20] They are depicted schematically in Figure 3.3.

1. The underlying circuits are genetically predetermined and designed to respond unconditionally to stimuli arising from major life-challenging circumstances.

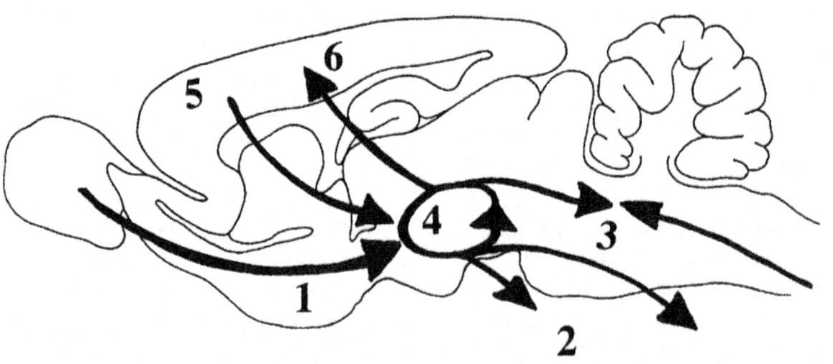

Figure 3.3. The various neural interactions that characterize all major emotional systems of the brain: (1) Various sensory stimuli can unconditionally access emotional systems; (2) emotional systems can generate instinctual motor outputs, as well as (3) modulate sensory inputs. (4) Emotional systems have positive feedback components that can sustain emotional arousal after precipitating events have passed. (5) These systems can be modulated by cognitive inputs and (6) can modify and channel cognitive activities. Also, the important criterion that emotional systems create affective states is not depicted, but it is assumed that arousal of the executive circuit for each emotion is a necessary condition for getting feeling states activated within the brain, perhaps by interacting with other brain circuits for self-representation, such as those that appear to exist in the midbrain periaqueductal and deep tectal circuits that interact with frontal cortical systems (see Chapter 16).

2. These circuits organize diverse behaviors by activating or inhibiting motor subroutines and concurrent autonomic-hormonal changes that have proved adaptive in the face of such life-challenging circumstances during the evolutionary history of the species.
3. Emotive circuits change the sensitivities of sensory systems that are relevant for the behavioral sequences that have been aroused.
4. Neural activity of emotive systems outlasts the precipitating circumstances.
5. Emotive circuits can come under the conditional control of emotionally neutral environmental stimuli.
6. Emotive circuits have reciprocal interactions with the brain mechanisms that elaborate higher decision-making processes and consciousness.

Of course, as mentioned, there is a seventh psychological criterion: The emotional circuits must be able to generate affective feelings, but this is hard to incorporate into the conceptual diagram. I will eventually develop the idea that affect emerges from the many interactions of emotional systems depicted in Figure 3.3 with primal neural mechanisms that represent "the self" (see Chapter 16), but let us first deal with the available facts concerning the various systems.

In addition to being the deep neural sources of psychic life, emotional circuits achieve their profound influence over the behavior and mental activity of an organism through the widespread effects on the rest of the nervous system. Emotive circuits change sensory, perceptual, and cognitive processing, and initiate a host of physiological changes that are naturally synchronized with the aroused behavioral tendencies characteristic of emotional experience. I will speak of these emotional systems in a variety of ways, using designations such as *executive*, *command*, and *operating* systems, to provide nuances of meaning that may be needed to conceptualize their overall functions. The use of the term *executive* implies that a neural system has a superordinate role in a cascade of hierarchical controls (i.e., the central "node" in Figure 2.2); *command* implies that a circuit can instigate a full-blown emotional process; *operating* implies that it can coordinate and synchronize the operation of several subsystems. Taken together, all of these components yield coherent psychobehavioral and physiological responses that constitute an emotional "organ system." This final term conceptualizes the fact that each system is composed of an anatomical network of interconnected neurons and endocrine, paracrine, and immune influences. As mentioned, certain components are shared by many emotional systems—for instance, a general cortical arousal function (which is partly based on brain norepinephrine and acetylcholine circuits, as described in Chapters 6 and 7) and general inhibitory functions that may help channel information (which are partly based on brain serotonin and GABA systems). The multiplicity of terminologies is not meant to imply that there are three different types of emotional organ systems; instead, each complex system, like the proverbial elephant being groped by the blind, can be "viewed" from different perspectives.

Even though psychologists have traditionally made a distinction between external (objective, third-person) events and internal (subjective, first-person) events, in functional brain research, especially with regard to processes that have ramifications in conscious awareness, this distinction must be questioned. To make progress in understanding how psychological processes emerge from brain functions, we will eventually have to judiciously combine first-person and third-person views of brain functions.

Indeed, we should always recognize that as far as psychological processes of the brain are concerned, everything after initial sensory integration is internal, while often seeming to remain external. As William James[21] put it,

> Subjectivity and objectivity are affairs not what experience is aboriginally made of, but of its classification. Classifications depend on our temporary purposes. For certain purposes it is convenient to take things in one set of relations, for other purposes in another set. In the two cases their contexts are apt to be different. In the case of our affectional experiences we have no permanent and steadfast purpose that obliges us to be consistent, so we find it easy to let them float ambiguously, sometimes classing them with our feelings, sometimes with more physical realities, according to caprice or to the convenience of the moment.

James went on to point out that it is quite natural for us to attribute feelings to external objects and events, even though they may in fact be part of our bodies: "Language would lose most of its esthetic and rhetorical value were we forbidden to project words primarily connoting our affections upon the objects by which the affections are aroused. The man is really hateful; the action really mean; the situation really tragic—all in themselves and quite apart from our opinion." Thus, from a cognitive perspective our feelings are deeply felt "opinions" and "attributions," but from the affective perspective they truly amount to distinct types of neural activities in the brain. This duality of viewpoints resembles some of the other famous dualities that other sciences have had to accept gracefully, for instance, the particulate and wave characteristics of electrons.[22]

In the present analysis, I will de-emphasize the obvious fact that emotions are aroused in us by various external events and instead will focus on the sources of feelings within intrinsic brain functions. Although the emotional tendencies of the brain were designed to respond to various types of real-world events, we must remember that they are not constructed from those events. Their essential and archaic nature was cobbled together during the long course of brain evolution so as to provide organisms ready solutions to the major survival problems confronting them. Figure 3.4 highlights the adaptive functions of the four most ancient emotional systems that have thus far been reasonably well characterized in neural terms.

Verbal Labels and a Neurologically Based Taxonomy of Emotional Processes

How did emotional organ systems emerge in the mammalian brain? As highlighted by the discussion of *Aplysia* behavior in the previous chapter, they probably arose from earlier reflexive-instinctual abilities possessed by simpler ancestral creatures in our evolutionary lineage. Gradually, through evolutionary modification and coordination of preexisting capabilities, executive systems emerged that were capable of providing an animal with greater behavioral coherence and flexibility in a variety of primal situations: (1) the search for food, water, and warmth; (2) the search for sex and companionship; (3) the need to care for offspring; (4) the urge to be reunited with companions after separation; (5) the urge to avoid pain and destruction; (6) the urge to express oneself vigorously with decisive actions if one's self-interests are compromised; (7) the urge to exhibit vigorous social interaction, and perhaps several others. It is reasonable to provisionally call the psychic states corresponding to these emotional urges *seeking*, *lust*, *nurturance*, *panic*, *fear*, *rage*, and *play*, respectively. Although these are not good scientific labels (because of the excess and often vague meanings of such vernacular terms), most alternatives are not much better (and, I believe, arguably worse). All the options we have are mere words with no intrinsic significance. The best labels should suggest that something very important, of a certain general type, is transpiring in the nervous system, and I will continue to utilize common vernacular labels since they are such a great aid to understandable communication that can help fertilize our search for further clarity. However, as explained in the next section, I will use such terms with a new twist.

Many animal behaviorists have asserted that subjective terms such as *anger* and *fear* are bad because they reek of *anthropomorphism*—the attribution of human mental qualities to animals. My previous analysis of such concerns asserted that

> it should be self-evident that the use of anthropomorphism in the study of mammalian emotions cannot be arbitrarily ruled out. Although its application may be risky under the best of circumstances, its validity depends on the degree of evolutionary con-

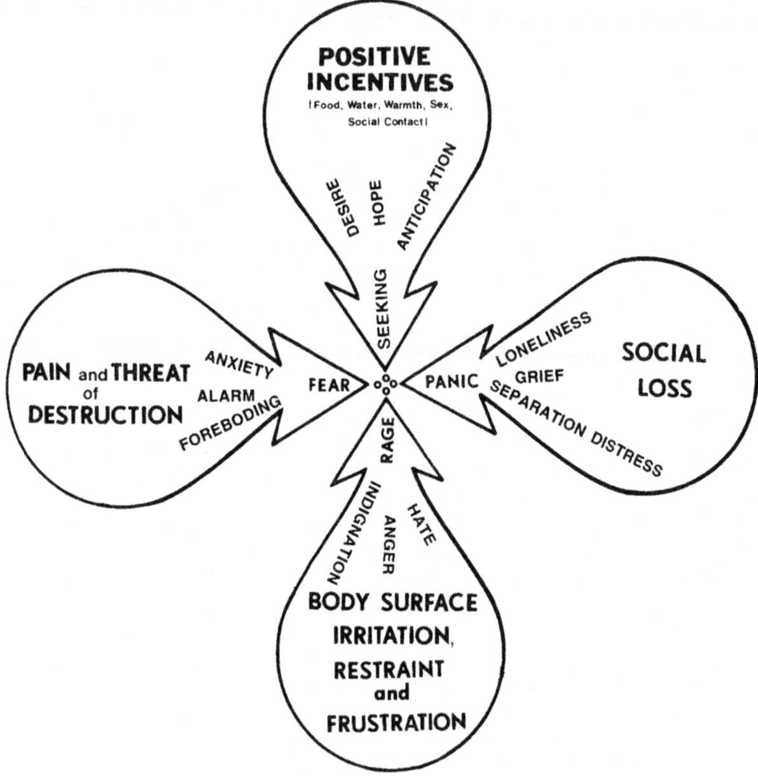

Figure 3.4. Various environmental challenges were so persistent during brain evolution that psychobehavioral tendencies to respond to such challenges have been encoded as emotional neural circuits within the mammalian brain. Hence, various external stimuli have the capacity to arouse specific emotional tendencies, but these emotional potentials exist within the neural circuits of the brain independently of external influences. Unregulated and excessive activities within these systems probably contribute to major psychiatric disorders. (Adapted from Panksepp, 1982; see n. 26.)

tinuity among brain mechanisms that elaborate emotions in humans and animals. Hence, the degree of anthropomorphism that can have scientific utility in mammalian brain research should be directly related to the extent that emotions reflect class-typical mechanisms as opposed to species-typical ones.[23]

The available evidence now overwhelmingly supports the conclusion that basic emotional processes emerge from homologous brain mechanisms in all mammals. Of course, emotional systems do not remain static during the life span of an organism—their infrastructures probably change as a function of development and individual experience—but we presently know regrettably little at that level of analysis, at least in the realm of brain research.[24]

Obviously, the ability of the human cortex to think and to fantasize, and thereby to pursue many unique paths of human cultural evolution, can dilute, mold, modify, and focus the dictates of these systems, but it cannot eliminate them. Since those wonderful human abilities are of secondary importance for understanding the deep nature of emotions, I have decided to use simple vernacular terms to discuss the affective lives of all mammals. However, it is important to be clear that the present aim is not to use such affective labels for emotional systems in explanatory ways but to use them merely as designators for coherently operating brain systems, having important internal and external consequences, that need to be clarified in order for us to understand emotions.

A Proposed Terminological Convention for Discussing Brain Emotional Systems

Short of holding an international convention to resolve terminological issues, the best solution may be to generate a chain of words that reflects the diversity of manifestations in which a specific brain system is involved. Thus, for the first system mentioned earlier, the "appetitive motivational system" that encourages animals to search for all resources, including food, water, and warmth, I once used the designator *curiosity/interest/foraging/anticipation/craving/expectancy system.*[25] This usage reflected my frustration with existing terminologies, but it would be cumbersome to formalize such chains of words as standard usage. Perhaps a good compromise would be to always use two descriptors, one behavioral and one psychological (e.g., *foraging/expectancy system* and *separation-distress/panic system*), to acknowledge that those two sources of information (i.e., first- and third-person perspectives) should always be used conjointly in the study of any basic emotional operating system of the brain.

However, I will utilize a new and simpler convention. Rather than chaining descriptors together, I will select a single affective designator written in UPPERCASE letters when it refers to one of the genetically ingrained brain emotional operating systems. This is used to alert the reader to the fact that I am using the term in a scientific rather than simply a vernacular way: I am talking about a specific neural system of the brain that is assumed to be a major source process for the emergence of the related vernacular terminologies but which in the present context has a more clearly restricted neuro-functional referent. In general, I will continue to use the labels I originally employed in the first formal neurotaxonomy of emotional processes,[26] but I have decided to relabel one, namely, "the expectancy system," even though the essential meaning of the concept remains unchanged. I do this because the original term I selected was deemed to be vague with respect to positive and negative expectancies. Thus, this "appetitive motivational system" will no longer be called the EXPECTANCY system but rather the SEEKING system (in Chapter 9, I will further discuss this change and contrast it with alternative terminologies for the underlying system that have been more recently employed by other investigators). The remaining systems will retain the original labels, but again the use of capitalization is designed to convey the fact that these are scientific terms and not just a loose form of folk psychologizing. Also, I will discuss several additional social-emotional systems that have been alluded to earlier (e.g., those related to sexual, maternal, and playful feelings and behavior processes), and here I will raise them to formal status within the emerging neuropsychological taxonomy of emotions. Thus, seven specific emotional systems will be fully discussed in separate chapters of this text.

A major opponent emotional process to SEEKING impulses arising from a brain system that energizes the body to angrily defend its territory and resources will be called the RAGE system. The brain system that appears to be central for generating a major form of trepidation that commonly leads to freezing and flight will be called the FEAR system. The one that generates feelings of loneliness and separation distress will still be called the PANIC system, even though this choice has caused a degree of critical concern since the term *panic* is also commonly used to designate intense states of fear. Unfortunately, SORROW or DISTRESS would have been just as debatable. My original reason for selecting the term PANIC was the supposition that an understanding of this neural circuit would provide important insights into the neural sources of the clinical disorder known as *panic attacks*. This position continues to be supported by existing evidence.[27] The additional systems for sexual, maternal, and playful feelings will be called LUST, CARE, and rough-and-tumble PLAY systems.

The preceding is not intended as a complete or exclusive list. Perhaps a social DOMINANCE system also exists in the brain, and as has been emphasized several times, surely there are intrinsic neural substrates for many other basic affective "motivational" feelings such as hunger, thirst, frustration, disgust, pain, and so on. For the time being, I will not capitalize these designators of affective feelings, since we do not know whether they are mediated by distinct types of brain organization, and since they are not the main focus of the text. There are also many higher human sentiments, from feelings of shame to those of sympathy, that are linked via social learning to the basic emotional systems. However, within the conceptual constraints that I have imposed on the present analysis (Figure 3.3), they will not be considered as major subcortical emotional operating systems.

Obviously, there are other ways to feel "good" and "bad" within the brain, and there are many specific types of "pleasures" and "aversions." Many of those that will not be presented as primary emotions here will be discussed in the context of various regulatory interactions in Chapters 8, 11, and 13. For instance, hunger interacts with the SEEKING system. Frustration is one way to activate the RAGE system, and LUST is obviously a multifaceted category.

Clearly, we cannot use most emotional words totally unambiguously, no matter how hard we try, which is probably the major reason modern neuroscience continues to avoid the issue of how feelings are organized in the brain. It is truly regrettable that both neuroscience and psychology have cultivated such neglect because of the pervasive semantic ambiguities that, until the neuroscience revolution, prevented us from forming adequate neurally based definitions for such concepts. However, when we begin to discuss the major emotional systems in brain terms, we should gradually be able to tackle the remaining ambiguities ever more empirically.

More important than quarreling about intrinsically ambiguous semantic distinctions (such as, is EXPECTANCY or SEEKING better? is PANIC or DISTRESS better?) is the recognition and study of the varieties of primitive emotional operating systems that exist in limbic and reptilian areas of the brain. And let me reemphasize: The most compelling evidence for the existence of such systems is our ability to evoke discrete emotional behaviors and states using localized electrical and chemical stimulation of the brain. For brain stimulation to activate coordinated impassioned behavior patterns (accompanied by affective states as indicated by behavioral approach and withdrawal tests), electrodes have to be situated in very specific subcortical (i.e., visceral/limbic) areas of the brain. But once an electrode is in the correct neuroanatomical location, essentially identical emotional tendencies can be evoked in all mammals, including humans.[28] For instance, we can energize SEEKING by stimulating very specific two-way circuits that course between specific midbrain and frontal cortical areas. We can evoke a similar form of exploratory behavioral arousal by activating the confluent dopamine system chemically with psychostimulant drugs such as amphetamines and cocaine in both animals and humans, as well as with various neuropeptides and glutamate in animals.

Although all emotional systems are strongly linked to behavior patterning circuits, it is important to emphasize that they do many other things, from controlling and coordinating the autonomic (i.e., automatic) functions of visceral organs to energizing the cortex to selectively process incoming information. Obviously, to be effective, emotional behaviors need to be backed up by various bodily and psychological adjustments. Sufficient evidence now indicates that the executive systems for emotions are also highly influential in generating subjective states in humans and comparable behavioral indices of affect in animals. Unfortunately, I will not yet be able to address this last issue for all of the emotional systems. The evidence is still quite modest for some systems, largely because few investigators are presently working on such important psychological questions.

The Blue-Ribbon, Grade A Emotional Systems

And how many basic command systems for emotionality have in fact been reasonably well identified? At least four primal emotional circuits mature soon after birth, as indexed by the ability of localized brain stimulation to evoke coherent emotional displays in experimental animals (Figure 3.5), and these systems appear to be remarkably similarly organized in humans. The four most well studied systems are (1) an appetitive motivation SEEKING system, which helps elaborate energetic search and goal-directed behaviors in behalf of any of a variety of distinct goal objects; (2) a RAGE system, which is especially easily aroused by thwarting and frustrations; (3) a FEAR system, which is designed to minimize the probability of bodily destruction; and (4) a separation distress PANIC system, which is especially important in the elaboration of social emotional processes related to attachment. Although I will focus on each of these systems in separate chapters, as an appetizer, let me briefly highlight these major "Blue-Ribbon, Grade A" emotional systems of the mammalian brain.

1. The SEEKING system (see Chapter 8): This emotional system is a coherently operating neuronal network that promotes a certain class of survival abilities. This system makes animals intensely interested in exploring their world and leads them to become excited when they are about to get what they desire. It eventually allows animals to find and eagerly anticipate the things they need for survival, including, of course, food, water, warmth, and their ultimate evolutionary survival need, sex. In other words, when fully aroused, it helps fill the mind with interest and motivates organisms to

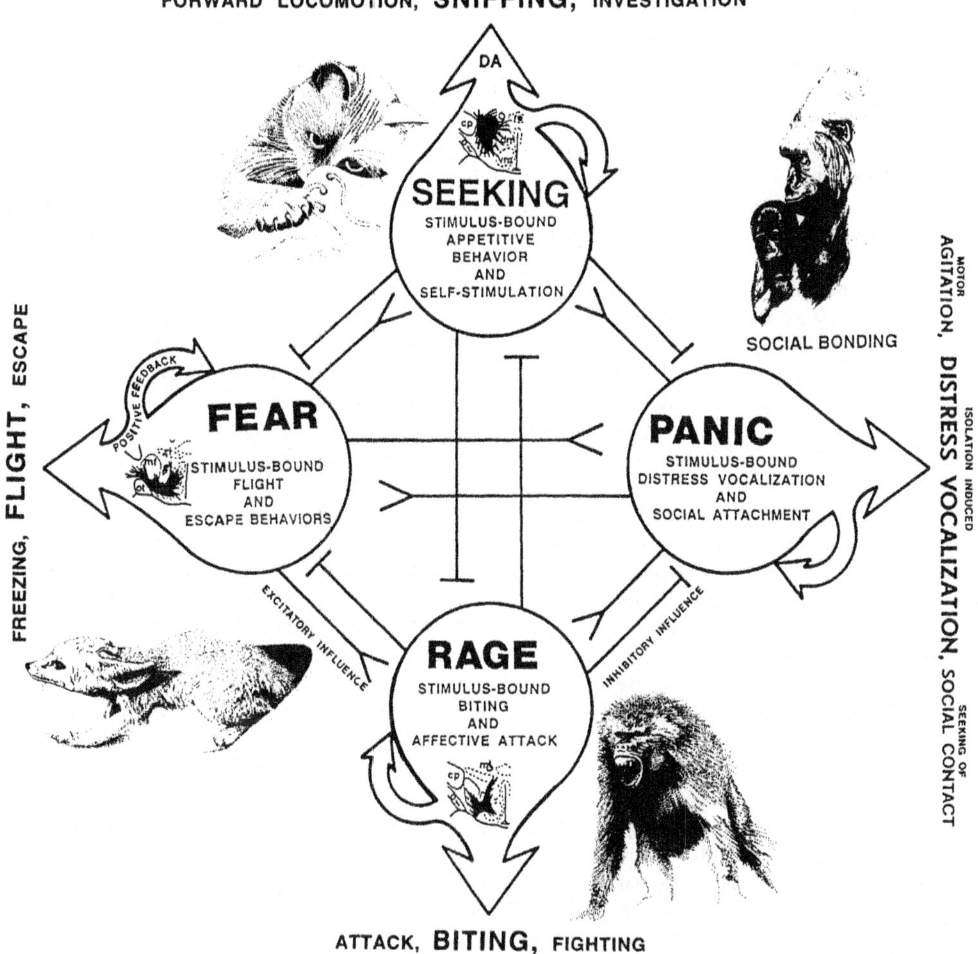

Figure 3.5. The major emotional operating systems are defined primarily by genetically coded neural circuits that generate well-organized behavior sequences that can be evoked by localized electrical stimulation of the brain. Representative behaviors generated by the various systems are indicated, and the approximate locations of the SEEKING, FEAR, and RAGE systems are depicted on a small frontal section through one side of the hypothalamus. As is evident, there is considerable overlap and hence neural interaction among systems. Some of the possible major interactions are indicated by the various interconnecting lines that suggest various excitatory and inhibitory influences among systems. (Adapted from Panksepp, 1982; see n. 26).

move their bodies effortlessly in search of the things they need, crave, and desire. In humans, this may be one of the main brain systems that generate and sustain curiosity, even for intellectual pursuits. This system is obviously quite efficient at facilitating learning, especially mastering information about where material resources are situated and the best way to obtain them. It also helps assure that our bodies will work in smoothly patterned and effective ways in such quests.

When this brain system becomes underactive, as is common with aging, a form of depression results. When the system becomes spontaneously overactive, which can happen as a result of various kinds of stress, an animal's behavior becomes excessive and schizophrenic or manic symptoms may follow—especially the "functional" forms of psychosis that can be treated with traditional antipsychotic medications (which all reduce dopamine activity in the brain), as opposed to the more chronic forms arising from brain degeneration (as indexed by ventricular enlargement).[29]

Neuroanatomically, the SEEKING system corresponds to the major self-stimulation system that courses from the midbrain up to the cortex, which has long been misconceptualized as a "reward or reinforcement system." In fact, as already mentioned, it appears to be a general-purpose neuronal system that helps coax animals and humans to move energetically from where they are presently situated to the places where they can find and consume the fruits of this world. A very important neurochemical in this system is dopamine, especially the dopaminergic mesolimbic and mesocortical dopamine circuits, which emanate from the ventral tegmental area (VTA) situated at the very back of the hypothalamus (Figure 3.6). These dopamine circuits tend to energize and coordinate the functions of many higher brain areas that mediate planning and foresight (such as the amygdala, nucleus accumbens, and frontal cortex—see next chapter) and promote states of eagerness and directed purpose in both humans and animals. It is no wonder that animals are eager to self-stimulate this system via indwelling electrodes. It now seems clear that many psychostimulant drugs commonly abused by humans, especially the amphetamines and cocaine, produce their psychic appeal by temporarily overarousing this emotional system. To some extent, other drugs such as opiates, nicotine, and alcohol also derive their hedonic appeal by interacting with this system (see "Afterthought," Chapter 6).

2. The RAGE system (see Chapter 10): Working in opposition to SEEKING is a system that mediates anger. RAGE is aroused by frustration and attempts to curtail an animal's freedom of action. It has long been known that one can enrage both animals and humans by stimulating very specific parts of the brain, which parallel the trajectory of the FEAR system. This system not only helps animals defend themselves by arousing fear in their opponents but also energizes behavior when an animal is irritated or restrained. Human anger may get much of its psychic "energy" from this brain system. Brain tumors that irritate the circuit can cause pathological rage, while damage to the system can promote serenity.

3. The FEAR system (see Chapter 11): A FEAR circuit was probably designed during evolution to help animals reduce pain and the possibility of destruction. When stimulated intensely, this circuit leads animals to run away as if they are extremely scared. With very weak stimulation, animals exhibit just the opposite motor tendency—a freezing response, common when animals are placed in circumstances where they have previously been hurt or frightened. Humans stimulated in these same brain areas report being engulfed by intense anxiety.

4. The PANIC system (see Chapter 14): To be a mammal is to be born socially dependent. Brain evolution has provided safeguards to assure that parents (usually the mother) take care of the offspring, and the offspring have powerful emotional systems to indicate that they are in need of care (as reflected in *crying* or, as scientists prefer to say, *separation calls*). The nature of these distress systems in the brains of caretakers and those they care for has only recently been clarified; they provide a neural substrate for understanding many other social emotional processes.

5. In addition to the preceding primitive systems that are evident in all mammals soon after birth, we also have more sophisticated special-purpose socioemotional systems that are engaged at appropriate times in the lives of all mammals—for instance, those that mediate sexual LUST (see Chapter 12), maternal CARE (see Chapter 13), and roughhousing PLAY (see Chapter 15). Each of these is built around neural complexities that are only provisionally understood. Sexual urges are mediated by specific brain circuits and chemistries that are quite distinct for males and females but appear to share some components such as the physiological and psychological effects of oxytocin, which also promotes maternal motivation. We now realize that maternal behavior circuits remain closely intermeshed with those that control sexuality, and this suggests how evolution gradually constructed the basic neural substrates for the social contract (i.e., the possibilities for love and bonding) in the mammalian brain.

As we will see, maternal nurturance probably arose gradually from preexisting circuits that initially mediated sexuality. Likewise, the mechanisms of social bonding and playfulness are closely intermeshed with the circuitries for the other pro-social behaviors. Because of the lack of hard data, I will focus more on the behaviors mediated by these circuits than on the associated subjective feelings. However, the neuroanatomical, neurophysiological, neurochemical, and neurobehavioral clarification of such emotional control systems is a prerequisite to addressing the underlying affective issues substantively.

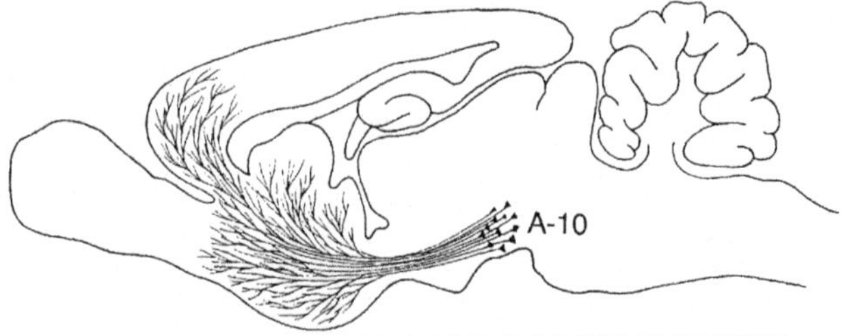

Figure 3.6. Schematic summary of the mesolimbic and mesocortical dopamine system on a lateral midsaggital view of the rat brain. This system allows the frontal cortex and the ventral striatum of the "reptilian brain" to process appetitive information effectively. The system mediates many forms of drug addiction and is also imbalanced in some forms of schizophrenia.

The Emotional Systems Are Evolutionary Tools to Promote Psychobehavioral Coherence

In sum, these basic emotional systems appear to rapidly instigate and coordinate the dynamic forms of brain organization that, in the course of evolution, proved highly effective in meeting various primal survival needs and thereby helped animals pass on their genes to future generations. Of course, most of animal behavior is directed toward effective survival, but contrary to the beliefs of early behaviorists, learning mechanisms are not the only brain functions that evolved to achieve those ends. While general-purpose learning mechanisms may help animals behave adaptively in future circumstances because of the specific life experiences they have had, emotional circuits help animals behave adaptively because of the major types of life challenges their ancestors faced in the course of evolutionary history. The instinctual dictates of these circuits allow organisms to cope with especially challenging events because of a form of evolutionary "learning"—the emergence of coordinated psychobehavioral potentials that are genetically ingrained in brain development. We might call these behaviors *evolutionary operants*. The inheritance of emotional command systems is probably polygenic, and the actual neural circuits that constitute each emotional organ system are obviously more complex than we presently understand. What follows in the ensuing chapters is a mere shadow of reality, but we are finally beginning to grasp the nature of these important brain functions that have, for too long, been ignored by psychologists. An understanding of these systems may prepare the way for a deeper understanding of many traditional psychological problems like the nature of learning and memory, as well as the sources of personality and psychopathology.

In addition to activating and coordinating changes in sensory, perceptual, motor, and physiological functions—which all appear to be suffused with poorly understood central neuroaffective states—the executive circuits for the basic emotions probably also help enable and encode new learning. This is accomplished by special-purpose associative mechanisms that are probably linked to fluctuating activities of each emotive system, and, as has been observed with all other forms of learning, the transmitter glutamate is a major player in all emotional learning that has been studied. As noted in the previous chapters, efficient learning may be conceptually achieved through the generation of subjectively experienced neuroemotional states that provide simple internalized codes of biological values that correspond to major life priorities for the animal. For instance, through classical conditioning (see Figure 1.2) emotionally neutral stimuli in the world can be rapidly imbued with emotional salience. Thus, memory coding and cognitive processes are closely related to emotional arousal, but emotionality is not isomorphic with those processes.

Before we can proceed to a discussion of the details of these emotional systems of the brain, it will first be essential to briefly summarize the successes of the "neuroscience revolution" upon which our future understanding of emotions and motivations must be built—including advances in our understanding of neuroanatomy (see Chapter 4), neurochemistry (see Chapter 5), and neurophysiology (see Chapter 6). Also, since developmental and aging issues are so important in present-day psychology, I would close this chapter by sharing my perspective on these topics. The following short essay will hopefully tie the many threads of thought we have covered in the first three chapters into a compact and coherent viewpoint.

The Ontogeny of Emotional Processes

A common question in developmental psychology is: What develops in emotional development? One approximate pictorial answer to this question was already provided in Figure 2.1. Each emotional system has an ontogenetic life course that we are beginning to understand at a neurobiological level. The answer which I have previously provided to this question went as follows:

> Traditional answers to this question will focus on the increasingly sophisticated interactions a child has with its world. From a psychological perspective, I would say that the main thing that develops in emotional development is the linking of internal affective values to new life experiences. However, in addition to the epigenetic processes related to each individual's personal emotional experiences leading to unique emotional habits and traits, there is also a spontaneous neurobiological unfolding of emotional and behavioral systems during childhood and adolescence. Some neuro-emotional processes are strongly influenced by prenatal experiences, for instance the ability of early hormonal tides to control the brain substrates of gender identity.
>
> Modern neuroscience is showing that the brain is not as unchanging a computational space as was commonly assumed. Neurochemical systems develop and remold at both pre- and post-synaptic sites throughout the lifespan of organisms. For instance receptor fields proliferate and shrink during specific phases of ontogenetic development, and they can show permanent changes in response to life events. Indeed, neurons in specific adult motivational systems can expand and shrink depending upon the environmental challenges and the resulting hormonal tides to which an animal is exposed. It is becoming ever increasingly clear that there is a dynamic interaction between environmental events and genetic events in the brain. With such complexities, it is a risky business to suppose that the stages of emotional and moral development that we see in

human children are simply due to the specific life experiences they have acquired. At the same time, it is foolhardy to push the biological view too far. Even with identical genetic backgrounds, there is a great deal of epigenetic diversity in the fine details of the nervous system. Only the general groundplans for brain connectivities are encoded within the genes, and probably quite indirectly at that (e.g., via expressions of various trophic factors). Neural growth is responsive to a large number of internal and external stochastic processes that lead to a diversity of detailed differences in every nook and cranny of the brain. But despite the infinite variety in the details, the overall plan of the mammalian brain has been highly conserved.

After birth, a great deal of neural unfolding remains to be completed in every species, and we can be reasonably confident that the maturation of specific neural systems does establish essential conditions for the unfolding of certain forms of emotionality. A few examples: 1) Social bonding (imprinting) processes are especially sensitive at certain times of life. 2) The separation distress system seems to exhibit increasing sensitivity during the initial phase of postnatal development, a long-plateau period, and a gradual decline during puberty. 3) Rough and tumble play exhibits a similar pattern. 4) Rats exhibit strong tendencies for maternal behavior during early juvenile development, at times comparable to those when human children are especially infatuated by dolls and play-mothering. 5) Parental tendencies are heralded by neurochemical changes, even genetic de-repression within the oxytocin system, which helps promote maternal intent. 6) And, of course, emotional aspects of sexuality mature at puberty under the sway of genetically controlled hormonal progressions, "developing" gender-specific impulses which were "exposed" as neurohormonal engrams during infancy.

Although there are many psychosocial specifics which develop concurrently, depending on the unique life experiences of individuals, the natural unfolding of neurobiological processes underlying emotionality should not be minimized. Indeed, we need to consider how the experiences of important life events feed back onto the structure of the underlying neural systems. For instance, does an enriched environment invigorate the exploratory systems of the brain? Do repeated experiences of social-loss in early childhood change the vigor and configuration of separation-distress systems? Answers to such compelling questions can now be achieved with certain long lasting neuronal markers (such as fluoro-gold) which can be administered at specific times of psychoneurological development, to see whether the morphological patterns in specific neuronal circuits are remodeled under the sway of specific environmental/emotional challenges. When we finally begin to do such experiments, we will truly be addressing the pervasive nature-nurture interactions that help mold the brain/mind throughout maturation.[30]

For relevant literature citations please refer to the original of the above, as well as several recent reviews that summarize the development[31] and aging[32] of emotional systems within the brain. As highlighted at the end of the quoted passage, this area is ripe for powerful new investigations of how the underlying neural substrates change as a function of normal neurobiological development, as well as individual experiences.

AFTERTHOUGHT: The Classic Neurological Theories of Emotion

During the past decade there has been a remarkable resurgence of interest in the psychology of emotions, and the books cited as suggested readings cover that vast cognitive literature. By comparison, neurological approaches to emotions are not well cultivated. This book seeks to correct that neglect, but in doing so it will focus heavily on a new and integrated view of matters at the expense of a great deal of past thinking in the area. Since past historical views will not receive as much emphasis here as they do in more traditional texts, I would at least briefly describe the four classic milestones in historical discussions of emotions from the biological perspective:

1. The James-Lange theory,[33] proposed over a century ago, suggested that emotions arise from our cognitive appraisal of the commotion that occurs in our inner organs during certain vigorous behaviors. This theory had a "gut appeal" for many investigators, since it makes it much easier to study emotional processes by studying peripheral physiological changes that can be easily monitored. And, of course, it is common to experience various forms of visceral commotion during emotions. It was a short step to assume that emotions are the cognitive readout of such visceral processes. This logical coup d'état circumvented critical brain issues (see Figure 3.2) and provided fuel for a great deal of relatively influential, but apparently misleading, research concerning the fundamental nature of emotions.[34] Although this "Jamesian" perspective has remained an especially attractive theory for cognitively oriented investigators who do not pursue neuroscience connections, neuroscientists severely criticized most of the major tenets of this peripheral-readout theory many years ago.

2. In 1927, Walter Cannon, a physiologist at Harvard, constructed a detailed, empirically based rebuttal to the James-Lange approach.[35] His key points were as follows (I will also briefly indicate, in italics, how Cannon's criticisms could be effectively countered using more recent data): (i) Total separation of the viscera from the brain by spinal cord lesions did not im-

pair emotional behavior. *However, the intensity of emotions was diminished somewhat by such manipulations, and now we also know that the viscera secrete many chemicals (especially hormones and neuropeptides) that may feed important information back to the brain indirectly.*[36] (ii) The viscera are relatively insensitive structures, and often very similar visceral changes occur in very distinct emotional states. *However, more recent evidence does suggest that the patterning of many visceral changes is modestly different among different emotions.*[37] (iii) Finally, Cannon noted that visceral changes are typically too slow to generate emotions, and artificial hormonal activation of organ activities (e.g., via injections of adrenalin) is not sufficient to generate specific emotions. *However, now we do know that injections of certain gastric peptides can rapidly produce emotional episodes. For instance, intravenous administration of cholecystokinin can provoke panic attacks.*[38]

Cannon proceeded to propose a brain-based theory, whereby specific brain circuits (especially thalamic ones) were deemed to be essential for the generation of emotions. Although we now know that other brain areas are generally more influential in emotionality than thalamic circuits (including the amygdala, hypothalamus, and central gray), Cannon did focus our attention on the psychobiological view. At present, it is undeniable that such a view will have to be a cornerstone for the scientific understanding of emotions, but the bodily processes emphasized by the James-Lange theory cannot be ignored. Indeed, bodily changes during emotions are so complex and extensive that there is plenty of room for many feedback influences onto central control processes from peripheral sources. The recent discovery of powerful interlinkages between the brain and immune processes provides new levels of interaction between peripheral and central functions. For instance, many of the *cytokines*—molecules that communicate between different immune compartments—have powerful direct effects on affective brain functions, and brain emotional processes modulate the intensity of immune responses.[39] Recent work suggests that the feeling of illness that we experience during a bacterial infection arises to a substantial degree from the release of interleukin-1, which activates various sickness behaviors and feelings by interacting with specific receptors within the brain.[40] We will probably discover similar neurochemical vectors for the feelings of tiredness and other forms of malaise, but the study of such linkages is just beginning. They could not have been even vaguely imagined 60 years ago when the classic brain theories of emotions were first being proposed.

3. In 1937, James Papez, a neuroanatomist at Cornell University, asserted that "emotion is such an important function that its mechanism, whatever it is, should be placed on a structural basis" and proceeded to delineate the central neuronal circuitry that he believed might mediate emotions.[41] Even though he did not clearly specify which emotion(s) he was concerned with, anatomically he was quite specific. He based much of his reasoning on early brain ablation experiments and the study of a brain disease that induces rage, namely rabies, which is known to damage the hippocampus. Papez suggested an interconnected series of brain areas that might subserve emotionality in general; this has come to be known as the *Papez circuit*. He envisioned how sensory input into the thalamus could be transmitted both upstream and downstream. He suggested that the anterior thalamus distributed emotional information to anterior cortices, especially the cingulate area, information from which was transmitted via the cingulum pathway to the hippocampus and then via the fornix to the mamillary bodies, which then distributed emotional signals back to the anterior thalamus (via the mamillothalamic tract), as well as downward to autonomic and motor systems of the brain stem and spinal cord (see Figure 3.7). These higher areas have been the focus of considerable emotional theorizing in recent years.[42]

The Papez circuit provoked a great deal of experimental work, but ultimately it turned out to be more of a provocative idea than a correct one. Although recent work has affirmed that the cingulate cortex is important for elaborating certain emotions, especially social ones such as feelings arising from separation and bonding,[43] the remaining brain areas of the Papez circuit are not essential executive components within emotional systems. Of course, many of these areas do participate in support mechanisms that interact with emotional processes. For instance, both the thalamus and the hippocampus help elaborate sensory and memorial inputs to emotional systems.[44] Apparently this hippocampal spatial analysis system helps integrate information about contextual cues that can precipitate fearful responses, such as being scared of environments in which one has received an electric shock.[45] This just goes to show that ultimately all brain areas participate in emotions to some extent, but here we will consider only those that seem to be central to the integrative-executive emotional processes and feeling states themselves.

4. In 1949, Paul MacLean elaborated upon Papez's theme[46] and helped firmly establish the concept of the "limbic system" as the focal brain division that must be investigated in order to understand emotionality. As detailed in the next chapter, he identified the medial surfaces of the telencephalic hemispheres (including cingulate, frontal, and temporal lobe areas—especially the amygdala) and interconnections with septal, hypothalamic, and central-medial brain stem areas as part of the neural landscape that constituted the "emotional brain." Although many modern neuroscientists disagree that the limbic system should be considered an anatomically and functionally distinct entity,[47] most agree that the brain areas highlighted by MacLean are essential substrates of emotionality. Moreover, an increasing number of investigators are beginning to appreciate that future progress will depend critically upon our ability

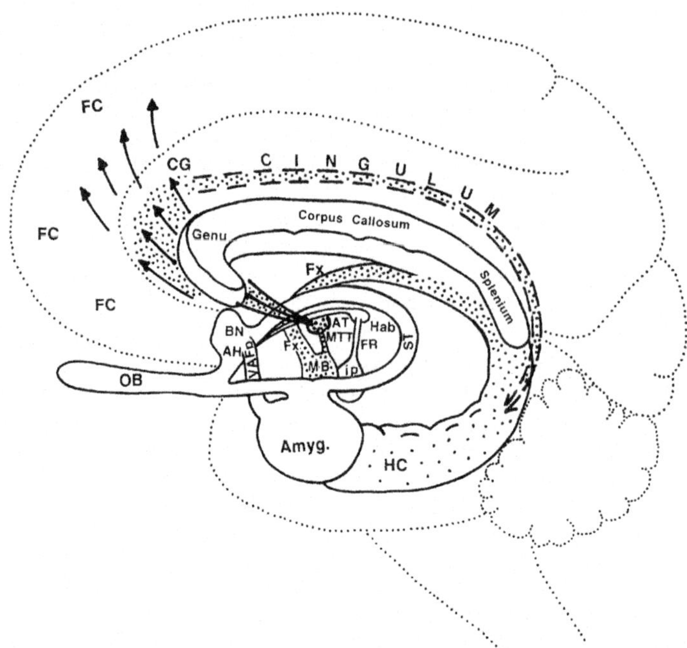

Figure 3.7. Schematic of the limbic system with the Papez circuit highlighted in stippling. FC: frontal cortex; CG: cingulate gyrus; OB: olfactory bulbs; BN: bed nucleus of the stria terminalis; AH: anterior hypothalamus; VAFp: ventral amygdalofugal pathway; Amyg: amygdala; HC: hippocampus; Fx: fornix; AT: anterior thalamus; MB: mamillary bodies; MTT: mamillo-thlamic tract; Hab: habenula; FR: fasciculus retroflexus; ip: interpeduncular nucleus.

to detail the neuroanatomical, neurophysiological, and neurochemical substrates of the psychobehavioral functions.[48] For this reason, the next three chapters will provide broad overviews of the foundation disciplines that are essential for making progress in the field. In the next chapter we will discuss neuroanatomy with a focus on the reptilian brain and visceral-emotional brain commonly known as the limbic system.

Suggested Readings

Birbaumer, N., & Ohman, A. (eds.) (1993). *The structure of emotions*. Göttingen: Hogrefe and Huber.

Christianson, S.-A. (ed.) (1992). *The handbook of emotion and memory*. Hillsdale, N.J.: Lawrence Erlbaum.

Darwin, C. (1872/1965). *The expression of the emotions in man and animals*. Chicago: Univ. of Chicago Press.

Fridja, N. H. (1986). *The emotions*. Cambridge: Cambridge Univ. Press.

Lazarus, R. S. (1991). *Emotion and adaptation*. New York: Oxford Univ. Press.

Mandler, G. (1984). *Mind and body: Psychology of emotion and stress*. NewYork: Norton.

Oatley, K., & Jenkins, J. M. (1996). *Understanding emotions*. Cambridge, Mass.: Blackwell.

Plutchik, R., & Kellerman, H. (eds.) (1984–1987). *Emotion: Theory, research, and experience*. 4 vols. New York: Academic Press.

Strongman, K. (ed.) (1991–1992). *International reviews of emotion research*. 2 vols. Chichester, U.K.: Wiley.

Tomkins, S. S. (1962–1963). *Affect, imagery, consciousness*. 2 vols. New York: Springer-Verlag.

4

Neurostatics

The Anatomy of the Brain/Mind

Whatever may be our opinions as to the relations between "mind" and "matter," our observation only extends to thought and emotion as connected with the living body, and, according to the general verdict of consciousness, more especially with certain parts of the body; namely, the central organs of the nervous system . . . made up of a vast number of little starlike bodies embedded in fine granular matter, connected with each other by ray-like branches in the form of pellucid threads.

Oliver Wendell Holmes, *Pages from an Old Volume of Life* (1863).

CENTRAL THEME

Many who have considered the matter believe that an understanding of psychological and behavioral processes must initially guide our understanding of the functions of the brain. Less well appreciated is the fact that understanding of the brain can highlight the nature of psychological processes. Intellectual commerce is always a two-way street. Recent discoveries about the brain have finally established a foundation for a mechanistic understanding of the mind. Numerous new techniques now exist to illuminate brain-mind relations, and the painstaking collection of new information continues at a fever pitch. The "neuroscience revolution" of the last few decades has enabled us to conceptualize human nature in dramatically new ways, and the debate is shifting from the issue of whether mind emerges from brain to how specific mental states, traits, and abilities arise from the brain. The ongoing breakthroughs are so important that even remote disciplines such as philosophy, economics, and political science are beginning to pay close attention to what the psychologically oriented neuroscientists are doing. All past progress in this quest has been premised on acceptance of the "neuron doctrine"—the recognition that individual neurons are the fundamental units that transfer information throughout the brain. Just as each human being has individual qualities as a receiver and transmitter of information, so too does each neuron have such qualities, both electrical and chemical. But a single neuron does nothing important psychologically by itself. Psychological processes emerge from the neurodynamic interactions of many interconnected neurons (i.e., circuits or neuronal networks), yielding many yet unmeasured and unimagined complexities. Foreseeable progress in this field will arise from our ability to relate functionally coherent circuit systems to primitive (i.e., genetically dictated) psychobehavioral tendencies. However, there is yet no consensus as to how we can best overlay psychological principles upon brain processes. One thing, however, is beyond doubt: It cannot be done without an adequate appreciation of the subject matter of this chapter—the complexities of neuroanatomy.

The Brain's Relations to the Mind

A central assumption of modern neuroscience is that all psychological functions ultimately emerge from the workings of the brain. Without specific brain activities there are no memories, no emotions, no motivations, no mind. Mind is considered as natural a function of brain circuit dynamics as digestion is of gastrointestinal actions, although the former is vastly more complex. The dualistic alternative—the notion of a disembodied mind that may parallel the functions of the brain but is not ultimately caused or restrained by those functions—has also been widely entertained down through the ages, but such metaphysical propositions no longer enjoy the respect of serious investigators (but see Appendix C). However, a variant of dualism continues—namely, the assumption that we can adequately understand psychological processes through the mere use of verbal symbols and simple measures, such as reaction times, without relying on brain research. This view still permeates most of academic psychology, including such recent variants as cognitive psychology.

To understand how mind emerges from brain functions, we must appreciate how the various neurons in different parts of the brain interconnect and intercommunicate. Since scientists have known of the existence of neurons for only a little over a century, it is little wonder that discussions of the human mind have been carried out for thousands of years exclusively on the basis of verbal concepts. That is a hard habit to break, but I trust the reader appreciates how little scientific insight concerning the *basic* sources of mind and behavior such analyses can provide. Words can only describe the contents of mind and its relation to environmental events, without ever providing adequate explanations of the internal functions that permit mental operations to proceed. Thanks to the neuroscience revolution, we are now able to study basic mind issues with neuroanatomical, neurophysiological, and neurochemical concepts. In this chapter, I will focus on neuroanatomy, while the other aspects are covered in the next two chapters.

It is impossible to do justice to the physical structure of the brain in the brief space available here, so my aim will be to promote an appreciation of this remarkable organ rather than comprehensive coverage. The attempt to master anatomical structures and the interconnections of the brain is an intimidating exercise for students. There is so much to learn, so much to visualize, and few have the intrinsic interest to master this difficult subject matter. However, when these facts are related to psychological issues, interest is often aroused to the point where we can begin to appreciate how mental processes emerge from the dynamics of various brain circuits interacting with the environment.

Neuroanatomical Homologies

Studying neuroanatomy entails an almost endless exercise in relating arcane nomenclatures to the topographic landmarks of a very complex organ. Brain structure brings to mind the wonderful intricacies of medieval cathedrals: A grand and stately order repeats itself, in general plan, from one mammalian species to the next. But variety is always there.

Fortunately, if one learns the subcortical neuroanatomy of one mammalian species, one has learned the ground plan for all other mammals. Indeed, by mastering the brain of one mammal, one immediately enjoys a good understanding of the subcortical neuroanatomy of most other vertebrate species. This is direct evidence for many structural homologies in the brain, which helps justify the belief that many brain functions are also homologous across species. Indeed, the most striking insight of many students when they first become entranced by neuroscience is the remarkable similarity between the organization of rat brains and those of humans. Such neuroanatomical and neurochemical homologies have been sufficient to convince many investigators that general principles governing human behavior can be revealed through brain research on other mammals, especially for the ancient subcortical operating systems that control arousal, attention, emotions, and motivations.

By comparison, overall cortical organization exhibits much greater variability among species. Accordingly, attempts to span cognitive issues, by trying to relate the higher psychic functions of humans to animal brain circuits, will be vastly more difficult, and perhaps impossible when it comes to our highest cortical abilities, the four "R's"—reading, writing, arithmetic, and rational thought. By comparison, the nature of reproductive emotional urges will be much better clarified by cross-species brain research. However, even though an understanding of humans' higher cortical functions cannot be achieved by studying rats, homologies do abound in the fine structural features of the cortex of most mammals, for instance, among the *columns*—the cylindrical functional modules of each animal's neocortex—as well as in the general input-output organization of the primary cortical projection areas that receive sensory messages and directly control movements. Similarities in cortical interconnectivities diminish markedly as one begins to compare the more complex secondary and tertiary association *cortices* where perceptions, as well as most cognitive and rational processes, are generated. In short, multimodal association areas of the cortex, where information from different senses is combined to yield concepts and ideas, are structurally similar in microscopic detail, but because of the types of exchange of information among an increasing number of areas, similarities between humans and other animals begin to diminish. The speech cortex is the most multimodal of them all, and there humans and other animals have most decisively parted ways (see Appendix B).

It is noteworthy that at the microscopic level there are two general types of cortex. The neocortex possessed by most mammals has neatly stratified "sheets" of six distinct cell layers, while a minority of mammals, primarily ancient creatures such as shrews and opossums, have a diffusely organized cortex, resembling that of birds, with less clear layering of cells than is evident in the neocortex of most mammals. Indeed, it comes as something of a surprise that our closest competitors for high intelligence on the face of the earth, the whales and dolphins, have this ancient form of cortex.[1] No one knows for sure whether this form of cortical organization can really generate the high levels of intelligence that many of us hope such creatures possess. Indeed, their frontal lobes—the region of the brain considered to be the seat of human foresight, insight, and planning—are comparatively small. However, before we take too much pride in our massive frontal lobes, which many believe are the repositories of our highest social feelings, such as sympathy and empathy and hence our sense of conscience, it should be pointed out that the frontal lobes of such ancient monotremes (i.e., transitional mammals) as the echidna (i.e., the spiny anteater of Australia) are also remarkably large, but there is little evidence that these animals are terribly bright.[2]

Although humans have the largest frontal lobes of any species, dolphins have a massive new brain area, the paralimbic lobe,[3] that we do not possess. The paralimbic lobe is an outgrowth of the cingulate gyrus, which is known to elaborate social communication and social emotions (such as feelings of separation distress and maternal intent) in all other mammals.[4] Thus, dolphins may have social thoughts and feelings that we can only vaguely imagine. Of course, intense social feelings are especially important for air-breathing mammals who must subsist in a demanding aquatic environment: If they faint, there is no chance of survival unless others come to their aid immediately.

In sum, a cross-species comparison of cognitions may well be a more difficult endeavor than studying the subcortically organized emotions and motivations. Brain scientists will probably have better success in providing a neuroscientific understanding of those psychological processes and biological values that emerge from brain areas we share most clearly with other species. From this vantage, a cross-species approach to affective neuroscience is more likely to reveal general principles of brain function than a comparative cognitive neuroscience.

An Introduction to the Anatomical Universe of the Brain

The construction of each mammalian brain is under the control of unfathomed genetically dictated rules that include developmental programs for the birth, proliferation, and migration of various neurons, programs for cell growth and extension (so that neurons in one area can connect up with those in another), and programs for selective cell death, or *apoptosis*, as it is now called, which selectively weeds out excess neurons to yield a well-carved and intricately detailed final product. These processes are controlled by various chemical gradients and path-guiding molecules that mediate cell "recognition" and "adhesion" and promote optimal patterns of neuronal growth. An especially exciting area is the discovery of many highly specific neuronal growth factors, and genetic deletion of some of these factors can yield animals that are deficient in specific sensory and motor abilities.[5] In addition to the genetic control of brain development, an animal's experience in its environment can have an equally important influence. In the present chapter, however, I will ignore many of these important issues, since they do not yet connect clearly with psychology. It is a daunting and controversial task to select a level of analysis that offers the best linkages to psychological issues, but I believe the neurochemically defined anatomical circuits discussed in Chapter 6 will prove most instructive. The student interested in a thorough treatment of neuroanatomy may wish to consult the texts by Brodal and by Nieuwenhuys, as well as several of the other neuroanatomy texts listed in the suggested readings at the end of this chapter.

Because our focus is on emotions, my anatomical discussion will concentrate on those subcortical processes of the visceral nervous system, or limbic system, from which the primal impulse for emotionality emerges. Less emphasis will be placed on the thalamic-neocortical axis of the somatic nervous system, which harvests information from our external bodily senses and guides our skeletal motor systems through the cognitive influences of appraisals, plans, and other representations of the outside world.[6] These two forms of information processing—visceral and somatic—can be considered to arise from two distinct regions within the brain (Figure 4.1). In addition, both somatic-cognitive and visceral-emotional processes converge on more ancient parts of the brain called the *basal ganglia*. This zone has been metaphorically called the *reptilian brain* because it is shared in a remarkably homologous fashion with even the lowest vertebrates. Although all three brain zones operate together, each contains a variety of distinct operating systems. This attractive concept, that there are three brains in one (Paul MacLean's "triune brain" concept portrayed in Figure 3.1), is supported by a variety of observations.[7] Although a debatable simplification from a strictly neuroanatomical perspective, MacLean's formulation provides a clear and straightforward way to begin conceptualizing the brain's overall organization. However, before discussing the details, let us consider some general functional issues that should be kept in mind when we think about neuroanatomy.

"Open" and "Closed" Systems of the Brain

We should always keep in mind a key conceptual distinction when we consider brain operating systems, namely, how "open" or "closed" are these systems in relation to environmental influences (Figure 4.2)? For instance, very simple reflexive behaviors such as yawning and eye blinking are typically considered to be "closed"—they operate in much the same way every time, with a characteristic time course and intensity. In humans, even such reflexive events are not completely closed and can be substantially modulated by environmental events. For instance, one can stifle a yawn, and even the intensity of the knee-jerk reflex is reduced when one is relaxed and increased when one is aroused (i.e., following exposure to erotic photographs or missing a few meals).[8]

Other brain systems, such as those that mediate emotional tendencies evoked by localized brain stimulation,

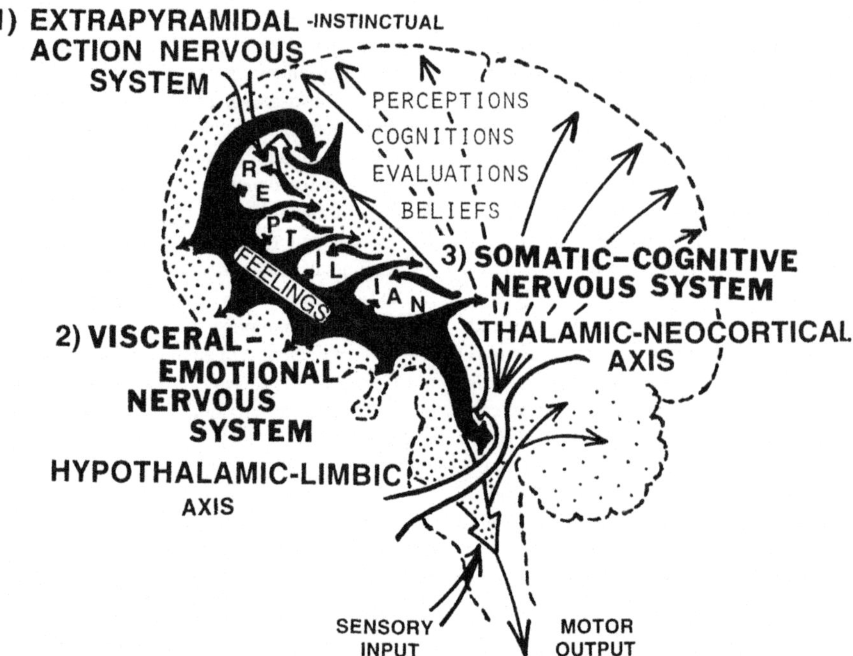

Figure 4.1. Schematic representation in the human brain of the major axes of visceral (hypothalamic-limbic axis—stream of feeling) and somatic (thalamic-neocortical axis—stream of thought) information processing. They converge on the reptilian brain, or basal ganglia. The dorsal streams of neural activity are related more to information coming from the external senses (vision, hearing, and touch), while the ventral-visceral streams of neural activity are related more to the chemical and internal senses (taste, smell, temperature, and various hormone and body energy and water detectors). Both streams of information converge on basic sensory-motor control programs of basal ganglia to generate behavior in which both somatic and visceral processes are blended to yield coherent behavior output.

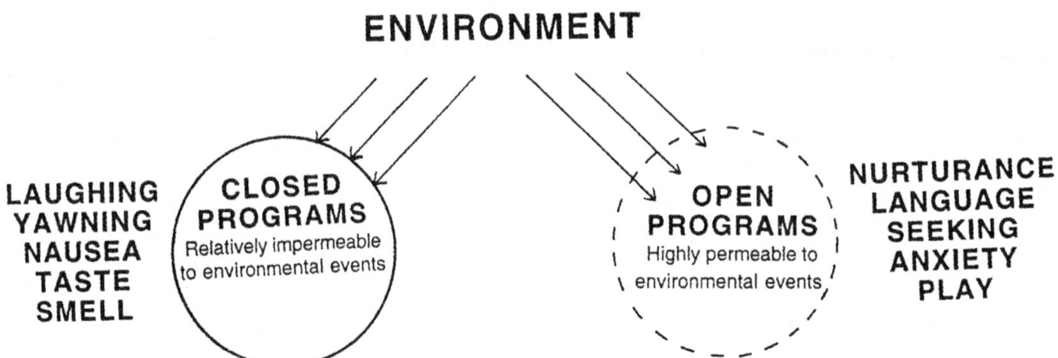

Figure 4.2. Schematic representation of closed and open programs of the brain. Environmental events trigger closed programs into fairly stereotyped actions such as yawning and laughing. Open programs are much more extensively modified by interactions with environmental events according to various principles of learning.

are more "open" to environmental events. As I will discuss in subsequent chapters, emotional circuits can be modulated by a diversity of environmental influences ranging from hormones to learning. Thus, even though many innate operating systems can arouse instinctual urges, all are subject to environmental modulation. Although the emotional systems are comparatively closed in lower mammals, they have probably been opened substantially in higher mammals by cortical evolution. For instance, even though humans can feel strong emotions, they do not have to share them with others if they do not so wish. All this emerges from the richness of neuronal interactions among evolutionarily unrelated brain systems. Nonetheless, the openness of these systems is modest in comparison to those located in the cortex, which associate and utilize information from the various external senses. The more open a brain program, the more the final output is controlled by nurture rather than nature.[9] Thus one of the most open programs in the brain is that which allows us to acquire language, but even this is under biological constraints (see Appendix B).

The Neuroscience Revolution and the Neuron Doctrine

Brain Tissues

The consistency of the living brain resembles that of an overripe peach, and its outward form does not readily provide hints to the nature of its internal organization. To yield a clear picture of its geographies, the brain needs to be hardened, or fixed (usually with formaldehyde), to the consistency of a hard-boiled egg, sliced into thin transparent sections, and stained in various ways to highlight specific structures. This whole process is called *histology*. Until this century, one could gather only vague hints about the brain's internal organization from the patterns of gray and white matter, which represent heavy densities of neuronal cell bodies (or *nuclei*) and clustered fiber pathways (or *tracts*), respectively. As noted at the beginning of this chapter, earlier observers likened the finer details of the nervous system to "starlike bodies" (now known to be nerve cells or neurons) and "pellucid threads" (now known as *axons* and *dendrites*), which are the transmitting and receiving branches of neurons, respectively (Figure 4.3). It was also noted that these structures were embedded in "fine granular matter" that we now call *glial cells*, the "housekeeper" cells of the nervous system, which provide essential metabolic and biophysical support for the information transmission functions of nerve cells. In addition to nuclei and tracts, the brain also contains a great deal of *reticular substance*, where neuronal cell bodies and neuronal fibers are not tightly clustered but interdigitate, in seemingly inextricable ways. These reticular areas are especially important for generating subtle psychological abilities because they integrate and combine many kinds of information via cascades of interconnections (or *circuits*). Indeed, many investiga-

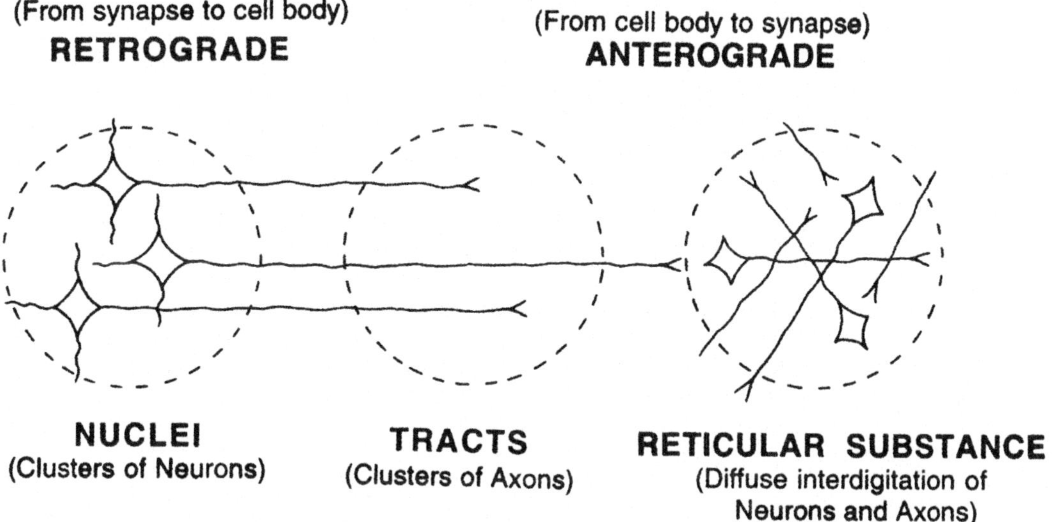

Figure 4.3. Neural tissue is composed of three general types of tissues: nuclei (or clusters of nerve cells), tracts (clusters of axonal fibers), and reticular substance (where the two interdigitate to such an extent that the pattern of interconnections is more difficult to discern). Anterograde (away from the cell body) and retrograde (toward the cell body) anatomical projections can now be studied with a host of neurochemical techniques, and the neurochemical character of individual neurons can be highlighted with immunocytochemical approaches.

tors believe that the most important kinds of psychointegrative processes are elaborated by reticular tissues; therefore, unraveling of the anatomical organization of reticular tissue is essential for understanding the neuronal infrastructure of basic psychological processes.

Of course, the intermeshing of these three types of tissues is very complex. Two photographic views of the rat brain sectioned at the level of the upper brain stem are depicted in Figure 4.4. On the left, the use of a cell body stain highlights the locations of major tracts and some nuclear groups, with most of the brain at this level being taken up by reticular-type tissue. On the right, a section through the same level reflecting dispersion of radioactive 2-deoxy-D-glucose (2-DG), a nonmetabolizable sugar that has been used to highlight neuronal functions (see Chapter 5), generally reflects the overall amounts of neuronal firing in various brain areas during a particular behavior. In this case, the animal was not doing anything special; it was simply left alone in its home cage. Clearly, there is little glucose uptake in tracts, and much less in the more ventral visceral structures than in the more dorsal thalamic-neocortical ones. This metabolic differentiation reflects a basic difference between limbic and somatic axes of the nervous system.

The Neuron Doctrine

Individual neurons are the fundamental units of information transfer in the brain. The classic technique that established the "neuron doctrine" of brain function was the Golgi stain. Camillo Golgi, an Italian histologist, developed a silver nitrate staining procedure at the end of the 19th century that could highlight the entire external structure of neurons. However, because

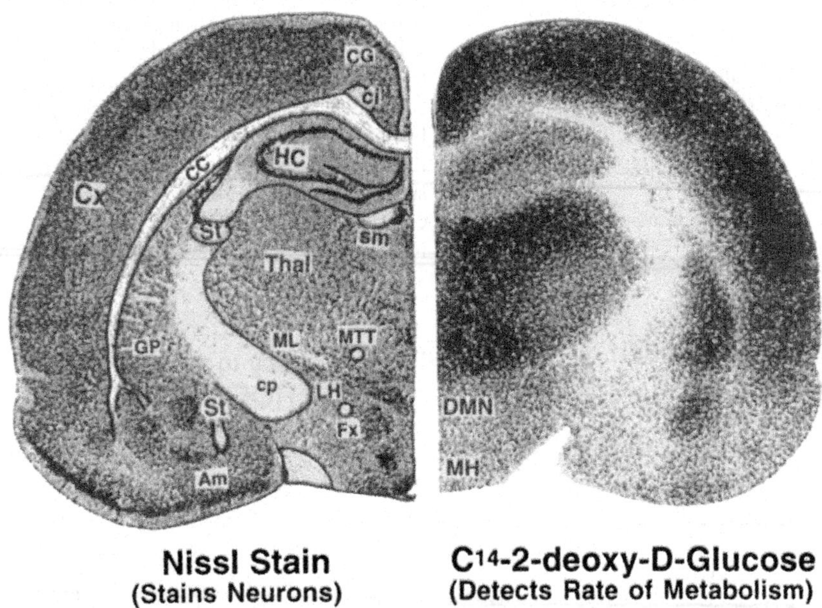

Figure 4.4. Two views of the rat brain highlighting different properties of brain tissues: on the left, cell staining using the Nissl procedure; on the right, the same brain section processed for radioactive 2-DG, which clearly highlights differences between somatic (thalamic-neocortical) and visceral (hypothalamic-limbic) areas of the brain. There are many anatomical, neurophysiological, and neurochemical distinctions between these zones of the brain, which clearly indicate that the dichotomy between the "thinking" and "feeling" parts of the brain is a fundamental distinction and not just a poetic metaphor. The greater mass of reptilian brain is anterior to this section, but the wedge between the lower wing of the corpus callosum (cc) and the descending motor fibers of the cerebral peduncle (cp) contains striatal tissue called the globus pallidus (GP). Other anatomical abbreviations are: Cx: cortex; CG: cingulate gyrus; ci: cingulum; HC: hippocampus; St: stria terminalis; sm: stria medularis; Thal: thalamus; ML: medial lemniscus; MTT: mammilo-thalamic tract; LH: lateral hypothalamus; Fx: fornix; Am: amygdala; DMN: dorsomedial nucleus of the hypothalamus; MH: medial hypothalamus.

of his incomplete microscopic analysis, Golgi reached the mistaken conclusion that the brain was a "synctium" —a network of continuously interconnected protoplasmic processes. It remained for Santiago Ramón y Cajal, the great Spanish neuroanatomist, to exploit Golgi's histological technique and demonstrate conclusively that neurons are discontinuous, communicating with each other at specialized junctions called *synapses*. Cajal also provided an unparalleled level of descriptive precision with his beautiful and meticulously detailed hand-drawn plates of neuronal patterns. His work remains the hallmark of excellence that neuroanatomists still seek to emulate.[10] It is a standing joke in the field that if anyone discovers a new substructure in the brain, they should check in Cajal's original work, since "if he didn't describe it, it does not exist." For making the internal terrain of the brain known to us, Cajal and Golgi jointly received Nobel Prizes in 1906, "in recognition of their work on the structure of the nervous system."[11]

This was an auspicious beginning for modern neuroscience. As Cajal stated, the neurons (or nerve cells) that he visualized were "the mysterious butterflies of the soul, the beating of whose wings may some day—who knows? —clarify the secret of mental life."[12] The Nobel Committee recognized the fundamental importance of the quest to understand the basic languages of the brain by continuing to reward those who have blazed new paths into the organ of the mind. For example, in 1986 Rita Levi-Montalcini was recognized for her discovery of nerve growth factor (NGF), one of a series of regulatory signals that guide the growth of nerve cells during early development.[13] Many other regulatory signals have been discovered since then.[14]

Individuals who have made seminal and lasting contributions to our understanding of basic brain functions have been so consistently recognized by the Nobel Committee during this century that one can now summarize the quest to understand the basic fabric of the mind by recounting their prizewinning accomplishments. First, let us briefly consider how neuroscientists have obtained better and more detailed anatomical road maps of the brain. In the future, it will be impossible to think creatively about the sources of basic psychological processes without being conversant with neuroanatomy.[15]

"Classic" Neuroanatomy versus the "New" Neuroanatomy

The Golgi stain is highly temperamental and stains only a small subset of neurons, perhaps the ones that are dying. In this way, it reveals the configuration of individual neurons. Dissection of pathways within reticular tissues proved to be especially difficult using classic techniques, such as the histological visualization of degenerating tissue (or *chromatolysis*) in distant parts of the brain after placement of small lesions in areas whose connectivities one wished to reveal. In trying to map out such degeneration patterns, one could not be sure whether the trajectory of systems that was revealed was due to the neurons that had been killed or to fibers of passage that had been concurrently damaged. The development of a new silver staining technique allowed visualization of individual degenerating fibers, which led to a small renaissance in neuroanatomy. However, by the late 1960s neuroanatomy had become a stagnant field. The available riches had been mined with those techniques, and there was little incentive for investigators to persist in the absence of new methodological advances. Around 1970, things started changing rapidly because of the development of new and powerful histological techniques for visualizing fine structures. The analysis of brain connections became a fresh and enthusiastic science.

So how did the new generation of neuroanatomists learn to trace the precise connections within the neural tangle of reticular substance? Just as our ability to see far out into the universe required the development of ever-better telescopes, so our ability to visualize the fine internal structure of the brain required development of tools that could follow individual neuronal threads through tightly packed jungles of brain tissue. In a sense, mapping neuroanatomy is similar to tracing roadways through a dense metropolitan area. Most roadways constructed by humans, however, are two-way streets, while all communication channels in the brain that have been constructed by evolution are *polarized*, sending information in only one direction. Thus, one needs separate techniques for identifying which roads leave specific brain areas and which ones enter them. Today a host of techniques can visualize nearly all aspects of the fine structures of the brain. We can see that individual neurons send their information via transmitting fibers, or *axons*, and receive incoming information at points known as *synapses*, via branching structures called *dendrites*. Without this knowledge, we could not relate psychological processes to specific brain circuits.

As emphasized previously, the new techniques were especially well designed to reveal the intricacies of reticular tissue in the brain. The three major problems in unraveling the architecture of reticular substance are: (1) Identifying where specific neurons send their information (via axons). This is the question of *anterograde connectivities*. (2) Identifying the point of origin of incoming messages conveyed to specific neurons (especially in complex information-processing areas). This is the question of *retrograde connectivities*—in other words, where are the neuronal cell bodies situated which transmit information to specific parts of the brain? (3) Determining the *chemical architecture*. How can we define the major neurochemical "personalities" of neuronal systems? All of these questions have been resolved by new technologies developed since 1970.

The Anterograde Question

A universal function of all cells is to manufacture proteins. To do this effectively, cell bodies have highly specialized uptake mechanisms for absorbing the constituent amino acid building blocks. In neurons, many proteins are conveyed toward synaptic endings of axons via specific transport systems consisting of *microtubules*. One can take advantage of such neuronal transport properties to highlight the trajectories of axons as they transmit information away from the cell body. This is done by (1) injecting radioactive amino acids, such as proline or leucine, and more recently many additional markers, into specific parts of the brain; (2) waiting several days for incorporation into protein synthesis and transport down the axon; (3) slicing the brain into thin sections; (4) photographing the sections by applying very sensitive film for anywhere from several days to several months (a technique called *autoradiography*); and (5) examining ribbons of silver grains produced by exposure to radioactivity. These grains indicate the trajectories of axonal pathways from neurons situated at the site of injection. Recently, additional nonradioactive fluorescent techniques have been developed to address similar questions.

The Retrograde Question

Synapses are specialized for thrifty use of their expensive information molecules. Since transmitters and enzymes require considerable energy to construct, presynaptic endings have specialized reuptake mechanisms that reabsorb many of the substances that are released into the synaptic cleft. One can take advantage of such specialized synaptic functions to highlight the locations of neurons that transmit information to specific parts of the brain. The general techniques are quite similar to those used to answer anterograde questions, but the indicator molecules and visualization approaches are usually quite different. One of the most commonly used molecules has been the plant enzyme horseradish peroxidase (HRP), but there are now a large variety of fluorescent dyes that can trace pathways even more brilliantly. Many of the early dyes (such as Evans blue and bizbenzimide) had the troublesome property of fading rapidly, but newer agents such as fluro-gold remain indefinitely inside the neurons where they have been transported. The fluro-gold technique allows us to ask profound questions, such as whether early experiences permanently affect neuronal development. For instance, we can determine how early social isolation can change the growth and degree of branching of brain circuits that mediate separation distress or other emotions. This experiment hasn't yet been done, but if early isolation does, in fact, cause permanent brain effects, then we may finally understand how the intensity and duration of early experiences help construct subsequent personality tendencies of humans and other animals.

Chemical Anatomy

Thanks to many detailed studies of the brain's chemical architecture, we can now add meaningful "color" to the static latticework of brain connectivities. The neurochemical personalities of whole neuronal systems have been revealed through a variety of histological recipes, the most universal of which is *immunocytochemistry*. In principle, the technique can visualize any chemical system of the brain. It relies upon the initial extraction and purification of a molecule of interest, followed by the exploitation of the immune response of experimental donor animals to generate specific-recognition molecules (antibodies). These antibodies are then extracted from their blood and used for the histological identification of target molecules on thin sections of brain tissue. In other words, once an investigator has a specific antibody for a given neurochemical, the antibody can be used in conjunction with a variety of visualization techniques to find the locations of that neurochemical within the apparent jungle of brain tissue. Obviously, this technique provides the most discriminating information when certain molecules are unique to a specific brain circuit. Visualization of molecules that are genetically expressed in all circuits provides little useful information about functionally specific circuits. Fortunately, there are many brain systems that appear to rely on very specific molecules for transmission of information. Through the use of immunocytochemical techniques, the fine architecture of many distinct chemical transmitter systems have now been revealed. Comparable techniques exist to identify where the receptors for specific transmitters are situated throughout the brain (see Chapter 6). As we will see in many subsequent chapters, some of these systems are responsible for specific types of affective and emotional experiences.

The General Topographic Map of the Brain: Global Categories and Structures

Unlike many other bodily organs, the gross anatomy of the brain is not very informative about the variety of brain functions. External configurations provide few clues to the subtlety of the dynamic internal processes. They offer only general geographic guidelines to orient us for the needed inquiries into deeper issues. In the presentation that follows, I will employ three didactic devices to clarify brain organization. First, I will summarize the overall gross morphology of the brain; second, I will focus on the characteristic segregation of primary sensory and motor functions in the brain; finally, I will focus on the "triune" organization in the brain, whereby three layers of mammalian brain evolution are recognized—reptilian (the basal ganglia), old-mammalian (limbic system), and neomammalian (neocortex).

An Overview of Brain Morphology

For our brief excursion into the external structures of the brain, let me start with a gross overview of a brain in extended or elongated form (Figure 4.5). During early development, the nervous system is a straight, hollow neural tube that lays out the basic rostral-caudal dimension of the developing neuroaxis. As neurons proliferate and migrate from the ventricular lining, the tube develops characteristic swellings. The major swellings lead to the classically recognized "continental" structures, from front (rostral) to back (caudal). At the very rostral end we have the forebrain, or *prosencephalon*, which undergoes further subswellings to form the cerebral hemispheres of the *telencephalon*, as well as two main subcortical zones of the upper brain stem, the thalamus and hypothalamus, which are jointly known as the *diencephalon*. These are followed by the midbrain, or *mesencephalon*, which remains relatively undifferentiated, and then by the lower brain stem or hindbrain, or *rhombencephalon*, which divides into the pontine-cerebellar area, or *metencephalon*, and the medulla oblongata, also known as the *myelencephalon*. Essentially, the bulk of information flows longitudinally up and down along the neuroaxis (i.e., along the rostral-caudal dimension), even though there are abundant radial connections throughout the neuroaxis.

As the expanding brain starts to fill the cranium, a number of bends, or *flexures*, emerge as the enlarging brain accommodates itself, "accordion fashion," to the round shape of the skull. The three major bends are the anterior *cephalic flexure* at the midbrain level, the *pontine flexure* farther down in the brain stem just below the cerebellum, and the *cervical flexure* at the lower brain stem. The complex shapes of the ventricles, which provide a central avenue for the transport of cerebrospinal fluid (which is a filtrate of the arterial blood), are due to the various rotations and flexures of the neural tube as it swells and bends to fit the inside of the skull. For instance, we can imagine the fourth ventricle being created like the splitting of a pea pod if it is bent in the direction of the seam. Also, the growth of the telencephalic swellings from the anterior sides of the neural tube gradually leads to a rotation of the cerebral hemispheres in backward and lateral directions. Because of this backward rotation of the telencephalic hemispheres over the diencephalon, the cerebral hemispheres lie directly over the thalamic part of the upper brain stem with no direct vertical connections between them. All connections loop

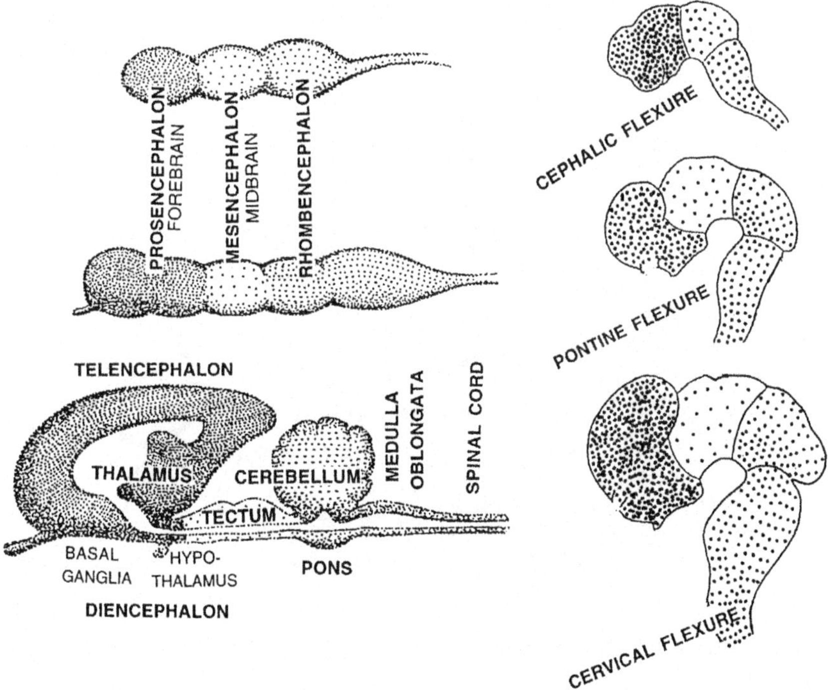

Figure 4.5. On the left are depicted the progressive swellings of the brain as a function of development. On the right, a more realistic depiction of the types of flexures and expansions that gradually lead to a mature appearance of the brain.

within these rotations of the neural tube; if one could unfold the brain, the simple longitudinal organization would again become evident.

The various stretchings and flexures of the neural tube have created cavities, four *ventricles*, at various points along the tube. In the forebrain, the cerebral hemispheres contain two *lateral ventricles*, which course downward to the middle of the brain to a single *third ventricle* situated right at the midline. The third ventricle connects via the narrow mesencephalic cerebral aqueduct to the *fourth ventricle* just under the cerebellum. The cerebrospinal fluid (CSF) that fills the ventricles is manufactured by specialized cells of the choroid plexuses that line the ventricles. The CSF is not only a route for the brain to get rid of its waste products but also a major conduit for hormonelike communication and coordination between distant brain areas. It now seems certain that information transfer in the brain is not simply synaptic but can also occur in a diffuse *paracrine* way, through local diffusion of neurochemicals.

The blood supply to the forebrain (Figure 4.6) is provided largely by the internal carotid arteries ascending from the heart to the base of the brain, where it forms the *circle of Willis*. The major cerebral arteries arise from the circle of Willis, with anterior midline structures of the forebrain receiving blood by the paired anterior cerebral arteries, the lateral surface of the forebrain being supplied by the middle cerebral arteries, and the back of the brain being perfused by the posterior cerebral arteries. The hindbrain and midbrain are supplied by the single vertebral artery that ascends along the ventral midline of the brain stem and extends radial arteries along its length. At the back of the hypothalamus, it joins the circle of Willis to provide a rich vasculature around the base of the diencephalon around the pituitary gland, which is a visceromotor, endocrine organ that controls the secretion of most hormones and hence the metabolism of the whole body.

Overall Functional Organization of the Brain: Sensory versus Motor Processes

Of course, a single neuron can do nothing important by itself. Brain functions emerge from the interplay of neuronal networks, and a long-standing hope of neuropsychology has been to relate psychological functions not only to specific brain structures but also to specific brain circuits. Indeed, the first "lawful relation" such as this was discovered early in the 19th century. It is called the *Bell-Magendie law* after the British and French scientists who discovered the principle at nearly the same time. This law simply asserts that sensory nerves enter the spinal cord toward the dorsal (back) side, while motor nerves exit from the ventral (front) side (Figure 4.7). This law has stood the test of time. In fact, it provides a general scheme of organization found throughout the brain: Sensory processes are generally more dorsally situated in the brain than are motor processes. A comparable segregation of sensory and motor processes is also apparent in the cortex, where motor processes are elaborated by the frontal lobe, while sensory processes are concentrated more posteriorly in the occipital (vision), temporal (hearing), and parietal (touch) lobes. Another organizational pattern is the medial location of visceral (and hence emotional) systems in cen-

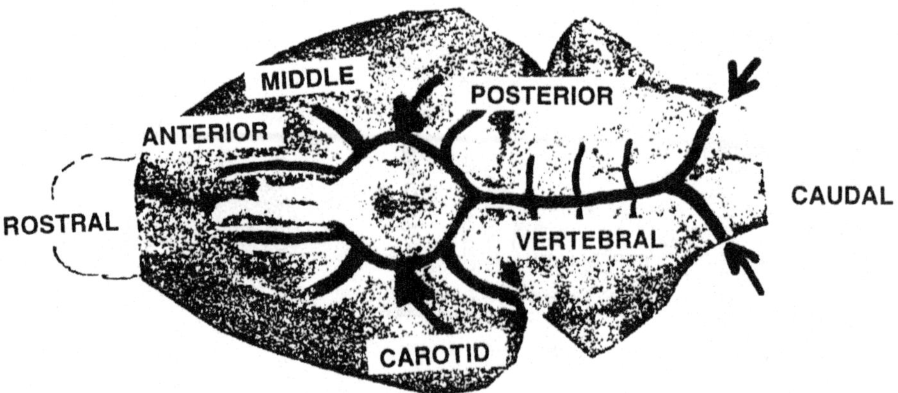

Figure 4.6. Blood supply depicted on the ventral surface of the rat brain. The rostral parts of the brain are fed by the carotid arteries entering the circle of Willis. The blood is distributed to each of the hemispheres by anterior and middle cerebral arteries. The brain stem is fed by the ascending vertebral artery on the base of the brain, and it also contributes to the perfusion of the back of the cerebral hemispheres via the posterior cerebral artery.

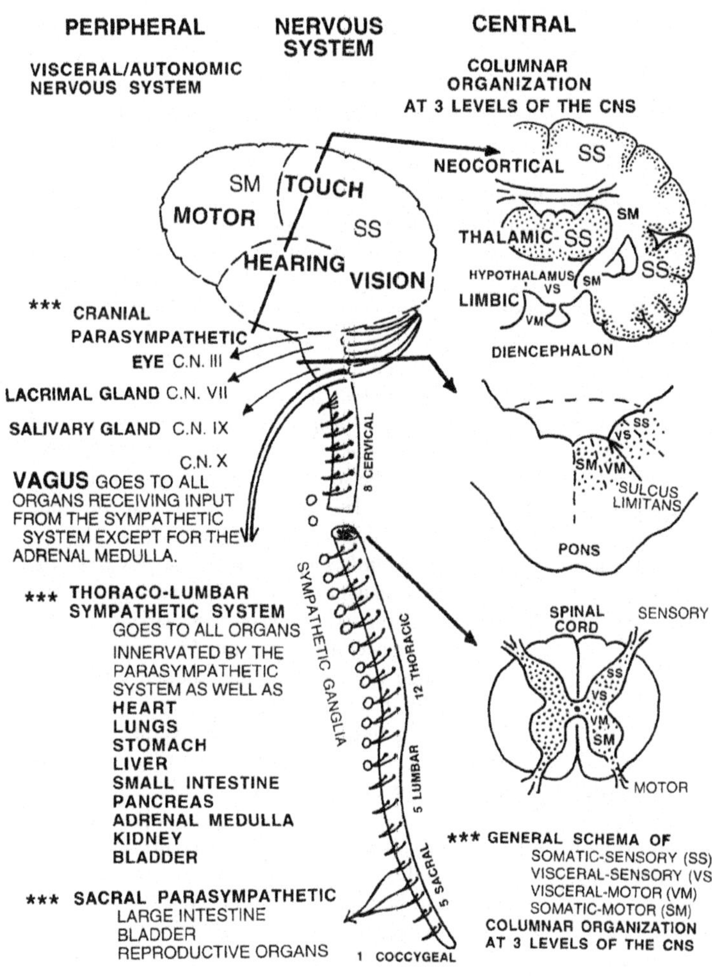

Figure 4.7. *Left:* A general summary of the nerves of the peripheral autonomic nervous system. The hypothalamus is generally considered to be the centrally situated head-ganglion of the autonomic nervous system. *Right:* Sensory and motor organization for somatic and visceral processes along the neuroaxis. The basic plan that is evident in the gray matter of the spinal cord from dorsal to ventral (i.e., somatic sensory [SS], visceral sensory [VS], visceromotor [VM], and somatomotor [SM]) is evident at all levels of the neuroaxis, with a section through the back of the diencephalon, the pons, and the spinal cord portrayed.

tral regions of the brain as compared with the lateral location of systems that control the exteroceptive senses and skeletomuscular body (soma).

Because new circuits have evolved by building on the outside of existing systems, a medial position indicates that visceroemotional processes are generally more ancient in brain evolution than somatic processes; as mentioned earlier, the latter are more closely related to cognitive representations of the external world. Although many thinkers dislike the distinction between affective and cognitive processes, this dichotomy is evident in brain organization. In general, the stream of cognitive activity emerges from the external senses, whence information is conveyed to and processed in the thalamus before being distributed to and reintegrated in the cortex. By contrast, emotional activity is intimately linked to visceral processes first elaborated in medial reticular networks of the lower brain stem, the regions found below the midbrain level, and also in the hypothalamus on the ventral part of the upper brain stem. Emerging from these locations, emotionality is then intermixed with higher levels of integration, including strong interactions with cognitive processes, in the higher reaches of the limbic system.

Let us further explore the distinction between affective and cognitive areas in the primitive organizational structure of the diencephalon (Figure 4.7). A variety of functional distinctions between visceral and somatic parts of the brain are apparent here. Thalamic tissue, on the dorsal portion of the diencephalon, collects information from the outside world. Its properties are quite distinct from those of hypothalamic tissue, located on the ventral diencephalon, which collects visceral information. Neurons in the thalamus fire rapidly, up to several hundred times per second, while hypothalamic cells are very slow by comparison, rarely firing more than a couple of times per second. (*Neuronal firing* and *action potentials*, which are central to the process of information transferral, will be discussed in the next chapter.) A comparable difference is apparent in the distinct metabolic rates of the two tissues. Thalamic circuits consume considerably more blood sugar, the sole and essential fuel for all brain activity, than do visceral hypothalamic circuits (see Figure 4.4).

The visceral zone of the hypothalamic-limbic region and the somatic zone of the thalamocortical system are also highly compartmentalized in terms of function, as indicated by distinct epilepsies that invade the two zones. Limbic epilepsies produce psychomotor fits but rarely cause full-blown convulsions, since their electrical storms tend to be restricted to the visceral parts of the brain. By contrast, grand mal seizures accompanied by full-blown, tonic-clonic convulsions are restricted largely to the somatic brain. It is also noteworthy that visceral parts of the brain have high concentrations of certain neuropeptide systems, while the somatic parts are typically impoverished in these same neurochemicals (see Chapter 6). In addition to these two major zones of the nervous system, there is a third—the *basal ganglia*, which contains the basic plans for many instinctual movements and other basic behavioral processes. Both cognitive and emotional information converges here before coherent behavior can occur. Let us focus more closely on this "triune brain" concept.

An Overview of the Triune Brain

How can one make a functionally meaningful picture from the massive intricacies of the brain? This barrier has long blocked the assimilation of neuroscience facts into our thinking about psychology. The complexity of the brain is so vast that one can easily get mired in details that prevent us from seeing the big picture.

One simplification that points us in the right direction is Paul MacLean's conception of the brain as a triune structure (of the type depicted in Figure 3.1).[16] MacLean divided a vast architecture into three layers of evolutionary development: (1) the ancient reptilian brain, which elaborates the basic motor plans animals exhibit each day, as well as primitive emotions such as seeking, and some aspects of fear, aggression, and sexuality; (2) the more recent old-mammalian brain, or limbic system, which increases the sophistication of basic reptilian emotions such as fear and anger, and most especially elaborates the social emotions; and (3) the most recent addition, the neomammalian brain, consisting largely of the neocortex, which elaborates propositional logic and our cognitive/rational appreciation of the outside world. This three-layered conceptualization helps us grasp the overall functional organization of higher brain areas better than any other scheme yet devised. Of course, exceptions can be found to all generalizations, and it must be kept in mind that the brain is a massively interconnected organ whose every part can find an access pathway to any other part. Even though many specialists have criticized the overall accuracy of the image of a "triune brain," the conceptualization provides a useful overview of mammalian brain organization above the lower brain stem.

The Basal Ganglia. The oldest zone, related closely to various midline structures of the brain stem, is the *reptilian brain*. This area deep in the brain appears to organize some fundamental aspects of instinctual motor capabilities in animals, such as postures and large axial movement patterns. MacLean (1990) clearly envisioned how this "reptilian" core of the brain may elaborate obligatory behavioral routines—the types of behavior patterns that reptiles still exhibit prominently in their day-to-day activity cycles. These include essential bodily functions such as elimination, seeking shelter, periods of hunting interspersed with inactivity, basking in the sun, and various social displays including courtship, aggressive challenges, and submissive displays. Reptiles perform the behaviors each day as if following some type of habitual master routine. They stop doing so if the so-called reptilian brain structures are damaged. The deep brain structures that constitute this part of the brain are, as a group, known as the *basal ganglia*, the *striatal complex*, or the *corpus striatum*. (Unfortunately, in neuroanatomy there are occasionally multiple names for essentially the same structures. This makes things especially confusing for novices, and a rite of passage occurs when one suddenly becomes comfortable with the multiple usages.)

The basal ganglia consist of many substructures, including the *caudate nucleus*, *globus pallidus*, *nucleus accumbens*, *entopeduncular nucleus*, *ventral tegmental area*, and *substantia nigra* (Figure 4.8). Occasionally, the *amygdaloid nuclei* are included in this category, even though this last structure is now more commonly considered to be part of the limbic system. The basal ganglia were originally conceptualized to be a slave of the cortical motor system, which transmits information to the body via large pyramidal cells. In reference to this, the striatal complex has sometimes been called the *extrapyramidal motor system*, but the functions of the reptilian brain are surely deeper and more mysterious than this term would suggest. The broader view was poignantly encapsulated by an early neurophilosopher who stated that the "royal road to the soul goes through the corpus striatum." In addition to such daily master routines as described earlier, it seems likely that basal ganglia circuitry elaborates a primitive feeling of motor presence, which may represent a primal source of "willpower." The more highly evolved brain regions must still utilize this system as a final output pathway for behavior. The major connectivities of the basal ganglia will be detailed later in this chapter.

The Limbic System. Surrounding this reptilian core and interdigitating with it at many points is the old-mammalian brain, which primarily elaborates ancient "family values" and other uniquely mammalian emotional tendencies (Figure 4.8). This intermediate layer interacts intimately with the visceral organs. It resembles a fringe around the cerebral hemispheres that mushroom from each side of the upper brain stem.

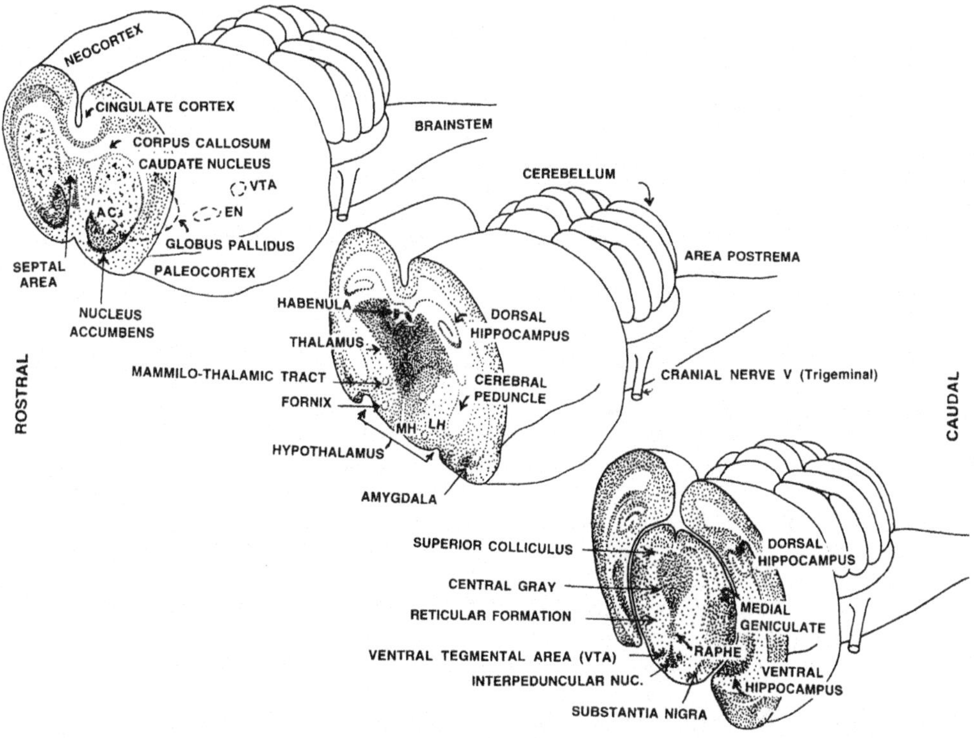

Figure 4.8. Three-dimensional depiction of the rat brain from the anterior lateral perspective. Each of the three frontal (or "coronal") sections depicts major subcortical structures of the reptilian brain and limbic system. The stippling on each section is indicative of the density of opiate receptors at these levels of the brain (for a full depiction of opiate receptors in the rat brain, see Figure 6.8).

Because of the backward rotation of the cerebral hemispheres within the cranium, this medial limbic region is endowed with several arching pathways, most prominently the *fornix* and *stria terminalis*, which, respectively, connect the hippocampus and amygdala to the hypothalamus. This part of the brain was first conceptualized as the *rhinencephalon*, or "nose brain," because of its intimate connections with the *olfactory bulbs*. Although olfactory influences still permeate this system, it has become clear that many specific emotional and motivational impulses are also intrinsically elaborated by neural systems that course through the limbic region. The utilization of olfactory functions to generate new behavioral systems may be an example of evolution elaborating upon old parts. For instance, animals seek out food with the exquisitely sensitive chemodetectors of their nose, and it seems that exploratory and appetitive motivational tendencies (which allow animals to anticipate positive events in the world) emerge from neural systems that encourage the use of the olfactory system.

The concept of the "rhinencephalon" was later supplanted by MacLean's concept of the "limbic system," a designation that has now become virtually synonymous with the concept of the "emotional brain." This concept has served as a useful generalization, although some anatomists find it vague in terms of its boundaries.[17] The major areas included in the limbic system are the *amygdala, hippocampus, septal area, preoptic area, hypothalamus*, and *central gray of the mesencephalon* (Figure 4.8). These zones of the brain are essential in elaborating a variety of emotional processes that characterize all mammalian species. In addition to providing modulatory control over behaviors elaborated by the reptilian brain, the limbic system helps generate the basic emotions that mediate various pro-social behaviors, including maternal nurturance, associated caressive behaviors, separation distress vocalizations, playfulness, and various other forms of competition and gregariousness. During the past two decades, we have come close to understanding the neuronal infrastructure that generates each of these specific emotional abilities, and each will be the focus of a subsequent chapter.

The Neomammalian Brain. Surrounding the ancient limbic system is the six-cell-layered neocortex, the crowning glory of brain evolution, which varies in amount and complexity among mammalian species. Please note that there are also more ancient limbic cortical areas, such as the archicortex and paleocortex, which have fewer cell layers.[18] By comparison, avian cortex, because of its lack of cell layering (as in ancient mammals) is not as visually self-evident. Avian higher cortical structures are diffusely organized anatomically (with no clear columnar formation), and their sensory projection areas, including key integrative areas such as the hippocampus, are more rostral in the brain due to a lack of backward rotation of the telencephalic hemispheres. On the other hand, the subcortical areas remain quite similarly laid out in birds and mammals: The cortex in both species is specialized for associating a diversity of sensations and innate ideas (such as a sense of causality and spatial referencing abilities) into perception, concepts, and attributions (Figure 4.8). It harvests information from the senses through specific thalamic relays and processes incoming information into neural representations of the world. This is the brain tissue we must study most thoroughly in our attempt to scientifically understand the rational mind and its ability to generate ideas.

All neocortical areas, at least in the majority of mammals that have a six-cell-layered neocortex, share a similar wiring plan based on cylindrical columns. Each area of the cortex is specialized to preferentially process certain types of information, and each cell layer within a column has precise interactions with other brain areas (Figure 4.9). Although much of the human cortex is multimodal, in that it gets information from many senses, it can only interrelate the types of information which its interconnectivities permit. Although the possibilities for new learning and new concept formation within the human cortex are vast, especially during youth, when cortical connections are more plastic (see Appendix B), they are not limitless. There *are* things our brains cannot imagine, and hence we have only a vague glimmer of what they may be.[19]

Intrinsic qualities of the human cortex give us greater powers of imagination than are available for other species. For instance, it is a highly sophisticated human concept to realize that other people have independent minds. Indeed, much of the subtlety of human behavior arises because we recognize that others are observing and appreciating the intent of our behaviors. In other words, humans have a "theory of mind"—an intrinsic tendency to try to read the minds of significant others around them.[20] There is some evidence that chimpanzees conduct some of their social affairs in similar ways,[21] but there is no extensive evidence of such abilities in other creatures. Presumably, an evolutionary prerequisite of such "mind-reading" tendencies in humans was the ability of ancestral animals to decode behavioral intentions; indeed, most mammals seem to have the rudiments of such abilities—especially in the emotional realm. It has been experimentally demonstrated that monkeys can decode the specific emotional vocalizations of other animals. For instance, vervet monkeys emit one of three distinct alarm calls for three types of predators—snakes, hawks, and cats. Other monkeys respond appropriately to taped recordings of these calls by scanning the ground, scanning the sky, and heading for the trees, respectively.[22] Even domestic chickens are able to decode the meaning of different types of alarm calls. They assume an erect position and scan the ground in response to "ground alarm calls," but they squat and hide, in apparent fear, to "aerial alarm calls," which are presumably differential warnings against the presence of predators such as snakes and raptors.[23] These abilities probably emerge from the highest, analytical reaches of their brains. Thus, even though there is very little evidence that the neocortex elaborates affective feelings, this tissue surely elaborates the appraisal processes that can trigger emotional responses.[24]

Although the highest brain areas will receive only modest attention in this book, it is again worth noting that the evolution of many neocortical functions may have been constrained by the emerging cognitive needs of preexisting limbic-emotional operating systems. In other words, as simple emotional responses were no longer adaptive in the competition for resources, the cortex assumed a critical role in evaluating and generating new behavioral plans to help sustain emotional and motivational stability, or homeostasis. Unfortunately, we really cannot analyze the historical paths of brain evolution.[25] Still, it seems likely that, in a deep evolutionary sense, many of the complex information-processing potentials of the cortex are servants (often unconscious, automatized servants) to the dictates of the affective forces that ruled behavior prior to cortical evolution. Consciousness seems to act only upon very well processed perceptual information as opposed to the many computations that go into the construction of percepts. Still, the neocortex provides an ever-increasing flexibility for the simpleminded dictates of the more primitive emotional and motivational systems (i.e., it tends to "open" the relatively "closed" subcortical systems to more subtle forms of environmental modulation).

The General Road Maps of the Triune Brain: Major Pathways

Starting from the cortex and working down through the limbic system to the basal ganglia and key components of the brain stem, I will trace the major paths of neural communication within the brain. My discussion of neuroanatomy will end at the midbrain (mesencephalic) level, because this is approximately where the circuits for behavioral spontaneity end. We know this because when the midbrain is disconnected from the lower brain stem, animals lose all ability to take care of their basic needs. They survive only in a vegetative state without the spontaneity and flexibility of behavior that are the hallmark of intact animals (see Chapter 3). In other words, they are no longer "active agents" in their environments.

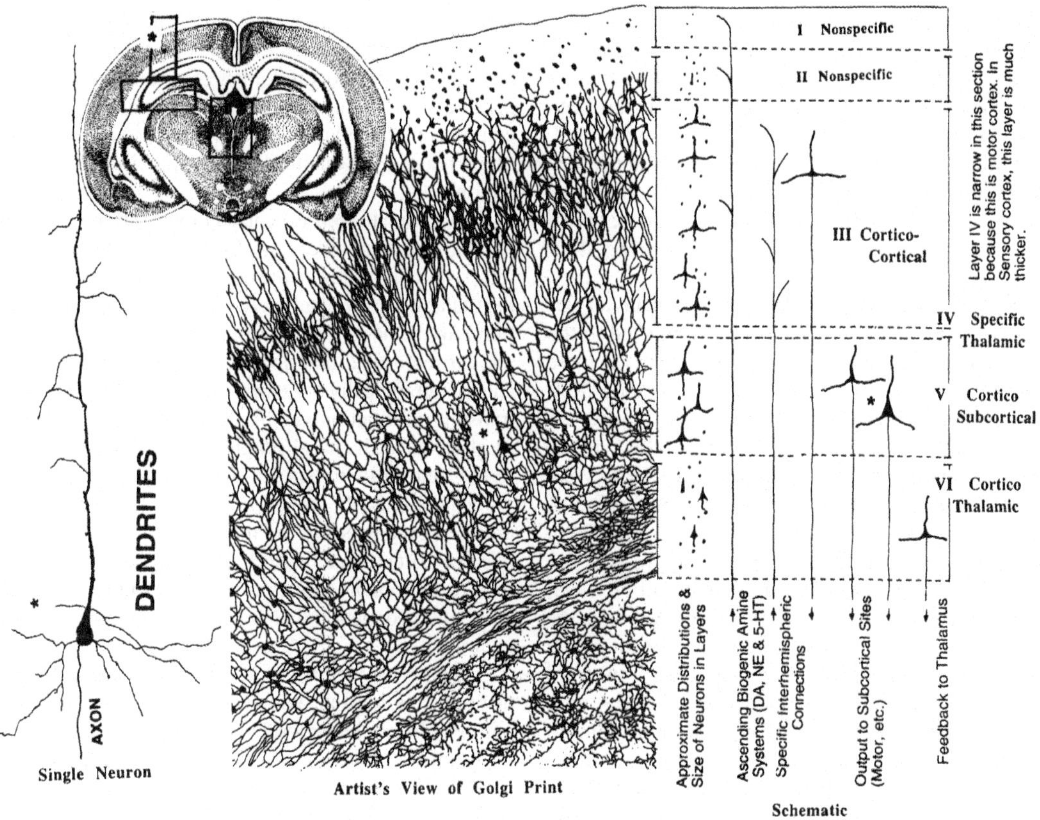

Figure 4.9. *Left:* General plan of cortical organization, with a single Golgi-stained neuron on the left. Can you find that neuron in the full cross section of cortex in the middle? It is indicated by an asterisk, and the location of that whole cortical section is depicted on the asterisk-highlighted coronal section of the brain. The other squares indicate approximate locations for the Fos immunocytographs depicted in Figure 15.7. *Right:* Summary of the six layers of cortex and their various connections to other brain areas. The nonspecific influences from biogenic amine systems such as those depicted in Figures 6.5 and 6.6 are concentrated in the topmost layers of the cortex. Layer III connects similar locations in the two hemispheres. Since layer IV is small in this section, it must be motor cortex. If this layer were large, it would be sensory cortex, getting input from the thalamus. Layers V and VI send information downward in the brain. About a thousand cortical neurons working together as a functional unit are called a *column*, which is hard to see in this view of the brain.

Behavioral spontaneity is possible only when the midbrain and hypothalamus are intact and remain connected to the lower brain stem. However, the behavior of such animals, in which more rostral tissue has been removed, is still quite disorganized and fragmented. Even though they do initiate spontaneous actions, they exhibit little behavioral flexibility and coherence. For instance, animals in this state will become more active when they are hungry, but they will not direct their activity effectively.

Organized and sequenced instinctual behavior occurs only when the basal ganglia are connected to the hypothalamus and brain stem. In other words, the mere removal of the neocortex does not lead to major deficits in instinctual behaviors, although such animals are certainly not very bright.[26] Experiments of this type, as well as localized brain-stimulation studies that evoke specific emotional behaviors, suggest that a series of emotional circuits exist within the limbic system. There are operating systems for exploration, aggressive defense, fear, and various social initiatives, all of which can be demonstrated at the midbrain level. Although the lower brain stem and spinal cord contain most of the sensory and motor nuclei that actually control outward behavior and accompanying autonomic changes, only the rudiments of behavioral spontaneity are found in these lower reaches. I will discuss some of these structures in subsequent chapters in conjunction with the individual emotional systems. Here I will focus only on the major circuits of the higher brain, which are the basic psychoneurological operating systems for behavioral spontaneity.

The Thalamic-Neocortical Axis

As mentioned earlier, the enlargement of the neocortex in recent brain evolution has resulted in expanding openness in circuits that were formerly closed, creating greater behavioral flexibility. The most obvious way to increase flexibility was by expanding the overall size of the cortex and the number of interconnections among its various subareas.[27] It should be noted that the number of neurons in the human neocortex is about 10 billion (10^{10}), and the number of synapses varies between 1,000 and 10,000 per nerve cell, yielding an estimated 10^{13} synaptic connections! This degree of complexity makes it improbable that we will ever understand all brain functions at the resolution of a single cell. We will have to create understanding out of larger segments of the brain. Indeed, as already mentioned, the modular unit of the neocortex is a *column*, a vertically oriented functional grouping of about 4,000 interconnected neurons with comparatively weak connections to immediately neighboring modules. These columns are strongly linked to other cortical modules and to lower brain areas by descending and looping connections. Coherently operating groups of neurons are called functional "networks" or "cell assemblies." An especially important point to remember is that even though the human brain has much more neocortex than other animals of comparable size, this is achieved by the addition of more columnar modules and their interconnections rather than by increasing the quality (i.e., complexity) of cortical columns.

In addition to well-organized inputs (afferents) from the thalamus and other cortical areas, the major inputs (efferents) of the cortex are descending circuits back to the thalamus, as well as massive dispersion of information into the basal ganglia (Figure 4.10). The output of the entire cortical mantle to the striatum is enormous and topographically organized, and most of its synapses transmit information via the simple amino acid known as glutamate. The basal ganglia send information back to the ventral thalamus via the output circuits of the globus pallidus, the *ansa lenticularis*. These messages are then processed by the thalamus and flow upward into the cortex once more. In this way, the "stream of thought" probably comes to be connected with basic daily plans for action that are encoded within the basal ganglia.

Cognitive information presumably has to percolate through this loop an undetermined number of times before coherent behavioral plans emerge. If the loop is experimentally broken, as can be done by placing neurotoxins into the caudate nucleus, animals' behavioral flexibility is compromised in ways that are just beginning to be documented. Indeed, in the human brain disorder known as *Huntington's disease*, this type of damage occurs for genetic reasons that have recently been identified.[28] In the brains of such individuals, excessive levels of endogenous glutamate may gradually destroy the basal ganglia. Although these patients eventually exhibit severe motor disabilities, their mental status is initially compromised by a schizoid type of disorder characterized by disjointed cognitive activity.[29] For instance, a person may remember all the steps in a favorite recipe but not be able to sequence them into a final product. Apparently, the flow of information through striatal-thalamic-cortical loops helps solidify behavior sequences based on various component parts. The cortex contains the component parts, but the striatum welds them into a coherent plan.

It is generally believed that complex factual memories (often termed *declarative* or *semantic memories*) are stored in the interconnections of the cortex, but many simple memories, such as motor habits, are controlled by subcortical circuits. For example, the basic motor memory for the classically conditioned eye-blink reflex (e.g., the anticipatory blinking caused by a tone that has been paired with a puff of air directed at an eye) resides within an ancient part of the cerebellum,[30] a structure that was traditionally thought to simply facilitate motor coordination but is now known to participate in many other processes, including emotional ones.[31] Even in the case of such basic learning, higher brain

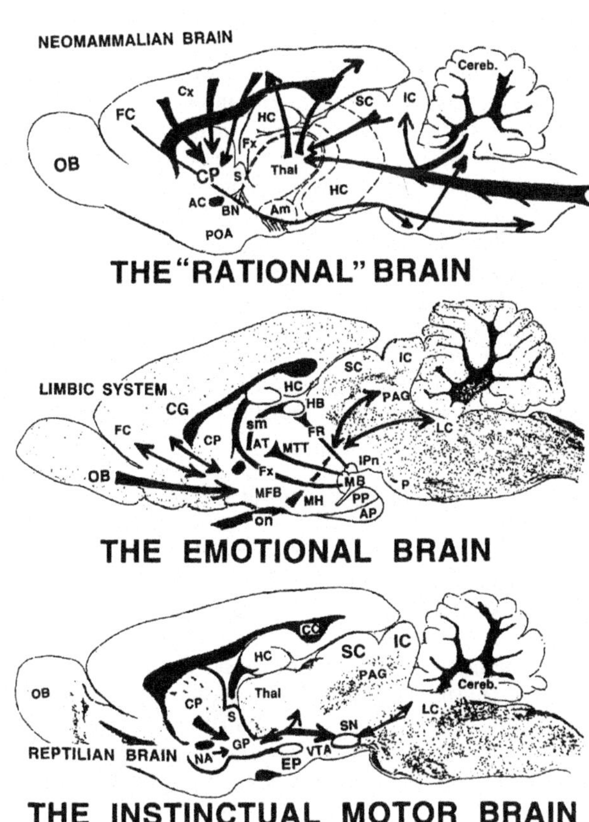

Figure 4.10. Major pathways of neomammalian, paleomammalian, and reptilian brain areas on mid-saggital views of the rat brain. Note that the neomammalian brain, or cortex (*top*), receives sensory input from the thalamus and sends most of its output to the basal ganglia (i.e., the caudate nucleus). On the bottom is the reptilian brain, which funnels its information to thalamus and lower brain stem motor nuclei. The limbic system (*middle*) has a series of complex arching pathways that integrate information from a variety of internal systems to coordinate emotional and motivated behaviors. AC: anterior commissure; AM: amygdala; AP: anterior pituitary; AT: anterior thalamus; BN: bed nucleus of the stria terminalis; CC: corpus callosum; CG: cingulate cortex; CN: caudate nucleus; CP: cerebral peduncle; FC: frontal cortex; FR: fasciculus retroflexus; FX: fornix; GP: globus pallidus; HB: habenula; HC: hippocampus; IC: inferior colliculus; IPN: interpeduncular nucleus; LC: locus coeruleus; LH: lateral hypothalamus; MB: mamillary body; MFB: medial forebrain bundle; MH: medial hypothalamus; ML: medial lemniscus; MTT: mamillothalamic tract; NA: nucleus accumbens; ON: optic nerve; PAG: periaqueductal gray; PB: parabrachial area; POA: preoptic area; PP: posterior pituitary; S: septum; SC: superior colliculus; SM: stria medullaris; SN: substantia nigra; Thal: thalamus; VTA: ventral tegmental area.

areas elaborate and reproduce one's cognitive knowledge of the conditioning. For instance, simple eye-blink conditioning is well represented within the hippocampus. However, this representation is not needed for the expression of "simple conditioning," where the unconditional stimulus (UCS) follows immediately on the heels of the conditional stimulus (CS). It is called upon only if there is a long interval between the CS and UCS. If one uses "trace" conditioning, where there is an interval between the CS and the UCS, the hippocampus becomes essential.[32] In discussing these brain functions, it is important to remember that several areas often participate in a single process. Indeed, the creation of redundancies, with multiple representation of processes through "distributed parallel processing," is the rule rather than the exception within the brain,[33] and even subtle and unstudied brain processes such as "the self" and the various emotions discussed in this book may become widely distributed in the brain (see Chapter 16).

Cortical control of primitive behaviors and basic emotions has been achieved in several ways. One way was for the cortex to extend emotions in time by allowing organisms to dwell on past and future events. Another pervasive solution was for the cortex to inhibit the actions of primitive instinctual systems situated in subcortical areas. For instance, all humans have circuits within their brains that can instigate intense rage, but it is rare for such impulses to control our outward behavior. However, if certain areas of the cortex are destroyed, these potentials are more likely to emerge as actions.[34] The cortex not only helps keep simpleminded impulses under control but presumably permits selective and refined expression of primitive tendencies. This makes our brains resemble old museums that contain many of the archetypal markings of our evolutionary past, but we are able to keep much of that suppressed by our cortical lid. Our brains are full of ancestral memories and processes that guide our actions and dreams but rarely emerge unadulterated by corticocultural influences during our everyday activities.

Connections of the Limbic System

Within the broad continuum of the limbic system, which includes hypothalamic and mesencephalic areas, there is a series of neurochemically coded pathways for the control of emotional and motivated behaviors. These pathways can be visualized only through the use of the immunocytochemical techniques summarized in Chapter 6. However, there are also larger, more visually distinct pathways that were discovered prior to the use of advanced mapping technologies. Such pathways give the limbic system its essential form, for they can be visualized with the naked eye (Figure 4.10). They include the *fornix*, the *stria terminalis*, the *ventral amygdalofugal pathway*, the *mamillothalamic tract*, the *habenulopeduncular tract*, and the *medial forebrain bundle*. These are the prominent landmarks that set off a vast amount of reticular substance where most information transactions transpire (Figure 4.10). They allow us to outline the overall geography of the limbic system.

These pathways include two major outputs of the amygdala. The arching stria terminalis, which was molded by the backward rotation of the developing cerebral hemispheres, sends descending information to a broad synaptic field extending from the *bed nucleus of the stria terminalis* to the *ventromedial nucleus of the hypothalamus*. The more direct *ventral amygdalofugal pathway* is located at the axis of telencephalic rotation and hence was not displaced by the backward expansion of the cortex. It provides direct input to the basal forebrain and anterior hypothalamus. In addition, a great number of pathways run through the corridor of the lateral hypothalamus, the best known of which is the *medial forebrain bundle* (MFB). This is the area where self-stimulation and a variety of stimulus-bound emotive behaviors can be obtained with greatest ease through localized electrical stimulation of the brain (ESB). Just medial to the MFB are many nuclear groups that process regulatory information about the body's metabolic and hormonal imbalances that may require the organism to interact with the outside world. This is achieved by interactions between various incoming sensory systems, including the external ones of smell and taste, intermixing locally gathered information about the body's metabolic and hormonal states (via interoreceptors) to yield generalized instinctual behaviors that are controlled by SEEKING circuits coursing through the adjacent lateral hypothalamic areas (see Figure 3.6 and Chapter 8 for details).

As mentioned previously, there are a great number of distinct neurochemically coded pathways, both ascending and descending, that project through the hypothalamus. These circuits ramify widely in the brain and provide the best opportunity we have at present to link specific types of psychoemotional processes to specific brain mechanisms. These emotional command systems resemble trees, with branches reaching into the higher brain areas to interact with perceptual and cognitive processes. The trunks reflect the ancient executive cores of each system, which are influenced by various bodily and simple perceptual states, and the roots lie in basal ganglia and brain stem areas, providing connections to various motor processes. Indeed, these discrete neurochemical pathways help generate and synchronize cognitive, physiological, behavioral, and feeling states within widely distributed areas of the nervous system. By viewing basic emotional systems in this way, we can appreciate why *categorical*, *componential*, and *social-constructivist* perspectives on the study of emotions need not compete but instead can work together. My preferred approach, the categorical one, can best characterize "trunk-line" issues concerning the organization of emotionality in the brain; the componential approach can identify how various fragments of experience are incorporated into emotional states; and the social-constructivist approach can describe how these systems contribute to cultural evolution and the cognitive interpretation of our great varieties of real-life experiences.

Connections of the Basal Ganglia

I have already discussed the cortical connections that feed into the basal ganglia. This massive flow of cortical information into the "reptilian brain" is repeatedly recirculated back to the cortex through the thalamus. The overall functions of the basal ganglia are under the control of one major "power switch"—ascending brain dopamine, which arises from cell groups in the ventromedial part of the midbrain. When dopamine is available, the basal ganglia conduct their functions efficiently. When dopamine activity is excessive—for instance, following administration of psychomotor stimulants such as amphetamine or cocaine, or under the pathological clinical condition of paranoid schizophrenia—then repetitive behavior patterns, persistent thoughts, and delusions begin to emerge. When dopamine is unavailable, as in Parkinson's disease or following excessive doses of antipsychotic drugs, all behavior is diminished, and displeasure sets in, along with a lack of energy. As dopamine systems ascend into the striatum, they divide into two distinct branches—the *nigrostriatal system*, which ascends from the *substantia nigra* to the *dorsal striatum* (also called the caudate-putamen complex), and the *mesolimbic/mesocortical pathways*, which ascend from the ventral tegmental area (VTA) to the *ventral striatum* (also called the nucleus accumbens) as well as to the frontal cortex (see Figures 3.6 and 8.1). Indeed, there are reciprocal descending connections between both the dorsal and ventral striatum and the respective mesencephalic cell groups. These reciprocating loops help protect the system from excessive arousal when it is perturbed by an overabundance of incoming stimulation. Each of the mesencephalic dopamine cell groups receives a diversity of inputs that probably convey information about general bodily states such as hunger, thermal imbalances, and other forms of stress.

Although the dorsal striatum receives many inputs from other brain areas, including amygdaloid nuclei and intralaminar thalamic nuclei, the most massive influence, as mentioned earlier, comes from the neocortex (Figure 4.10). Nonetheless, it should be remembered that this input is not obligatory for normal striatal function, since the overall motor bearing of simple mammals, such as rats, is not grossly disturbed by neocortical lesions: Decorticate animals continue to exhibit their instinctive behavior patterns. It is noteworthy that this is not the case for humans, except very young ones who have not become dependent on higher processes. Comparable neocortical damage in humans has severe motor effects, namely paralysis, suggesting that adult human brain functions are more dependent on neocortical functions than the brains of lower mammals.

The major pattern of connections of the ventral striatum (Figure 4.10) is similar to that of the dorsal striatum except for the fact that higher inputs arise from the limbic/visceral cortices, including *frontal*, *cingulate*, and *olfactory cortices* and *periamygdaloid areas*, rather than those of the somatic neocortex (Figure 4.10). This motor outflow is also similar, except that it is focused on the *ventral tegmental area* rather than the adjacent *substantia nigra*, which receives greater input from the dorsal striatum. It is generally thought that the ventral striatal system is one of the major avenues through which affective processes are blended with basic motor tendencies. A more detailed discussion of such issues will be undertaken in Chapter 8.

The Mesencephalon and Lower Brain Stem: Executive Systems for Behavioral Output

Within the midbrain, we find the lowest level of integration for most of the emotional operating systems that we will discuss. Most emotional command systems make strong connections with midline visceral structures—the central gray around the cerebral aqueduct (also called the *periaqueductal gray*) and surrounding reticular tissues. It is within these zones that we find the lowest integrative centers for the coherent emission of rage and defensive behaviors (see Chapter 10), for fear (see Chapter 11), for separation distress (see Chapter 14), for exploratory urges (see Chapter 9), for sexual urges (see Chapter 12), and for the experiences of pleasure and pain. These lowermost structures of the emotional "trees" are absolutely essential for spontaneous engagement with the world. When they are even moderately damaged, animals become behaviorally sluggish, and with extensive damage, a comatose state is common. Ascending systems at this level of the neuroaxis include basic circuits for maintenance of vigilance and sleep states (see Chapter 7). As we proceed laterally from these central structures, we are confronted by the somatic nervous system—with ascending sensory processes and descending motor processes. Although damage to these areas can impair certain skills, it does not typically compromise an animal's tendency to be a spontaneously active creature. As discussed in Chapter 16, it is probably within these central mesencephalic reaches of the brain stem that we will eventually find the primal neural representations of "the self."

Two areas of the brain are especially interesting in any attempt to discuss subtle concepts such as the primordial "self." At the very roof (or tectum) of the brain stem, we find two sets of moundlike, twin structures called the *corpora quadrigemina*—the more caudal (tailward) twins being the *inferior colliculi*, which process auditory information, and the more rostral (headward) twins being the *superior colliculi*. The latter are primarily engaged in processing visual information, although their deeper layers also contain maps for auditory and somatosensory space and certain motor control functions, especially the spontaneous eye movements needed for rapid orientation during pursuit. The mesencephalic *central gray* is situated just below the colliculi; as mentioned, this tissue contains basic neural components for many emotional processes, including fear, anger, sexuality, pleasure, and pain. The superior colliculus is especially interesting because it is here that we begin to get a glimmer of the first evolutionary appearance of a sophisticated representation of self. This might be expected simply from the fact that this part of the brain contains multimodal sensory systems designed to elaborate simple orientation responses. In other words, these systems may provide a sense of presence for the animal within its world. How this is achieved is an especially intriguing story that will be continued in the last chapter of this book.

In sum, to appreciate brain functions, one cannot avoid the intricacies of neuroanatomy. To provide an overall picture of the key brain areas that will be of concern throughout this text, I have constructed a simple stereotaxic atlas of the rat brain depicted in the three major planes of Euclidian space (Figure 4.11). For a similar depiction of opiate receptors in the brain, see Figure 6.8. Of course, for the mind to be woven on the living loom of the brain, there also has to be the dimension of time. Mind consists of the dynamic temporal flow of information through the networks provided by the anatomical connectivities of the brain. However, we must remember that there are also other channels of information flow, including paracrine ones for the diffusion of neurochemistries, some of which act nonsynaptically, and perhaps still others that we do not yet fully appreciate.

The Hierarchical Organization of the Brain

The brain is a hierarchical system (see Figure 2.2). Higher functions can operate only on the basis of lower

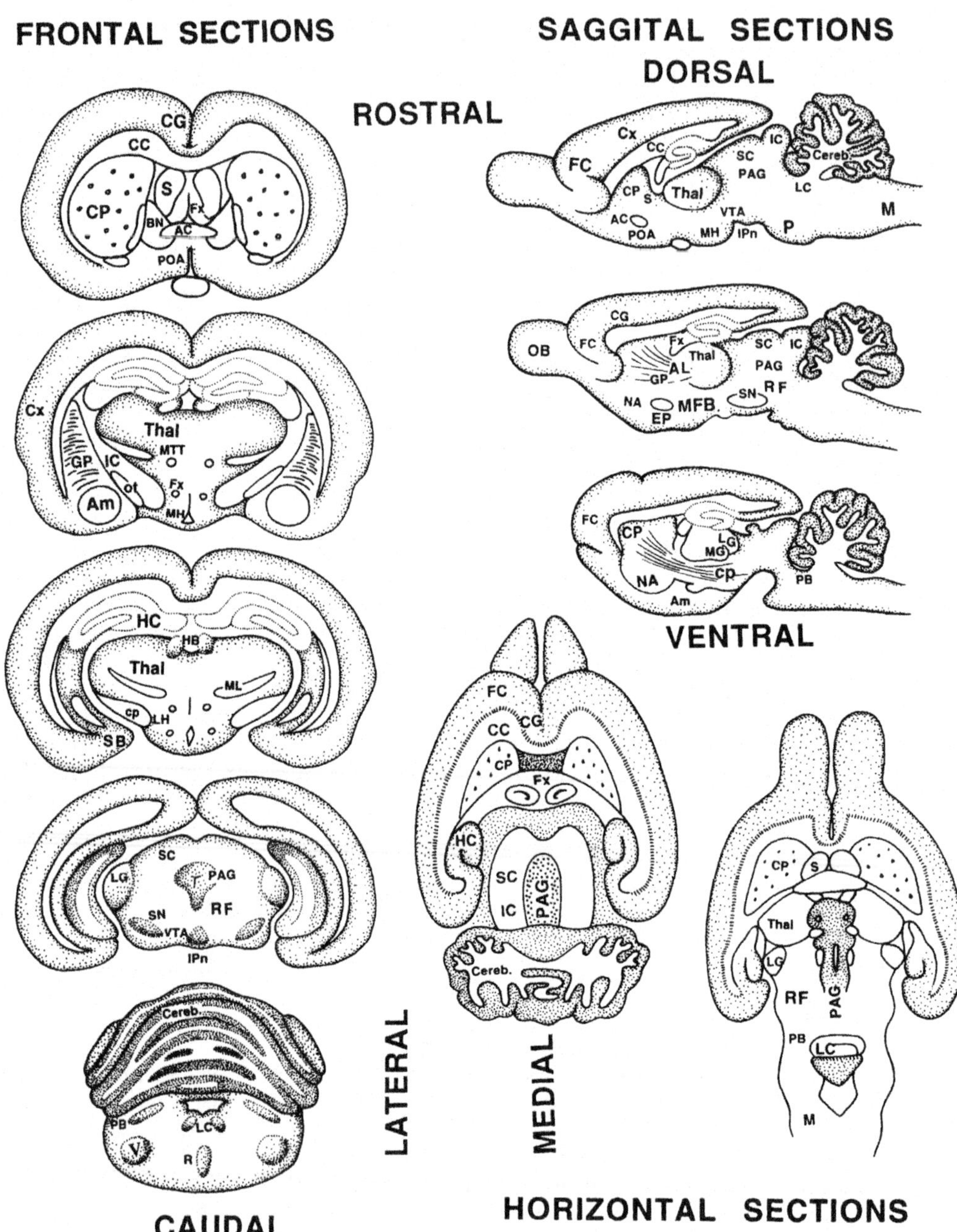

Figure 4.11. Stereotaxic atlas of the rat brain in three coordinates. These are actual tracings from photographed brain sections. Anatomical designations are: AC: Anterior Commissure; AL: Ansa Lenticularis; Am: Amygdala; BN: Bed Nucleus of the Stria Terminalis; CC: Corpus Callosum; Cereb: Cerebellum; CG: Cingulate Cortex; CP: Caudate-Putamen; cp: Cerebral Peduncle; Cx: Cortex; EP: Entopeduncular Nucleus; FC: Frontal Cortex; Fx: Fornix; GP: Globus Pallidus; HB: Habenula; HC: Hippocampus; IC: Inferior Colliculus; ic: internal capsule; IPn: Interpeduncular Nucleus; LG: Lateral Geniculate; LH: Lateral Hypothalamus; LC: Locus Coeruleus; M: Medulla; MFB: Medial Forebrain Bundle; MG: Medial Geniculate; MH: Medial Hypothalamus; ML: Medial Lemniscus; MTT: Mammilothalamic tract; NA: Nucleus Accumbens; OB: Olfactory Bulb; ot: optic tract; P: Pons; PAG: Periaqueductal Gray; PB: Parabrachial Area; POA: Preoptic Area; R: Raphe; RF: Reticular Formation; S: Septum; SB: Subiculum; SN: Substantia Nigra; SC: Superior Colliculus; Thal: Thalamus; V: Motor nucleus of cranial nerve five; VTA: Ventral Tegmental Area.

functions; but quite often lower functions can operate independently of higher ones. Since the lower functions are essential, it is understandable why brain stem damage is generally more debilitating than cortical damage. Higher functions are typically more *open*, while lower ones are more reflexive, stereotyped, and *closed*. For instance, the basic vital functions of the brain—those that regulate organic bodily functions such as respiration—are organized at very low levels. Higher levels provide increasingly flexible control over these lower functions. For instance, the higher brain stem (especially the hypothalamus) and the nearby structures of the basal ganglia allow animals to generate behavioral spontaneity and the various complex behaviors that help adjust activity in relation to bodily needs. The highest cortical levels, which surround these ancient structures, allow complex patterns of incoming information to be stored and imbued with affective and other types of meaning. To use our computer analogy from Chapter 1, the lower functions resemble read-only memory (ROM) "operating systems," which are essential for computers to do anything coherent, while the higher functions resemble random-access memory (RAM) space where increasingly complex computations can be done. As more RAM space becomes available, the same operating systems can accomplish more and more. The relative abundance of RAM-like space in humans helps explain the complexity and sophistication of human abilities. However, if we wish to understand the fundamental sources of our human emotions and motivations, we will have to focus our efforts primarily on the subcortical operating systems that we share with other animals.

AFTERTHOUGHT: Three Historical Milestones in Our Neuroanatomical Understanding of Emotion

The token chapter on emotions in most neuroscience texts typically summarizes a few classic findings. Here, I present thumbnail sketches of three such discoveries in the area of neuroanatomy. In Chapter 5, I will similarly describe key work from the neurophysiological perspective, and in Chapter 6 from the neurochemical perspective. This will provide a succinct summary of some of the most widely acknowledged neuroscience contributions to our understanding of emotions during this century.

1. The first "breakthrough" was the recognition that the basic urges for emotionality are situated in deep subcortical areas of the brain. Surgical removal of the cerebral hemispheres (i.e., decerebration) as well as certain cortical regions makes animals temperamental, with prominent bouts of rage in reaction to minor irritations.[35] Since such animals do not always direct their temperamental energies correctly (to appropriate targets), their emotional displays were often deemed to be "pseudoaffective." This usage reflected the opinion that the animals didn't actually experience internal affective states corresponding to the observed emotional behaviors. This position was not justified. The lack of directedness may have simply indicated that the animals were disoriented. More recent work, as summarized in Chapters 8 to 15, suggests that affective experiences do emerge from the arousal of the subcortical circuits that are released by decerebration. The subcortical localization of the basic brain systems for such emotional outbursts eventually led to the concept of a limbic system, which still guides most of the neuroanatomical work on emotionality.

2. The second set of key findings was that removal of several discrete brain areas, including the temporal lobes, the frontal lobes, the septal area, and the ventromedial hypothalamus, dramatically modified emotionality in animals and humans in characteristic ways. Temporal lobectomy made animals hypersexual, hyperoral, and less fearful—the so-called Klüver-Bucy syndrome, which is also evident in humans.[36] This is largely due to destruction of the underlying amygdaloid complex. While frontal lobe lesions made animals more placid, they also exhibited strong tendencies for simpleminded emotional outbursts when thwarted. Humans with such brain damage seem to live intensely in the present, without much thought about the past or future. They tend not to plan ahead. Septal lesions produced hyperemotional and hyperaggressive animals, as did ventromedial hypothalamic lesions. Animals subjected to the latter remained persistently savage, while the rage of septal animals diminished markedly as a function of time since brain damage.[37] Indeed, septal-lesioned animals often become friendlier than normal.[38] These emotional changes are so replicable from experiment to experiment that they affirm the existence of stable subcortical brain substrates for the generation of emotionality.

3. From the present vantage, the most important historical contribution is a set of studies, using electrical stimulation of subcortical areas of the brain in cats, that were conducted by Walter Hess in Zurich, Switzerland, during the second quarter of this century.[39] These studies indicated that one can obtain a variety of emotional behavior patterns by electrically stimulating specific parts of the brain, especially the hypothalamic zones of the diencephalon and the central zones of the midbrain. The coordinated emotional behaviors that were activated suggested the animals were experiencing emotional states. Animals could be induced to act angry, fearful, curious, or hungry, as well as nauseous, by stimulation of this "head-ganglion of the autonomic nervous system," as Hess called it. This eventually led to the recognition that animals craved stimulation of certain brain sites: They would self-stimulate circuits such as the MFB, which courses through the lateral diencephalon. In contrast, they despised stimulation of other nearby sites, including anterior and ventrolateral

hypothalamic sites, as well as many zones of the mesencephalic perventricular gray.[40] This suggested that "pleasure approach" and "distress avoidance" were elaborated by specific brain circuits. Presently a few investigators are working out the anatomical and neurochemical details of these circuits, and this work now provides the deepest insights into the intrinsic emotional nature of the mammalian brain. For initiating this seminal work, Walter Hess was awarded the Nobel Prize in 1949 "for his discovery of the functional organization of the interbrain as a coordinator of the activities of the internal organs." Hess's work continues to inspire lines of investigation that are bringing us ever closer to a lasting material understanding of emotionality in both humans and animals.

Suggested Readings

Braitenberg, V., & Schulz, A. (1991). *Anatomy of the cortex.* New York: Springer-Verlag.

Brodal, A. (1981). *Neurological anatomy in relation to clinical medicine* (3d ed.). New York: Oxford Univ. Press.

Crosby, E. C., Humphrey, T., & Lauer, E. W. (1962). *Correlative anatomy of the nervous system.* New York: Macmillan.

Curtis, B. A., Jacobson, S. J., & Marcus, E. M. (eds.) (1972). *An introduction to the neurosciences.* Philadelphia: Saunders.

Haymaker, W., Anderson, E., & Nauta, W. J. H. (1969). *The hypothalamus.* Springfield, Ill.: Thomas.

Luria, A. R. (1966). *Higher cortical functions in man.* New York: Basic Books.

Morgane, P. J., & Panksepp, J. (eds.) (1980). *Handbook of the hypothalamus.* Vol. 1, *Anatomy of the hypothalamus.* New York: Marcel Dekker.

Nauta, W. J. H., & Feirtag, M. (1988). *Fundamental neuroanatomy.* New York: Freeman.

Nieuwenhuys, R., Voogd, J., & van Huijzen, C. (1988). *The human central nervous system* (3d ed.). Berlin: Springer-Verlag.

Shepherd, G. M. (1983). *Neurobiology.* New York: Oxford Univ. Press.

5

Neurodynamics

The Electrical Languages of the Brain

The brain is waking and with it the mind is returning. It is as if the Milky Way entered upon some cosmic dance. Swiftly the head-mass becomes an enchanted loom, where millions of flushing shuttles weave a dissolving pattern, always a meaningful pattern, though never an abiding one: A shifting harmony of sub-patterns.

Sir Charles Sherrington, *Man on His Nature* (1940)

CENTRAL THEME

The view of the brain as an "enchanted loom" is one of the most famous images of the nervous system in operation. To some extent it is an elegantly simple picture: Individual neurons convey information via a universal electrochemical process, speaking to other neurons in chemical dialects. But the simplicity is deceptive. It only provides the beginning of understanding as far as psychology is concerned. The study of the electrical responses of individual neurons has yet to give us a credible picture of the intrinsic neurodynamics of the mind. There is a yet unfathomed internal harmony to brain functions, with many neural systems working together to produce mind. One of the best ways to approach the operations of the brain holistically and in real time is via electroencephalographic (EEG) measures, which can monitor the joint dendritic activities of large ensembles of neurons. A shortcoming of this technique is its inability to reveal the deep functions of the intact human brain. One of the most difficult problems is that the brain has so many endogenous subcortical functions (i.e., ones that were constructed through evolutionary selection rather than within the individual life experiences of an organism), and we cannot readily study such processes in humans using electrical recording procedures. In animals, we can demonstrate the role of specific subcortical circuits in various psychobehavioral processes via various interventions, but the dynamic electrical codes that operate within these circuits are difficult to decipher using objective procedures. There is a massive spontaneity of neuronal activity throughout the brain. It is as if we were confronted by many hieroglyphics, with no Rosetta stone. Although early theorists thought the machinery of the brain was only set into action by external stimuli impinging on the organism, we now know that, in addition to harvesting information from the various senses, the brain also has many internally generated activities that provide information from the ancestral past, thereby creating the innate functions of the mind. This is reflected in the ability of artificial brain stimulation to evoke coherent emotional behavior patterns and associated feeling states.

The Dynamics of the Brain "Computer": From Action Potentials to Behavior

The essence of psychological matters lies hidden within the microscopic neurochemical and neuroelectrical interrelations of many regions of the brain. There is no psychology without action potentials, synaptic potentials, ion channels, and a multitude of neurotransmitters and neuromodulators. The complex interactions of all of these neurophysical processes intertwine dynamically to yield the magic of psychological and behavioral processes. In analogous fashion, information processing in modern microcomputers is achieved through the microstructure and electrical properties of various component parts, dynamically interconnected by the central processing unit (CPU) in ways that permit them to behave as if by magic. But in the brain, each neuron has its own CPU!

As we have already seen, computer terminology can only serve as a metaphoric shorthand for discussing a number of neural processes, and we should remember that the similarities are more superficial than revealing. As in the case of an actual brain, the surface appearance of computers provides few insights into the magic that these electronic "brains" generate via the controlled flow of information. In fact, when one compares the underlying processes of brains and digital computers, there are only modest relationships between the two. While computers obey a few rigid logical rules, biology carries out many subtle functions created by aeons of evolutionary selection. Brain rules do not follow the simple constraints of digital logic; rather, they reflect processes that have been refined for the multiple purposes of adaptive fitness. Some hints about these rules, and their constraints, can be obtained from the study of computers, especially modern "neural-net" computers that concurrently process several streams of information.[1] However, the true mechanisms of mind can only be understood by studying the electrical activities of interacting ensembles of neurons within living brains, in conjunction with the behavioral activities that living organisms undertake.

The study of neural pathways (see Chapter 4), without a thorough consideration of their functions, is mere anatomy—albeit it constrains what brain circuits are capable of doing! The material fabric of the brain comes to life through a study of its dynamic activities—electrophysiological, neurochemical, behavioral, and psychological. These diverse levels of operation are interrelated within the brain in ways that remain poorly understood, although great progress has already been achieved in relating electrophysiological and neurochemical levels to behavior. More modest linkages have also been achieved in correlating the biophysical and molecular levels with psychological processes.[2]

Monitoring the Electrical Languages of the Brain

Neurons convey information in one direction only—from cell body down the axon, toward the dendrites and cell bodies of other neurons—as an intermittent flow of electrical impulses (Figure 5.1). Such neuronal firings consist of progressions of electrical "waves" or *action potentials*, constituting a frequency-type code of information that flows from the axon hillock down the axon to the synapse. In other words, each firing of a neuron is essentially similar to all other firings (resembling the turning on and off of digital switches in computers), and it is the amount and pattern of firings that distributes information throughout the brain.[3] But this digital-type information is periodically converted into graded analog signals: At *synapses* the barrages of frequency-modulated (FM) neuronal firings are converted into various chemical languages that generate an amplitude-modulated (AM) signal. This is achieved via the release of chemical transmitter substances that act on receiving elements known as *receptors*, situated on neuronal membranes on the other side of the synaptic cleft. Postsynaptically, the two main electrical messages conveyed by neurons are "fire more," which is called *excitation*, and "fire less," which is called *inhibition*, but there are many distinct neurochemical ways this can be achieved (see Chapter 6).[4]

The magnitude of the postsynaptic signal is dependent on the quantity of neurotransmitter released at each synapse. In addition, many complex properties of the

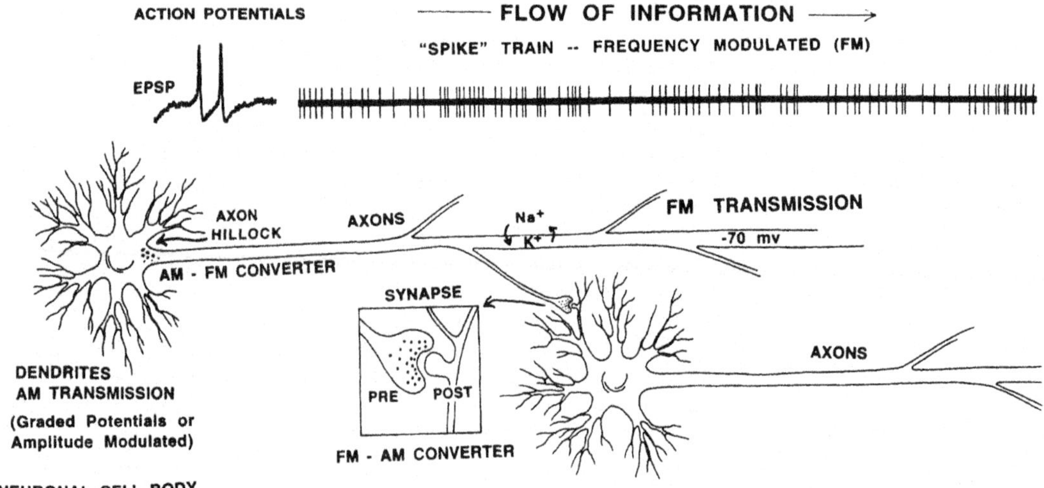

Figure 5.1. Schematic representation of information processing in two interconnected neurons. The flow of information is from left to right. *Top*: Two enlarged action potentials are depicted, followed by a typical FM spike-train that one might see in a "single-unit" recording. At the synapse (*middle insert*), the FM signal is converted to an AM signal via the release of transmitters. The cell body transmits an AM signal, which is converted to neuronal firing, or an FM signal, where the axon exits the cell body (i.e., at the "initial segment" or "axon hillock"). FM: frequency modulated; AM: amplitude modulated.

postsynaptic membrane also determine the magnitude of the graded electrical signal induced in the dendrites and cell body, or *soma*, of each receiving neuron. These properties include the number of available receptors and cascades of postsynaptic biochemical reactions. When the graded signal reaches a certain threshold at a sufficient number of excitatory synapses, a sensitive area on the nerve cell begins to fire. This zone, at the emergence of the axon from the soma, is called the *axon hillock*. In electrical terms, firing means that the electrical charge around the membrane rapidly shifts from internal negativity to positivity in a process called *depolarization*, which is mediated by ions (i.e., positively or negatively charged atoms). Inhibition, on the other hand, consists of graded resistance of postsynaptic elements to excitatory influences. Thus, neurons "speak" to other neurons via one-way communication channels situated at synaptic clefts, with chemically based amplitude codes. The induced excitatory signals are again converted to frequency codes at the axon hillock and transmitted to other neurons in the form of discrete electrical waves of constant size. Each of these waves is called an *action potential*. At the next synapse, the FM information in these action potentials is again converted to variable amplitude codes through the variable release of transmitters and summated conversion of the converging packets of chemical information into synaptic potentials.

The acquisition of this awesome knowledge was a long time coming, but it has been amply rewarded with Nobel Prizes. Still, we should wonder whether an analysis of pre-synaptic events or postsynaptic events will prove more informative for unraveling psychological processes. Of course, both need to be studied, but one could argue that we will make more progress in understanding emotions and other mental processes by focusing our efforts on the analysis of the graded postsynaptic (also called dendritic) events that can be recorded off the human scalp noninvasively using EEG and electromagnetographic procedures.[5] Using such techniques, we can monitor the activities of large ensembles of neurons in real time from many sites off the craniums of individuals performing psychologically interesting tasks. The summated electrical waves from thousands of dendritic potentials at each electrode site provide a fuzzy estimate of the information processing that is occurring in the underlying brain circuits. Since this technique can be implemented non-invasively and at a fairly global level of analysis—namely, the coordinated activities of ensembles of neurons in real time—the EEG is presently the best way to proceed in the neural analysis of mental processes. But before expanding on that argument, let us look at some historical antecedents that have brought us to our present level of sophistication.[6]

For new students of brain sciences, the classical findings in neurophysiology are as important to appreciate as more recent advances. The possibility that information in the nervous system is electrically transmitted was introduced by the 18th century physiologist Luigi Galvani (1737–1798), who was able to induce movements in frog legs by the application of electricity to their nerve trunks. That the mammalian nervous system is electrically excitable was confirmed and extended by many other investigators, including some ghoulish work around 1870 by two German physicians, Fritsch and Hitzig, on soldiers with head injuries on Prussian battlefields. They could induce movements by electrically stimulating areas of the human brain just anterior to the central sulcus that we now know as motor cortex. However, it was not until 1926 that Lord Adrian in England actually measured the nature of the electrical transmission within a nerve fiber.[7] Thereafter, electrical transmission of information was rapidly recognized as a universal property of all neurons. Adrian found that neuronal firing consisted of an all-or-none electrical change known as an *action potential* (even though electrophysiologists are now prone to say they analyze "spikes" from "single units," which is a shorthand way of saying they are studying the action potentials of individual neurons). The "all-or-none" electrical response means that each action potential is essentially the same size, and hence information is conveyed along the axon by frequency modulation as opposed to amplitude modulation as occurs in the dendrites and cell bodies. Characterization of the action potential was recognized as a momentous scientific discovery, which would have profound implications for our eventual understanding of mind. It was widely believed that the primary "language" of neural tissue had finally been revealed. At present, however, many scholars believe that ensembles of neurons may have their own *intrinsic* as well as perhaps *emergent* properties, so that the analysis of circuits may be more important for clarifying most psychological issues.

At the time Lord Adrian was making the first direct measurements of neuronal firing in frog nerves, Sir Charles Sherrington was outlining how simple motor acts, such as spinal reflexes, might be constructed by the interplay of excitatory and inhibitory synaptic processes. Indeed, although others, including Freud, had suggested that there might be information transfer points between neurons, Sherrington coined the word *synapse* to describe the discontinuities between nerve cells that could be inferred from studying reflexes via a phenomenon now called *synaptic delay,* which indicates that information transfer across synapses is slower than along nerve fibers. In 1932, Adrian and Sherrington were jointly honored by the Nobel Prize Committee "for their discoveries regarding the function of neurons."

Indeed, the history of these prizes reveals the esteem the scientific community has had for those who revealed the basic functions of the brain. Even relatively modest contributions were rewarded at times. For example, in 1944, Erlanger and Gasser received a prize "for their discoveries regarding the highly differentiated functions of single nerve fibers" in recognition of their demonstration that large-diameter nerve fibers conduct action potentials more rapidly than small-diameter fibers. Soon thereafter it was also discovered that axons that are well insulated with a fatty sheath called *myelin* transmit information even faster than unmyelinated fibers of the same size. This is because the ionic changes that cause neuronal firing can leap rapidly from node to node, between successive tiny locations along the axon where the myelin insulation is absent at the so-called *nodes of Ranvier*. This form of rapid conduction was named *saltatory conduction* (from the Latin *saltatio*, meaning "leaping").

Although the action potential is now well established as the fundamental and universal language of nervous systems, it took several investigators many years to work out the details of how neuronal firing actually occurs. In 1963, John Eccles, Alan Hodgkin, and Andrew Huxley shared a Nobel Prize "for their discoveries concerning the ionic mechanisms involved in excitation and inhibition in the peripheral and central portions of the nerve cell membrane." To make an important story very short, Huxley and Hodgkin discovered that the action potential occurs when cascades of positively charged ions flow along the length of the axonal membrane of the neuron in a wavelike fashion from the cell body to the synapse (where, as already mentioned, they induce transmitter release). Normally, the inside of a neuron is slightly negatively charged because of the proteins that are manufactured there. This is called the *resting membrane potential.*

Neuronal firing, or depolarization, consists of an influx of positively charged sodium ions (Na^+), which are present in much higher concentrations outside the cell. Immediately thereafter, the slightly larger positively charged potassium ions (K^+), present in higher concentrations inside the nerve cell, rush out to reestablish a resting, nonfiring state. Not surprisingly, this is called *repolarization,* an essential condition for the neuron to fire again. In other words, when a neuron fires, a positive Na^+ current enters the cell, and promptly thereafter the resting membrane potential is reestablished by a positive K^+ current flowing out of the cell. Repolarization tends to overshoot the resting level, assuring that action potentials flow in only one direction—from axon hillock toward the synapse. These ionic shifts occur only in a small area surrounding the membrane rather than throughout the cell body, and they occur through specific ion pores, or channels.

It is remarkable that these changes can occur up to hundreds of times per second in certain highly responsive neurons, which are most abundant in the sensory and thalamic-neocortical, "cognitive" regions of the brain. Other neurons rarely fire more than a few times per second. These slower-paced types are abundant in the emotional or hypothalamic-limbic regions of the brain. The reptilian brain is one of the few areas in the higher reaches of the brain where there is an abundance of neurons that do not fire at all unless the right environmental stimulus comes along.[8] In a metaphoric sense, their activity resembles the sluggish arousal patterns of many lizards.

At the synapse, the frequency-coded language of action potentials is converted to graded signals in the postsynaptic neuron. This is a consequence of the convergence of a variety of chemical transmitters. Each *neurotransmitter* or *neuromodulator* constitutes a synaptic language, conveying specific types of electrical messages. Taken in mass, some systems may broadcast distinct psychobehavioral tendencies throughout the nervous system (as detailed in Chapter 6). Originally it was thought that each nerve cell could utilize only a single transmitter (the so-called *Dale's law*), but that has proved to be an incorrect assumption. In fact, most neurons contain several types of molecules for information conveyance. One of these, the primary neurotransmitter, directly controls neuronal firing by inducing changes in ionic conductance across the membrane. Others, typically called *neuromodulators*, comprise an enormous class of molecules known as *neuropeptides*, which tend to modulate the intensity of the neurotransmitter effects, regulating the flow and patterning of action potentials within the brain. As we will see repeatedly, the neuropeptides are presently among the best candidates for creating emotional specificity in the brain, and we can envision this process as being achieved through the selection of various potential patterns of neural activity.

The actual release of neurotransmitters and modulators from presynaptic endings by incoming action potentials is instigated by a fairly homogeneous process—the inflow of calcium ions (Ca^{++}) into the presynaptic ending—as Nobel laureate Bernard Katz originally demonstrated in his work on the highly accessible synaptic junction between nerve and muscle (i.e., the *motor end plate*). At this synapse the transmitter acetylcholine, released from motor nerves from discrete *vesicular packets*, generates muscular contractions via Ca^{++} influx. The fact that muscular contraction and synaptic transmission are both triggered by the entry of Ca^{++} into cells highlights a wonderful example of how evolution utilized the same general principle for several different purposes. As assumed by the early investigators, it was eventually demonstrated that Ca^{++} entry was achieved through a specific *ion channel*, and this finding has been amply confirmed by subsequent research.[9]

When neurotransmitters interact with specific receptor molecules situated on postsynaptic membranes, various types of graded electrical changes are evoked in the postsynaptic neurons. It was Sir John Eccles who characterized the precise electrical changes that occur when one neuron speaks to another across the synapse via the various chemical languages that convey messages of excitation or inhibition (see Figure 5.1). His work indicated that receiving neurons generate graded inhibitory postsynaptic potentials (IPSPs) and excitatory postsynaptic potentials (EPSPs), which arise from the summation of many discrete minipotentials. These minipotentials reflect the release of vesiculor transmitter packets from presynaptic endings. Depending on the joint impact of many of these converging inputs on a postsynaptic neuron, an increasing negative charge (usually via chloride or Cl– inflow) yields inhibition. In other words, an increase of internal negative charge or potassium outflow makes neurons resistant to firing. Conversely, a decrease in internal negativity produces excitation, which, if the electrical depolarization passes a threshold level, leads to ionically driven action potentials proceeding down the axon toward synapses. Eccles also demonstrated that the frequency of the transmitted action potentials is related to the total amount of converging electrical pressure, or summation, exerted on the receiving cell by many synapses. A single neuron typically receives input from thousands of synapses. Because of such studies, it is now generally accepted that mind reflects the ultracomplex but organized flow of electrically coded information among the circuits of the brain. Much of the patterning of this information is controlled by endogenous, epigenetically refined brain processes. The natural patternings of these systems are the "inner causes" of behavior that behaviorism eschewed.

The next large breakthrough in our understanding of how neurons "speak" was the identification of the exact mechanisms by which various ions cross neuronal membranes. Although it had long been assumed that ionic currents move across the nerve cell membrane through specialized ion channels, it took some clever technology to demonstrate this process objectively. In 1991, two German neuroscientists, Erwin Neher and Bert Sakmann, received Nobel Prizes for developing an exquisitely fine procedure known as the *patch-clamp technique* for studying how individual ion pores actually operate.[10] A detailed understanding of such minute processes should lead to a new generation of medications for various brain disorders. Indeed, *calcium channel blockers* such as nimodipine have now been approved for reducing secondary brain damage that typically follows the primary brain injury arising from strokes.[11] In addition, neuroscientists have suggested a technique for early evaluation of a person's potential for Alzheimer's disease by monitoring for decreased potassium channels in samples of skin.[12] Until the advent of modern brain imaging procedures, such brain degeneration could not be biologically detected until postmortem brain analysis. To understand why skin serves as a good test tissue, we might recall that in evolutionary terms, the source of the nervous system is the embryonic ectoderm. In other words, brain is specialized skin tissue. This also explains why cells are so much more tightly packed in the brain than in most other organs of the body. They originate from tissue that was designed to interact with and protect us from the outside world. In a sense, the brain—or neuroectoderm—does that in very unique ways.

Most physiological psychology and neuroscience texts cover neuronal processes in very fine detail, with mathematical explanations to highlight precisely what goes on, including the famous *Nernst equation*, which describes how neurons actually develop asymmetrical distributions of electrical charge (i.e., ions) inside and outside their cellular membranes. The study of these types of molecular mechanisms continues to be a very active field of neuroscience inquiry, but we will not dwell further on such details here. That level of knowledge does not yet relate well to the current task, which is to address the nature of basic brain operating systems and their relations to emotional processes. We will focus instead on those brain electrical and metabolic activities that have been correlated most clearly with psychological and behavioral issues.

EEG Studies versus Single-Unit Studies in the Analysis of Psychological Processes

In sum, there are two general types of electrical activity that must be considered in the analysis of neurons: (1) a large number of graded synaptic potentials that converge on dendrites and neuronal cell bodies from many inputs, and (2) all-or-none action potential outputs that run the length of axons (Figure 5.1). Both can inform us about changing brain activities during specific psychobehavioral conditions. The first can tell us how a neuron integrates inputs, and the second how it integrates outputs. The study of graded dendritic potentials *in individual neurons* is more difficult than the study of action potentials because the former can be captured only through the difficult technique of intracellular recording, in which the point of an electrode must enter a neuron, while the latter can be measured with extracellular procedures that are technically easier to implement. Of course, the direct recording of single-cell activities always requires the implantation of fine electrodes directly into brain tissue, which makes such a technique unacceptable for routine human studies, although it has occasionally been used in conjunction with brain surgeries performed for other medical purposes. Graded potentials, on the other hand, are summated from millions of neurons and may be measured quite readily by large subcortical electrodes or, more commonly in humans, from electrodes on the surface of the intact skull. This is the brain activity that is measured in EEG recordings, and it is the only relatively inexpensive and noninvasive technique that can monitor the ongoing neurodynamics of the human brain at speeds that parallel mental activities.

While single-unit studies can tell us how a specific cell is behaving in a certain context, summated synaptic potentials recorded by EEG allow us to estimate how large ensembles of neurons coordinate their activities in the course of an actual psychobehavioral process. Because a single neuron is considered to be the basic unit of the nervous system, behavioral neuroscientists prefer the apparent precision of single-unit analyses for their animal studies, even though the EEG may, in fact, provide more compelling information about global brain functions that can be linked more easily to large-scale psychological processes, ranging from cognitive activities to emotional responsivities. Although it can be debated whether a study of *dendritic potentials* (or inputs to neurons) or the study of *action potentials* (the outputs of neurons) provides greater insight into the integrative psychobehavioral functions of the nervous system, the EEG obviously has more potential for harvesting the neurodynamics of the human brain. There are good reasons to believe that the detailed analysis of dendritic potentials from large cell assemblies (i.e., a systems analysis) can provide important neuropsychological insights more readily than a focus on the action potentials of individual cells. By analogy, the study of whole muscle movements yields greater insights into the patterns of behavior than a study of the electrical activities of individual muscle fibers. One great success story has been how EEG recording revolutionized sleep research during the second half of the 20th century (see Chapter 7).

A critical dilemma in animal brain research is how to orient EEG recording electrodes within the brain in such a way to maximize observation of distinct neural systems in action. Some electrode configurations and locations are bound to yield more noise than useful signal due to the massive overlap of interdigitating systems. There is no such problem when one records from a single cell, but now the difficulty is fathoming how activities of individual neurons reflect the critical properties of coherently operating neural networks. Although the raw EEG, as classically used in epilepsy research, provided relatively little insight into the psychological functions of the brain, new multielectrode and computational approaches can now be deployed to yield remarkable new insights that the older techniques could not.[13] Of course, both EEG and single-unit techniques have been exceedingly important for the development of neuroscience. In the following I will highlight how these two techniques have been used to clarify several psychological problems.

Single-Unit Studies

Because of our understanding of the basic electrical languages of the brain, we can now inquire how neurons in various brain areas respond to world events. Single-unit studies have provided detailed maps of all the major sensory and motor projection areas of the brain, yielding a preliminary scheme of how perceptions and actions are constructed.

The initial great achievements of single-unit studies were in the sensory realm, revealing the codes of *visual feature detectors* for the first time. It is now clear that vision is constructed from the interplay of many discrete neuronal functions, including systems that decode motion, static form, dynamic form, and, of course, color.[14] David Hubel and Torsten Wiesel were the first to demonstrate that neurons in the visual cortex are tuned to receive such specific types of information as the orientation of lines and edges and their movements in specific directions. These highly tuned sensitivities are thought to constitute the basic neuronal grammar of vision. For their insightful and seminal work, the Nobel Committee honored Hubel and Wiesel in 1981 "for discovering how sight stimulation in infancy is tied to future vision and how the brain interprets signals from the eye." Roger Sperry was concurrently honored "for his research into the specialized functions of each side of the brain" (see Chapter 16 and Appendix C). The details of neurophysiological processes have continued to be a topic of major interest among neuroscientists, and the factual riches are so vast it would require more space to do them justice than is available here.[15]

Comparable analyses have allowed investigators to decode many other sensory and perceptual functions of the brain, as well as the details of motor processes. Motor systems have been more difficult to map, because the experimenter does not have as much stimulus control in the experiment. Instead, one must follow the flow of brain and behavioral change concurrently, in the hope of identifying which brain areas initiate and integrate behavioral responses. The best results have been obtained when animals are placed in well-structured situations requiring a stereotyped motor response. A commonly used test requires monkeys to work for juice by twisting a "joystick" type of manipulandum, so that either flexor or extensor muscles are selectively activated in the arm. One remarkable finding of such research has been that the frontal cortex and basal ganglia elaborate motor plans,[16] and that one specific area of the brain, the *supplementary motor area* (SMA), seems to always participate in the initiation of movement, and hence intentionality.[17] Neuronal activity in the SMA predictably precedes voluntary motor actions. Indeed, one modern-day dualist, Nobel Prize–winner Sir John Eccles, following in the footsteps of Descartes, who posited a brain/mind interface in the pineal gland (see Appendix C), has suggested that the SMA is a major brain area where "mind" and brain interact.[18] Most monistically oriented investigators consider this hypothesis far-fetched or even nonsensical, but no one has yet provided a coherent neural explanation for the primal source of intentionality within motor systems. Perhaps an answer to this question requires a much better understanding of the neural substrates of "self-representation" than has yet been developed (see Chapter 16).

Only recently have investigators started to apply single-unit electrophysiological recording procedures to the more subtle aspects of mental organization. A few dedicated investigators have implemented these difficult techniques in the study of central integrative functions, providing a glimpse of where specific psychological subtleties begin to emerge. For instance, reinforcement processes appear to imbue neutral stimuli with positive values along a neural continuum that runs from the vicinity of ventral tegmental dopamine systems, through the lateral hypothalamic self-stimulation zones, to basal forebrain nuclei and the orbitofrontal cortex (see Figure 3.6 and Chapter 8).[19] We also know that temporal cortical neurons compute facial recognition from the flow of well-processed visual information,[20] and it is noteworthy that many nerve cells are responsive to emotional facial expressions. For instance, certain higher-order perceptual cells (sometimes called "grandmother cells") extract information related to social dominance, such as a raised chin.[21] We are also learning which neurochemical systems—such as dopamine, norepinephrine, serotonin, and acetylcholine—are active during various sleeping, waking, and other behavioral states. While norepinephrine and serotonin cells "sleep" when we sleep, dopamine neurons remain prepared to fire at high rates during all of our various vigilance states, and all of the above neurochemical systems exhibit increased firing during emotionally aroused waking states (sees Chapter 7 and 8). The many successes of the single-unit approach are too numerous to summarize here. They are primarily responsible for revealing which neural systems participate in the construction of representations from incoming sensory stimuli and which neurons guide motor outflow.

However, the technique has told us rather little about how intrinsic behavioral tendencies are actually constructed from the interactions of the many intrinsic neural systems that reside in the "great intermediate net" (which is a wonderful catchphrase suggested by neuroanatomist Walle Nauta for all of those poorly understood intervening processes between sensory inputs and motor outputs that we will focus upon in this text). In this context, it is noteworthy that many neurons can generate their own firing endogenously, often in an oscillatory fashion.[22] This suggests that many neuropsychological functions are of essentially endogenous origin—for instance, the tendency of babies to move their limbs and bodies in repetitive, stereotyped ways. Such intrinsic brain functions are reflected in the persistent, ongoing electrical waves of EEG recordings.[23] The fluctuations in the frequency and amplitude of these signals reflect the interactions of internal and external events converging in the brain. Although the EEG has generally been deemed to provide undesirably fuzzy signals of brain activity, recent computational approaches, implemented through the power of modern high-speed computers, add new promise to this old technique. One recent breakthrough is the observation of very rapid 40-Hz EEG oscillatory bursts that may highlight brain functions related to psychological processing of stimuli, as well as perhaps consciousness itself.[24]

Global EEG Measures of Brain Electrical Activity

EEG brain waves were first noted by Hans Berger, a German psychiatrist, in 1929. He found that when people were resting with their eyes closed, their brain waves went up and down in rhythms of about 10 cycles per second; he called this the *alpha rhythm.* Berger also noted that these resting waves disappeared when people opened their eyes and attended to the world. This phenomenon, called *alpha blocking*, is now known to be caused by a shift of the dominant frequency of the EEG into what is called the *beta* range. This type of faster brain activity, called *desynchronization*, reflects the fact that neurons under the electrode are no longer firing in phase (i.e., in close temporal conjunction with each other) but appear to be working more independently. In other words, the dominant frequency of ongoing EEG waves (usually described in hertz [Hz], or cycles per second) gives us a measure of how the brain is processing information. When the waves are synchronized in high-amplitude, slow patterns, we can assume that neurons are firing in synchrony and the cortex is not processing detailed information. When the waves become desynchronized in low rapid patterns, nearby neurons are operating more independently, and the cortex is typically in an aroused, information-processing mode.[25] This relationship does not necessarily hold for all brain areas, and the pattern is actually reversed in regions such as the hippocamus where theta waves mark active information processing.

At present, five general categories of brain waves are recognized in humans. The slowest rhythm is *delta* (0.5–3 Hz), which generally tends to reflect that the subject is sleepy (see Chapter 7). The next is *theta* (4–7 Hz), which has been related to meditative experiences, unconscious processing, and some negative emotional effects such as frustration.[26] However, as mentioned, theta reflects active information processing in certain brain areas such as the hippocampus (HC). When this rhythm occurs in the HC, an organism is typically exploring and the HC is presumably elaborating thoughts and memories.[27] This rhythm is also characteristic of the HC during rapid eye movement (REM) sleep (see Chapter 7). The brain's relaxed, or "idling," rhythm is *alpha* (8–12 Hz), which provides an excellent reference measure for detecting changes in brain arousal. In other words, the ongoing electrical energy in the alpha range can be used as a baseline for detecting how various brain areas become aroused during specific cognitive tasks and emotional situations. *Beta* rhythm (typically 13–30 Hz) is generally considered an excellent measure of cognitive and emotional activation. Finally, oscillations above beta are usually considered to be in the *gamma* range (i.e., more than 30 Hz); they are presently thought to reflect some of the highest functions of the human brain, such as perceptual and higher cognitive processes.[28] With modern computational techniques, one can easily segregate the various frequency bands (through a mathematical procedure called *Fourier analysis*); one can estimate the power (or amplitude) within the component waves and highlight their coherence (i.e., synchronization) at different brain sites.

Individuals differ greatly in the characteristic types of brain wave parameters they exhibit. For instance some have a great deal of alpha and others comparatively little; others are rich in theta while most are not. The manner in which these fairly stable differences relate to personality has not been determined, but one possibility is that those with a great deal of alpha tend to be "laid-back," concept-oriented people, while those with a predominance of beta are more "action-type," detail-oriented people. Other personality relationships have been suggested, but more work must be done before such ideas can be accepted.[29] EEG techniques have been most valuable in allowing neurologists to study various brain disorders, the most prominent being epilepsy, which can be monitored with scalp electrodes, since seizures are accompanied by rhythmic, high-amplitude delta waves that are never seen during normal states of consciousness.

There is reason to hope that modern EEG procedures, which can simultaneously measure small shifts in the distribution of power within graded *dendritic potentials* from many different sites on the cranial surface, can provide much better estimates than did earlier approaches of how psychological processes are organized in the brain. Recent advances in computer technology have made complex multielectrode analyses of brain electrical activity feasible. Modern computers can easily sift highly informative signals from background electrical noise through the use of sophisticated filtering and computational procedures.

One of the first averaging procedures to be developed was the evoked potential (EP), which monitors brain activity immediately after the repeated presentation of brief stimuli. One can obtain the glimmer of interesting neuropsychological effects when this procedure is used in conjunction with the so-called *oddball procedure*, whereby brain responses to two types of variably presented auditory stimuli are monitored, one tone being frequently presented and the other one rarely. For instance, a 1000-Hz tone may be presented 80% of the time, while a 2000-Hz tone is present 20% of the time. The rarer stimulus generates a much stronger brain response, especially a positive-going wave at about 300 milliseconds after stimulus onset. The oddball response pattern can even be detected to an unexpected "absence" of stimuli. Accordingly, this has been named the *P300 response*, which is widely believed to reflect active attentional processing of novel stimuli,[30] while others think that it is merely a neuronal punctuation mark signaling the completion of a psychologically meaningful unit of processing.[31] Unfortunately, EPs are effective detectors of predictable changes in brain activity for no more than the first second following the presentation of each stimulus, after which the ongoing intrinsic variability of endogenous brain activity tends to overwhelm any meaningful signal (i.e., the signal-to-noise ratio declines rapidly).

The use of comparable signal averaging procedures on selected frequency components of the EEG is now allowing investigators to circumvent this temporal problem. For instance, one can now follow small electrical changes across the cortical surface for many seconds during a cognitive task by observing how the power (i.e., the voltage, or height, of brain waves squared) in various EEG frequency domains changes after experimentally presented events.[32] Another important measure is that of coherence, or temporal correlation, between brain waves recorded from distant sites. If brain waves are moving together rather than independently, in the absence of an epileptic seizure, it is assumed that those areas are coordinating their activity. For instance, one of the highest levels of brain-wave coherence ever observed has been from musicians mentally rehearsing their compositions.[33]

A variety of powerful new findings are emerging from such modern EEG studies. For instance, various investigators are attempting, with considerable success, to track simple thoughts and associations in the cortex by cross-correlational analysis of electrical activity from up to 128 electrode sites.[34] Several investigators have developed computational procedures for representing waves of electrical activity across the cortical surface by using bands of colors, which allows one to get a real-time "feel" for the tidal changes in brain activity during psychological activities.[35] One promising approach of this type is a variant of the alpha-blocking phenomenon that Hans Berger originally described. To detect small changes in alpha blocking, one can average many trials of the same experience. This *event-related desynchronization* (ERD) represents repeated arousal shifts from the resting alpha state with respect to specific environmental events. In the same way, one can map the patterns of *event-related synchronization* (ERS) to provide an estimate of which brain areas are processing less information during psychological activity.[36]

Investigators have been able to detect characteristic brain changes in a variety of simple cognitive tasks such as verbal categorization. When subjects are requested to decide whether visually presented words belong in one category or another, ERD changes predictably occur during the stages of cognitive processing—starting with an initial arousal of the visual cortex, followed by arousal of the anterior speech areas, and then the supplementary motor cortex as the individual begins to behave.[37]

Do specific cortical EEG changes accompany emotions? This area of brain research is poorly developed due to the difficulty of reliably inducing emotions in laboratory situations (although some intriguing work is summarized in the "Afterthought" of this chapter). To evaluate this possibility with the ERD procedure described earlier, many years ago I sought to become adept at an emotional exercise developed by Manfred Clynes, called "sentic cycles," whereby one can bring emotional arousal under voluntary control.[38] In this exercise one evokes such emotions as anger, sadness, love, joy, and reverence by voluntarily simulating specific dynamic expressions. In 1989 an ERD-topographic analysis was done on my EEG rhythms while I systematically and repeatedly evoked these feelings. ERD measures were also taken while I experienced no particular feeling at all. The results were striking. Each emotion produced marked and complex changes in ERDs within the alpha band in many brain areas, indicating that alpha power decreases in distinct regions and in distinct temporal patterns for each emotion.[39] Such results indicate the powerful effects that feelings can have on higher brain activities, but before we can reach definitive conclusions, a great deal of work remains to be done on the different types of situations that elicit emotional responses.

A clinical situation in which the ERD technique has shown promise is presented in Figure 5.2. Normal and autistic children viewed a photograph of their mother in flashes lasting one quarter of a second. The normal children exhibited a brain arousal (i.e., an ERD response) pattern to this stimulus, but the autistic children exhibited the opposite (i.e., an ERS). However, two hours after being treated with the opiate receptor antagonist naltrexone, the autistic children started to exhibit mild arousal to the same stimulus.[40] In this context, it is worth noting that EEG is one of the few techniques that can be used routinely in identical ways in both animal and human research. This can be claimed for no other modern brain-imaging techniques (largely because of the cost involved). Thus, EEG analysis remains a potentially powerful procedure for evaluating how animal and human brains handle both cognitive and emotional information. Changes observed in humans can be modeled in animals, where there is a real possibility of working out the details of the underlying neural mechanisms.

The new EEG approaches are supplemented by a variety of other techniques that can analyze such factors as cortical blood flow and electromagnetic changes in the brain. These research tools are just beginning to be implemented for the analysis of emotions.[41] Like the cranial-surface EEG method typically employed in hu-

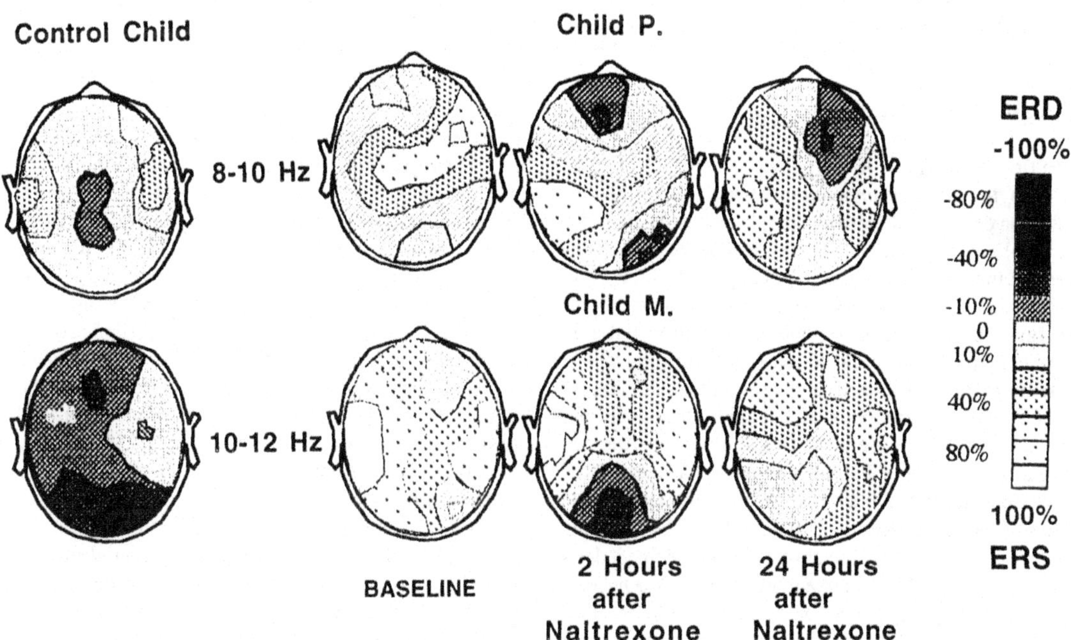

Figure 5.2. Event-related desynchronizations (ERDs, darker) and event-related synchronizations (ERSs, lighter) during quarter-second exposure to mother's picture on the skull surface of a normal child and two autistic children. Power changes in both upper (10–12 Hz) and lower (8–10 Hz) alpha bands are depicted for the control child, but only the more responsive band for each is depicted for the autistic children. In Child P., opiate receptor blockade with naltrexone (0.5 mg/kg) induced arousal in left frontal and right occipital cortical areas; this effect was still evident a day later when the child was still exhibiting clinical improvement. In Child M., there was increased arousal in the high alpha band only in the occipital cortex, which was accompanied by increased visual attention, but this effect did not outlast the acute drug effect. (Adapted from Lensing et al., 1994; see n. 4.).

mans, these procedures can only detect changes on the surface of the brain. To understand the neurodynamics of basic emotions and motivations at their source, one must also monitor subcortical activities. Until recently, that could only be done with depth electrodes (routinely used only in animals), but a variety of three-dimensional, brain-imaging techniques (including the PET and MRI approaches described subsequently) are beginning to be used to analyze emotional changes in the human brain.[42] Unfortunately, their current cost tends to make them prohibitive for animal research, and their temporal resolution is poor compared with the EEG. Most of these techniques take snapshots of the brain over fairly long segments of time, which precludes any real-time dynamic analysis, but even these problems are being solved through the development of functional MRI.

New Views into the Brain

A key question in psychobiology has been: How might we visualize the patterns of the dynamic processes that transpire throughout the brain? Only recently have tools been developed to allow investigators to estimate the subcortical locations and degrees of neuronal dynamics as a function of psychological and behavioral states.

The 2-DG Technique

The first technique of this type was *2-deoxy-D-glucose (2-DG) functional brain mapping*, which traces the distribution of a special type of sugar, 2-DG, that cannot be metabolized. The rationale for this technique arose from the fact that all neurons use blood sugar (D-glucose) as their major source of fuel. Since neuronal firing is an energy-consuming process, one can obtain visual evidence of changes in neural activity by *autoradiographic* determination of radioactive glucose uptake and distributions in brain subregions. Since rapidly firing neurons consume more glucose, such autoradiographs (as depicted on the right of Figure 4.4) give us a snapshot of how much sugar had been consumed in the various regions of the brain. However, since ordinary blood sugar (i.e., D-glucose) is fully metabolized within cells, it does not provide a good integrative marker. What was needed to make the technique work was a form of glucose, like 2-DG, that would linger within cells without being excreted. In this way investigators could estimate which areas of the brain were active under which behavioral circumstances.[43]

This technique has been quite useful for analyzing certain brain functions, especially sensory and motor processes and the effects of many pharmacological challenges,[44] but it turned out to be less effective for resolving the geography of functional systems within the "great intermediate net" unless one used direct localized electrical stimulation of the brain. In fact, after a period of great hopes, it did not provide significant new insights into the circuits of reticular tissue where many emotional brain systems are intertwined. The pictures that the 2-DG technique yielded were rather fuzzy anatomically, providing, at best, a vague functional map of the brain. The lack of resolution for analyzing emotional processes may have been due either to massive interdigitation of diverse systems or to nearby opponent processes (such as inhibitory and excitatory systems) that may cancel out the visual image of each other's effects. However, there were some successes. For instance, as summarized in Figure 5.3, the trajectory of self-stimulation systems was visualized during application of electrical stimulation of the brain (ESB).[45] Neural areas that participate in imprinting were also identified in the avian brain.[46] Although the approach remains somewhat disappointing in its ability to clarify psychologically interesting brain functions, it did provide the conceptual basis for the development of dramatic new ways to image the living brain in humans—the technique called *positron-emission tomography (PET) scanning*.

PET Scans

During the past decade, remarkable progress has been made in our ability to visualize what is going on inside the living human brain. A major breakthrough was the discovery by Allan Cormack and Godfrey Hounsfield of a noninvasive way to obtain pictures of internal structures. In 1979, they received the Nobel Prize "for the development of a revolutionary X-ray technique, computer axial tomography scan." Although this initially provided a three-dimensional static view only of anatomical structures, the computational procedures employed for these *computer-assisted tomography (CAT) scans* were soon used by others to develop techniques for visualizing *dynamic* biochemical changes within the brain. After intravenous injection of various short-lived radioactive, positron-emitting molecules, especially variants of 2-DG sugars, investigators can gauge the local activities of individual brain regions by monitoring the patterns of radioactive emissions around the skull. These PET scans employ sophisticated mathematical triangulation procedures similar to those used in CAT scans to computationally reconstruct images of various planes of the brain (for orientation, see the three major planes of the rat brain in Figure 4.11). In turn, these reconstructed sections depict the differential densities of isotopes within subregions of the brain, giving us ballpark ideas of which brain areas participate in which psychobehavioral processes.[47]

The PET technique was first used to study rates of brain sugar metabolism, based on the logic of 2-DG studies in animals. This technology has now been refined to monitor the activities of specific neurochemical systems inside the living brain. PET scans can now

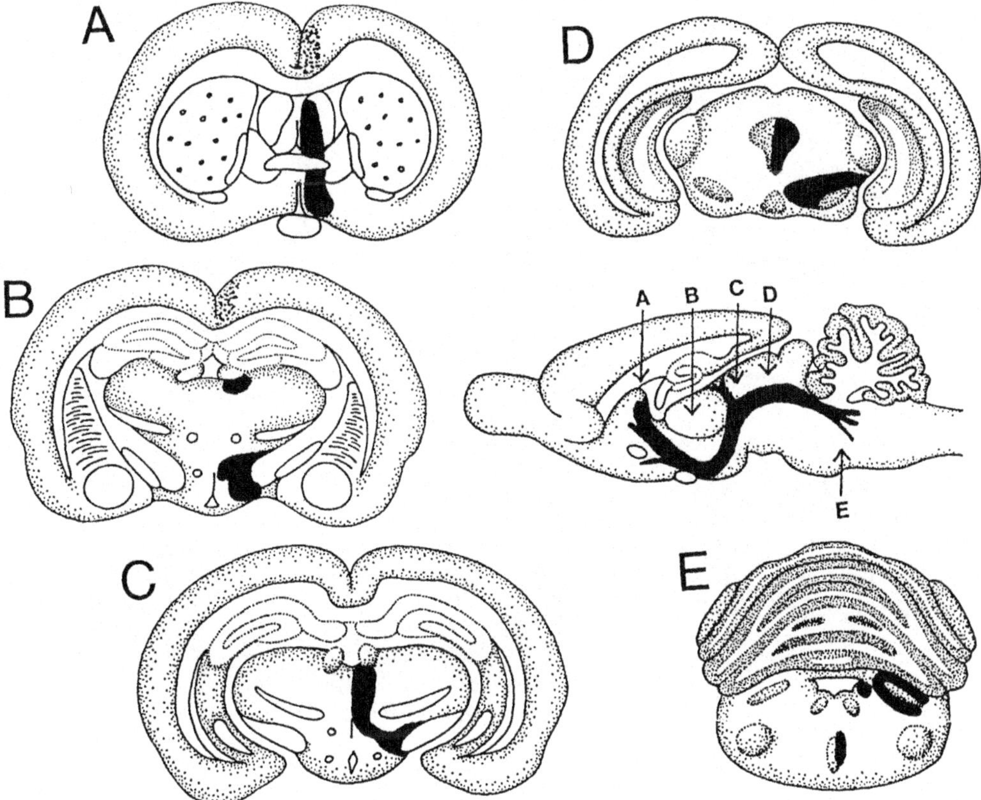

Figure 5.3. Summary of major increases in brain metabolism as reflected by uptake of ^{14}C-2-deoxy-D-glucose (2-DG) during "rewarding" electrical stimulation of the lateral hypothalamic area. The electrode site was approximately at the level of section B, within the dark area indicating elevated glucose uptake. (Adapted from Roberts, 1980; see n. 45.) For anatomical locations, see labels on the corresponding sections depicted in Figure 4.10.

highlight what is happening at specific synaptic fields. Such procedures have verified that in Parkinson's disease there are deficits of dopamine activity in the basal ganglia[48] and that the brains of schizophrenics have excessive receptors for this same transmitter.[49] The changes in brain activity during panic attacks and in obsessive-compulsive disorders, depression, and several other psychiatric disorders have now been visualized.[50] For instance, individuals with obsessive-compulsive disorder tend to show excessive activity in frontal lobe areas (Figure 5.4). One of the shortcomings of these techniques has been the relatively long time window for observing brain activities. One has to harvest data for a minimum of several minutes during each run, although with certain isotopes the time has been brought down to about 10 seconds, which is still much too long to follow the flow of ongoing cognitive activities in real time. For that, the EEG is still the procedure of choice, for it has a resolution that can follow brain activity in real time. However, there is one other technique that is rapidly overcoming this technical problem.

Magnetic Resonance Imaging

For a while now, *magnetic resonance imaging* (*MRI*) has been providing finer pictures of the internal anatomy of the living brain than could be imagined at the beginning of the neuroscience revolution in the mid-1970s. In this procedure, the magnetic properties of specific brain constituents are monitored/reconstructed into three-dimensional anatomical images. A variant of this technique, known as *MRI spectroscopy*, has recently been harnessed to monitor the dynamic activities of specific neurochemical systems. Coupled to on-line video imaging equipment, related procedures provide "moving pictures" of neuronal activity (as indexed by brain tissue oxygenation) throughout the brain to the geographic precision of a pinhead. This variant is called *f*MRI, where the *f* stands for *fast* or *functional*. So far the technique has been largely used to validate classic neurological findings, such as the location of various sensory, motor, and association cortices, but it is rapidly becoming a major investiga-

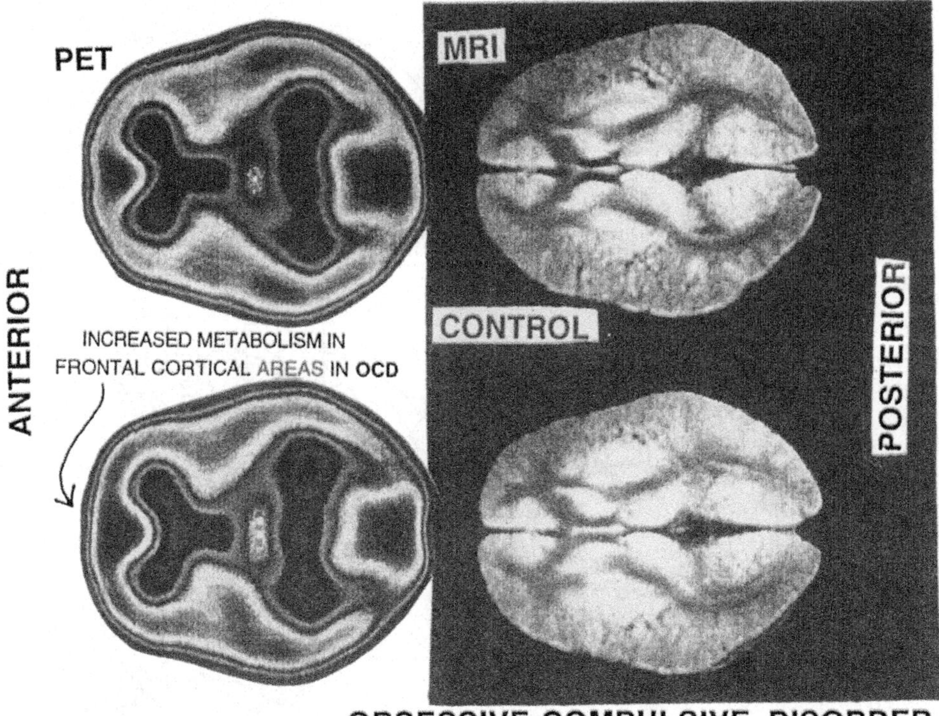

Figure 5.4. Horizontal PET (positron emission tomography, *left*) and MRI (magnetic resonance imaging, *right*) images through the brain of normal individuals and those exhibiting obsessive-compulsive disorder. The MRI scans indicated that no structural differences were evident. However, the functional PET scans of brain glucose uptake indicate hypermetabolism in medial frontal areas of the brain where behavioral plans are generated. Each reflects computer-averaged images from 10 individuals. These images were kindly provided by Dr. Gordon Harris of the New England Medical Center. (A full description of these findings is in Harris & Hoehn-Saric, 1995; see n. 50.)

tive tool, and recently the role of the amygdala in human fear has been confirmed.[51]

These developments have given unprecedented assurance that brain/mind relations can finally be studied in humans. Some specialists have even suggested that such approaches may eliminate the need for animal brain research in psychology. But this is far from true. These procedures cannot yet reveal most of the critical neurochemical activities that control behavior, and their resolution for brain stem functions is still rather poor. In addition, many of the processes we need to understand cannot be brought under sufficiently tight experimental control in human studies. For instance, we cannot activate discrete emotional systems using electrical and chemical stimulation procedures in humans.[52] To understand the emotional brain, animal research will be essential for a long time. Recently, several very powerful techniques have been developed for visualizing brain processes in animals. However, these will never be applicable for human research, for they require removal of the brain from the cranium soon after behavioral tasks are completed so that special types of histology can be performed on the tissues.

The Promise of New Techniques

Although measurement of electrical and metabolic activities in the brain can provide powerful markers of brain areas that are active during specific psychological and behavior states, they offer only limited information on the overall geographic trajectories of the brain's emotional circuits. It would be ideal if analytical techniques could be developed to distinguish coherently operating brain circuits in action within the animal brain. At present we must use other means to estimate the locations and neurochemical constructions of the basic emotional operating systems. Fortunately, several powerful new techniques have recently become available for use in animals. The anatomical techniques described in the following, which focus on neuronal DNA expression, may finally begin to answer functional questions in a definitive fashion.

When certain neurons change their rate of firing, their DNA rapidly expresses new growth-regulatory genes called *proto-oncogenes*.[53] Since some of these genes are turned on when neurons begin to fire vigorously, their products have now been used to identify the neuronal fields that are active during specific behavioral states. In other words, one can use the DNA products from these genes—various RNAs and proteins—as markers for the sets of neurons that participate in a specific psychobehavioral process. So far, the most widely used marker has been for the protein from the gene known as *cfos*. The expression of this gene can be measured directly with the techniques of *in situ hybridization*, which will be described in detail in Chapter 6. Alternatively, one can localize changes in the protein end product of the gene (Fos) via traditional *immunocytochemical* procedures. With such techniques one can record the changes of all of the neurons in the brain at once. For a photo depiction of the types of activity that can be visualized with this technique, see Figure 15.7, which depicts Fos changes in the brain during rough-and-tumble play.

So far this procedure has confirmed many of the findings about brain-behavior relations that were made with more primitive techniques such as brain lesioning. For instance, during male sexual behavior, many neurons begin to express *cfos* in the preoptic area of the hypothalamus, and it has long been known that damage here severely compromises the sexual motivation of male rats. This is not the place to summarize the many intriguing results that are emerging from the widespread use of this technique, but another interesting example is provided in the "Afterthought" of this chapter.

In general, current advances in understanding brain functions are being driven by the development of new techniques and technologies.[54] This will be even more evident in the next chapter when we come to the analysis of chemical dynamics in the brain. However, there is still a great deal of room for new conceptualizations to guide the novel use of old techniques. As mentioned, this type of emerging sophistication is transforming the EEG analysis of brain activity. This classic technique is now being combined with novel conceptualizations of brain activity, as extracted with mathematical descriptions of ultracomplex neuronal interactions within the brain. As summarized in the next section, recent descriptions of "nonlinear dynamics," commonly called "chaos" analysis, are allowing investigators to grasp how conscious perceptual processes may be embedded within EEG signals.

Chaos in the Electrical Activities of the Brain

To understand complex processes, it is often necessary to simplify matters as much as possible. Parenthetically, this was one of Descartes's four rules for pursuing knowledge: "to think in an orderly fashion when concerned with the search for truth, beginning with the things which were simplest and easiest to understand, and gradually and by degrees reaching toward more complex knowledge, even treating, as though ordered, materials which were not necessarily so."[55] However, sometimes a technique comes along that allows you to deal directly with the complexity of nature. One of the most impressive successes along these lines has been the development of mathematical procedures that can trace orderly progressions in seemingly random and unpredictable systems. Chaos theory has now been able to provide insights into the orderly patterns that operate in a variety of seemingly random processes.[56] A main characteristic of such systems is that initial conditions are very important for the eventual patterns that emerge, while seemingly small influences can have far-reaching consequences. Following even mild perturbations, chaotic systems can fall into new, seemingly unpredictable, states of organization. However, it can be demonstrated that the seeming random patterns are in fact still governed by "attractors"—systemic properties that generate complex but repetitive patterns. Such approaches are having a growing impact on the analysis of complex physiological systems, including brain electrical activities.[57]

To give a better feel for the nature of "chaotic" but orderly activity in the brain, Walter Freeman has provided a striking image, which, as he forewarns, is somewhat oversimplified:

> I sometimes like to suggest the difference between chaos and randomness by comparing the behavior of commuters dashing through a train station at rush hour with the behavior of a large, terrified crowd. The activity of the commuters resembles chaos in that although an observer unfamiliar with train stations might think people were running every which way without reason, order does underlie the surface complexity: everyone is hurrying to catch a specific train. The traffic flow could rapidly be changed simply by announcing a track change. In contrast, mass hysteria is random. No simple announcement would make a large mob become cooperative.[58]

Investigators have now demonstrated that EEG recordings exhibit new chaotic patterns as brains make sense of incoming stimuli. Some have suggested that these patterns may reflect fundamental ways in which the brain works. Walter Freeman has been at the forefront of this work, demonstrating that meaningful olfactory stimulation in thirsty rabbits—namely, odors that have been associated with significant events such as delivery of water—induce chaotic neural activity on the surface of the olfactory bulbs. Neural ensembles begin to fire in complex 40-Hz oscillatory patterns, which is consistent with the idea that the overall patterns are controlled by various attractors within the brain. In other words, a specific type of reverberatory pattern reflects the construction of a meaningful perceptual state in the brain. Indeed, Freeman has suggested that coordinated interactions of different brain areas are sustained by a dynamic cross talk that is essential for meaningful communication in the brain and perhaps for perceptual awareness to occur. In other words, when higher cortical areas re-represent the oscillatory patterns induced within the olfactory bulbs, animals begin to understand the fact that the sensory cues are predicting forthcoming rewards. When such cross talk is prevented by damaging the neural connections between the bulbs and the secondary oscillations in the cortex, animals begin to lose their apparent appreciation of the meaning of the olfactory stimuli.[59]

These bold ideas have profound implications for our understanding of how the brain may elaborate affective consciousness. As a first approximation, it might be suggested that the various basic emotional circuits of the brain can serve as potential "attractors" for distinct types of neural activity in other parts of the brain. Thus, when an organism becomes emotionally aroused, neural ensembles throughout the brain may become captivated into certain repetitive firing patterns, thereby promoting the retrieval of a variety of stored memories and other brain processes relevant for each emotional state. Chaos theory may also suggest ways in which small environmental events, such as a change in tone of voice or a mere glance, can modify mood.[60] Through the influence of emotional attractors, organisms may rapidly shift into any of a variety of waking states depending on rapidly changing environmental events. Although this type of analysis will be essential for understanding how emotions are reflected in the electrical activities of the brain, we are presently remote from being able to formally characterize emotions in such terms.

AFTERTHOUGHT: Neurodynamics of Emotional Processes

How have the dynamic procedures described in this chapter been used to highlight the nature of emotionality within the brain? Although progress has been slow, let us note three of the most promising lines of inquiry—one derived from epilepsy and brain-stimulation studies, one from EEG analysis of brain states during emotional episodes, and one from the use of PET scans.

1. It is well known that epileptic foci in the limbic system are characterized by emotional changes in humans. For instance, one common type of seizure occurs in psychomotor epilepsy, with its source typically being situated in the temporal lobes. In addition to a host of bodily feelings, usually visceral changes, just prior to an attack, individuals often experience an "aura," a preseizure state characterized by various affective feelings. Most commonly observed are feelings of desire, fear, anger, and affection, as well as both dejected and ecstatic feelings.[61] These changes are reminiscent of those that investigators have been able to induce by localized electrical stimulation of the brain (see Chapter 3). This suggests that limbic seizures may activate the basic brain systems of emotionality in ways resembling direct activation of the underlying brain circuits with ESB or via environmental events that trigger emotional episodes.

It is known that individuals with temporal lobe epilepsy tend to develop characteristic personality disorders.[62] For instance, one of the most famous historical cases is that of the great Russian novelist Fyodor Dostoyevsky (1821–1881), who developed a chronic seizure disorder following his arrest for participating in socialist intellectual activities in the middle of the 19th century. After being taken to the place of execution, presumably to be shot, he was given a reprieve at the last moment (a form of emotional terror the czar sometimes used to keep creative people in line). Unfortunately for Dostoyevsky, but fortunately for world literature, the ensuing post-traumatic stress disorder that developed during his exile in Siberia was manifested, for the rest of his life, by what we now recognize to be an acquired temporal lobe seizure disorder. The accompanying neuropsychological changes promoted powerful feelings of ecstatic delight and demonic despair that permeated much of Dostoyevsky's anguished life and literary output.

It is noteworthy that similar experimentally induced epilepsies can also produce permanent personality changes in animals. In an experimental procedure known as *kindling*, animals are induced to exhibit epileptic states by the periodic application of localized electrical stimulation to specific areas of the brain. The term *kindling* comes from the gradual induction of this permanent brain sensitivity. The amygdala, an emotion-mediating brain area, is an ideal site for kindling studies, since seizure activity can be induced here most rapidly. The procedure consists simply of applying a burst of brain stimulation through indwelling electrodes for a period of one second, once a day, for a week or two. After the first brief ESB, nothing special happens, unless one observes the EEG, where one will note a momentary seizure immediately after the brain stimulation. This induced epileptic fit gets larger and larger as the days pass, and after a few days, the ESB begins to provoke brief periods of outright convulsive activity. After a week or so, the brief stimulation produces a full-blown motor fit, unambiguous both behaviorally and in the poststimulation EEG. Thereafter, the animal will always have a seizure when it receives this burst of brain stimulation. Gradually even other stimuli become capable of triggering seizures, especially loud sounds and flashing lights.[63]

Kindling can also be induced by giving animals seizure-inducing drugs every several days or even very loud auditory stimulation, which provokes fits in certain sensitive strains of animals.[64] The induction of these epileptic states reflects a functional reorganization of the nervous system, since no structural changes have been found to result from kindling procedures. If one follows the development of auditory kindling with *cfos* procedures, one initially finds cell activation only in deep areas of the auditory system in the lower brain stem; but when the animal is finally kindled, neuronal activation is evident in widespread areas of the limbic system.[65] Thus, kindling induces a permanent change in the functional organization of the brain, without any changes that are clearly evident at the structural level.

Do kindled animals exhibit changes in emotionality similar to humans with limbic psychomotor fits? Most definitely. Although relatively little work has been done on this most interesting issue, the emotional personality of these animals seems to change as they become kindled. Cats tend to become temperamental and irritable.[66] In female rats, we have observed a form of "nymphomania": Normal female rats come into estrus (or sexual receptivity) for only a couple of hours every four days, but after kindling many females remain in constant estrus. They are willing to have sex with males at all times. It is as if their hormonal receptivity cycle has been locked in overdrive.[67] The fact that one can obtain these types of chronic personality changes in animals suggests that emotional systems undergo chronic changes in activity as a result of certain types of experiences. Indeed, a variant of this procedure, called *long-term potentiation* (LTP), has become a popular model for memory research. In LTP, a permanent change in neuronal firing is induced in the hippocampus by repeated activation with electrical stimulation.[68] It has been shown that changes in LTP parallel changes in memory—those manipulations that reduce LTP diminish memory formation, and those that increase LTP facilitate the learning of new associations.[69] In other words, the mechanisms of memory are related to those of epilepsy!

Might it be that certain psychiatric disorders emerge from such permanent changes in the brain? For instance, post-traumatic stress disorder (PTSD), common in individuals who have experienced such prolonged emotional trauma as exposure to extreme violence and danger, is characterized by permanent personality changes, including frequent moods of intense fear and anger. Antiseizure medications such as carbamazepine are quite effective in reducing the severity of PTSD. Such agents also block the development of kindling in animals.[70] Thus, there seems to be a deep relationship between these seemingly different phenomena. Indeed, as summarized next, there appear to be relationships between certain forms of brain activity and emotional responsivity.

2. Many people have tried to divine the presence of emotional and other personality traits from the characteristic patterns of EEG exhibited by different individuals. It is clear that people often have distinct types of EEG patterns, but definitive conclusions are difficult to derive from the empirical literature. However, one consistent theme with regard to emotionality and EEG changes has recently been emerging. Several laboratories have now demonstrated that happy feelings, even sustaining a voluntary but sincere smile, will induce arousal (alpha blocking) in left frontal areas of the brain,[71] while unhappy feelings, including disgust, will evoke larger arousal in right frontal areas.[72] Indeed, individuals who are prone to depression tend to exhibit more right frontal arousal than those who are not.[73] These patterns can be observed even in babies. Indeed, infants who exhibit the highest arousal in right frontal areas tend to be the ones who are most likely to cry in response to brief periods of maternal separation.[74]

These brain changes are consistent with the emotional changes that have commonly been observed in humans following right and left hemisphere strokes (also see Chapter 16). The right hemisphere becomes aroused in response to negative emotions, and damage here typically has few negative emotional consequences; often, patients remain cheerful despite the severity of their problems. On the contrary, comparable damage to the left frontal areas, which become aroused in response to positive emotions, can cause catastrophic emotional distress, and such patients are more prone to become despondent and depressed.[75] Presumably this is because they have lost the use of brain areas that mediate positive emotionality. Indeed, as mentioned earlier, the brains of depressed individuals exhibit less arousal of the left frontal areas than normal individuals. It will be interesting to see whether their depressions can be elevated using biofeedback techniques aimed at increasing the resting level of left frontal cortical EEG arousal. Indeed, even more direct interventions may work. We can activate the intact brain using *rapid transcranial magnetic stimulation* (rTMS), and several investigators have been able to alleviate drug-resistant forms of clinical depression by selectively stimulating the frontal cortex just on the left side of the brain (see Chapter 16).

3. The most compelling evidence for subcortical localization of emotions in normal individuals presently comes from PET scanning studies. Several such studies have provided remarkable images of localized functional changes in the brain during a variety of activities, ranging from simple sensory bombardment to cognitive tasks.[76] Especially exciting is the visualization of some emotional processes. Although the results remain preliminary, it has been found that people prone to panic attacks exhibit overactivity in their right para-

hippocampal regions, where cognitive information from the cortex presumably enters emotional networks.[77] During feelings of happiness, the brain tends to exhibit a reduction of neuronal activity, while with feelings of sadness such activity is increased.[78] So far, these techniques have only yielded arousal patterns in relatively high brain areas during emotional episodes, and it remains perplexing that arousal of primitive brain stem systems that have long been implicated in emotional organization in animal work is rarely evident. This may be due to the fact that such techniques are not especially effective in detecting the arousal of compact brain zones where functionally opposing circuits are closely interdigitating. Clearly, other direct measures of the neurodynamics of emotional states will need to be developed if we are ever to move from the intellectual arena of theoretical conjectures to definitive empirical approaches in this important area of inquiry.

Suggested Readings

Brunia, C. H. M., Mulder, G., & Verbaten, M. N. (eds.) (1991). *Event-related brain research.* New York: Elsevier.

Diksic, M., & Reba, R. C. (eds.) (1991). *Radiopharmaceuticals and brain pathophysiology studied with PET and SPECT.* Boca Raton, Fla.: CRC Press.

Liebet, B. (1985). Unconscious cerebral initiative and the role of conscious will in voluntary action. *Behav. Brain Sci.* 8:529–566.

Maurer, K., & Dierks, T. (1991). *Atlas of brain mapping.* Berlin: Springer-Verlag.

Nunez, P. L. (1995). *Neocortical dynamics and human EEG rhythms.* New York: Oxford.

Pfurtscheller, G., & Lopes da Silva, F. H. (eds.) (1988). *Functional brain imaging.* Toronto: Hans Huber.

Posner, M. I., & Raichle, M. E. (1994). *Images of the mind.* Scientific American Library. San Francisco: Freeman.

Skarda, C. A., & Freeman, W. J. (1987). How brains make chaos in order to make sense of the world. *Behav. Brain Sci.* 10:161–195.

Verleger, R. (1988). Event-related potentials and cognition: A critique of the context updating hypothesis and an alternative interpretation of P3. *Behav. Brain Sci.* 11:343–428.

Walter, W. G. (1953). *The living brain.* New York: W. W. Norton.

6

Neurodynamics
Neurochemical Maps of the Brain

The intention is to furnish a psychology that shall be a natural science: that is, to represent psychical processes as quantitatively determinate states of specifiable material particles, thus making those processes perspicuous and free from contradiction. . . . The neurons are to be taken as the material particles.

Sigmund Freud, *Project for a Scientific Psychology* (1895)

CENTRAL THEME

We have progressed remarkably far in the hundred years since Freud penned his materialistic thoughts as a young man in his late 20s. However, rather than neurons, the most important "material particles" we must now investigate are the many types of molecules that serve as neurotransmitters and receptors, which convey information from one neuron to another. On the basis of this knowledge, a neurobiological revolution has transformed psychiatry, and new discoveries will yield more powerful and specific medicines than have ever been available before. Without a thorough knowledge of transmitter "particles," this would not be possible. The first neurotransmitters were discovered some four decades after Freud expressed his great hope for a scientific psychology, and now several dozen major systems have been well characterized. Many more remain to be discovered. We are beginning to understand how attention, emotions, and motivations, as well as perceptions and memories, are constructed through the synaptic chemistries that mediate information transmission in the brain. Information transfer *within* a single neuron is an electrical process, but at synapses the electrical language of the brain is momentarily converted into chemical *transmitter* languages. After transmitters cross the synaptic cleft and interact with specific receptor molecules, the neuronal messages are passed onward in cascades of biochemical events that convert the various chemical dialects back to electrical ones. Neuroscientists use *immunocytochemical* techniques to visualize the chemical languages of neuronal circuits, relying on "detective-like" antibodies to identify and localize specific brain chemicals. This technique can also be used to visualize the locations of various receptor fields, but a more commonly used technique is *receptor autoradiography*. In fact, we now have tools to visually examine the exquisitely patterned distributions of nearly all chemical systems of the brain. We can even describe where and when new peptide chemistries are *transcribed* from DNA using a technique called *in situ hybridization*. We can also measure the release of many neurotransmitters within specific parts of the brain in behaving animals. Finally, we are now in a position to understand how primitive emotions arise from specific neurochemistries of the mammalian brain. This information is leading to a revolution in our conceptualization of human nature.

DNA: The Source of Mental Life

The central dogma of molecular biology is summarized in Figure 6.1. It asserts that all the information we need to construct a mammalian body, whether of man or mouse, is contained in the approximately hundred thousand genes of mammalian DNA. Individual genes, small segments of DNA, contain instructions for the manufacture of specific proteins. This is how individual organisms vary: DNA is identical within the nucleus of each and every cell of any one individual, but it differs in subtle yet important ways from one human individual and one mammalian species to the next. Some have genes for blue eyes, some for hazel eyes, and so on. Genes interact with each other in powerful ways that remain poorly understood, and most psychological traits are due to these interactions, not to the effects of single genes. Still, the nucleus of every cell of every mammalian species has essentially the same amount of DNA, and very similar genes, which is why all mammals ex-

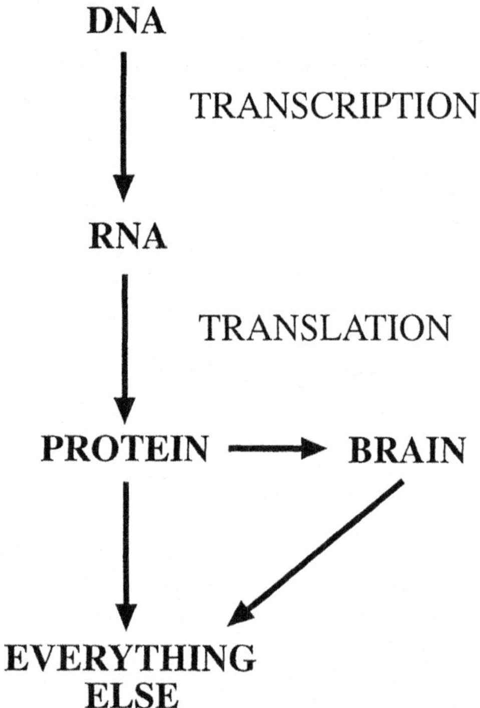

Figure 6.1. Summary of the current "central dogma" that underlies the analysis of all biological processes, including those that mediate basic psychobiological processes. The only major concept missing from this schematic is the environment, and these influences permeate all phases of these transactions.

hibit extensive homologies throughout their brains and bodies. It is remarkable to ponder how human uniqueness and our special cognitive complexities emerge from this massively shared heritage (see Appendix A).[1]

Indeed, our newfound understanding of the progression of events from DNA to a fully developed organism is the most profound scientific story of the 20th century (Figure 6.1). It goes like this: In every cell, the sole function of DNA is to manufacture RNA; the sole role of RNA is to manufacture proteins (chains of amino acids); and the role of proteins is to do everything else. This "everything else" is a vast potentiality that emerges from interactions with the world—including the universe of biological, social, and cultural complexity that stretches up to the highest reaches of human achievement. DNA can only accomplish its appointed task in receptive environments. Genetic and environmental potentials "go together like a horse and carriage," to borrow a phrase from a popular song of long ago: "You can't have one without the other." Although identical twins have similar IQs even if reared apart, that estimate of heritability would diminish if one was reared in the lap of intellectual luxury, while the other was brought up in a closet. In short, we only inherit brain/mind potentialities.

In supportive environments, the many differences among species, as well as among the various cells of our bodies, arise from the fact that different cells express different genes at different times. For instance, your kidney may employ 20% or so of the available genes in each of its cells, and muscle cells use about the same proportion, but each is specialized for its appointed task by the specific patterns of genes they have come to employ during tissue differentiation. Overall, the brain expresses more of its genetic potential, estimated at about 50%, than any other organ of the body. This allows it to be the most complex and most plastic organ in the known universe. Here I will not detail our enormous knowledge about genetic mechanisms but will highlight key neurochemistries made possible by DNA.[2]

First, let us summarize how DNA unreels its genetic story from a repetitive code of four nucleotides that are joined together in pairs: *Adenine* is joined with *thymine*, and *cytosine* is joined with *guanine* as a *double helix* like a long spiraling zipper. When the base pairs of DNA "unzip," they join with the related bases of *RNA*—adenine with *uracil*, thymine with *adenine*, cytosine with *guanine*, and guanine with *cytosine*, to form *messenger RNAs* that join up with intracellular structures known as *ribosomes* to manufacture all bodily proteins and peptides, which are long and short chains of amino acids, respectively. Amino acid sequences are dictated by *triplet codes* on RNA—that is, successive three-base segments of RNA represent the successive amino acids that are to be incorporated into the elongating peptide chains.[3]

The conversion of DNA to RNA is called *transcription.* The conversion of RNA to proteins is called *translation*. Often the initial product of genetic expression is a large "mother protein" from which many additional molecules are produced by *posttranslational processing,* whereby specific enzymes cut protein chains between specific amino acids. These enzymes are complex proteins whose linear structures are coded in DNA sequences, but they must be folded into three-dimensional structures before they can function properly to maintain the economy of the body. Although enzymes do not actively transmit information in the brain, they are the clerks that manage every transaction that makes the transmission of neural information possible. Thus, all mental functions rely critically upon the background work performed by enzymes.

A Brief Synopsis of Neurotransmitter and Receptor Synthesis

The manufacture, or *anabolism*, and destruction, or *catabolism*, of molecules in the body are under the control of a host of enzymes, each with its own precise job. Enzymes promote three general types of biochemical transactions in the construction of synaptic neurotransmitters and neuromodulators: (1) Many of the brain's neuromodulators are short proteins called *neuropeptides*, which are clipped from larger "mother proteins" by specific *cleavage enzymes*. (2) Other brain molecules, such as acetylcholine (ACh), the first synaptic transmitter ever discovered, are produced when even larger molecular fragments from various brain chemicals are joined through the assistance of specific anabolic enzymes. (3) Many other transmitters are simply amino acids that have been enzymatically modified in minor ways, such as the addition of a hydroxyl (OH) group here or the removal of a carboxyl (COOH) group there. This is how the neurotransmitters dopamine, norepinephrine, and serotonin—which figure so heavily in current biological psychiatry—are manufactured.

Most transmitters are destroyed soon after release by specific catabolic enzymes, or by reuptake processes, which remove the transmitter from the synapse. For instance, ACh is inactivated by the enzyme *acetylcholinesterase*, or *cholinesterase* for short. In the following, we will consider the "marriage" and "divorce" processes of ACh synthesis and degradation in detail (Figure 6.2).

In other words, ACh arises from the enzymatically mediated "marriage" of the nutrient choline and the acetyl group (CH_3CO) from acetyl CoA, a widely distributed molecule of the body produced by general energy metabolism (Figure 6.2). The enzyme that presides over this marriage is called *choline acetyltransferase*, or *ChAT* for short. As mentioned, the degradative enzyme that breaks this union back into the two component parts is cholinesterase. The cascade of events represented here for ACh typifies the processes of all other brain transmitter systems. All brain transmitters require specific *synthetic* (or *anabolic*) *enzymes* for their construction, and there are also a host of *degradative* (or *catabolic*) *enzymes* to help assure that transmitters are inactivated soon after they have conveyed their messages to receptors.

Receptors must also be manufactured, but they are somewhat more stable components of synaptic information transfer processes. Receptors linger for days, concentrated in the viscous lipoprotein fluid that constitutes synaptic membranes, before they are recycled and replaced with new receptors. In comparison with transmitters, receptors are gigantic, often with many biologically active sites. The long chains of amino acids that constitute receptors typically thread in and out of synaptic membranes many times. For example, ACh receptors exhibit seven such crossings, which are called *transmembrane domains*. A remarkable number of receptors have similar transmembrane domains, which reflects the fact that they have shared a long evolutionary history. Since invertebrates typically also have homologous receptors, they must have first emerged in brain evolution a very long time ago. Indeed, we can estimate divergence times of species by counting up the number of amino acid changes that are contained in receptors, as well as all of the other long proteins of the body (for a brief explanation of such biological clocks, see Appendix A). In sum, during evolutionary diversification, many ancient receptor lines have been conserved. Genetic diversification has yielded a variety of specific receptor subtypes in each receptor family, but many started their evolutionary journey from a common ancestral form.[4]

Thus, the varieties of receptors now found within the mammalian brain are awesome. Not only does each transmitter have its own receptor, but most have multiple subtypes. For instance, at present over a dozen receptors are known to receive messages from the transmitter serotonin, and identification of the functions of

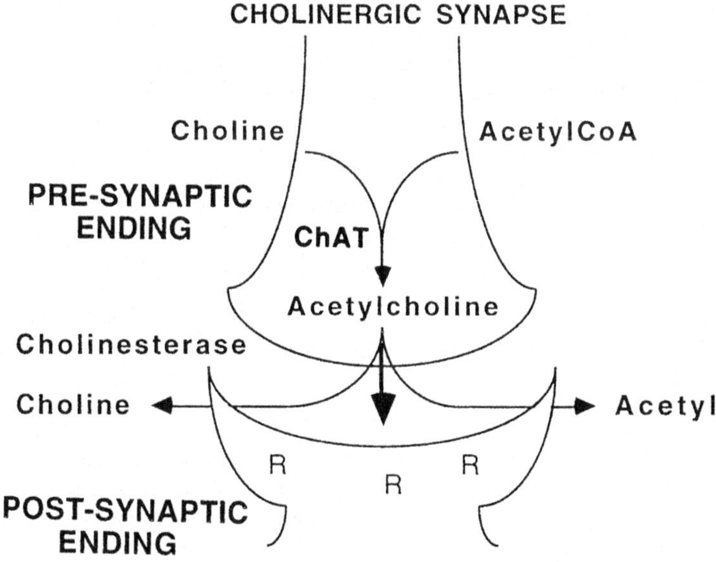

Figure 6.2. Summary of the major neurochemical processes that characterize acetylcholine (or cholinergic) synapses in the brain. Choline and acetyl CoA are joined into ACh via the mediation of the enzyme choline acetyltransferase (ChAT). After synaptic release, ACh is degraded into choline and acetyl via the enzyme cholinesterase R-receptor.

each subtype is an active area of inquiry because serotonin figures in virtually all psychiatric disorders. In addition, the brain contains receptors for many peripheral hormones, including testosterone, estrogen, and cortisol. It also contains receptors for many immune system intermediaries such as the *cytokines.* However, for our introductory purposes, I will briefly focus on ACh receptors before proceeding to detail how transmitters are constructed in the brain.

ACh receptor subtypes are divided into two classes, *nicotinic* and *muscarinic*, because of their distinct actions in the body. In general, the muscarinic receptors modify visceral activities, while nicotinic receptors activate skeletal muscles. This dichotomy tends to support the distinction between visceral-emotional and somatic-cognitive processes, as discussed in Chapters 4 and 5. At the time of this writing, five varieties of muscarinic and seven types of nicotinic receptor subtypes are known. Their differential functions have not been adequately deciphered because the molecular tools for such work are just being developed through the manufacture of artificial molecules that are selective receptor *agonists* and *antagonists*—namely, molecules that can selectively *activate* or *block* the individual receptor subtypes. Although the study of receptor multiplicity is a very active area of inquiry, for most systems the complexity is not yet well interfaced with emotional issues. Accordingly, I will focus on presynaptic chemical processes, where a more substantial body of data for the chemical coding of emotions and motivations already exists.

In presynaptic endings, all transmitters follow certain common rules. Most are packaged in *vesicles*—small, membrane-covered "cargo vessels"—that not only protect transmitters from catabolic enzymes but also allow synapses to dump a substantial number of transmitter molecules into the synaptic cleft at one time. The process of transmitter release is initiated by calcium entry into the presynaptic terminal as a result of arriving action potentials. The released transmitters bind to postsynaptic as well as presynaptic receptors, thereby inducing complex cascades of intracellular events that modify the electrical activities of the receiving cells. Synaptic activity can be terminated by a variety of mechanisms, including (1) active *enzymatic degradation* of transmitters, (2) specific presynaptic *reuptake* or *transporter* mechanisms that extract transmitters from the synaptic cleft and return them into the presynaptic ending, where they can be either degraded or recycled into vesicles, or (3) *passive dissipation* (i.e., diffusion) and slow degradation, which appears to be the most common form of degradation for the many peptide neuromodulators that help create motivational and emotional specificity within the brain.

An understanding of how the various transmitter molecules operate at synapses is essential for understanding the psychological functions of the brain. The synthetic and degradative pathways for such molecules, their regional localizations within the brain, as well as interactions with postsynaptic receptor molecules are essential elements of processes whereby mind and behavior emerge from brain matter. It is noteworthy that no neurotransmitter or neuromodulator has been discovered in humans that is qualitatively different from those found in other mammals. In fact, all mammals share remarkably similar anatomical distributions of most neurochemical systems within their brains. However, there are also distinctions in systems between different animals and species, which help explain their personality differences. One of the most dramatic contrasts observed so far is within brain oxytocin systems (see Chapter 13 and Figure 14.10) of various species. However, we will have to avoid such details here and instead focus on those discoveries that provide the broad foundation for current thinking about the neurochemical dynamics of the living brain.

The Discovery of Synaptic Chemistries, Old and New

Chemical transmission of information at synapses was first substantiated by Sir Henry Dale and Otto Loewi, and the Nobel Committee rewarded them promptly in 1936 "for their discoveries regarding the chemical transmission of the nerve impulse." The transmitter they discovered was *acetylcholine.* Many others have followed; among the most thoroughly studied are the relatively small molecules norepinephrine, dopamine, serotonin, and gamma-aminobutyric acid (GABA), which are simple modifications of amino acids. The scientists who discovered how these transmitter substances are synthesized, secreted, and degraded paved the way for the revolution in psychiatry sparked by the discovery of drugs that could modify emotional disorders through specific actions on neurons. Indeed, in 1970 Julius Axelrod, Ulf von Euler, and Bernard Katz were recognized by the Nobel Committee "for their discoveries concerning the humoral transmitters in the nerve terminals and the mechanisms for their storage, release and inactivation." As a group, these investigators provided the first detailed information about the neurochemical mechanisms of synaptic transmission.

Until the early 1970s, only the handful of neurotransmitters mentioned above were well known. Since then there has been an explosion of discoveries, among the most spectacular being a group called *neuropeptides.* Neuropeptides are short chains of amino acids, usually ranging from 3 to 40; the brain contains at least several hundred different kinds. Many appear to provide specific control over basic psychological functions such as appetite, stress, and discrete emotions, including separation distress and maternal and sexual feelings (see Chapters 12 to 14). The discovery and characterization of neuropeptides were made possible by the development of new analytic techniques, and Rosalyn Yallow received a Nobel Prize in 1977 "for the development of radioimmunoassays of peptide hormones." In that same year, Roger Guillemin and Andrew Schally, who capitalized on Yallow's new techniques, were jointly recognized "for discoveries concerning the peptide hormones of the brain." These pioneers led the way in neuropeptide research with the isolation and characterization of the first brain peptide, a three–amino acid chain of glutamate-histidine-proline, commonly called thyrotrophin releasing hormone (TRH).

TRH initiates the cascade of events that induces the thyroid gland to secrete thyroxine and thereby to increase the body's metabolic arousal, but it is also expressed in widespread neural systems of the brain. Many peptide systems have now been discovered; their historical progression is summarized in Figure 6.3. Many of the peptides that were first identified as hormones of the body (e.g., oxytocin, vasopressin, prolactin, angiotensin, and ACTH) have now been found to be transmitters or modulators within brain circuits. Discovering their psychoneural functions is one of the most exciting current chapters of brain research. They are especially important for emotion research since some, especially the endogenous opioid peptides, are already known to modify feeling states in humans and corresponding behavioral changes in animals.

Logically, it could have been possible for evolution to build brains that relied on a single transmitter, just

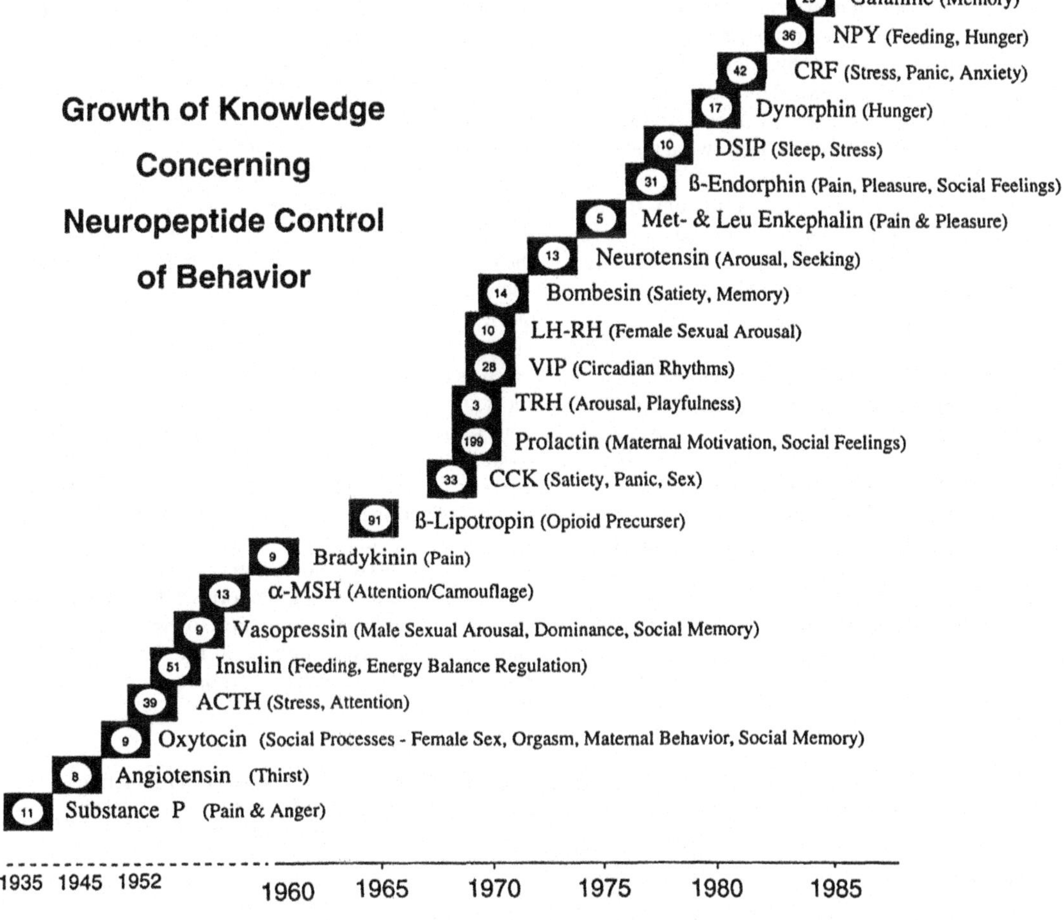

Figure 6.3. Time line of the discovery of major neuropeptides that participate in various brain functions related to the control of behavior and various emotional and motivational processes. Progress was slow in the beginning (dotted line) but sped up enormously around 1970. The numbers inside squares indicate the number of amino acids in each of these neuropeptides.

as computers are based on a single, electrical type of information carrier. To some extent that did in fact happen, because simple amino acid transmitters such as GABA and glutamate do participate in every behavioral, physiological, and cognitive process that has been studied. However, evolution has also created a vast number of neurochemical languages whose functional codes, most of them still undeciphered, are beginning to provide special avenues of insight into brain/mind interrelationships. There is a great deal of neuropeptide specificity in the coding of behavior, and it is esthetically pleasing to note that we often observe a correspondence between the peripheral functions of these neuropeptides and their role within the brain (Table 6.1). For instance, in the periphery, insulin controls metabolic dispersion of nutrients, while in the brain it helps mediate satiety (see Chapter 9). Likewise, in the periphery, the hormone angiotensin promotes water retention in the kidney, while in the brain it promotes thirst. Thus, many neuropeptide languages highlight the tendency of evolution to reutilize existing elements for new tasks that are harmonious with previous functions. However, this useful principle is a double-edged sword that needs to be wielded carefully.

When evolution uses existing functions for new purposes, the end result is typically called an *exaptation.* For instance, the use of gill arches to construct jawbones was such a transition. The use of some of those bones to construct the inner ear is another classic example. Thus, adaptations are exaptations if one can demonstrate an evolutionary progression based on the transformation of preexisting parts to new uses. Obviously, this issue can be a troublesome one for deriving functions by arguments of homology. Although we cannot do much about this potential dilemma, we should always remain alert to the possibility that what we might be tempted to interpret as a functional homology might actually be an exaptation that is far removed from the ancestral function. If that is the case, no special cross-species functional generalization can be derived. Thus, arguments by homology must always be evaluated empirically. Although it is common for exaptation to yield more complex functions, in the molecular realm it often yields diversification and simplification of preexisting parts.

Many of the larger proteins and peptides can be broken down into smaller fragments, some of which may retain neural activity, in a process called *posttranslational processing*. This may eventually prove important for understanding how moods are modulated by molecular events. There is some evidence that a molecule with one function can yield a molecular fragment with new functions, sometimes related to the old function, sometimes not. For instance, oxytocin, which mediates various pro-social processes, including maternal behavior and the inhibition of separation distress (Chapters 12 to 14), can yield a tripeptide called PLG (proline-leucine-glycine), which mediates none of the above but has antidepressant effects.[5] From one perspective, one might say there is no continuity between these functions; from another, one might argue that since depression is most commonly precipitated by social loss, the antidepressant effect of PLG is congruent with the brain functions of oxytocin. In short, there are bound to be many surprises in such analyses, and because the fertility of logic is always constrained by the truth of our premises, we will be able to twist our reasoning to either detect or deny various evolutionary relationships. Since the bottom line is that we simply cannot go back to trace such historical paths of inheritance, our evolutionary stories are useful only to the extent that they can generate fruitful empirical predictions.

Among recent neurochemical surprises, perhaps the most unexpected has been the identification of the gaseous transmitters such as *carbon monoxide* and *nitric oxide* (which, please note, is not the same as "laughing gas," or nitrous oxide). Nitric oxide has a remarkable number of peripheral functions, from promoting breathing to blood circulation. In the brain, the hottest idea is that such gaseous transmitters may be especially important for the elaboration of memories.[6] Besides conveying information in the brain, nitric oxide is quite toxic in excess and may participate in the development of various neurodegenerative disorders such as Alzhei-

Table 6.1. Relationships between Some Neuropeptides and Their Peripheral and Central Functions

Peptide	Peripheral Function	Central Function
Angiotensin	Control of blood pressure	Thirst and water intake
LH-RH	Preparation of sex hormones	Sexual readiness
Oxytocin	Birthing and milk letdown	Maternal acceptance and readiness
CRF	Activate adrenal stress response	Central elaboration of stress
α-MSH	Dispersion of pigment for camouflage	Hiding, fear and attention
TRH	Metabolic arousal	Brain arousal, play (?)
Vasopressin	Kidney water retention	Memory retention Behavioral persistence Male sexual behavior
Somatostatin	Inhibit growth hormone	Inhibit all behavior

mer's disease. Thus, what is good in small quantities may be harmful to the brain in large amounts.

Another neurotransmitter that is neurotoxic in excess is the simple amino acid *glutamate*. Glutamate is also important for the proper mediation of memory and cognitive processes, but being the single most important excitatory transmitter in the brain, it is actually involved in everything an organism does. However, when secreted in excessive amounts, it damages receptive neurons. This may be one of the causes of such neuropsychiatric disorders as Huntington's disease. Such findings may soon be translated into new treatments for people with related brain problems.[7] In animal models, some effects of stroke can already be alleviated with glutamate receptor antagonists, and it is possible that administration of such drugs at the right time can forestall the onset of Huntington's disease. However, more recently investigators have also found that underactivity in this system may be neurotoxic, producing brain damage that resembles the changes seen in schizophrenia.[8] With these powerful molecules, medicine will have to carefully weigh the costs and benefits that can be produced by different doses of the available glutamatergic agents.

Let me close this section by making some general comments about the many drugs that are currently used to modify neurochemical systems. We now have a great number of agents, especially for the nonpeptide transmitters, to modify various neurochemical processes at virtually all stages of synaptic transmission: Some drugs modify synthesis, degradation, and actions of transmitters at receptors. Others modify vesicular packaging of transmitters, synaptic reuptake/transporter mechanisms, and the efficacy of transmitters when they act upon postsynaptic as well as presynaptic receptors. Nonetheless, most of the brain neuropeptide systems that elaborate emotions and moods cannot yet be manipulated with synthetic drugs. Given orally, most peptides are digested like meat, and so do not enter the brain.[9] Even if they gain access to the bloodstream by injection, they usually have considerable difficulty passing through the various blood-brain barriers (BBBs) that control the flow of molecules from the circulation into the brain. Indeed, this shielding of the brain from circulating molecules is true for most other transmitters, including serotonin, dopamine, and norepinephrine. Thus, the search for new pharmaceuticals that imitate the effects of neuropeptides and are sufficiently lipid-scluble to gain entry into the brain is an active area of inquiry.

Nature has already provided us with some molecules of this type. Certain well-known alkaloid drugs, such as morphine and heroin, derive their power over human and animal feelings by interacting with a specific type of peptide receptor, the *mu*-receptor, that normally receives messages from the endogenous brain opioid *ß-endorphin*. In other words, morphine and heroin, which are chemically different from opioid peptides, mimic these endogenous addictive molecules.[10]

Because of the great medical and societal interest in opiate addiction, molecules have also been developed, such as naloxone and naltrexone, that block the *mu* receptor and hence block the rewarding effects of opiates. Because of the availability of such receptor antagonists, we now have considerable evidence that opioids participate in pleasure and related emotional processes of the mammalian brain. As we will see in Chapters 8 and 14, brain opioids promote the development of food and social preferences. However, there are no drugs that can activate most other neuropeptide systems following peripheral administration. In the absence of such pharmacological tools, practically the only way to study neuropeptide functions is to observe physiological and behavioral changes following direct placement into brain tissue. Consequently, animal research remains essential for understanding the role of these interesting molecules.

On the Neurochemical Coding of Psychobehavioral Processes

Psychobiologists are interested not only in discovering functions within specific brain areas but also in identifying the trajectories and neurochemical characteristics of the underlying circuits. Since all brain functions are ultimately subserved by chemically controlled changes in interneuronal communication, it is crucial to delineate the functions of the many neurotransmitter systems that exist in the brain. The chemical coding of specific brain processes will eventually provide many useful ways to manipulate brain substrates for beneficial medical and, no doubt, questionable recreational and cosmetic ends.[11]

A perplexing feature of psychopharmacological research has been the remarkably wide spectrum of behavioral and physiological effects that certain drugs exert. It is not uncommon for a single neurochemical system, or a single psychoactive drug, to have effects on nearly every behavior that is measured. For instance, the list of behavioral functions that brain serotonin does *not* modify is very short, containing no items, whereas the list of functions serotonin *does* affect includes everything the animal does.[12] Essentially the same conclusion holds for ACh, dopamine (DA), norepinephrine (NE), glutamate, and GABA. This indicates that many transmitters can exert global effects on brain and psychological functions, but there are some consistent patterns with regard to the direction of change. For instance, facilitation of serotonin typically suppresses behavior, while drugs that promote DA, NE, and ACh activity typically facilitate behaviors. As would be expected of molecules that modify moods and emotions, such changes modify everything an animal does. By comparison, steroid and peptide neuromodulators often have more precise behavioral and emotional effects,[13] even though it must be remembered that specific emotional changes can often produce a diversity of secondary consequences.

To make conceptual sense of such wide-ranging effects, we may occasionally need to climb to higher theoretical ground from which a panoramic overview can help put things in perspective.[14] Although this approach involves the ever-present danger of oversimplifying complex issues, it has the advantage of offering clear and testable behavioral predictions that may be interfaced with psychological concepts. To some extent, theoretical risk taking is essential for advancing our understanding of brain functions. Following this factual summary of neurochemical systems, I will devote the rest of the book to such neurotheoretical conceptualizations.

Neurochemical Systematics

For organizational purposes, I will categorize brain *neurotransmitter systems*[15] into four categories: (1) amino acids that undergo only minor modification when employed as transmitters, (2) the enzymatically modified amino acids, known as the *biogenic amines*, (3) the chains of amino acids known as neuropeptides, and (4) a miscellaneous group including ACh and a variety of other items. For instance, as mentioned, there are gaseous transmitters, ones that may emerge from fatty acids, and it remains possible that certain common metabolic intermediaries such as glucose may also participate in information transmission in the brain.[16] These latter items will not receive much attention here, since most do not yet interface clearly with emotional issues.

1. The simplest, and perhaps most abundant, items are the amino acid transmitters. The main excitatory transmitter, whose task is to initiate neuronal firing, is *glutamate*, essentially the same substance commonly used to add flavor to foods, especially in oriental cooking. There is reason to believe it participates in virtually all brain functions, with memory being the focus of much current research.[17] It is tempting to speculate that in the "primordial soup" in which life on earth presumably originated, glutamate was one of the most useful and abundant nutrients available. Early cells developed a sense for it, a "taste" if you will, which eventually allowed it to serve as a neurotransmitter in brain circuits. Glutamate is the most common and abundant excitatory transmitter in the mammalian brain, and it is usually synthesized from the precursor amino acid, glutamine. Conversely, its metabolic product, GABA, is the most abundant inhibitory transmitter in the brain, and it functions as widely as glutamate. However, in contrast to glutamate, which is abundant throughout the body, GABA is not a widely distributed amino acid, essentially existing only within the brain. There it is synthesized from glutamate via a single decarboxylation step that is mediated by the enzyme *glutamic acid decarboxylase*. Because of this tight metabolic interconnection between brain glutamate and GABA, brain inhibition and excitation can be efficiently balanced through the regulation of the intervening enzyme.[18]

Because these amino acid transmitters are so widely distributed in the brain and participate in so many vital functions, they are difficult to study using peripheral administration of pharmaceutical agents—simply too many behavioral functions are disrupted to obtain meaningful results. Following peripheral administration, many of these amino acids are excluded by various BBBs from entering into brain functions.[19] Thus, much of the functional information about these amino acids has to be obtained by direct manipulation of local brain systems (i.e., by microinjection of these agents into specific brain areas via small cannulae) or through the administration of specific amino acid receptor antagonists.

2. A second series of well-studied transmitters consists of enzymatically modified amino acids called *biogenic amines*. In addition to a variety of trace amines and histamine, the most prominent transmitters of this class are DA, NE, and serotonin (which is commonly called 5-HT because of its chemical name 5-hydroxytryptamine). The first two are derived from the six-carbon ring of tyrosine, a catechol-type structure, and hence, as a subclass, are called *catecholamines*. Serotonin, on the other hand, is derived from the double-ring, or indole, structure of tryptophan and hence is called an *indoleamine*. The specific molding that these precursor amino acids must undergo to become neurotransmitters is summarized in Figure 6.4. For both catecholamines and indoleamines, the first step is hydroxylation through the addition of an OH group, yielding L-DOPA and 5-HTP, respectively, followed by decarboxylation through the removal of a COOH group, yielding DA and 5-HT, respectively. In certain neurons, DA can be further processed into NE via another hydroxylation that is mediated by an enzyme called *dopamine-ß-hydroxylase*, or *DßH*. It is the presence of this last enzyme that makes a DA-synthesizing neuron an NE neuron! Thus, when NE synthesis is inhibited with *DßH* inhibitors, NE neurons become DA neurons until the enzyme inhibitor wears off. In two groups of neurons of the lower brain stem, NE can be further converted into epinephrine by the addition of a methyl group. However, epinephrine is a comparatively minor transmitter in the brain, although it is secreted abundantly in the periphery by the adrenal medulla, serving as a major stress hormone that recruits metabolic resources from liver glycogen stores. In the brain it seems to have a similar effect—dramatically increasing intracellular energy utilization.

As with the amino acid transmitters, brain levels of biogenic amines cannot be effectively modified by peripheral administration of those transmitters; however, the first two precursors in the metabolic chain, namely, L-DOPA and 5-HTP (see Figure 6.4), can cross the BBB and, under appropriate conditions, do increase transmitter synthesis. This is called the *precursor loading strategy*, and it is especially effective in neurological disorders such as Parkinson's disease, in which DA neurons have started to degenerate more rapidly than normal.[20] Administration of L-DOPA can restore lost functions. However, one might ask how DA restoration could occur if the relevant DA neurons have degenerated. One potential explanation is that following administration of L-DOPA, serotonin neurons, whose axons reach the same locations as those of DA neurons, begin to manufacture DA. This may be due to the fact that the decarboxylation—the second step in both DA and 5-HT synthesis—is mediated by the same enzyme, namely, *aromatic amino acid decarboxylase*. Since L-DOPA can cross the BBB and is taken up by serotonin cells, these cells begin to manufacture DA. This does not take place under ordinary circumstances because L-DOPA is manufactured only in dopamine cells and hence is not normally present in the circulation. By a similar flow of events, brain 5-HT can be increased by ingesting the immediate precursor 5-HTP, but again, 5-HT will now also be synthesized in catecholamine cells.

Can biogenic amines also be increased by giving the precursor amino acids? Yes, at least in the case of serotonin. Under normal physiological conditions, the availability of the precursor amino acid is the *rate-limiting step* for serotonin synthesis, which means we can increase brain 5-HT substantially through dietary consumption of tryptophan.[21] On the contrary, the availability of *tyrosine hydroxylase* is typically the rate-limiting step for catecholamine synthesis, which means that the precursor loading strategy typically does not produce substantial increases in brain levels of DA and NE under normal dietary circumstances. However, dietary deprivation of tyrosine, along with its precursor *phenylalanine*, can reduce brain catecholamine levels substantially. The same is true, of course, for tryptophan deprivation. In general, organisms that do not have enough tryptophan in their diet are hyperexcitable, while those without adequate tyrosine and phenylalanine are withdrawn and behaviorally sluggish.[22] Our ability to modify other neurochemistries by dietary means is an important way to control a variety of brain functions that can potentially increase the quality of life without the use of drugs.[23]

3. Third, there is an enormous group of peptide neurotransmitters/modulators made up of chains of amino acids that are typically cleaved from much larger "mother peptides." Prominent items in this group are (i) various brain opioids, such as the endorphins, enkephalins and dynorphins, all of which are derived from different genes; (ii) the various peptide hormones of the pituitary gland, namely, oxytocin, vasopressin,

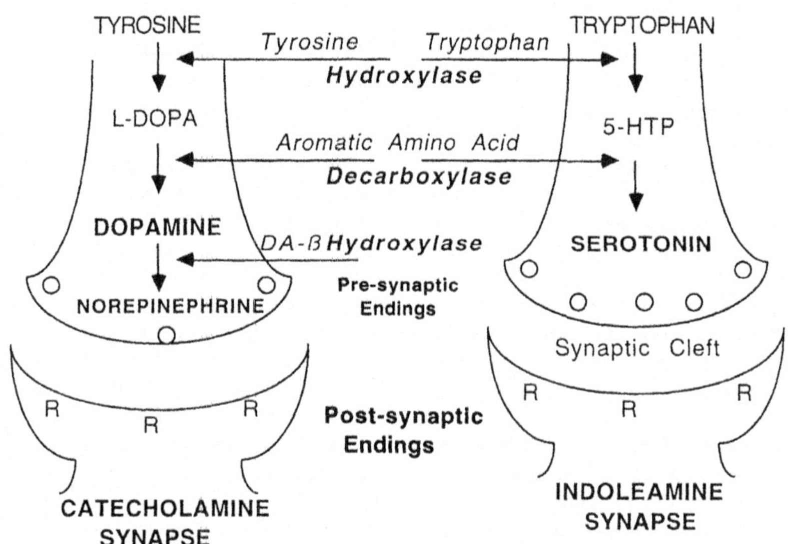

Figure 6.4. Summary of the synthesis of catecholamine transmitters (dopamine and norepinephrine) and the major brain indoleamine transmitter (serotonin). Both synthetic pathways start via the enzymatically mediated hydroxylation of the respective amino acid substrates (tyrosine and tryptophan), followed by a decarboxylation step that is mediated by a shared enzyme. Dopamine can be hydroxylated further to form norepinephrine. Since both L-dopa and 5-HTP can be taken up into neurons from the circulation, administration of these substrates can lead to the manufacture of serotonin in catecholamine neurons and the manufacture of dopamine in indoleamine neurons.

ACTH, and prolactin; (iii) various hypothalamic releasing agents—CRF, LH-RH, TRH—which control the release of pituitary hormones; (iv) various gastric peptides, including CCK, bombesin, and VIP; and (v) a large variety of other peptides, including several that have no clear peripheral functions, such as galanin, substance P, CGRP, NPY, and many others (for an explanation of abbreviations and dates of discovery, see Figure 6.3). The likelihood that discrete chemical coding of behavior exists for these substances is high (see Table 6.1).

In short, unlike the much smaller and more ubiquitous biogenic amines and amino acids, neuropeptides are the most promising candidates for mediating specific behavioral and psychological functions. Unfortunately, there is one great problem in studying their functions. Peptide systems cannot be readily manipulated by peripheral means. Peptides, like all other proteins, are typically broken down (digested) in the stomach and liver and do not enter the brain intact. Even if they could enter the bloodstream from the stomach (as some fragments do), most cannot pass through the BBB. However, it is noteworthy that some rather large peptides such as prolactin do have active uptake mechanisms from the circulation to the brain. In any event, to study the cerebral functions of most neuropeptides in intact organisms, one must administer them directly into the brain via cannulae, which essentially precludes meaningful work in humans, although in some instances intranasal administration can be used to circumvent these problems. However, because nature has created a few nonpeptide molecules with the required structural characteristics to act on the relevant brain receptors, some peptide systems can be modified by peripherally administered drugs. As already mentioned, the best-known examples are opiate alkaloids derived from the opium poppy (*Papaver somniferum*), which are absorbed from the periphery and exert effects similar to the endogenous brain opioid ß-endorphin.

As with all neurochemical systems, complexity is the rule rather than the exception. For instance, for the opioid peptides there are three distinct neurochemical families, the *endorphins*, *enkephalins*, and *dynorphins*, all of which emerge from larger peptides synthesized by specific genes. These opioid peptides have distinct brain distribution patterns and act upon different receptors, called *mu*, *delta*, and *kappa*, respectively.

4. Finally, there is a series of miscellaneous items, such as *acetylcholine*, that do not fall into any coherent category. Another such item would be the purine transmitter *adenosine*, which may be a natural sleep-promoting sedative system in the brain. Indeed, caffeinated drinks yield their arousal effects largely by blocking adenosine receptors, which are concentrated in the thalamus.[24] In addition, brain activity can be modulated by circulating steroids such as cortisol, testosterone, estrogen, and progesterone via specific receptor interactions.[25] It has also become clear that various fatty acid intermediates, such as prostaglandins, and immune system factors, such as interferons and cytokines, can modify brain activities.[26] There are undoubtedly many other neurochemical systems that remain to be identified in the vast menagerie of brain chemicals. Please remember that almost half the 100,000 types of genes that we possess are expressed within brain tissues. Even though only a small subset are information molecules, we have not yet come close to compiling an exhaustive list.

All known transmitter molecules generate their functional effects by interacting with specific receptor proteins concentrated in synaptic zones. This means that many psychoactive drugs produce their effects by taking advantage of the brain's natural information channels. Indeed, in those instances where powerful psychoactive drugs have long been derived from traditional plant sources (e.g., morphine, cocaine, caffeine, and nicotine), receptors for brain chemical systems have typically been discovered before the endogenous molecules that interact with those receptors. This sequence was first exemplified by the discovery of opioid receptors in 1972 and of the endogenous neuromodulators, or ligands, for those receptors in 1975.[27] Comparable success was soon achieved for the receptors upon which psychostimulants such as amphetamine and cocaine act, and they have now turned out to be ones that control DA reuptake into presynaptic endings.[28] However, the identification of the endogenous molecules, or ligands, that act on other "drug receptors," such as those that receive antianxiety drugs of the benzodiazepine class, or the "angel dust" and marijuana receptors, have been more tortuous scientific journeys.[29]

More recently, thanks to advances in biochemistry, many peptide transmitter systems have been identified prior to the receptors for those systems. The discovery of such transmitters in the brain has typically been made possible through powerful general-purpose tools such as *immunocytochemistry*, which can be used to localize all peptides within the brain.[30] The localization of neurochemical systems in the brain not only provides basic information concerning the anatomical organization of those systems themselves, but scientists can also obtain useful clues concerning the potential functions of those neurotransmitters from anatomical patterns. Comparable techniques exist for the identification of receptor fields within the brain. This is typically achieved via the autoradiographic analysis of the regional brain binding of radioactive forms of the various transmitter agents.

The images generated in this way are enormously complex and remarkably beautiful. Accurate analysis of how the various neurochemical systems participate in psychological functions is obviously very difficult. Other techniques that can be used to estimate neurotransmitter utilization in the behaving animal will be summarized at the end of this chapter. First, however, I will provide a synopsis of the general anatomies and psychobehavioral functions of the key neurochemical systems of the mammalian brain.

Acetylcholine: An Attentional/Action System

As already mentioned, ACh was the first neurotransmitter to be identified. This discovery occurred when investigators were still debating whether neurons communicated with each other directly via electrical changes, as argued by proponents of the "spark school," or via chemical intermediaries, as proposed by adherents of the "soup school." In Berlin, Otto Loewi used remarkably simple methods to demonstrate that the theory of chemical transmission was the more substantive hypothesis. He found that electrical stimulation of the vagus nerve in frogs reduced heart rate by means of a chemical intermediary. In an elegant cross-perfusion experiment, Loewi was able to transfer a heart rate–lowering factor from one heart to another via an aqueous medium. He called this unknown material *Vagusstuffe* ("vagusstuff"), and Sir Henry Dale proceeded to demonstrate that the active ingredient was ACh. However, now it is also known that some synapses are strictly electrical, requiring no chemical intermediary, but they are quite rare.[31]

The definitive anatomical mapping of ACh systems has been achieved by immunocytochemical approaches directed toward its synthetic and degradative enzymes. Immunocytochemical analysis of choline acetyltransferase (ChAT) activity is generally deemed to provide the more definitive maps because the breakdown enzyme, cholinesterase, is also contained in non-ACh neurons. This work has indicated that discrete ACh nuclei exist throughout the nervous system—from small cells scattered around the cortex to clusters of long-axoned ones in the basal forebrain and various brain stem areas. For the present purposes, we will consider only the six largest ACh neuronal groups in the brain (Figure 6.5)—four in the basal forebrain that control cortical and hippocampal functions, and two in the midbrain that control thalamic and hypothalamic functions.[32] The distribution of *cholinergic* (Ch) receptors in the brain is even more widespread.[33]

Cholinergic (which is a shorthand way of saying that

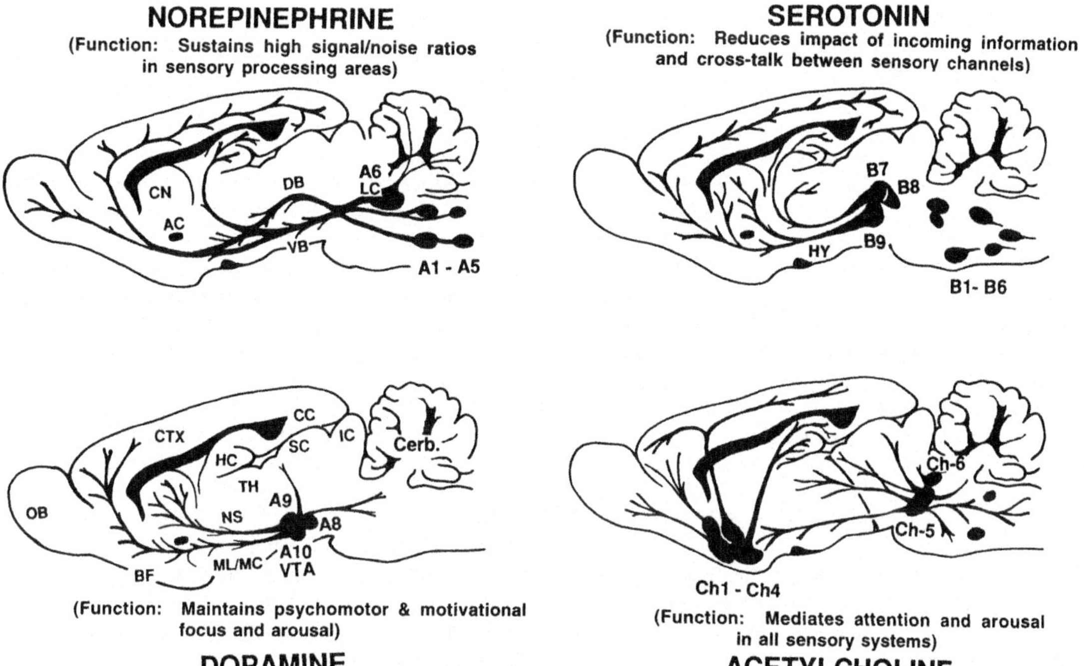

Figure 6.5. Parasaggital depictions of the dispersions of acetylcholine and biogenic amine (dopamine, norepinephrine, and serotonin) systems in the rat brain. LC: locus coeruleus; DB: dorsal noradrenergic bundle; VB: ventral noradrenergic bundle; CN: caudate nucleus; AC: anterior commissure; OB: olfactory bulb; CTX: cortex; BF: basal forebrain; HC: hippocampus; TH: thalamus; SC: superior colliculus; IC: inferior colliculus; NS: nigrostriatal pathway; ML/MC: mesolimbic and mesocortical pathways; HY: hypothalamus. "A" designations indicate major norepinephrine and dopamine cell groups; "B" designations indicate major serotonin/raphe cell groups; "Ch" designations indicate major cholinergic cell groups.

something is related to ACh) systems have the ability to control much of the brain's activity and appear to be executive systems for broad psychobehavioral functions such as waking and attention. There are six major cholinergic cell groups, designated Ch-1 to Ch-6, with many other more sparsely localized cells through many other parts of the brain. One high-density cluster in the basal forebrain (Ch-4) extends its axons throughout the cortex and is especially important for sustaining higher information processing. This system, along with other nearby ACh neuron clusters, commonly degenerates in Alzheimer's disease. The two major cell clusters in the mesencephalon (Ch-5 and Ch-6) facilitate thalamic information processing. In addition, most of the major somatic motor nuclei of the lower brain stem, such as that of cranial nerve V, the trigeminal nerve, which controls biting, clenching, and chewing, as well as cranial nerve VII, which controls facial movements, exhibit high-density cholinergic innervation. Scattered ACh neurons within the pontine reticular fields appear to contribute to the regulation of vigilance states, especially the onset and EEG arousal of REM sleep, via long ascending pathways to reticular fields of the thalamus and hypothalamus. Many smaller cell groupings, such as the small interneurons scattered throughout the striatum and cortex, appear to provide local control over more discrete functions, presumably local arousal processes of these brain areas.

Because of their widespread distributions, one can appreciate the difficulties in ascribing unitary behavioral functions to ACh systems. This is why pharmacological studies, in which drugs that modify cholinergic systems are given systemically, yield such a wide array of behavioral effects that they are difficult to interpret with a single concept. Still, most investigators agree that the neuropsychological constructs that best subsume cholinergic functions are attention or arousal. Further, it is also a system that facilitates action tendencies. When placed in specific subareas of the brain, ACh (or longer-acting cholinergic drugs, such as carbachol, which simulate ACh effects) can provoke numerous forms of behavioral arousal such as increased aggression, drinking, and vocalization.[34] Administration of *muscarinic* ACh receptor blockers, such as *atropine* or *scopolamine*, can reduce memory abilities, attention, and practically all forms of motivated behavior. On the other hand, if one blocks peripheral nicotinic receptors, the predominant variety of ACh receptor found at neuromuscular junctions, by administration of curare (the South American Indian dart poison), a flaccid paralysis develops rapidly. Death soon follows unless artificial respiration is provided. There is now abundant evidence that the nicotine consumed during smoking can also facilitate cerebral information processing, and this may be one reason people become addicted to cigarettes.[35]

After being released into the synapse, ACh is broken down into its precursors by cholinesterase. Many insecticides and nerve gases used in chemical warfare work by inhibiting this enzyme, which would lead to a massive buildup of ACh, which could impair movement because of the induction of a rigid paralysis at nicotinic neuromuscular ACh receptors. Excessive ACh levels at muscarinic receptors precipitate many dangerous autonomic symptoms that can also lead to death. The antidote that soldiers carry for such emergencies is a drug to counteract excessive ACh activity—namely, atropine—which itself is a potent poison if taken in sufficient quantities. In other words, the strategy involves trying to balance the effect of one poison with another.

In the right amounts and under the right conditions, these dangerous drugs can be useful medicines. For instance, when my son was just 2 years old, he accidentally consumed many of the eye-catching red berries of the plant commonly known as deadly nightshade or belladonna. By the time we had taken him to the hospital to get his stomach pumped, his heart rate had increased substantially. He was also becoming delirious and exhibited a hot, dry flushing of the skin—all anticholinergic symptoms of belladonna poisoning. The active ingredient of the plant is scopolamine, which blocks muscarinic ACh receptors and can lead to a compensatory overarousal of the sympathetic nervous system. Following stomach pumping, the recommended antidote was the cholinesterase inhibitor physostigmine, which elevates endogenous ACh levels so the receptor blockade can be overcome. Of course, in the process of pitting of one poison against another, one must administer just the right dose to achieve the desired cholinergic balance. Accordingly, I kept an eagle eye on everything being done to help my son in our local emergency room. The nurses made a simple decimal-point error and were about to inject my son with ten times the dosage his pediatrician had prescribed by phone. Standing firm against the nurse's insistence that I should behave as a passive bystander, I vehemently objected to their injecting my son with the amount that was in the syringe. Finally, they agreed to recalculate and quickly discovered their error. If I had not been there with the type of knowledge contained in this chapter, and experience with simple dose computations, my son might have died.

A small amount of physostigmine can also be a good medicine in various disorders where there is not enough ACh activity in the nervous system—for instance, myasthenia gravis, a disease characterized by abnormally rapid development of muscular weakness and fatigue during the course of the day. Eventually, affected individuals even have difficulty swallowing and commonly die from suffocation. We now know that this is an autoimmune disease, in which an individual generates antibodies to his or her own nicotinic ACh receptors, the receptors that mediate all of our skeletal-muscular movements.[36] Physostigmine can improve motor abilities by making more ACh available at these understaffed synapses. Likewise, Alzheimer's disease is partly due to the destruction of ACh systems in the brain (Ch-1 to Ch-4), and thus it is not surprising that physostigmine, and other more modern cholineserase inhibitors such as Tacrin® (which is approved for the treatment of Alzheimer's), can improve memory in these individuals, since it allows their low ACh levels to be stretched farther. Unfortunately, such drugs are rather short-acting and have many side effects. A more promising avenue for treating this devastating brain disorder is to find a molecule that can stimulate the relevant ACh receptors, which remain intact even though their presynaptic elements have degenerated. Animal data indicate that one specific subtype of muscarinic receptor must be targeted for extra stimulation, namely, the M1 variety.[37] Although there are now many experimental drugs available that can selectively activate the M1 ACh receptor, considerable testing still needs to be completed before they can be made available for human use.

Biogenic Amines: Central State Attentional Controls

The revolution in biological psychiatry of the past 40 years has been based, more than anything else, on the discovery of drugs that affect brain DA, NE, 5-HT, and the less well understood histamine systems, which, as already mentioned, are collectively called the biogenic amines. The metabolic and neural pathways that operate via these biogenic amines are now well understood, and we have a vast number of drugs to manipulate them rather precisely. Daniel Bovet received a Nobel Prize in 1957 for his seminal work on the development of drugs that affect these systems. In 1970, Julius Axelrod became a Nobel laureate for his detailed work on how the nerve terminals of biogenic amine systems operate. Thanks to these and other investigators, our detailed understanding of these systems is impressive, and we have excellent ideas to explain why many of these drugs help people with psychiatric problems. For instance, antipsychotic drugs reduce activity in DA systems, various antidepressants can increase synaptic activity of all three systems, and the antimanic drug lithium may exert its effect by regulating excessive brain NE activity. However, it must be remembered that most drugs have several effects on the brain, and it is sometimes difficult to sift the true therapeutic causes from the many other effects.[38] For the present purposes, however, let us consider the catecholamines and indoleamines separately, since they appear to exert functionally antagonistic effects on the brain.

Central Catecholamines: Arousal Systems of the Brain

In the previous chapter, I described some aspects of the organization of brain DA systems. DA is just one of a triumvirate of related transmitters that arise in sequence from the amino acid tyrosine (Figure 6.2). NE and epinephrine are the other major transmitters. The striking anatomical organization of catecholamine systems was first revealed in the 1960s by a group of Swedish histochemists who developed fluorescent procedures for highlighting the location of these transmitters in the brain. Their results were fully confirmed by subsequent immunohistochemical studies on the various synthetic enzymes (e.g., tyrosine hydroxylase and dopamine-ß-hydroxylase). Up to 15 discrete NE and DA cell groups, designated A1 to A17, have been discovered, scattered like islands in an archipelago, from the lower to upper reaches of the hypothalamus, with A16 being in the olfactory bulbs and A17 in the retina (which is still part of the central nervous system). The lower ones (A1 to A7) contain NE, and all the higher ones contain DA. Finally, the two lowermost catecholamine cell groups (designated C1 and C2) contain epinephrine. Each of these nuclei contains anywhere from a thousand to several thousand neurons. It has been estimated that the total number of DA neurons in the rat brain may be about 20,000, while the NE groups have only about a quarter of that number. However, these small numbers belie their influence, which is remarkably widespread in the brain.

Since some of the most rostral and caudal cell groups are quite small, I will focus on the larger ones, with long axons that control much of the brain's activity, which are situated from the pons to the caudal hypothalamus. These cell groups, from A6 to A10, transmit information to many areas of the brain (Figure 6.5). The three rostral nuclei of this intermediary group manufacture DA, and there are two especially famous regions there. The most lateral one, A9, which arises from the part of the midbrain known as the *substantia nigra pars compacta*, send axons largely to the dorsal striatum (caudate nuclei) via the nigrostriatal tract. The more medial group, A10, which is part of the *ventral tegmental area* (VTA), innervates the ventral striatum (nucleus accumbens) and frontal cortex via the *mesolimbic* and *mesocortical* tracts, respectively. Compared with DA systems, which restrict their outputs to the reptilian brain (i.e., the basal ganglia) and frontal cortex, the projections of the caudally situated NE systems are more widespread.

The ability of these systems to control widespread areas of the brain is especially well highlighted by the best-known NE cell group, the *locus coeruleus*, the A6 cell group, which controls higher brain activity via the *dorsal NE pathway*. This group sends inputs to the cortex, hypothalamus, cerebellum, lower brain stem, and spinal cord—exerting global control over brain activity. The more caudal groups innervate the hypothalamus and limbic system via a *ventral NE pathway*. As far as we know, all of these neurons contain internal pacemaker mechanisms to maintain spontaneous activity requiring no incoming influences.[39] This does not mean they are unresponsive to input. For instance, NE cells are exquisitely sensitive to environmental stimuli, especially powerful emotional events.[40] Clearly, these brain systems control holistic aspects of brain functioning rather than discrete behavioral processes. Accordingly, their functions are better expressed in psychoneural rather than mere behavioral terms.

It is tempting to speculate that epinephrine may have been the first catecholamine to have a major neural function since it is situated in the lowermost, primitive parts of the brain, and its axonal influence only reaches up to the hypothalamic level. On the basis of the assumption that more caudal structures are more ancient, it is reasonable to assume that the evolution of NE neurons preceded the evolution of those that contain DA. As summarized schematically in Figure 6.6, a functional theme seems evident in the evolutionary progression of this system, reflecting, once again, the tendency of natural selection to adapt, or more precisely *exapt*, preexisting parts to new functions. Since one of the major peripheral functions of epinephrine is to control the rate of metabolism (it is one of the most powerful hormones to stoke up the intracellular furnace by increasing breakdown of glycogen and oxidative metabolism), the functions of NE and DA may reflect successive refinements on this ancient arousal function. Existing evidence suggests that NE promotes sensory arousal, while DA promotes motor arousal.[41] As we would expect from such functional considerations, NE terminals are concentrated in sensory projection areas of the cortex, while DA terminals are more prominent in motor areas.[42]

In short, these systems mediate the alerting, arousal, and efficiency of information processing. In this role, catecholamines probably influence performance in a classic inverted U-shaped fashion: Behavior increases from the initial point of arousal up to a certain level and then diminishes as excessive arousal begins to preclude behavioral flexibility. This relationship is commonly called the *Yerkes-Dodson law*.[43] Thus, with excessive DA activity, animals begin to exhibit repetitive behavior patterns known as *stereotypies*; with low NE activity, they tend to perseverate on a task despite changes in stimulus contingencies (presumably because of attentional deficits). Without adequate cortical NE, organisms are also prone to act impulsively rather than deliberately. The common childhood condition known as attention deficit disorder (ADD, or *hyperkinesis*, as it used to be called) is partly due to low brain NE activity. These children seem excessively active and unable to stay on task in classroom settings. For a long time it was perplexing that psychostimulants, such as amphetamines that can facilitate both NE and DA arousal in the brain, tend to reduce the hyperactivity of such children. How could an arousal-promoting drug reduce behavioral overactivity? The resolution of this apparent paradox is actually quite simple. The children have too little cortical arousal, which permits their subcortical emotional systems to govern behavior impulsively.[44] When cortical arousal is facilitated with psychostimulants, ADD children are able to better utilize their attentional abilities to stay on task. In other words, ADD kids resemble decorticate animals, which are also hyperactive

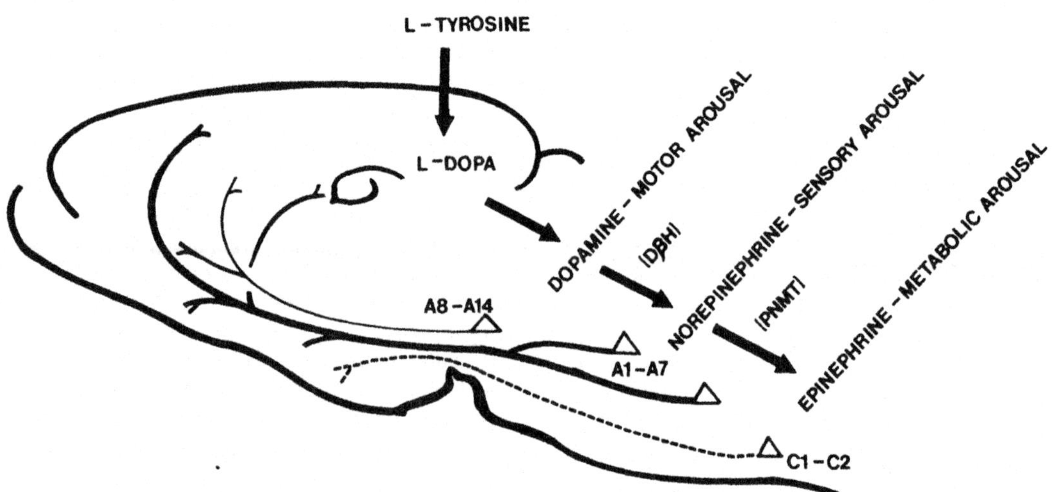

Figure 6.6. Schematic representation of the possible evolutionary progression of catecholamine arousal systems in the brain, with the most ancient epinephrine groups mediating metabolic arousal, the more recent norepinephrine cell groups mediating sensory arousal, and dopamine systems mediating psychomotor arousal. DßH: dopamine-ß-hydroxylase; PNMT: phenethylamine-N-methyl-transferase. (Adapted from Panksepp, 1981; see chap. 3, n. 25.)

and jump rapidly from one activity to another. Thus, we must always remember that behavioral arousal is not a unitary construct. It has many forms.

One might wonder at this juncture how arousal induced by ACh may differ from that which results from NE activity. Although the psychological answer is not yet clear, the neurophysiological one is becoming apparent. NE dampens the background "noise" or cortical neural activity irrelevant to a given task. This makes the influence of specific incoming signals more prominent in the cortex—namely, the ratio of the signal to background noise is increased.[45] On the other hand, ACh actually appears to be a gatekeeper for incoming sensory signals into the thalamus and cortex.[46] From this, one might expect that with high NE activity, organisms can better process information that already has access to the cortex, while high ACh activity might allow more information to come to bear on the solution to a problem. Under normal circumstances, both processes probably go together.

Indoleamines: Rest and Relaxation Systems of the Brain?

A detailed description of brain serotonin systems was also achieved first by the Swedish histochemists Falck and Hillarp, who first visualized the catecholamines. Their findings have now been amply confirmed and extended with immunohistochemical visualization of both serotonin and tryptophan hydroxylase. The neurons that manufacture serotonin are clustered in specific brain stem areas, and they have been divided into nine nuclei, which were given "B" designations. All serotonin nuclei are situated at the very midline (or seam) of the brain indicating that they are very ancient in brain evolution. They are generically called the *raphe nuclei* (which in French means "seam"). The axons of the lowermost cell groups (B1–B6) are restricted largely to the pons and medulla, with most of the pathways descending into the lower brain stem and spinal cord. B8 provides local controls to the midbrain as well as the cerebellum. Those systems will not receive much attention here. The more rostral systems, including B7, also called the *dorsal raphe nucleus*, and B9, the *medial raphe nucleus*, have extensive ascending axonal projections that parallel the ascending catecholamine projections and also control higher brain activities in rather global ways all the way from the midbrain throughout the higher reaches of the cortex. In general, B7, the dorsal raphe, tends to control dorsal brain activity in the hippocampus and neocortex, while B9 controls ventral brain activity in the hypothalamus, limbic system, and striatum. These neurons, just like NE ones, also have endogenous pacemakers, and their activity fluctuates systematically as a function of sleep-waking cycles (see "Afterthought," Chapter 7). Unlike NE cells, however, their activity is more modestly affected by environmental events, requiring quite stressful stimuli to jog them into a faster firing rate.[47]

There are good reasons to believe that this system mediates a relatively homogeneous central state function. All motivated and active emotional behaviors, including feeding, drinking, sex, aggression, play, and practically every other activity (except sleep), appear to be reduced as serotonergic activity increases.[48] However, the conclusion that serotonin mediates behavioral inhibition is tempered by the discovery of a vast diversity of distinct serotonin receptors. At this writing, the number of 5-HT receptors stands at 15. When serotonin acts on certain receptors, emotional behaviors such as anxiety (as measured by behavioral inhibition) increase, but when other receptors are involved, emotionality is reduced.[49] Why such complexity exists on the postsynaptic side, with comparative simplicity at the presynaptic side, remains perplexing. In other words, these systems release a single transmitter, 5-HT, rather globally in the brain, but this substance can operate on a vast number of receptors with apparently very different functional properties. One possible way to make sense of this is that at the various synaptic fields, serotonin release is also controlled by local presynaptic mechanisms (i.e., via axoaxonic synapses). Through such local controls, it is possible to have regionally restricted release of 5-HT onto only a subset of serotonin receptors.

The Neuropeptides: Systems for Psychobehavioral Specificity

At one time, neuroscience accepted a law, called *Dale's law,* which asserted that each neuron contains a single transmitter. Then it was discovered that many neurons contained the "classic" neurotransmitters, such as ACh and the biogenic amines, as well as a diversity of neuropeptides. Many of these colocalized neuropeptides may not be transmitters in the sense that they directly induce excitatory and inhibitory postsynaptic potentials. In other words, they do not directly control depolarization, which causes neuronal excitation, and hyperpolarization, which causes neuronal inhibition; rather, they may be modulators that control the intensity of neuronal responses. The discovery of the vast array of neuropeptide circuits has added a dramatic new dimension to our understanding of the chemical coding of behavior. For the first time, a series of neuroactive molecules truly appears to exert control over specific physiological and behavioral functions. Some have well-restricted anatomical trajectories, but many can affect widespread areas of the brain via *paracrine* routes, namely, by means of diffusion through brain tissue with the help of the ventricular system. I will focus on many neuropeptide systems throughout upcoming chapters. For now, let us simply introduce four systems that will figure prominently in our discussions. An overview of the anatomical dispersion of ß-endorphin, corticotrophin releasing factor (CRF), cholecystokinin (CCK), as well as a pair of related peptides known as oxytocin and vasopressin, is provided in Figure 6.7.

1. Most of the ß-endorphin within the brain arises from a clustered group of neurons within the medial hypothalamus. These neurons can also express α-melanocyte stimulating hormone (αMSH) and adrenocorticotrophic hormone (ACTH), which generally have behavioral effects diametrically opposite to those of ß-endorphin.[50] In other words, these hormones facilitate negative emotional arousal, while the endorphins reduce them. For an overview of opioid receptors, see Figure 6.8.

2. CRF neurons are concentrated in two nuclei, the paraventricular and supraoptic nuclei, which project to the anterior pituitary to control ACTH release from anterior pituitary cells. CRF axons emerge from these cells, as well as from many others scattered in the anterior hypothalamus/bed nucleus of the stria terminalis, and project throughout the medial periventricular areas of the brain stem. A high concentration of terminals is found on the NE cell group A6 (the locus coeruleus), where it promotes a general form of brain arousal. The ß-endorphin and CRF systems seem to have a yin-yang relationship in the brain. CRF activates a general stress response, with many specific emotional repercussions, whereas ß-endorphin promotes an anti-stress response and an overall calming of negative affective arousal.[51]

3. Quite specific social-emotional processes appear to be mediated by oxytocin and vasopressin. Oxytocin promotes a female-typical tone of calm nurturance, while vasopressin conveys a message of male sexual persistence and aggressive assertiveness (see Chapter 12). Along with ß-endorphin and CRF, these systems are prominent in specific subcortical areas of the brain but are poorly represented in the cortex.[52]

4. There are others, such as CCK, which operate prominently in both cortical and subcortical neuronal areas. This peptide, widely considered to be a satiety transmitter in the body, is now receiving considerable attention as a potential mediator of panic attacks (see Chapter 11).[53] This highlights the care we need to take in trying to interpret various behavioral effects. Surely

ß-ENDORPHIN

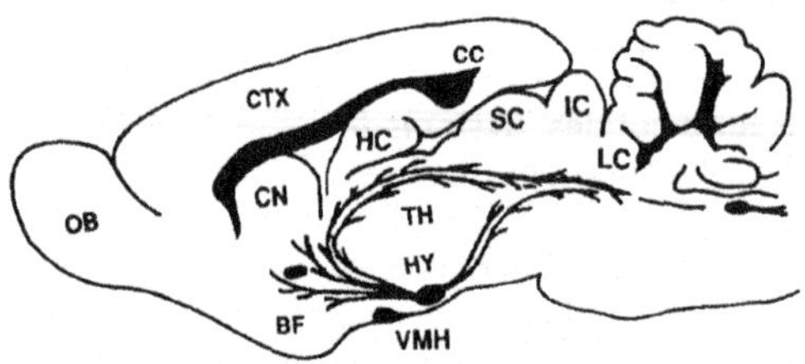

(Function: Counteracts homeostatic imbalances; creates pleasure)

CORTICOTROPHIN RELEASING FACTOR

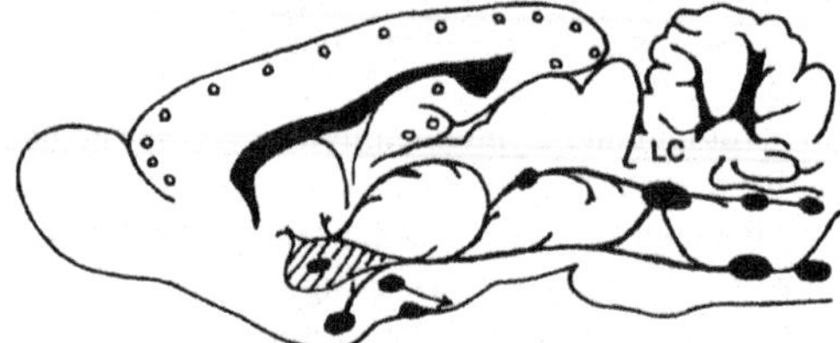

(Function: Promotes effects of stress and negative emotional stimuli)

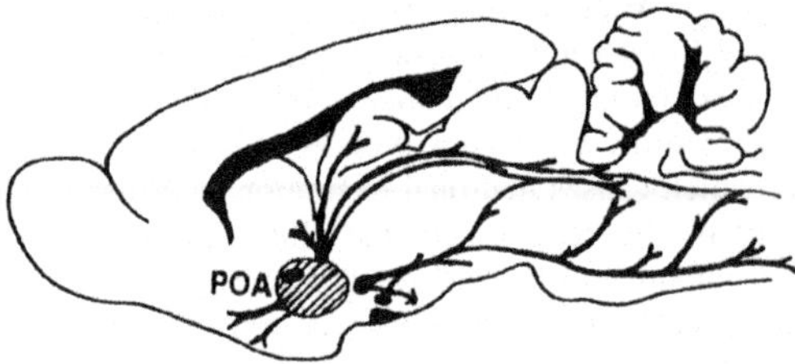

VASOPRESSIN/OXYTOCIN

(Functions: AVP promotes male-typical persistence; Oxytocin, female-type nurturance and acceptance)

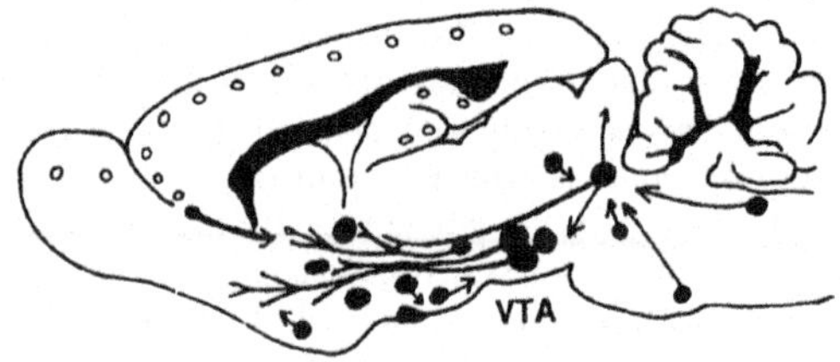

CHOLECYSTOKININ

(Functions: Regulation of emotional systems: feeding, sex, exploration, anxiety, and pain)

Figure 6.7. Parasaggital depiction of the dispersions of four major neuropeptide systems. LC: locus coeruleus; DB: dorsal noradrenergic bundle; VB: ventral noradrenergic bundle; CN: caudate nucleus; AC: anterior commissure; OB: olfactory bulb; CTX: cortex; BF: basal forebrain; HC: hippocampus; TH: thalamus; SC: superior colliculus; IC: inferior colliculus; CC: corpus callosum; POA: preoptic area; VTA: ventral tegmental area. Small circles in the cortex indicate the presence of local interneurons for CRF and cholecystokinin systems.

panic can reduce food intake without being a natural control system for energy regulation in the body. Thus, it is clear that we can easily misinterpret simple behavioral changes if we do not fully consider the affective nature of the animal mind!

Amino Acid Transmitters: Transmitters for the Basic Programs

The anatomies of simple amino acid transmitter systems—such as glutamate, aspartate, glycine, and GABA—have been quite difficult to study not only because they are widespread in the brain but also because most of the molecules participate in various aspects of general cellular metabolism. Since these transmitters appear to mediate a large number of essential behavioral and physiological processes in the brain, it is simply very difficult to study their functions in specific psychobehavioral systems using peripherally administered pharamacological agents.

For instance, glutamatergic transmission may be an essential ingredient in most incoming sensory systems. Also, descending glutamate systems from the whole neocortical mantle into the basal ganglia probably control every thought, every perception, and every emotional attribution that the brain can make. For several years, glutamate transmission through its various receptor subtypes (the main ones being NMDA [N-methyl-D-aspartic acid], kainate, and AMPA [α-amino-3-hydroxy-5-methylisoxasole-4-propionic acid]) has been the hottest neurochemical system for understanding learning, memory, and consciousness.

The simplest amino acid neurotransmitter is glycine, but unlike glutamate, it usually serves inhibitory functions in the brain. For instance, within the brain stem, glycine exerts inhibition over a wide range of motor processes. One of the most powerful ways to increase startle is to pretreat an animal with the glycine antagonist strychnine. A little more of this poison will cause convulsions. However, it is noteworthy that there is another glycine receptor in the brain, which functions in higher regions to control the intensity of glutamate transmission. This may prove to be an especially effective site for facilitating cognitive activity. A series of recent studies have found that high doses of glycine can ameliorate some of the cognitive disorganization that characterizes schizophrenia.[54]

Likewise, GABA is widely distributed in the brain. Indeed, it is the most common transmitter in inhibitory interneurons that exerts local homeostatic control within neuronal circuits. Small regional shifts in GABA inhibition may be one of the major ways specific behavior patterns and psychological functions may be selectively initiated in various parts of the brain. As with glycine, if we globally reduce GABA in the brain, animals exhibit seizures, and most antiseizure medications facilitate GABA activity. Thus, the most cogent way to study the role of GABA in specific behaviors would be via regional brain manipulation of GABA synaptic activities, by local intracerebral administration of drugs. For instance, blockade of GABA receptors within the hypothalamus can markedly increase fear,[55] but the same manipulation in most other brain areas will not. Indeed, this principle applies to all of the amino acid transmitters. One should be highly suspicious of psychobehavioral studies that employ peripherally administered agents that globally modify activity in these systems. This is simply not the way these brain systems normally operate, and hence they cannot be studied effectively using peripheral routes of drug administration. Only central administration into specific brain areas can clearly inform us about the normal mental, emotional, and behavioral functions of these transmitters. But even at such levels of analysis, the overlap of antagonistic psychobehavioral systems can make investigations difficult.

The Promise of New Molecules

In addition to the molecules that control the dynamic transfer of information in the brain, there is also a host of recently discovered molecules that establish the neural connections upon which information is transmitted on the complex neuronal highways and interconnections of the brain. These connections are sometimes grossly severed, as in spinal and head injuries, but there are also many children who are born with neurodevelopmental disorders in which brain disconnections are more subtle. Although the symptoms of some of these disorders can be ameliorated with medicines that act upon the neural systems already discussed, none can presently be adequately rectified. There is hope, but only hope, that some of these brain problems will eventually be treatable with new generations of medicines that act upon the biochemical systems that govern the growth of interconnections within the developing brain. Let me briefly discuss these molecules in the context of the childhood disorder known as autism, which is accompanied by complex cognitive and emotional problems, many of which arise from defects in the connectivities of the brain.

As recent work has clearly indicated, many children with autism have a brain disconnection syndrome, especially between cerebellar and limbic zones with other higher brain areas.[56] In other words, neural systems that should be working in close unison appear not to have developed normal synaptic interchange in various brain areas that control socialization, communication, and imagination. What might be able to restore the connections? Certainly no human surgeon is likely to ever have the skill to restitch the fine neural cloth of the brain, but there is now hope that we will eventually find molecules that might be able to do the job. The reason for optimism along these lines is the massive recent progress in identification of various growth factors and their receptors in the brain.

A class of molecules called *neurexins* are neural recognition molecules that exist as proteins on nerve membranes and help guide the construction of the nervous system.[57] During posttranslational processing of these proteins, thousands of variants may be created that could confer biochemical identities to various types of neurons. Another class of molecules called *netrins* provide guidance for the growth of axons.[58] Some of these molecules can also repel other axons, presumably to increase the likelihood that brain connections are made precisely.[59] But let us here focus on the *neurotrophins*, a class of nerve growth factors that seems most likely to enter clinical practice in the near future.

A series of complex peptide molecules have now been identified that govern the maturation and development of specific neural systems. They go by such fancy names as nerve growth factor (NGF), brain-derived neurotrophic factor (BDNF), epidermal growth factors, fibroblast growth factors, glial-derived growth factors, insulin-like growth factors, and many others. These molecules control very specific growth processes in the brain, and they can also protect neurons against various forms of toxicity. For instance, BDNF and NGF can protect cerebellar granule cells and Purkinje cells.[60] These are the types of neurons known to be deficient within cerebellar tissues of many autistic children, raising the possibility that certain growth factors may have been lacking during certain periods of development.

This remarkable episode in neuroscience started with the initial discovery, in the late 1940s, of a factor in neural tissue that could specifically promote growth of nerves of the autonomic nervous system. The pioneer was a young Italian scientist working at Washington University in Saint Louis during World War II, and the molecule she discovered was called nerve growth factor (NGF). Rita Levi-Montalcini was awarded the Nobel Prize for this work. NGF has already been used extensively to restore some function in damaged ACh systems of the animal brain (i.e., the systems that are especially deficient in Alzheimer's disease), but so far, therapeutic effects in human trials have been limited. Infusion of NGF into the brain of some Alzheimer's patients has led to modest restoration of function, but not of sufficient scope for that specific therapy to become routine. However, we now know that BDNF has a much stronger effect on the growth of those neurons than NGF and may prove to be more effective in treatment of Alzheimer's. In any event, the cholinergic targets for NGF are known to be important in all aspects of attention and cognition, and recent work suggests that many of the other neurotrophins modulate learning and memory in these circuits.[61]

It presently seems that each of the newly discovered nerve growth factors or neurotrophins exerts its effect on specific neural systems, many of them sensory ones that are known to be deficient in autistic disorders. Each of the NGF-like neurotrophins works through specific membrane receptors that share a family resemblance, and all operate through the so-called *Trk* (pronounced "track") receptors, because they are derived from the tyrosine kinase receptor superfamily. These include *TrkA*, which receives the NGF message; *TrkB*, which receives the BDNF and neurotrophin-4 messages; *TrkC*, which receives the neurotrophin-3 signal, and so forth.

One recent noteworthy feat is the biochemical construction of a pan-neurotrophin, which can interact with all three receptor sites,[62] but this peptide still has to be delivered directly into the brain to achieve broad-ranging nerve growth effects. An equally remarkable feat has been the production of various "knockout" mice in which the genes for each of these receptors have been deleted from their genetic libraries; the consequences have been thought-provoking for all of us who are interested in the possible sources of autistic disorders.

Mice missing these genes exhibit very specific neurological deficits, many of them resembling sensory problems commonly encountered in autistic children. For instance, mice missing the *TrkA, TrkB* , and *TrkC* genes grow up with severe pain sensitivity and somatosensory and auditory deficits.[63]

Could it be that autistic children have internal deficiencies in some of these growth factors? At this point we do not know, since the levels have never been measured (and for various reasons the assays are not presently feasible), but this is bound to be a productive line of inquiry. There is a reasonable chance that one day we will be able to treat the specific neurological problems of an autistic child with these miniature surgeons—or perhaps "architects" would be a better analogy. Researchers have recently developed permanent nerve growth factor delivery systems through gene transfer to carrier cells that can be transplanted into the brain to facilitate restoration of specific neurochemical systems, such as cholinergic innervation from the septal area to the hippocampus.[64]

None of this knowledge is yet close to clinical practice—certainly not for poorly understood disorders such as autism. The initial clinical trials will target disorders in which the underlying neuropathologies are reasonably well understood—disorders such as Alzheimer's, Huntington's, and Parkinson's diseases, and various rare single-gene genetic disorders in children. These powerful growth-control molecules must be studied more closely and then tamed before they help us restore health and normality to broken brains.

Currently, the best help we can provide for autistic children are various forms of education that can also increase neuronal plasticity in yet unknown ways. One of the oldest findings in the field is that sensory enrichment can increase cortical growth by increasing the size and number of neural interconnections.[65] It seems quite possible that scientifically yet unproven therapeutic approaches such as sensory integration therapy[66] and auditory integration training[67] exert many of their effects by stimulating various growth-promoting molecules to increased efforts on behalf of neural growth in the brains of autistic children. It is known that various neurotrophic growth effects in the brain are dependent on neuronal activity.[68] Although we do not yet know for a fact that neural plasticity and neural growth are promoted by rich sensory experiences in autistic children, the probability is so high that it is foolish for parents not to provide as much sensory-motor and related cognitive-affective stimulation for their children as is possible.

The extent to which the molecules described here exert effects on the growth of emotional systems in the brain remains unstudied. However, considering the fact that all other neural systems that have been studied, mostly within the somatic thalamic-neocortical axis, exhibit use-dependent changes, we can anticipate that specific growth-control molecules also exist for the various visceral emotional command circuits discussed in this text.

The Promise of New Neurochemical Techniques

Ultimately, the most definitive information about the neurochemical control of behavior has to emerge from our ability to specify which neurochemical systems are active in the brain under specific psychobehavioral circumstances. Accordingly, progress in our materialistic understanding of neuropsychic processes will depend on the development of new approaches to study neurochemical changes in living animals. Until recently, only pharmacological manipulations of living animals and measurement of neurochemistries in brain subareas of animals no longer living could afford a glimpse of how various brain chemistries control behavior. As already mentioned, refined assays can now be done using immunocytochemical procedures on thin tissue sections, which allow one to estimate whether specific cells have been involved in specific behaviors. In addition, recently developed techniques allow investigators to estimate the chemical changes that transpire between neurons within the living animal. Although some of these techniques are still being developed and refined, they are worth noting, for our future insights will depend largely on the wider-scale implementation of such experimental approaches.

Push-Pull Approaches

The first way investigators tried to determine what was being released at synaptic interfaces was by placing fine concentric double-barreled cannulae (essentially two stainless steel syringe needles, one inside the other) into specific parts of the brain and pushing in fluid through one channel while pulling out fluid at the same rate from the other channel. The recovered fluid was then assayed for levels of neuroactive molecules using any of a variety of analytic techniques, especially high-performance liquid chromatography (HPLC), which can readily segregate molecules of various sizes and electrical charges. In some more recent approaches, the collection of brain fluids is done through dialysis membranes, which consist of fine cellophane having very tiny pores that allow molecules of only a certain size to pass through into the collection fluids, simplifying the assay procedures.[69]

In Vivo Voltametry

Many neurotransmitters can be oxidized by the imposition of electrical currents, and the electrical potentials generated during such procedures can be used to identify which types of molecules are being released at the electrode sites. Although there has been much controversy over which molecules these techniques actually measure, they have recently become an especially effective tool for determining the conditions under which the biogenic amines are released within the brain. Some provocative results will be shared in Chapter 8.[70]

Subtractive Autoradiography

A technique that has not yet come into common use is the administration of radioactive transmitters or drugs, which bind to synaptic receptors in living animals as they perform certain behaviors, followed by autoradiography, in order to estimate whether levels of receptor binding vary as a function of the actions animals have performed.[71] The assumption is that if a specific brain chemical system is activated it should occupy a proportion of the available receptor sites, leaving fewer sites available for binding the externally administered ligand. Reduced binding would highlight zones of the brain where specific neurochemical systems were active.

A useful aspect of this approach, as well as the following one, is its ability to provide "snapshots" of changes throughout the brain. Serial sections, as depicted in Figure 6.8, indicate that opiate binding is widespread, which clearly indicates that brain opioids are involved in a large number of functions. Some key anatomical areas are highlighted in the figure for didactic purposes.

In Situ Hybridization

This has become a powerful technique for determining how the genetic expression of transmitters and other brain chemicals is modified by past experiences.[72] Ongoing genetic expression is a dynamic process, highly responsive to an animal's specific history. The technique relies on the availability of DNA *probes* that can

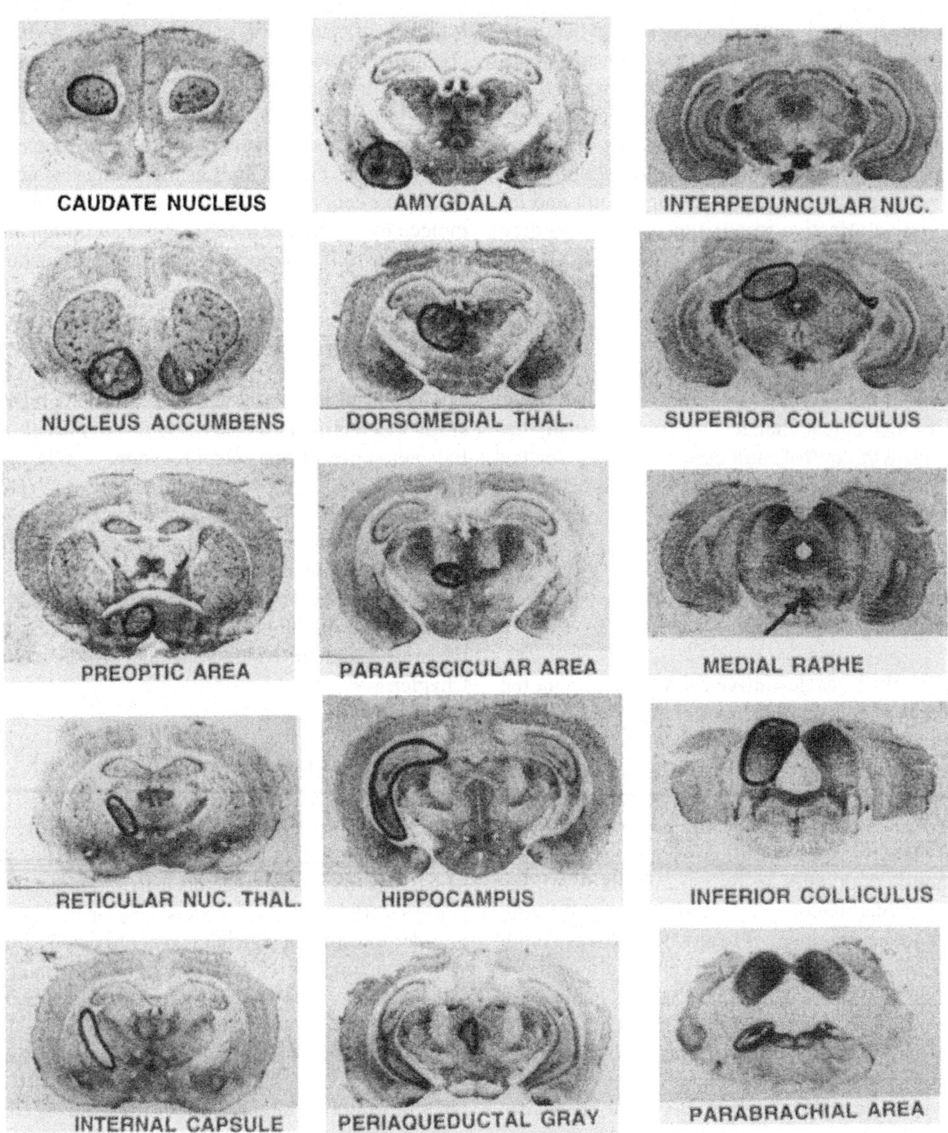

Figure 6.8. Frontal sections of autoradiographs depicting tritiated diprenorphine binding in the rat brain. The most anterior is the upper right, and the most posterior is the lower left. Can you find some of these brain areas on the other anatomical depictions in Chapter 4 (Figures 4.4, 4.8, and 4.10)? To help in using anatomical nomenclature, each section has one major brain area highlighted. (Adapted from Panksepp and Bishop, 1981; see n. 71.)

identify the location of corresponding mRNA segments within tissues. When the gene for a specific neuropeptide has been identified, a complementary segment of DNA can be constructed. This can serve as a recognition molecule to localize expression of that gene in tissue, since the DNA probe will bind to the corresponding RNA molecules that have been transcribed within a cell. This technique has been used to effectively demonstrate that the birthing process and subsequent maternal behavior can activate oxytocin systems in the brain. Perhaps this has answered the age-old question of where mothers find the psychological strength to begin mothering so soon upon the birth of their first child, although they may have doubted their competence to be mothers before receiving that genetic boost in confidence. As we will see in Chapter 13, oxytocin is a brain system that controls nurturance and probably facilitates the affective dimension of human emotional experience called acceptance.

The nature of the organic systems that control psychological processes can finally be revealed by such technical approaches. And so Freud's early vision, cited in the epigraph for this chapter, is coming to pass: Many psychological processes, including our basic emotions, are finally being explained by "specifiable material particles."

AFTERTHOUGHT: The Neurochemistry of Some Emotional Processes

Just as I covered three major lines of evidence concerning the nature of emotions from neuroanatomical and neurophysiological perspectives in the previous two chapters, here I focus on three of the best-developed lines of neurochemical evidence. I provide (1) a synoptic review of how modern psychoactive drugs modify psychiatric disorders, (2) a very brief description of advances in our understanding of drug craving and addiction, and (3) an overview of the brain "stress response" and other issues related to the peripheral autonomic nervous system.

1. Most of the medicines used in current psychiatric practice emerged from our understanding of the neurochemical systems depicted in Figure 6.5. It is remarkable how many of the successes of biological psychiatry have arisen from our ability to manipulate just a handful of neurochemical systems,[73] but that is because these systems are so widespread in the brain, affecting all brain functions in fairly predictable ways—catecholamines facilitating the energization of affective responses (both positive and negative), and serotonin systems generally decreasing negative affective responses and behaviors, even though positive responses can also be diminished.

Of the drugs currently used to alleviate depression, some prolong the synaptic availability of biogenic amine transmitters, while others slow degradation. In the former class are the many tricyclic antidepressants that can facilitate norepinephrine, serotonin, or dopamine reuptake at synapses. More recently, other specific reuptake inhibitors have been developed, perhaps the most famous being the selective serotonin reuptake inhibitors (SSRIs). Representatives of the other major class of drugs inhibit the enzyme monoamine oxidase (MAO) that normally helps degrade biogenic amines following release. MAO inhibitors are less commonly used than the reuptake inhibitors because they have more side effects, such as the increased toxicity of certain foods that are high in the amino acid tyramine. However, recent developments (e.g., discovery of several forms of MAO in the brain) have yielded some safer and more specific drugs of that class. Some of them, such as *phenelzine*, are also quite effective for other disorders, such as "social phobias," the strong discomfort that some people feel during social interactions. Others like *deprenyl* have been found to increase life span in animals.

The class of drugs known as *antipsychotics* generally dampens DA activity. Since there are several different DA receptors, modern work has sought to more specifically target the D_2 receptors, which are present in abnormally high quantities in the schizophrenic brain. Most antipsychotics are receptor *blockers*, which means that they prevent dopamine from having normal physiological interactions with its receptor. Other drugs that stimulate receptors are called *agonists*; such drugs can promote schizophrenic symptoms. For instance, the indirect agonists such as cocaine and amphetamines can induce sufficiently strong paranoid symptoms that psychiatrists have difficulty distinguishing them from the real thing.

Most modern *antianxiety agents* interact with their own receptor, a benzodiazepine receptor, which can facilitate GABA activity in the brain. More recently, some totally new types of antianxiety agents have been discovered, such as *buspirone,* which interact with serotonin receptors. With the revelation of the role of many other neuropeptides in the genesis of anxiety, perhaps specific anxieties, it is likely that even more specific antianxiety agents will be developed in the future.

Many investigators presently believe that functional psychiatric disorders result from neurochemical imbalances (i.e., lack of regulation) among many transmitter systems as opposed to a pathology in a single one, so there may be many ways to restore overall balance. The recent discovery of a large number of neuropeptide transmitter and receptor systems has opened the door to the development of a new generation of psychiatric medicines, which may be able to modify distinct mood and behavioral states. Take the case of *bulimia*, in which individuals show abnormal binge-and-purge feeding patterns. A brain peptide called neuropeptide Y (NPY), when placed directly into the brain, can induce animals to eat copious amounts of food. This peptide is also elevated in the cerebrospinal fluid of individuals who exhibit bulimia. If there is a causal relationship between the two, one would predict that NPY receptor antagonists might ameliorate bulimia in humans. To the contrary, NPY receptor agonists might precipitate bulimia. These provocative ideas cannot be tested in humans because drugs do not yet exist that can cross the BBB and exert these actions on NPY receptors. But such molecules may soon be developed, and then we will be able to systematically evaluate how this peptide controls human moods and behavior.[74]

2. A milestone in our understanding of neuropsychic causes of drug abuse was the observation that animals, like humans, can express a strong desire for certain pharmaceutical agents, especially opiates and amphetamine-like psychostimulants. These studies are now bringing us close to an understanding of the neurochemistry of human and animal pleasure and cravings.[75] A detailed understanding of the brain chemistries that permit these drugs to produce their effects (e.g., the brain opioid and ascending dopamine systems, which arise from A10 cell groups of the ventral tegmental area; Figure 6.5), has

opened up a Pandora's box—or a treasure chest, depending on your perspective—of ways to modify the moods and emotions of humans by pharmaceutical means. For a summary of opioid receptor distributions, see Figure 6.8.

Down through the ages, two of the most emotionally attractive types of drugs have been narcotics, such as morphine and heroin, and psychostimulants, such as cocaine and more recently the amphetamines. We now understand why people and animals are strongly attracted to voluntarily self-administer these agents. The drugs interact with specific receptors in the brain that normally help mediate various pleasures and psychic excitement.

Although there are many environmental and psychosocial reasons for people to take such drugs, ultimately the only reason there is heroin addiction is because the brain contains *mu*-opiate receptors. These receptors normally control an animal's urges to maintain various brain and bodily balances (i.e., homeostatic balance) via feeding, sexual/social behavior, and so forth. The psychic reflections of doing "the right thing biologically" are feelings of satisfaction and pleasure (see Chapter 9). Which of the many brain opiate systems actually mediate this subjective feeling is not well understood, but animals will self-administer opiates directly into various parts of the brain. The most effective locations are in the brain stem, near the central gray of the midbrain, and the ventral-tegmental area, where the A10 mesolimbic DA cells are situated.

Cocaine and amphetamine produce their psychic appeal via this same system—namely, by increasing DA availability at synapses of the mesolimbic circuit. If this system is damaged, self-administration of psychostimulants declines. One of the normal functions of this system is to energize appetitive behavior (see Chapter 8). Thus, it is no wonder that humans develop a strong craving for these drugs, since the normal function of the underlying brain system is to facilitate a generalized form of appetitive behavior. Through the availability of psychostimulant drugs, animals can directly activate the brain systems that normally motivate them to explore and investigate their world and to vigorously pursue courses of action. When they get into the vicious cycle of self-stimulating this system, everything else in the world decreases in their value hierarchy. The psychic appeal of cocaine seems to be mediated by the dopamine reuptake site, since knockout mice without this receptor do not appear to desire psychostimulants.[76] Also, it should be noted that the euphoria and craving that are induced by elevated DA at synapses apparently are due to interactions with one type of receptor (D_2) rather than the other major variant of the dopamine receptor (D_1).[77]

It is likely that certain addictive behaviors in humans, such as compulsive gambling, are strongly controlled by internal urges that are generated by dopamine chemistries. One of the key questions in controlling these addictions is how to diminish the craving for these agents once the desire to do so has been established. Recently, investigators have been able to reduce cocaine intake in animals by inducing them to generate antibodies to cocaine.[78]

3. Psychologists have traditionally had a difficult time generating a satisfactory definition of "stress." In psychobiology, it is much easier: Stress is anything that activates the pituitary-adrenal system (the ACTH-cortisol axis). Everything that is typically considered to be a stressor in humans generates this brain response.[79] The overall response is now well understood (Figure 6.9). A variety of neuroemotional influences converge on cells of the paraventricular nucleus (PVN) of the hypothalamus, which contain CRF. These neurons, via axons descending toward the pituitary, can trigger ACTH release from the pituitary. ACTH, which is released into the bloodstream, seeks out target tissue in the adrenal cortex, where it triggers the release of cortisol. Cortisol helps promote energy utilization in the body, and obviously more bodily resources need to be used in all stressful situations. This peripheral system is aroused in response to essentially all emotional stressors. As we will see in Chapters 11 and 14, the central CRF pathways within the brain help organize and coordinate various negative emotional responses.

Cortisol also feeds back onto brain tissue, where there are specific receptors for the steroid hormone, especially in the hippocampus (which controls cognitive processing), as well as on the CRF neurons of the PVN. Cortisol normally exerts an inhibitory effect on the PVN cells and thereby regulates the intensity of the stress response. In many individuals with depression, this self-regulatory, negative feedback mechanism no longer operates properly. Stress responses do not diminish normally once a stressful episode is over. The clinical test used to evaluate the patency of this negative feedback mechanism is the dexamethasone suppression test (DST). This entails injecting an individual with dexamethasone, a potent synthetic form of cortisol, and observing whether his or her endogenous cortisol level is reduced. If not, the feedback loop is not working properly and there is a good chance that the individual is clinically depressed. Although the failure of the DST can have other causes, commonly the response does return to normal as the depression lifts.

The feedback of cortisol onto hippocampal tissues also modifies cognitive abilities relevant to stress. Exactly what cortisol does there is not certain, but it may help promote cognitive strategies to cope with stressors. However, this feedback mechanism is also subject to imbalances. The neurons that contain the cortisol receptors can tolerate only so much stimulation. If cortisol secretion is sustained at excessive levels, the metabolic resources of hippocampal neurons become depleted and

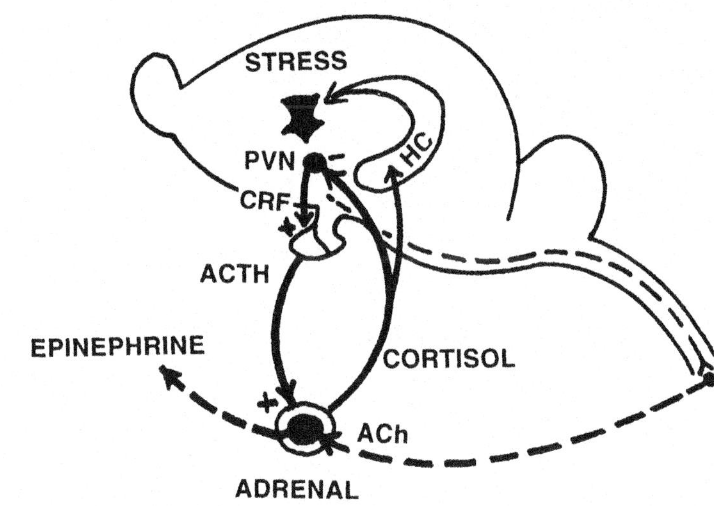

Figure 6.9. Summary of the pituitary-adrenal (solid lines) and sympathoadrenal (dotted lines) stress response systems. The pituitary-adrenal response is instigated by stress releasing corticotrophin releasing factor (CRF) from the paraventricular nucleus of the hypothalamus (PVN), which triggers release of ACTH from the anterior pituitary, which releases cortisol (or corticosterone in rats) from the adrenal cortex. Cortisol then activates bodily metabolism and feeds back into the brain to directly control its own activities in the PVN as well as to higher brain areas that provide adaptive psychological responses to stress, such as the hippocampus (HC).

die prematurely. In short, a sustained stress response can kill certain brain cells! At present, we know that this neurotoxic effect can be produced in both experimental laboratory animals and those confronting real-life stressors in the wild, and that comparable changes can occur simply as a function of aging.[80] Since brain cells are not replaced, this can pose a serious problem for subsequent cognitive abilities.[81]

Although the pituitary-adrenal stress response has greatly clarified the nature of stress, there are obviously many other aspects to the overall response. For instance, a second major limb of the stress response is via a neural pathway arising from the hypothalamus and descending to the spinal cord, which, via "sympathetic" efferents, activates the release of epinephrine and norepinephrine from the adrenal medulla (Figure 6.8). These hormones help to break down liver glycogen rapidly and make abundant blood sugar available for the stressed organism.

Indeed, practically all visceral organs and many other brain and immune responses are recruited during stress. I will not attempt to summarize these lines of evidence in this text, since they are well covered elsewhere,[82] but it is worth highlighting the fact that the peripheral autonomic nervous system has long been recognized as the output system for emotions. Now, however, we appreciate that there is also a separate *visceral*, or *enteric, nervous system* that is critical for elaborating organ responses during emotions,[83] This nervous system consists of an endogenous plexus of nerves that line the gastrointestinal system and other organs; they are rich in various neuropeptides, which have some influence back into the brain via reafferent neural and humoral routes. However, most important from the present perspective, the brain itself contains many similar neural systems spread throughout the limbic system and related brain areas that govern the central integration of emotional responsivity. Although the peripheral issues are of great importance as potential measures of emotionality, as well as for understanding psychosomatic disorders that arise from overtaxed emotional responses,[84] the more basic and crucial task is to explore the central brain systems that mediate emotionality.

Suggested Readings

Bousfield, D. (ed.) (1985). *Neurotransmitters in action.* New York: Elsevier.

Cooper, J. R., Bloom, F. E., & Roth, R. H. (1995). *The biochemical basis of neuropharmacology.* New York: Oxford Univ. Press.

Costa, E., & Greengard, P. (eds.) (1969–1984). *Advances in biochemical psychopharmacology*, vols. 1–39. New York: Raven Press.

Feldman, R. S., & Quenzer, L. F. (1984). *Fundamentals of neuropsychopharmacology.* Sunderland, Mass.: Sinauer.

Ganten, D., & Pfaff, D. (eds.) (1990). *Behavioral aspects of neuroendocrinology: Current topics in neuroendocrinology*, vol. 10. Berlin: Springer-Verlag.

Iversen, L. L., Iversen, S. D., & Snyder, S. H. (eds.) (1975–1984). *Handbook of psychopharmacology.* Vols. 1–18. New York: Plenum Press.

Leonard, B. E. (1993). *Fundamentals of psychopharmacology.* Chichester, U.K.: Wiley.

Meltzer, H. Y. (ed.) (1987). *Psychopharmacology: The third generation of progress.* New York: Raven Press.

Nieuwenhuys, R. (1985). *Chemoarchitecture of the brain.* Berlin: Springer-Verlag.

Simonov, P. V. (1986). *The emotional brain.* New York, Plenum Press.

PART II

Basic Emotional and Motivational Processes

In the preceding chapters, we have seen the great esteem that Nobel Committees have had for major advances in our basic understanding of how the brain functions. Most of the recognition has gone to individuals who have worked out mechanisms that have broad implications for understanding neural actions. By comparison, the pursuits of individuals who have worked on the integrative functions of the whole brain have not been comparably lauded. The work of Hess was an exception. When recognition for integrative work was offered again, it went not to the behaviorists who had been working on the nature of learning but to the ethologists who had been working on the spontaneous behavior patterns of animals. In appreciation of the fact that an understanding of instinctual processes is of first-order importance for understanding brain functions, in 1973 the Nobel Committee recognized the work of Konrad Lorenz, Nico Tinbergen, and Karl Von Frisch, the founding fathers of modern ethology "for their discoveries concerning organization and elicitation of individual and social behavior patterns."

The work of these ethologists has generated lasting understanding of behaviors in our fellow animals. Lorenz characterized the rapid imprinting or social attachment processes that emerge between mother geese and their offspring soon after birth. He also found that under artificial conditions this type of social bonding or preference would develop for members of other species, including Lorenz himself. Tinbergen demonstrated that animals are prepared to respond in stereotyped ways to certain aspects of their environments. For instance, young seagulls would beg for food by pecking the feeding spot on the bills of inanimate models that barely resembled the beaks of their parents. He also demonstrated that such "sign stimuli" also existed in stickleback fish, which exhibited aggression simply toward the bulging red belly of a model fish. Von Frisch was the first to work out the innate communication system of another species, namely, the ability of honeybees to inform other members of their hive about the location of food sources by performing a "waggle dance." In fact, the ethological tradition represented by these works goes back to the 1872 classic *The Expression of the Emotions in Man and Animals*, in which Charles Darwin promoted analysis of the various emotional behavior patterns animals and humans exhibit in nature, a tradition that is being pursued vigorously to this day through the analysis of facial expressions of emotions in humans and postural expressions of emotions in animals.

For a while, ethology, this uniquely European tradition of studying animal behavior, provided a credible alternative to the traditions started by American behaviorists, such as J. B. Watson and B. F. Skinner. While behaviorism pursued the general research strategy of observing the learning behavior of animals in artificial environments, the ethologists sought to clarify how animals spontaneously behaved in their natural environments. For many years, ethologists and behaviorists quarreled over which was the proper approach.

We now recognize that each was partially right. Ethology deals more effectively with the relatively "closed programs" of the brain, and behaviorism deals better with the more "open programs" that permit behavioral flexibility via new learning. The two finally started to come together when it was realized that the so-called misbehavior of organisms (see Chapter 1) arose from the fact that in the midst of difficult learning tasks, animals would often tend to revert to their instinctual behavioral tendencies. Likewise, it was gradually recognized that animals are "prepared" to learn certain things more easily than others. In other words, evolution had constructed different animals to subsist best in different environments.

Although both traditions provided many new and lasting "laws of behavior," until quite recently, neither tradition tried to link itself to the other or to brain research. Both now recognize that their scientific future is limited if they do not cultivate connections to neuroscience, and so the powerful new disciplines of neuroethology and behavioral neuroscience have emerged. Mainstream psychology is also slowly coming to realize that it must pay closer attention to the nature of the brain in order to make progress in understanding the causes of basic psychological processes.

It is becoming increasingly clear that humans have as many instinctual operating systems in their brains as other mammals. However, in mature humans such instinctual processes may be difficult to observe because they are no longer expressed directly in adult behavior but instead are filtered and modified by higher cognitive activity. Thus, in adult humans, many instincts manifest themselves only as subtle psychological tendencies, such as subjective feeling states, which provide internal guidance to behavior. The reason many scholars who know little about modern brain research are still willing to assert that human behavior is not controlled by instinctual processes is because many of our operating systems are in fact very "open" and hence very prone to be modified by the vast layers of cognitive and affective complexity that learning permits. Still, the failure of psychology to deal effectively with the nature of the many instinctual systems of human and animal brains remains one of the great failings of the discipline. The converse could be said for neuroscience.

Instinctual operating systems of the brain must underlie sophisticated human abilities. For example, the general urge and ability of young children to pick up language is instinctual (i.e., based on specific brain operating systems that are coming to be well understood; see Appendix B). Of course, these genetically provided abilities are remarkably "open" and hence permeable to many environmental influences, so that the end results exhibit incredible diversity of external forms in the real world. However, diversity is always supported from below by a variety of shared mechanisms. When the underlying brain programs are damaged in adults, language abilities are predictably impaired. As linguist Noam Chomsky has forcefully argued, there is a "deep linguistic structure" in the human brain, which unfolds spontaneously during early development, giving a distinctive human stamp to all human languages around the world. Here I will begin to analyze the proposition that human emotions are controlled likewise—by the deep structure of emotional circuits that we still share with other animals. The best way to understand these emotional systems in human brains is to analyze the corresponding emotional behavior patterns generated by animal brains.

Before discussing the details of some of the emotive systems in animal brains, let me first summarize the perspective developed so far. The basic emotions appear to arise from executive circuits of the brain that simultaneously synchronize a large number of mental and bodily functions in response to major life-challenging situations. Although many emotional nuances can be "socially constructed" by the human mind, usually designed by the textures of specific human cultures, the affective strength of the basic emotions arises from intrinsically "motivating" neurophysiological properties of genetically ordained subcortical emotive systems.

Since brain emotive systems were designed through evolutionary selection to respond in prepared ways to certain environmental events, it often seems from our "mind's-eye" perspective that world events are *creating* emotions as opposed to just *triggering* evolutionarily prepared and epigenetically refined states of the brain. In fact, many of the feelings and behavioral tendencies that characterize the basic emotions reflect, more than anything else, the intrinsic, genetically prepared properties of brain organization. Although the underlying emotional circuits influence and guide learning, their initial adaptive functions were to *initiate, synchronize*, and *energize* sets of coherent physiological, behavioral, and psychological changes that are primal instinctive solutions to various archetypal life-challenging situations. The subjective experience of emotions presumably allows organisms to code the value of environmental events so as to facilitate the expression of various learned behaviors.

In the second part of this book, I will discuss five types of emotional and motivational systems that all mammals share. I discuss (1) the concept of "state control systems" as highlighted by an analysis of the sleep-waking mechanisms in the context of which all behavior has to occur; (2) how SEEKING circuits for *interest, curiosity*, and *eager anticipation* help generate expectations and direct animals to the positive rewards to be had from the environment; (3) how those systems help maintain physical "drive" states, such as water and energy balance, which need to be regulated, in part, by behavioral means via interaction with specific environmental "incentives"; (4) RAGE circuits for *anger* and *impassioned aggression* that help counter irritations, frustrations, and other threats to one's freedom of action; and (5) various FEAR and anxiety circuits that help protect an animal from physical harm. Although there are many other social-emotional and motivational systems in the brain, as summarized in the final third of this text, the systems covered in this section provide a solid cross-species foundation for the complexities to follow.

7

Sleep, Arousal, and Mythmaking in the Brain

Dreams tell us the way we really think and feel, not the way we pretend we think and feel. We can blind ourselves and fool ourselves while we are awake, but not while we sleep. Through our dreams we have access to vast stores of memory, amazing depths of insight, and common sense as well as to resources of creative thinking, which offer us a richer and more productive life.

G. Delaney, *Breakthrough Dreaming* (1991)

CENTRAL THEME

Shakespeare proposed one possible function of sleep when he suggested that it "knits up the raveled sleeve of care." A great number of functions have now been attributed to sleep and dreaming, but few have been definitively demonstrated with the tools of science. One thing is certain, though. Each day our lives cycle through the master routines of sleeping, dreaming, and waking. All our activities are guided by the age-old rhythms of nature, and many neural mechanisms assure that we remain in tune with the cycling of days and nights across the seasons. Our brains contain endogenous daily rhythm generators and also, perhaps, calendar mechanisms that respond to monthly lunar cycles, as well as the transit of the seasons. Brain scientists have been especially eager to study the mechanisms that control these processes, and our various states of vigilance have been pursued vigorously thanks to highly objective electroencephalographic (EEG) procedures to monitor the brain in action. During waking, the EEG is typically full of low-amplitude, high-frequency beta waves, which indicate that the brain is processing information. As one goes into quiet sleep, which deepens through several stages, the cortex exhibits increasingly large high-amplitude slow waves. This reflects a brain state where very little active processing is transpiring. Slow wave sleep (SWS) is typically followed by a highly activated form of sleep, accompanied by cortical arousal (more energized than the waking EEG), a flaccid muscular paralysis (atonia), and rapid eye movements accompanied by vivid dreaming (i.e., rapid eye movement [REM] sleep). It is generally believed that SWS reflects ongoing bodily repair processes, while dreaming sleep reflects active information reintegration within the brain. Although we do not know for sure what the various sleep stages do for us, aside from alleviating tiredness, we do know a great deal about the brain mechanisms that generate these states. All of the executive structures are quite deep in the brain, some in the lower brain stem. To the best of our knowledge, however, the most influential mechanisms for SWS are higher in the brain than the active waking mechanisms, while the executive mechanisms for REM sleep are the lowest of the three. If we accept that caudal structures are generally more primitive than rostral ones, we are forced to contemplate the strange possibility that the basic dream generators are more ancient in brain evolution than are the generators of our waking consciousness. In this chapter, we will try to resolve this paradox by focusing on possible interactions between dreaming processes and ancient emotional systems of the brain.

The Varieties of Consciousness: To Sleep, Perchance to Dream

The brain goes through various "state shifts" during both waking and sleep. Surprisingly, it has been more difficult for scientists to agree on the types of discrete states of waking consciousness than on those that occur during sleep. This is because there are relatively unambiguous EEG indicators for various sleep states. Neuroscientists are more enthusiastic about pursuing brain vigilance states that can be objectively distinguished, and the EEG clearly discriminates three global vigilance states of the nervous system—waking, SWS, and dreaming or REM sleep. SWS can be further divided into several stages—light SWS to deep SWS in animals, with four SWS stages typically being recognized in humans. Since the nature of SWS staging is not critical for our purposes, it will not be detailed further.

Although the waking states have typically not been subcategorized, it eventually may be possible to do so by focusing on the many different emotional and mood states organisms can experience. Once we better understand the various affective states and develop objective brain indicators for them, we may come to agree that distinct waking states can exist within the brain. At present, however, we understand the brain generators for the two major sleep states—SWS and REM—better than those for the various waking systems. In this chapter, I will focus on their neural underpinnings and the various theories that have been put forth to explain their existence. I will also pay special attention to the relations between REM and the brain mechanisms of emotionality.

The sleep state that fascinates everyone most is dreaming. Some call it REM sleep; others call it activated sleep or paradoxical sleep. There are many theories about the role of REM sleep in the brain economy, ranging from those that suggest it helps construct memories to those that would have us believe it helps destroy useless memories. Unfortunately, there are more ideas than definitive knowledge in the field.[1] Indeed, I will share a new theory in this chapter, which is as likely to be true as any other. But before I proceed to the details, let me first share a few dreams that may help highlight the underlying psychodynamics and then proceed to the neurodynamics of dreaming. The two dreams I will relate have not been selected for any special heuristic value; they are simply the most recent ones that my spouse and I shared with each other as I was about to write this chapter. First, my wife's dream in her own words:

> First, I am in a large institutional shower room putting some caustic treatment on my hair—peroxide or a straightener—and I know I must get it rinsed out quickly, not just because it will burn my skin, but because I already know that I am in the midst of urgent circumstances which may require flight and escape. Then the scene shifts to a large office, like editorial rooms of city newspapers as depicted in the movies. It's located at the end of a long hallway of what appears to be an institutional building—a hospital, perhaps. I am in the office with two or three people, an Asian couple and one or more weakly defined members of their family; other people are also around. It is daytime. My hair is now dry and I'm dressed for work. Suddenly we "know," or find out somehow, that two armies are approaching our vicinity, and we may become surrounded by a fierce battle. Somehow I know that it is the Union and Confederate armies of the Civil War, although everything visual in the dream corresponds to our contemporary times. For example, I see the Asian woman talking on a cellular phone. I urge her to find out from whomever she is speaking to the direction of the armies' approach; I feel that we must leave immediately to avoid getting entrapped by the battle. Helping and protecting these foreign guests seems to be my responsibility. While talking on the phone, the woman learns that one of her young female relatives (maybe a sister or niece) has just been awarded the "Nobel Prize for Birdwatching" because she sighted a rare "chipping bunting" for the first time in over 60 years! Suddenly, it becomes clear that this young woman is with us, and I feel even greater urgency to get us all safely out of the building so that the Nobel laureate will not be captured by hostile forces.
>
> We hurry down several corridors, having great difficulty finding a route of escape, until I decide we must crawl out a window on the first floor. Several obstacles, mostly chairs, are in front of the window and have to be moved. Finally, I clear the way and show the others how to climb out. After successfully leading the way, I am very concerned by how long it is taking them to follow.
>
> I drop down to the ground and hide in a large bush waiting and calling in an urgent whisper for the others to follow. I see that I am now located in the backyard of my childhood home, but this does not surprise me. The others are very slow, and I keep urging them. I feel a great deal of anxiety and carefully keep my gaze lowered, so that the scouts of the approaching armies won't catch any gleam from my eyes. I see, however, that my daughter is near me, cleverly hiding in the next bush, following my example. She was not with us inside. I don't know who, if anyone, follows me as I move away from the building. I'm satisfied that someone at least—my daughter—made it outside. I walk through a forest toward a railroad (similar to the one near my childhood home), keeping a careful watch for advance scouts of the approaching armies. I wake up.

Perhaps Freud, Jung, or some other famous dream interpreter would have had a fine time with this, but let's admit once more—we do not yet know, scientifically, what function the dream serves in our cerebral homeostasis. No one really knows if there is any deep and profound symbolic meaning in dream content. It could simply be a random by-product of the brain's attempt to restabilize its circuits or clear its memory banks of useless clutter. We do not know whether the dream is an extraneous glimmer (an epiphenomenon) of a critical brain process that we do not fully comprehend or a meaningful reflection of the functionally important shuffling of our cognitive and/or emotional files that has true implications for our personality and cognitive structures. It is sad to say that we know more about the brain mechanisms that control the physiological changes that are aroused during REM sleep than about the neuro- and psychodynamic balances that arise from dreaming.

However, several universal characteristics seem evident in my wife's dream. Not only is it full of emotion,[2] but it has incorporated recent cognitions into a new schematic pattern. The hair-washing episode in her dream is reminiscent of one in the movie *Malcolm X* that we had recently seen. Surely having recently sat through the poignant weeklong PBS *Civil War* series had something to do with the overall setting although it may have also represented the conflict she had recently experienced with university administrators. Perhaps the Asian woman in the dream was somehow related to my wife's hopes of being hired by the Foreign Service around the same time. Also, not long before this dream, a species of bird from Europe that had never been sighted in America had mistakenly migrated across the Atlantic and was being eagerly pursued by birdwatchers up and down the Atlantic seaboard, but instead of existing species such as *chipping sparrows* and *painted buntings*, here we have a new composite species, the nonexistent "chipping bunting." It is almost as if we are seeing new ideas being created and old worries being blended in the crucible of the brain.

But some have also thought that dreaming is the crucible of madness, and they may well be right. Many have suggested that schizophrenia reflects the release of dreaming processes into the waking state. Several investigators have tried to prove this hypothesis, but solid evidence has been elusive. Schizophrenics do not exhibit any more REM than normal folks, except during the evening before a "schizophrenic break," when REM is in fact elevated.[3] Of course, this turning point can be recorded only in individuals who have episodic schizophrenic breakdowns. This suggests that the emotional "energies" that are aroused during the initial florid phase of schizophrenia may be released within the dreaming process.

There may also be commonalities between schizophrenia and the unique electrical events (i.e., *PGO spikes*) that occur during dream periods (which will be described more fully later). For now, let us just imagine them as bolts of "neuronal lightning" shooting through the brain. These massive nerve discharges do not occur during normal waking states, but similar types of electrical events have been recorded from deep limbic areas of the schizophrenic brain.[4] The only other conditions in which this electrical signature of the dream has been regularly observed during the waking state are in organisms under the influence of LSD or when brain biogenic amines are rapidly depleted and serotonin synthesis is concurrently decreased by pharmacological means.[5] Indeed, there may be a deep neurophysiological commonality between the dream, the LSD experience, and schizophrenic hallucinations—even though the former two are largely visual, while the latter is largely auditory. In fact, all three states share low brain serotonin activity (see the "Afterthought" of this chapter for more detail on this intriguing matter).

In any event, the dream is a place of fantasies—a place where we sometimes live within our wishes and within cherished, as well as dreaded, memories of the past. And so, in my wife's dream we see how the old important memories of childhood emerge unexpectedly (but not with any accompanying surprise) from some deep recesses of the mind, perhaps as hidden wishes for the securities of times long past. When one is in danger, one should seek the safety of home! And among all the new faces, dear old ones often join us without much warning. My wife's daughter suddenly appears, and she may feel better to be continuing on her perilous journey with her beloved child by her side. I have also dreamed about my own daughter, Tiina, during the past few years. Let me briefly share one that I had a few nights before I sat down to write this chapter early in the 1993 school year. Tiina should have been entering college that fall.

> I am standing at a professorial podium looking at several dozen students sitting in scattered groups around the auditorium—groups of girls on the left with a few guys scattered around and a group of four happy-looking black male students on the right, all with very fancy dreadlock hairdos. There is no one I explicitly recognize, although some of the girls look a bit familiar. All of a sudden, a girl enters through a back door, and I recognize her immediately, Tiina, my daughter; a feeling of joy fills me, for it seems I have not seen her for such a very long time. She smiles and waves to me in acknowledgment (in her very characteristic and endearing way). More gracefully than I have ever seen before, almost as if floating, she comes toward the front and sits down alone just in front of the group of Afro-American students. I am so happy to see her, but after a while the students behind her begin to tease her, and with no show of ill will she simply gets up and moves to a seat closer to the front. She looks radiant, a bit older than I remember her. All of a sudden the auditorium meeting is finished, and I am milling in the front with some students, all the while trying to catch a glimpse of Tiina. I can't see her anywhere. I become panicky and start to push through what is now a crowd. All of a sudden I realize she is dead, but I do not think that realization was in the dream, but in the panicked moment that I woke up as I went into a cold sweat. Everything in the dream is vividly engraved in my mind. I can't shake the dream for hours. . . . It influences my mood for days.

At that point in time, my precious daughter, Tiina, who had a large, culturally diverse range of friends, had been dead for two and a half years, killed in a horrible car accident along with three friends (Stephanie, Maggie, and Kevin). A drunken driver being pursued by a careless policeman careened into their car. I have had many horrible dreams (as well as thoughts and feelings, of course) about this accident and its horrendous aftermath.[6] Tiina would have been starting college that year, and she was on my mind as I watched the many bright and eager new students traversing the campus. Tiina is dead, yet in my dreams she is often still alive. In some corner of my mind, the past exists unchanged! Maybe Freud was partly right in saying that all our dreams, if we understand their hidden meanings correctly, reflect "wish fulfillments" or "complexes" (emotional tender spots) that arise from our innermost desires and deepest fears. In the dream, emotional realities may stand up to be counted as the less important details and pretenses of our conscious lives fade with the onslaught of sleep. Great and small hopes for the future lie side by side within the brain along with the awful realities of the past.

There seem to be two distinct worlds within our minds, like matter and antimatter, worlds that are often 180 degrees out of phase with each other. Indeed, as is discussed more extensively later, the electrical activity of the brain stem during dreaming is the mirror image of waking—the ability of certain brain areas to modulate the activity of others during waking changes from excitation to inhibition during REM.[7] In other words, areas of the brain that facilitate behavior in waking now inhibit those same behaviors. Many believe that if we understand this topsy-turvy reversal of the ruling potentials in the brain, we will better understand the nature of everyday mental realities, as well as the nature of minds that are overcome by madness.

What a strange thing, this dreaming process, that has now been the focus of more scientific inquiry than any other intrinsic mechanism of the brain. In terms of the EEG, it looks like a waking state, but in terms of behavior it looks like flaccid paralysis. Indeed, perhaps what is now the REM state was the original form of waking consciousness in early brain evolution, when emotionality was more important than reason in the competition for resources. This ancient form of waking consciousness may have come to be actively suppressed in order for higher brain evolution to proceed efficiently. This is essentially a new theory of dreaming. It is remarkable that with the number of ideas that have already been proposed, there is still room for more. But maybe that is, in fact, what dreaming provides—an endless variety of ideas, especially when life is stressful and we need to entertain new alternatives. Indeed, it is a demonstrated fact that the amount of dreaming sleep goes up when organisms are confronted by stressful, emotionally challenging situations.[8] I will elaborate upon existing theories toward the end of this chapter, but I will first present some important factual details concerning the nature of sleep and dream generators in the brain.

Sleep and Waking as Active Functions of the Brain

Before certain critical experiments were done, it was thought that the waking state was sustained by the bombardment of the brain by incoming stimuli from the senses and that sleep ensued only when stimulation from the environment was sufficiently diminished. It is now clear that the brain has active mechanisms for the induction of waking (arousal and attention), as well as distinct endogenously active mechanisms for the induction of SWS and REM. During SWS, which is normally an essential neural gateway for entry into REM (except in cases of narcolepsy, where organisms fall directly from waking into REM), the cortex is gradually captivated by deepening tides of slow waves, which, as mentioned, are commonly subcategorized in human sleep research into four stages that reflect the gradual deepening of sleep. SWS is interspersed with periods of activated REM sleep, so that, as the night progresses, the episodes of SWS get shorter while REM episodes get longer.[9] Children exhibit much more REM than older people, and deep SWS also diminishes markedly with age.[10]

When neuronal action potentials are analyzed during the three states of vigilance, we generally get a picture of waking activity as accompanied by a great deal of spontaneous neural activity, with only some cells being silent, waiting for the right environmental stimulus to come along. This generally yields a fast, low-amplitude *beta* pattern of electrical activity on the cortical surface. In SWS, the total amount of neural activity in most parts of the brain, such as the cortex, diminishes marginally, but there is a large redistribution of firing. Many neurons in the thalamic-neocortical axis begin to fire synchronously, yielding sleep spindles (an oscillatory waveform characteristic of oncoming SWS) and delta waves, as if cortical zones are under the influence of a powerful new executive system that diminishes attention.[11] In fact, many of these brain changes arise from rhythmic pacemaker neurons that appear to be situated in old nonspecific reticular (i.e., intralaminar) areas of the thalamus. There are also other brain areas, especially in the basal forebrain and anterior hypothalamus, from where cortical slow-wave activity can be promoted. Repetitive electrical stimulation of these parts of the brain in awake animals readily induces sleep, and a very specific site in the ventrolateral preoptic area has recently been identified as a potential SWS generator.[12]

During REM sleep, most of the brain exhibits slightly more neuronal activity than during waking, with storms of intense activity sweeping through certain areas of the brain. However, many neurons that are most active during waking (e.g., norepinephrine [NE] and serotonin [5-HT] neurons) cease firing completely during REM (see the "Afterthought" of this chapter). PET scan images of the brain during dreaming highlight clear arousal in the limbic system, especially the amygdala. Indeed, many emotion-mediating areas of the brain "light up" during REM, but one surprise has been that the prefrontal areas, which generate active plans, remain quiescent, as they do during SWS.[13]

One area of the brain—namely, the hippocampus—exhibits highly synchronous rhythmic theta activity during REM. During waking, this type of hippocampal synchronization (also known as *theta rhythm*, which is common when animals are exploring their environment) usually indicates that the circuits are systematically encoding information (i.e., translating recent experiences into long-term memories).[14] Does this reflect a similar process transpiring during REM, even though it is well known that we have great difficulty consciously remembering our dreams? Perhaps this is not a paradox, if the theta activity during REM reflects information processing that is allowing transient memory stores to become integrated into subconscious behavioral habits. Perhaps the dream theories of Freud and Jung, which suggested that dreams reflect unconscious and symbolic emotional forces affecting an individual, may still hold some basic truths, even though they are hard to evaluate empirically and have been criticized by many.

Although we do not presently know exactly how memories are consolidated during REM, we can anticipate that the hippocampus will be in the middle of the neuronal action. After all, the hippocampus is the brain area that is well established to be a mediator between short- and long-term memories, and it goes into a characteristic *theta* state during REM. Also, it is now clear that the types of information processing that were undertaken by the hippocampus during waking are rerepresented during the endogenous dynamics of the REM state.[15]

The REM state is usually categorized into two components (1) the tonic or sustained components of REM, like the pervasive muscular relaxation (atonia) that keeps organisms from acting out their dreams, and (2) the phasic components, which are reflected in the many muscular twitches (i.e., dream actions) that break through the atonia. During these twitches, the brain is bombarded by endogenous bolts of neural "lightning" called *PGO spikes* (since they are especially evident in the visual system represented in the *pons*, *lateral geniculate bodies*, and *occipital cortex*). During these neural storms, organisms remain recumbent (in a state of muscular atonia) because of a massive inhibition, probably induced by the amino acid transmitter glycine, exerted on the motor neurons that control the large antigravity muscles of the body.[16] Later I will describe the behavior of animals in which this atonia mechanism (situated just below the locus coeruleus, which is situated at the pontine level of the brain stem) has been damaged, whereupon animals begin to act out the emotionality of their dreams. The massive PGO neuronal discharges are accompanied by REMs, bodily jerks, and muscular tremors that break through the motor inhibition and often resemble fragments of motivated/emotional behaviors (e.g., weak barks and snarls in dogs, with slight running movements of the paws, which presumably reflect their dream content).

Although this "activated" or "paradoxical" phase of sleep has been most commonly called REM sleep, the initials could just as well stand for *rapid ear movement* sleep, for there are corresponding muscular twitches in the auditory apparatus of the middle ear, as well as in many other parts of the body.[17] For instance, in olfactory creatures such as rats there is a lot of whisker twitching and sniffing during REM—a behavior that is normally seen during exploration of the environment and investigation of objects (see Chapter 8).[18] Males have a high probability of having erections during REM periods, humans almost continuously,[19] and rats only periodically.[20] Usually the most vivid, affectively laden dreams occur during REM episodes; they are especially intense during the gales of PGO spikes. The occasional dreamlike reports that occur during SWS (as noted in selective awakening studies in the laboratory) are sedate by comparison.[21] One common misconception is that nightmares, night terrors, and sleepwalking occur during REM sleep; in fact, they typically emerge during the deepest SWS (i.e., stage 4, or delta, sleep).[22]

The architecture of sleep staging is not random but reflects an underlying order that remains poorly understood. The average rate at which animals cycle through a full set of stages (i.e., the average REM-to-REM interval) is called the basic rest-activity cycle (BRAC). It is directly related to the metabolic rate of animals, with smaller creatures having short BRACs (e.g., 20 minutes on the average for cats) and larger animals having longer cycles (90 minutes on the average for humans).[23] The question of whether the BRAC can also be detected in waking activity has been resolved for both of these species. For instance, if one obtains a continuous ongoing measure of behavior during waking (as can be done by having animals work for a brain stimulation reward), cats exhibit a 20-minute rhythm in the rate of responding.[24] Likewise, it has been found that if one unobtrusively observes humans, they tend to show invigorated periods of facial grooming (e.g., touching the face, including nose picking) approximately every 90 minutes.[25] These rhythms, which are shorter than a day (*ultradian*), are embedded within daily (*circadian*) rhythms, as well as in longer cycles (*infradian*) such as the ones that govern monthly and annual cycles. The manner in which sleep and the various waking routines are embedded within the circadian rhythm has come to be understood in considerable detail.

The Master Clock of the Brain and Melatonin

Elucidation of the brain mechanisms that control the daily 24-hour circadian rhythm has been a great success story. The major pacemaker mechanism for the daily clock is situated in paired, circular groupings of neurons called the *suprachiasmatic nuclei* (SCN), which, as their name implies, are situated directly behind the eyes above the optic chiasm (Figure 7.1).[26] The neurons in this nucleus not only maintain their firing rhythm for approximately 24 hours after being disconnected from all other brain areas but also continue to cycle for some time when removed from the body and kept in tissue culture.[27] In rats, the peak of SCN neuronal activity is during the daytime (when animals are typically resting), which suggests that the nucleus operates primarily by actively inhibiting many behavioral control systems.[28] Indeed, despite the discovery of other potential SWS generators in the ventrolateral preoptic area, it may still be that the outputs of this nucleus and others promote SWS during anterior hypothalamic stimulation. The multiple output pathways from the SCN control practically all behavioral rhythms that have been studied, from feeding to sleep. Under constant environmental conditions, the two SCN can sometimes become desynchronized, yielding two independent free-running rhythms, which are normally either slightly longer or shorter than 24 hours. Damage to one SCN reestablishes a single free-running rhythm.[29] When both nuclei are destroyed, however, animals scatter their behavior rather haphazardly throughout the day instead of maintaining a cyclic routine of daily activities.[30] However, rhythmic behavior can be restored in such animals by transplanting neonatal SCN neurons into their brains.[31] Generally, light is a powerful time setter (*zeitgeber*) for the SCN. Even a brief pulse of bright light given once a day will synchronize rhythms under constant 24-hour lighting conditions.[32] However, activity in the nucleus is coordinated by a variety of additional influences, ranging from caffeine intake to the pineal hormone melatonin.

One can entrain the free-running rhythms typically observed under constant environmental conditions by administering melatonin at a set time each day.[33] Within the pineal gland, melatonin is normally synthesized from serotonin in two enzymatic steps: with the aid of the enzymes *N-acetyltransferase* (NAT) and *hydroxyindole-O-methyltransferase* (HIOMT). Melatonin is typically released into the circulation of most mammals when illumination diminishes and they are preparing for sleep. Melatonin reduces SCN activity directly by acting on the high density of melatonin receptors situated throughout the nucleus (Figure 7.1).[34] Investigators are still discovering what a remarkable molecule melatonin is; it not only serves as a powerful inducer of SWS but also synchronizes circadian rhythms and beneficially regulates a variety of other bodily processes, including growth and puberty. It has been reported to alleviate anxiety and to modify depression (some individuals become less depressed, but in others depression is increased),[35] and can even inhibit cancerous tumor growths when taken in the late evening, the time of day when it is normally secreted.[36] It can increase life span by about 20% under special conditions in experimental animals.[37] It exerts a global control over the brain, and, more than any other natural agent presently known, can serve as a safe and highly effective sleep-promoting agent.[38] During the past few years, as information about this remarkable hormone has become increasingly available to the public, there has been a great increase in use, since it is available without prescription in many countries. Although cautious investigators are fond of indicating that the long-term consequences of melatonin use

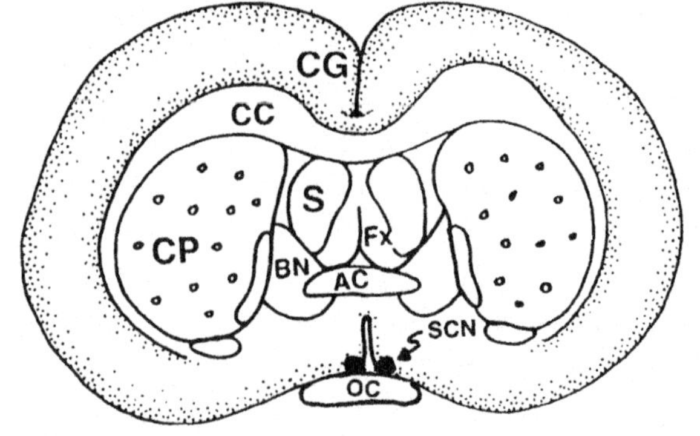

Figure 7.1. Giving radioactive melatonin to rats very nicely highlights the locations of the suprachiasmatic nuclei (SCN) of the hypothalamus that control practically all circadian rhythms exhibited by animals. Quite a similar picture is obtained, except much of the rest of the brain is also dark, when animals are given radioactive 2-DG during their sleep phase (i.e., the light-phase of the circadian illumination cycle). In other words, the nucleus is most active when behavior is inhibited. Anotomical designations: CG: cingulate gyrus; CC: corpus callosum; CP: caudate-putamen; S: septal area; BN: bed nucleus of the stria terminalis; Fx: fornix; AC: anterior comissure; OC: optic chiasm.

are not known, blind people have now taken it on a regular basis for over a decade to stabilize their circadian rhythm with no ill effects.

Although melatonin is a remarkably safe and effective endogenous sleep-promoting molecule, the brain contains a large variety of others.[39] About 30 have been identified, but it remains unclear which are the natural inducers of sleep. Right now, certain molecules of the *interleukin* class, which are part of the immune response that can help inform the nervous system about bodily problems, appear to be especially potent sleep-promoting agents, as is a recently discovered lipid that builds up in the brains of cats that are deprived of sleep.[40] Also, a sedating, adenosine-based transmitter system is heavily represented in the thalamus and the rest of the somatic nervous system.[41] Caffeine is a natural antagonist for the adenosine receptor,[42] which helps explain why people can sustain arousal with beverages like coffee, and why some people have great difficulty sleeping following consumption of caffeinated beverages.

Brain Mechanisms of Sleep and Arousal

Clarification of the active brain mechanisms that control sleep and waking represents one of the great accomplishments of psychobiology. It has also provided the main rationale for accepting that the brain is spontaneously active with a variety of distinct internally generated vigilance states. In order to identify the critical brain areas that mediate the major states of consciousness—namely, waking, SWS, and REM—investigators transected (sliced) the living brain (usually cats) at various anterior-posterior locations to determine whether the front or back was still able to mediate these states.

Before summarizing the results of these highly invasive experiments, let me emphasize that they do not tell us anything about how many brain areas actually participate in normal sleep-waking states. They only tell us where in the brain essential generators for these states might be situated. Thus, the finding that executive structures for a brain state such as REM are situated in the lower brain stem does not eliminate the potential importance of higher brain areas for the dreams that organisms experience. In fact, dreaming and REM can be dissociated in the brain. For instance, psychologically disturbed people who were subjected to *frontal lobectomies* during a bygone era of psychosurgery (the 1940s and 1950s) continued to exhibit normal physiological indices of REM sleep, but they reported no dream content when woken from REM.[43] Thus, the physiological indices of REM are not always accompanied by psychic experiences of dreaming, which suggests that dreaming is a higher brain function, while the ability to get into this state is a lower brain function.

The Waking Systems

The initial identification of the brain zones that are primarily responsible for governing sleep and waking was achieved by radical transections of the brain stem at various levels (Figure 7.2).[44] The higher brain, disconnected from the sensory inputs of the body, is quite sufficient for maintaining the normal cycling of sleep-waking states. An animal crippled in this way, with the spinal cord separated from the rest of the brain, is called the *encephale isolé* preparation. Such quadriplegic animals still exhibit normal BRACs within their EEG records but not, of course, in their bodily behaviors. If transections are made in the brain stem at the high midbrain level, in a procedure called the *cerveau isolé* preparation, animals become comatose, and their forebrains remain in almost continuous slow-wave activity. Only after many weeks of recovery will *cerveau isolé* animals exhibit some modest return of EEG desynchronization suggestive of some waking activity, while EEG indicators of REM sleep never return to brain areas anterior to the cut. However, the lower brain stem of such animals continues to exhibit a spontaneous cycling between waking and activated sleep, implying that basic mechanisms for both waking and REM exist in brain areas below the *cerveau isolé* cut—that they both lie below the rostral half of the midbrain. In discussing additional cuts between these foregoing ones, it will be important to remember that in the *cerveau isolé* preparation only 4 of the 12 cranial nerves remain attached to the forebrain—namely, the olfactory bulbs (I), optic nerves (II) for two major channels of sensory input, and oculomotor (III) and trochlear nerves (IV) for eye movements.

A most remarkable finding was that by moving the cuts slightly farther back from the classic *cerveau isolé* transection, one eventually obtains animals that exhibit a great deal of waking-type EEG activity in the forebrain, without any indication of REM in those higher brain areas.[45] Even more remarkably, this can be achieved without allowing any additional sensory input into the forebrain. In other words, with a cut that is still just anterior to the entry point of the fifth cranial nerve—namely, the trigeminal, which conveys facial sensations into the brain stem—the forebrain comes to exhibit a great deal of waking EEG activity.[46] The spontaneous appearance of EEG indices of waking in this *midpontine pretrigeminal* preparation suggested to early investigators that a spontaneous generator for the maintenance of waking resides within a narrow zone of brain stem near the mesencephalic-pontine junction. Because the midpontine pretrigeminal cut did not allow any additional sensory influences into the forebrain, it was concluded that the basic waking mechanisms of the brain do not require sensory input from the body to sustain arousal. It is apparent that the small wedge of brain stem between the *cereveau isolé* cut and the midpontine pretrigeminal cut contains an endogenous pacemaker for the generation of waking.

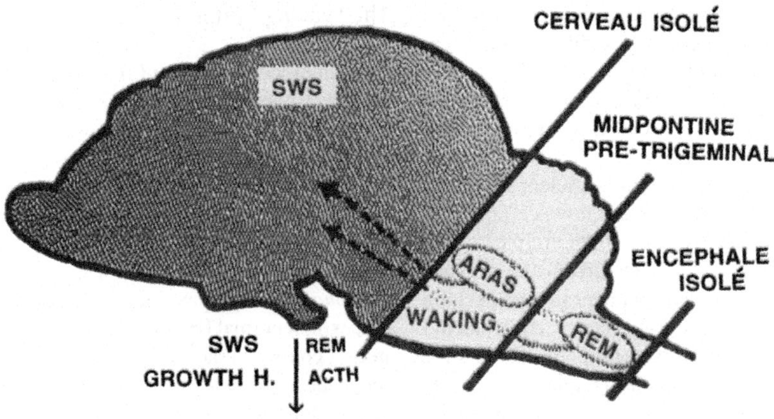

Figure 7.2. Overview of the types of brain transections that led to the general locations of major waking, SWS, and REM systems within the neuro- axis. For instance, with the midpontine pretrigeminal cut, waking and SWS were left in the forebrain, while the potential for REM was only manifested in neural and bodily systems below the cut. When the cut was slightly further rostral, through the midbrain (i.e., the *cereveau isolé* cut), the forebrain remained perpetu-ally in the darkness of SWS, while tissue below the cut cycled between waking type arousal and activated sleep states. Also, note that growth hormone secretion from the pituitary occurs in conjunction to SWS episodes, while ACTH secretion is entrained to REM periods.

In additional work, when this reticular zone of the brain was electrically stimulated in sleeping animals, the animals woke up immediately. These findings led to the classic idea that the brain has an ascending reticular activating system (ARAS) to generate waking arousal.[47] Although such global concepts as the "limbic system" and ARAS have been scorned as gross oversimplifications by subsequent generations of investigators, those conceptualizations should be respected for the powerful advances they represented in their time. Only successive approximations can guide our search for substantive knowledge concerning the many other intrinsic brain functions, especially the emotional ones, that remain to be studied within the "great intermediate net."

The other remarkable characteristic of the midpontine pretrigeminal preparation was that while waking returned to the forebrain, the brain stem below the cut retained the potential for generating REM sleep. This was clear since the body, which is under the control of neural tissue below the cut, showed periods of atonia accompanied by the phasic changes characteristic of activated sleep.[48] This confirmed that the basic brain systems for waking and REM sleep could be anatomically distinguished. Further, because of its more caudal location (which suggests increasing primitiveness), the executive circuitry for the REM mechanism seemed outwardly more ancient than the waking ARAS mechanisms. Although this perplexing issue has rarely been addressed in the literature, it does raise the seemingly absurd possibility that the essential trigger circuits for dreaming emerged before waking during the long course of brain evolution. As will be discussed in more detail later, this paradox provides a clue to the fundamental nature of REM arousal within the mammalian brain.

But first, several major questions concerning the nature of the waking mechanism need to be resolved. The most important is: Does the aroused EEG in the forebrain of the pretrigeminal animal truly reflect the presence of a functional waking consciousness? For instance, is the pretrigeminal cat aware of its surroundings and capable of integrating events going on around its paralyzed body? This could only be answered by the ability of such an animal to exhibit new instrumental learning within its isolated forebrain. This was an especially difficult question to answer, since such a forebrain can experience only vision and smell and can communicate with the world only through its eyes (since only the oculomotor and trochlear motor nerves remained connected to the forebrain). It would have been absurd to try to achieve learning in such animals through the administration of traditional rewards such as food, water, warmth, and touch, since the incoming nerves for these sensations lie well below the cut. In other words, taste, which comes in via cranial nerves VII, X, and XI (the facial, vagus, and glossopharyngeal nerves, respectively), and the sensations of warmth and touch, which arise largely from the spinal cord, had been surgically disconnected from the forebrain processes of consciousness that investigators wished to analyze. Hence, one could only use olfactory and visual stimuli from the outside world as potential rewards to modify instrumental movements of the eyes—reinforcement channels that are not commonly used to study animal learning. Rather than attempting such difficult experiments, investigators decided to evaluate the efficacy of central "reward" evoked by stimulation of the lateral hypothalamus—which, because of its anatomical trajectory, should have remained intact in the isolated forebrain (see Chapter 8). It turned out that pretrigeminal cats readily learned to move their eyes to self-administer rewarding hypothalamic stimulation.[49] Thus, we may conclude that their waking EEG was probably accompanied by conscious awareness. The alternative, of course, is that animals can learn such responses without any consciousness.

Another key question was the precise nature of the waking mechanism that was situated within the rostral pons between the *cerveau isolé* and *pretrigeminal* cuts. A partial answer to this appears to be the existence of two cholinergic cell groups in this area, namely, Ch-5 and Ch-6, which operate in tandem with the nearby locus coeruleus, the large norepinephrine cell group (A6) (see Figure 6.5). These nuclear groups are all situated at the pontomesencephalic tissue that was added to the telencephalic part of the *cerveau isolé* preparation by the pretrigeminal cut (Figure 7.2). It is well established that these ascending neural systems participate in cerebral arousal and attention, but there are also several additional arousal mechanisms, such as dopaminergic, histaminergic, glutamatergic, and various neuropeptide systems situated even farther up in the brain stem. However, those higher systems alone do not seem able to maintain waking consciousness within the isolated forebrain. What is needed for waking consciousness is the influence of the aforementioned cholinergic and noradrenergic innervation of the forebrain. The *cerveau isolé* surgery severs the ascending axons of both of these systems.

It is now certain that the cholinergic cell groups situated near the rostral pons are a central feature of the ARAS. These attention-promoting sytems can control activity in many anterior brain areas, as well as in many areas in the lower brain stem, including cranial nerve nuclei.[50] In short, brain stem cholinergic systems open neural gateways that promote the processing of sensory information within widespread areas of the brain during waking, especially via sensory information channels that course through the thalamus. One can induce clear facilitation of neural activity in ascending sensory pathways of the thalamus by electrical stimulation of the brain stem cholinergic cell groups. The effect also substantially outlasts the stimulation. For instance, one second of stimulation to nerve group Ch-6 can increase the excitability of thalamic systems for up to six minutes,[51] which suggests that such stimulation, in addition to releasing ACh, also releases neuromodulators that sustain the short-term arousal provoked by ACh. If one blocks the effects of cholinergic systems by administering muscarinic receptor antagonists such as atropine or scopolamine, one can generate powerful slow wave activity in the cortex. This can occur without induction of behavioral sleep! Such animals are awake even though they appear disoriented. Indeed, they are in a confusional state with often horrid hallucinations, if human subjective experience can be accepted as a guide for understanding the animal mind.

It is now well accepted that during reduced cholinergic activity in the brain, attentional and memory consolidation capacities of both humans and animals are severely compromised. Indeed, many of the cognitive problems of Alzheimer's disease are due to deterioration of these neurochemical systems, especially of the rostral basal forebrain cholinergic cells (cell groups Ch-1–Ch-4).[52] In short, the widespread cholinergic systems of the forebrain and brain stem are essential for sustained waking arousal and attention of higher brain areas in broad and nonspecific ways. As will be discussed later, there is also reason to believe that the more scattered cholinergic neurons farther down in the brain stem are essential for the arousal of REM sleep. This finding suggests that some kind of neurobiological continuity exists between REM arousal and waking arousal within the brain. It is possible that the widely scattered ACh neurons that now govern the phasic aspects of REM originally mediated a more emotional form of waking in our ancestral species.

The role of NE neurons in sustaining waking behavior seems more modest than that of cholinergic systems. Destruction of NE cell groups deepens SWS and increases REM sleep.[53] Although sleepiness and tiredness are increased by depletion of brain NE systems, this system appears to control selective attention rather than the overall capacity for normal waking consciousness. When one observes the actual effects of NE release on sensory processing within the cortex, one finds that there is an amplification of signal-to-noise ratios, which is effected more by a reduction of the seemingly random background chatter (i.e., neural noise?) rather than an amplification of incoming sensory signals.[54] Thus, while cholinergic cell groups intensify all sensory signals headed for the cortex, NE may focus attention on specific components of the world.

NE cells typically respond to any novel sensory event, but these effects habituate fairly quickly;[55] however, the changes are more sustained if the environmental events have substantial emotional impact. For instance, a cat's locus coeruleus becomes very active when the cat is confronted by a barking dog.[56] Some have suggested that the NE system of the locus coeruleus is a specific emotional system promoting fear,[57] but there is little evidence for such affective specificity. To the best of our knowledge, NE participates to some extent in all cognitive and emotional activities, pleasant as well as unpleasant ones.

Brain Mechanisms of Slow Wave Sleep

Since cholinergic cell groups of the basal forebrain help mediate attention and memory formation, a reduction in their activities will promote SWS. However, this effect by itself does not seem to be sufficient to put an organism to sleep, even though anticholinergics used to be the most common active ingredient in over-the-counter sleep medications. The same can be said for reductions in brain NE activity. Other factors must contribute to the equation before sleep can solidify. Perhaps a certain amount of adenosine or GABA activity has to build up. As already mentioned, arousal of specific preoptic nuclei within the anterior hypothalamus is highly effective in promoting SWS, and those neurons contain GABA. In sum, there is probably no single SWS generator in the brain. Many factors can reduce brain arousal. As with so many other functions, SWS is multiply and perhaps hierarchically controlled within the brain.

Historically, one biogenic amine system has been recognized as a facilitator of SWS: the serotonin-containing raphe neurons of the brain stem. But it is unlikely that this is an active sleep-promoting system as opposed to one that normally participates in generating calm behaviors during waking. Electrophysiological analysis has never demonstrated increased raphe cell firing during the onset of sleep. Indeed, raphe neurons actually fire less during the transition from waking to SWS,[58] so we must consider their activity in the context of the whole spectrum of ongoing brain changes. For instance, perhaps mild serotonin activity may be especially relaxing in the presence of diminished ACh or NE tone. In any event, pharmacological facilitators of serotonin activity are typically quite powerful sleep-promoting agents: The serotonin precursors, tryptophan and 5–hydroxytryptophan, markedly promote SWS, as do serotonin-releasing drugs such as fenfluramine and serotonin reuptake inhibitors (especially certain tricyclic antidepressants such as amytriptiline, which also has especially strong anticholinergic effects).[59] It is unlikely that all of these forms of induced sleep resemble the natural process. Finally, it should be reemphasized that one metabolic product of serotonin—namely, melatonin—is a remarkably powerful promoter of natural SWS. Indeed, melatonin-induced sleep seems deeper than normal sleep, which may explain why those who take it sometimes get by with less overall sleep each night. Unfortunately, the increased deepness cannot be measured with surface EEG recordings.

It is noteworthy that all of the manipulations that increase serotonin availability at synapses uniformly and markedly reduce REM sleep, even though people who initially start to take melatonin often describe more vivid dreams. As will be discussed later, it may well be that one function of REM sleep is to rejuvenate the serotonin system; if the availability of serotonin is pharmacologically amplified at synapses, animals do appear to have a reduced need for REM sleep.

While facilitation of serotonin activity can increase SWS, depletion of serotonin can reduce the amount of SWS, as one might expect.[60] Inhibition of serotonin synthesis with the tryptophan hydroxylase inhibitor parachlorophenylalanine (PCPA), promotes insomnia and hence increases arousal (although there are remarkable and still unexplained species differences in this effect, with cats being much more severely affected than rats or humans).[61] In sum, the overall regulation of SWS is complex, and many additional factors contribute to sound sleep, ranging from a wide variety of neuropeptides such as delta sleep–inducing-peptide (DSIP) as well as some metabolic products of GABA such as gamma-hydroxybutyrate.[62]

Brain Mechanisms of REM Sleep: Is Dreaming Older Than Waking in Brain Evolution?

As mentioned earlier, following a pretrigeminal brain stem transection, basic waking mechanisms exist above the cut while neurons that turn on REM sleep remain below the cut (Figure 7.2). Further transection studies indicate that the REM executive mechanism resides within the lower pons, since a cut between the pons and the medulla leaves the REM mechanism in rostral brain areas.[63] There are several distinct REM functions within this general zone of the brain stem, since a cut right through the middle of the pons tends to impair the integration of REM, leaving the mechanisms for atonia above the transection and those for the phasic components below. With such damage, the coherence of the REM state disintegrates. The area of the brain that maintains the tonic functions of REM such as atonia is situated just below the A6 NE nucleus of the locus coeruleus, while the phasic mechanisms are situated in the dorsolateral pontine reticular formation. When these respective areas are individually lesioned, the tonic and phasic components of REM are selectively attenuated.[64] Both systems for REM are built to a substantial extent around cholinergic neural influences. Placement of drugs that promote ACh activity into these lower brain stem regions can trigger REM sleep episodes.[65]

In this context, it is noteworthy that many of the *giant cells of the reticular tegmental fields* (the so-called FTG neurons) exhibit dramatic bursts of firing during REM sleep. It is generally thought that they contribute substantially to the phasic components of REM. It has been noted that these same cells mediate rapid orientation movements during waking, indicating that their activities are not simply confined to REM, but this does not minimize their importance for helping generate the neural storms of REM (e.g., PGO spikes).[66] Indeed, from the perspective that the ancient REM mechanisms originally contributed to an ancient form of waking arousal, the continued participation of such cells in some primitive orienting reflexes makes considerable sense.

Although both waking arousal and REM arousal have strong cholinergic influences, it is noteworthy that the REM state is no longer just a waking state masked under the massive motor relaxation of atonia; it is a distinct brain state. The entire brain stem appears to make a dramatic "180-degree state-shift" during REM: The reticular formation begins to actively promote inhibition as opposed to excitation.[67] This has been demonstrated by analyzing the effects of reticular stimulation on the jaw-closing reflex aroused by direct activation of the motor nuclei of the trigeminal (i.e., the motor component of cranial nerve V). In the waking state, prior reticular stimulation facilitates the biting reflex, but during the REM state, stimulation applied to exactly the same sites inhibits the reflex. This startling finding indicates that the function of certain reticular zones is diametrically reversed during dreaming sleep, and this contributes to the massive motor inhibition that characterizes REM sleep.

As noted previously, it is remarkable how far down in the brain stem the executive mechanisms for REM sleep are situated: The heart of the major concentration of REM-initiating neurons lies caudal to the ARAS waking mechanism. Brain mechanisms that evolved earlier are typically lower within the neuroaxis and in more medial positions than more recent additions. Are we to believe that REM mechanisms are somewhat older than waking ones? However unlikely this may seem on the face of it, the above brain localizations coax us to consider such an absurdity.

We should note that although REM is an ancient brain function in mammals, to the best of our knowledge, fish and reptiles exhibit no such state. REM sleep is also rudimentary in birds, occurring only in brief and infrequent episodes.[68] Indeed, one ancient egg-laying mammal, the echidna (the marsupial spiny anteater of Australia, which has a number of unusual brain features such as enlarged frontal lobes and no corpus callosum), apparently exhibits no REM sleep.[69] Using this evolutionary context as a background, it is unlikely that REM evolved de novo within the lower brain stem of early mammals. It seems more reasonable to assume that the brain mechanisms that now mediate REM in essentially all mammals once subserved some other type of brain function in ancestral creatures. Indeed, from a range of facts summarized earlier, we might surmise that what is now known as the REM mechanism originally controlled a primitive form of waking arousal. With the evolution of higher brain areas, a newer and more efficient waking mechanism may have been needed, leading to the emergence of the ARAS. The more ancient form of arousal may have been gradually overridden and relegated to providing a background function such as the integration of emotional information that seems to occur during dreaming. People who hold dream experiences in great esteem may be correctly affirming the importance of the affective information that is encoded through our ancient emotional urges for the proper conduct of our waking activities.

If this is true, what type of waking was mediated by the ancient system that now mediates dreaming? One reasonable possibility, suggested by the high affective content of most dreams, is that what is now the REM sleep mechanism originally mediated the selective arousal of emotionality. Prior to the emergence of complex cognitive strategies, animals may have generated most of their behavior from primary-process psychobehavioral routines that we now recognize as the primitive emotional systems—such as those covered in this middle part of the text. In other words, many of the behaviors of ancient animals may have emerged largely from preprogrammed emotional subroutines. These simpleminded behavioral solutions were eventually superseded by more sophisticated cognitive approaches that required not only more neocortex but also new arousal mechanisms to sustain efficient waking functions within those emerging brain areas.

As the new thalamocortical cognitive mechanisms evolved, the old emotional arousal system may have assumed the subsidiary role of doing computations on the environmental relationships that had transpired during waking, especially those with a strong emotional content. In other words, the REM system may now allow ancient emotional impulses to be integrated with the newer cognitive skills of the more recently evolved brain waking sytems. This could help explain many striking attributes of REM sleep, ranging from its heavy emotional content to its apparent functions of enhancing learning and solidifying memory consolidation, which will be discussed later in this chapter.

Is Sleep Essential for Survival?

Researchers have no problem suggesting an overall function for waking. It is the state during which organisms gather the fruits of the world needed for survival, avoid dangers, and spend time together propagating the species. Because of cultural evolution, especially the effective development of agriculture, modern humans also have time left over for the pursuit of many creative activities. By comparison, the psychological functions of sleep are not so evident, and even though there is much speculation, no proposed function has yet been demonstrated unambiguously. Still, a general assumption of most investigators is that SWS and REM sleep states serve distinct functions in the body and brain. Obviously, with a phenomenon as complex and pervasive as sleep, there are bound to be several correct answers to functional questions, depending on one's levels of analysis. Indeed, since sleep systems operate at so many different levels of the brain and body, we must avoid the temptation to take unitary theoretical perspectives too seriously. Just like eating serves many functions, ranging from social functions to the assimilation of macro- and micronutrients, the stages of sleep are bound to have many ramifications for the lives of organisms.

Still, the most basic question is whether sleep is necessary for survival. At one time it was widely believed that animals did not really require REM sleep, and the need for SWS could not be properly evaluated since it cannot be selectively eliminated (i.e., by blocking access to SWS we also block access to REM). Nonetheless, work using a devilishly clever methodology for total sleep deprivation and prolonged selective REM deprivation eventually yielded some unambiguous findings. Sleep is essential for life![70] Rats were housed on circular island platforms surrounded by water. The platforms were divided in half by an immovable partition, and an experimental animal and a yoked (i.e., tightly matched) control animal were allowed to live on each side of the partition. The floor began to rotate whenever the experimental animal fell asleep, as determined by EEG criteria. The EEG of the yoked control animal had no such effect. If the experimental animal did not wake up, the rotation gradually pushed it, but usually not the control, into the surrounding water, which certainly did provoke arousal. The experimental rats began to die approximately two weeks following the initiation of total sleep deprivation and five to six weeks after the beginning of selective REM deprivation (even if the total amount of dunking received by experimental and yoked animals was strictly controlled). The yoked controls who lived on the other side of the periodically rotating platforms, but whose EEGs did not govern rotation, continued to thrive. In short, control animals remained healthy, because their sleep was only modestly disrupted by the rotation of the platform.

The precise reason the experimental animals died remained elusive for a long time. Their inability to sustain thermoregulation may have been a major cause. Indeed, they ate more than normal, while still losing weight. Apparently, they were unable to properly store and utilize energy. Their ultimate death may reflect an immune system collapse; recent work suggests that many of the animals deprived of sleep may eventually die of a bacterial infection of the bloodstream.[71] Thus, they may be succumbing to a chronically sustained stress response. Although these experiments seem cruel, they have provided definitive evidence that sleep does help sustain the health of the body. However, the specific brain functions of SWS and REM sleep have remained more elusive.

Sleep and Its Basic Bodily and Brain Functions

One way to view sleep is within the context of the many bodily changes that transpire during the various vigilance states. Specific hormonal changes tend to occur during specific components of sleep and waking cycles. For instance, during waking, the release of insulin is linked to the act of eating—being secreted in proportion to the amount of energy consumed that needs to be tucked away in fat stores (see Chapter 9). These stores eventually need to be distributed for tissue repair, and apparently the body prefers to concentrate many of its restorative activities into periods of SWS when the body is not being used vigorously. Thus, many now believe that SWS is a permissive period for tissue repair processes.[72]

One impressive line of evidence that SWS does restore bodily functions is the fact that secretion of growth hormone (GH) from the anterior pituitary is tightly linked to SWS onset. Usually there are several pulses of GH during the night, with the largest one occurring during the early periods of SWS, which are typically the longest of the night, with secondary secretions during subsequent SWS periods (Figure 7.3). Further, the amount of GH secretion during the initial SWS period is positively related to the metabolic status of the animal, being larger in well-fed animals than in hungry ones.[73] This permits especially accurate redistribution of available energy resources during sleep. As an important corollary, this suggests that brain tissue can directly gauge overall energy intake during the day. If this is the case, a most reasonable location for the energy-sensitive brain tissue would be in the ventromedial hypothalamus, directly above the pituitary stalk, where GH secretion is regulated. A great deal of research now indicates that this is indeed the case (see Chapter 9). Since GH promotes tissue repair, especially of muscles, we can also appreciate why work and physical exercise would tend to promote SWS.

The secretion of GH during SWS is critically dependent on the occurrence of SWS episodes. If SWS is disturbed, so is GH secretion.[74] Also, since GH can increase subsequent REM periods,[75] sleep disruptions that block GH secretion can have effects on subsequent sleep staging. In childhood, GH promotes linear bone growth, so the strong GH-SWS relationship may help explain why certain children fail to thrive in emotionally disturbing environments. Indeed, the syndrome of *psychosocial dwarfism*, which arises from chaotic family circumstances, often leads to disturbed sleep patterns, which then lead to diminished GH secretion in the afflicted children.[76] When emotional stress levels are decreased by placement into more stable and supportive environments where the children can sleep well again, they resume their growth.

The direct dependence of GH on the presence of SWS poses no major problems for world travelers or shift workers. When sleep patterns change, the pattern of GH secretion adapts promptly. This is not the case for other hormonal rhythms, such as pituitary adrenocorticotrophic hormone (ACTH) secretion, which is entrained to REM sleep but not actually triggered by REM episodes.

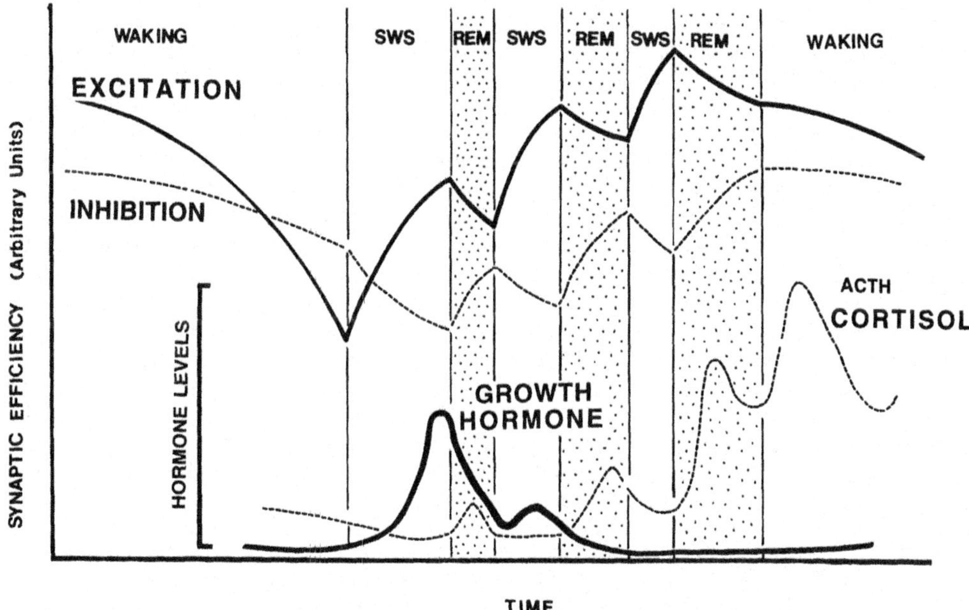

Figure 7.3. Patterns of hormone secretion (*bottom*) and possible neurochemical changes (*top*) as a function of cycling stages of SWS and REM. Different phases of sleep probably promote different types of brain and body restoration. It is possible that the successive phases of SWS and REM help regulate overall excitatory and inhibitory potentials in the brain so as to sustain a balance of neurochemistries to help mediate coherent behaviors during waking. (Adapted from Panksepp, 1981; see n. 99.)

REM periods, like SWS periods, have their own hormonal signatures, the most prominent one being the preferential secretion of ACTH (Figure 7.3).[77] This, of course, triggers the secretion of the glucocorticoid cortisol from the human adrenal gland (see Figure 6.8). During normal sleep, such "stresslike" hormone secretions intensify with each successive REM period as the night progresses. There is reason to believe that these secretions gradually prepare the body for waking activities by facilitating catabolic activities—promoting energy utilization in the body. Adrenal glucocorticoids do this by facilitating *gluconeogenesis* (the production of glucose from protein) and also by producing some insulin resistance in body tissues, making more energy available to the brain, which, unlike other bodily tissues, does not require insulin to utilize glucose efficiently. Presumably then, REM-related cortisol secretion helps to extract available body energy stores for promoting waking activities. It is not far-fetched to assume that ACTH pulses may also serve as a natural alarm clock that gradually helps wake us when the body is ready once more to exhibit efficient waking behavior.

However, ACTH secretion is only a passive servant that comes to be coupled to REM episodes. In other words, the circadian rhythm of ACTH secretion is not causally controlled by our REM periods. The real master is the biological clock in the SCN. Hence, ACTH secretion does not shift rapidly following major shifts in sleep patterns. For instance, a 12-hour shift (i.e., as if you had traveled to the other side of the earth) requires up to two weeks for full readjustment.[78] This helps explain why one tends to feel sluggish and strange following a reversal of sleep-waking patterns (as in shift work or with jet lag). The body is no longer distributing its resources at the regular time, so mental abilities cannot properly match environmental demands. Judicious administration of bright light and melatonin prior to jet travel can help the biological clock synchronize faster.[79] For instance, if you are traveling from the United States to Europe (leading to a "phase advance" in bodily rhythms), small amounts of melatonin, taken on several successive evenings prior to departure, approximately an hour earlier each time, can markedly speed up clock readjustment on reaching your destination. Getting a lot of bright light early in the morning also helps considerably.

Also relevant to its role in emotionality, ACTH is one of the prime hormones that allow the body and brain to cope with stress (Figure 6.8). It is secreted from the pituitary in response to practically any stressful situation, regardless of the cause.[80] As discussed at the end of the previous chapter, the pituitary adrenal stress response is initiated by physical or psychic stressors that can gain access to the corticotrophin releasing factor

(CRF) neurons of the hypothalamic paraventricular nucleus (PVN). Part of this activation arises from ascending NE systems which synapse on the PVN (but this cannot be the cause of CRF secretion during REM, since NE neurons are silent at that time). In any event, activated PVN neurons trigger the release of ACTH from the anterior pituitary (see Figure 6.8). The adrenal glucocorticoids that are thereby released feed back onto the PVN and exert a negative feedback or braking effect on the further release of CRF.[81] Parenthetically, since CRF controls several anxiety-related emotions in the brain (see Chapters 11 and 14), the concurrent release of this peptide within the brain during REM may promote the emergence of emotionally aversive dream content.

It is noteworthy that this hormonal feedback loop is broken in certain psychiatric disorders that are commonly accompanied by sleep disturbances. For instance, depressed individuals often do not exhibit a suppression of cortisol secretion in response to administration of glucocorticoid hormones such as dexamethasone (hence a diagnostic test has been developed that is called the *dexamethasone suppression test*, as discussed in Chapter 6).[82] In fact, many depressed individuals exhibit excessively high secretions of ACTH and cortisol during REM sleep in the middle of the night. This tends to waken them in the early morning hours.[83] Also, it is important to note that some of the feedback effects of adrenal steroids, such as cortisol, on the brain may worsen depression. For instance, it is not uncommon to observe depression during steroid therapy for other disorders, even though some individuals also exhibit mania or elation.[84]

From this perspective, it is not too surprising that artificial prevention of REM sleep or total sleep deprivation can counteract depression as effectively as any of the available antidepressant drugs.[85] Presumably this is achieved, at least in part, by blocking hormone secretions that accompany REM, and perhaps through the overall reduction of neurochemical changes that normally result from sleep. Indeed, it remains possible that many antidepressant drugs exert at least part of their therapeutic effects indirectly by suppressing REM. It is well established that drugs that block the uptake of biogenic amines from the synaptic cleft (i.e., the tricyclic antidepressants and selective serotonin reuptake inhibitors) are all quite potent inhibitors of REM. However, it remains to be empirically demonstrated that the antidepressant effects of these drugs arise from their effects on REM-related brain processes.

The Potential Adaptive Functions of REM Sleep

A remarkable number of ideas have been generated concerning the possible functions of REM sleep. They include rather improbable items such as providing an exercise period for "binocular coordination," "drive discharge," and even "periodic arousals from sleep for enhancing predator detection" (even though it is evident that predators typically exhibit more REM sleep than do prey species).[86] An especially creative albeit improbable theory, generated by Nobel Prize–winner Francis Crick, the codiscoverer of the structure of DNA, suggests that REM is a permissive period for the forgetting of excess memory traces.[87] In other words, REM dumps excess memories that might otherwise inundate the brain with useless "cognitive litter." Although it might explain the bizarre, apparently random, spilling of information into dream consciousness during REM, the theory has practically no credible support at the present time.

There are any number of more plausible hypotheses related to the possible role of REM sleep in the control of developmental processes and information processing. The idea that REM sleep may have a special influence on early development arose from the observation that young animals exhibit the greatest amount of REM sleep, followed by a systematic decline with age. Accordingly, REM may provide an opportunity for certain critical but as yet undetermined processes to transpire in the growing brain. One of the foremost investigators of how the brain controls sleep has posited that REM sleep may facilitate the activation and exercise of genetically determined behavior patterns.[88] Jouvet suggested that REM sleep resembles a "burn-in" process comparable to that used by computer manufacturers to assure that all components are operational and thereby to minimize failure rates. In other words, REM may facilitate the transmission of instinctual behavior patterns from genetically specified neuronal codes into the efficient dynamic activities of brain circuits.

Although the idea is provocative, it has proved difficult to confirm, and at present it has no clear empirical support. In our own lab, we tested Jouvet's idea by preventing REM sleep in young rats soon after birth with the drug chlorimipramine (a tricyclic antidepressant drug that selectively blocks serotonin reuptake and can essentially eliminate REM sleep for long periods of time).[89] This treatment was continued for slightly over three weeks throughout the period of early development, after which the animals were evaluated on their readiness to indulge in rough-and-tumble play, a relatively complex instinctual behavior pattern that juvenile rats exhibit even in the absence of relevant early social experience (see Chapter 15). We observed only a marginal tendency for the REM-deprived animals to be deficient in play. Generally, their play was normal, but there were mild changes in some behaviors, such as a slightly slower development of stable dominance patterns. In any event, these findings provided no clear support for Jouvet's intriguing hypothesis.

Of course, the high level of REM during early development may be related to new information processing and neuronal growth, a massive task for young organisms, rather than to any "burning in" of brain circuits. Since REM sleep has been implicated in memory consolidation and protein synthesis, it would logically be expected to be high during early life.[90] There is widespread agreement that REM does have some special role in the processing of learned information, even though the empirical findings have often been confusing. REM increases following some, but not all, learning tasks. REM deprivation following learning tends to undermine memory consolidation for some types of learning but not for others. Investigators have sought to make sense of this puzzling array of results by suggesting that REM is only involved in the solidification of complex memories but *not* in the consolidation of memories for which the nervous system is fully *prepared* by evolution.[91]

A variant of the preceding is that REM allows the basic emotional circuits of the brain to be accessed in a systematic way, which may permit emotion-related information collected during waking hours to be reaccessed and solidified as lasting memories in sleep. REM periods may allow some type of restructuring and stabilization of the information that has been harvested into temporary memory stores. During REM, neural computations may be done on this partially stored information, and consolidation may be strengthened on the basis of reliable predictive relationships that exist between the various events that have been experienced. The dream may reflect the computational solidification process as different emotionally coded memory stores are reactivated, and the web of associated relationships is allowed to unreel once more and to coalesce into long-term memories and plans, depending on the predominant patterns of reevaluation. The highest statistical relationships between events that regularly reappear together may be selected as putative causes for emotional concerns in the real world, and hence stored in long-term memory to be used as anticipatory strategies on future occasions when similar circumstances arise. In other words, REM may generate what cognitively oriented investigators call "attributions." For instance, we may solidify certain assumptions about causal influences in the world through the REM process, but it is certainly possible that the perceived relationships are, in fact, delusional. This may help us see the potential relations between dreaming, schizophrenia, and more everyday forms of madness.

If REM arousal mechanisms are in fact the descendants of ancient arousal mechanisms for energizing emotional states, this view would help explain many striking characteristics of dreaming, from its pervasive emotionality to the fact that the executive generators are situated remarkably deep within the brain stem. From this vantage, REM may be a selective time for complex emotion-laden information patterns encountered during waking to be reprocessed into long-term affective memory stores. More than anything, these new stores may contribute to the unconscious, subconscious, or preconscious habits and personality development of the animal, which may help explain the amnesia we typically exhibit for our dreamwork. It may help solidify our emotional strengths as well as our weaknesses. Of course, this view (which resembles those of Freud and Jung) also remains with little empirical support. It is fair to say that despite thousands of excellent studies, we remain on the near shore of a definitive understanding of this fascinating brain process.

REM Sleep, Emotionality, and Learning

The relationship between dreaming, emotionality, and learning is widely recognized, and, as mentioned earlier, it is possible that REM reflects the ancestral brain "residue" of an ancient waking system that served to selectively arouse emotional processes. Indeed, there are still many relationships between dreaming and emotions. As previously indicated, the amount of REM sleep is routinely elevated after organisms are confronted by new environments and stressful situations. This is also true for early development, when the world is new and emotions are raw. As noted, animals exhibit more REM when they are young than at any other time of life. Presumably these effects arise from the fact that encounters with a great deal of new information and intensification of emotional patterns can, in some presently unknown way, feed back on the basic REM generators of the brain stem. It is becoming clear that REM is intimately involved in emotions and new information processing, but REM does not facilitate all forms of learning.

The imposition of REM deprivation after a learning task does not impair the consolidation of simple emotional memories (like one-way avoidance of electric shock, which resembles running away from a predator).[92] These simple tasks are very easy for animals to learn since they are concordant with the natural dictates of their emotional systems (i.e., it requires no great cognitive skill to run away from approaching danger). In other words, animals appear to be evolutionarily *prepared* to learn such simple emotional tasks. The same amount of REM deprivation severely compromises learning of complex emotional tasks that are not prefigured in the animal's evolutionary history, such as "two-way avoidance," which requires continual movement back and forth between safe and danger zones of a test chamber. In the natural world, such devilish situations do not normally arise. A safe area does not turn into a danger area, and back to a safe area again, over and over, within the span of a few moments. Only the cleverness of behavioral researchers has brought these nightmarish circumstances into a rat's life. Without posttraining REM sleep, rats take very much longer to master such emotionally difficult tasks. Apparently they cannot extract the meaningful, but counterintuitive, relationships that exist in the situation. Exposure to two-way avoidance learning tasks also markedly elevates the amounts of posttraining REM that rats exhibit, while simple one-way avoidance learning yields no comparable elevations.[93]

The relations between REM and emotionality have been demonstrated most clearly by studies in which the atonia mechanisms situated just below the locus coeruleus have been damaged.[94] Instead of becoming immobilized during REM, such animals act out their dreams. This provides our clearest porthole into the nature of animal dreams and affirms that the REM state is laden with emotional storms. Cats exhibit only four major behavior patterns—exploration, fearfulness, anger, and grooming behaviors. It is almost as if the phasic REM mechanisms were repeatedly, but in some as yet uncharted order, activating the executive machinery for instinctual brain processes related to emotionality. Not only does this work affirm that REM sleep is intimately related to the emotional machinery of the brain, but it also indicates that the psychic, hallucinatory components of dreaming are activated by the phasic REM mechanisms (PGO spikes and the bursting of FTG cells) rather than by the atonia mechanism.

Although dream content is closely linked to PGO generators, one must ultimately make a distinction between phasic REM generators and the hallucinatory dream content of REM sleep. The human dream probably arises from the many higher brain systems upon which the PGO spikes impinge. As mentioned earlier, people who have had frontal lobectomies still exhibit normal amounts of the objective indicators of REM sleep, but they lose the dream content that normally accompanies the state (or at least any memory thereof). When such individuals are woken from REM, they describe no vivid experiences, only gray emptiness. This could be interpreted as an illogical and perplexing finding, since the frontal areas consist largely of motor association cortex. Does this observation tell us another important thing about REM—that much of the dream content that we experience is critically dependent on the motor side of our higher brain apparatus rather than on the sensory side? Although this may seem unlikely on the surface, we should remember that the frontal cortex contains neural circuits that help elaborate intentions, plans, expectancies, and probably some of the higher affective aspects of consciousness (see Chapter 16). Perhaps without these hopes and fears for the future, the sensory side of the brain simply does not become fully activated during REM. Perhaps motor planning mechanisms are necessary to retrieve sensory-perceptual images from more posterior cerebral areas. It is also noteworthy that the frontal areas of the brain rather than the posterior sensory areas are more strongly innervated by the diverse subcortical emotional systems that are discussed throughout this book. However, this view of dream organization does have one serious flaw: Recent PET scanning data indicate that the prefrontal cortex is relatively quiescent during REM (see note 13).

Focusing on the higher reaches of the brain gives us a more realistic view of the ultimate complexity of the neural substrates of dreams. Since the cognitive and emotional challenges that animals experience tend to increase subsequent REM, there are bound to be regulatory feedbacks from higher areas back to the brain stem REM generators. Indeed, the possibility of such linkages has been suggested by experiments in which the neocortex is destroyed. Removal of the neocortex in cats has profound effects on sleep; both REM and SWS are dramatically reduced,[95] probably because of the removal of tonic inhibitory influences that normally allow the subcortical systems to function in a well-ordered fashion.

We can be certain that the executive mechanisms for sleep have not been truly disrupted by such brain damage. If these hyperaroused animals (remember, decortication releases subcortical impulses) are sedated with barbiturate anesthetics, both SWS and REM return to normal levels.[96] The inhibition within the brain stem is sufficiently restored by these anesthetics to allow the primitive executive mechanisms to operate efficiently once more. This suggests that higher brain influences can feed back upon the executive machinery of the lower brain stem. This point is further highlighted by the fact that various waking experiences can either increase or decrease the amounts and types of sleep animals exhibit. At present, we have no clear evidence how that is achieved. Such issues are closely related to the largest unresolved question of sleep research: What are the precise functions of the various sleep stages in brain homeostasis?

Possible Neurochemical Functions of REM

It is generally agreed that sleep stages have some type of restorative effects on the neurobiological functions of the brain. The most common hypothesis has been that they allow certain transmitters to be rejuvenated. The most well-developed idea has been that brain NE is restored during REM.[97] Even though no support has been found for this idea when brain levels of NE are measured, it is possible that REM selectively facilitates synaptic efficacy. In other words, REM may control NE postsynaptic receptor regulation, and it has been found that during waking, when NE systems are active, brain NE receptor sensitivity does decline. Conversely, during REM sleep, when NE neurons cease firing, there is an up-regulation of receptors, promoting restoration of normal synaptic transmission.[98] Parenthetically, these findings do seem paradoxical from the perspective that REM deprivation can alleviate depression (i.e., some antidepressants also facilitate NE activity), but it is no doubt the case that REM helps restore many other neurochemical systems, including presumably some that intensify negative affect. Also, it is possible that REM helps solidify affectively negative cognitions, which can then intensify depressive episodes.

I favor an alternative neurochemical viewpoint that sees REM as providing a period of relatively selective rejuvenation in the synaptic efficacy of the serotonin (i.e., 5-HT) system,[99] with no clear hypothesis whether this is achieved through increases in presynaptic availability of the transmitter, postsynaptic receptor sensitivity, or other changes such as differential synaptic reuptake of amines. This hypothesis is based on the rather obvious resemblances between the spontaneous behavioral tendencies of serotonin-depleted animals and those that have been selectively deprived of REM sleep. These animals do not appear tired but instead exhibit frantic energy. In a phrase, such animals are behaviorally *disinhibited*: They are more active, more aggressive, hypersexual, and generally exhibit more motivational/emotional energy than "REM-satiated" animals. In short, they appear to be manic. Little wonder that REM deprivation alleviates depression.

We have tested the serotonin rejuvenation proposition fairly straightforwardly. First, we selected a physiological response, thermoregulation, which is quite sensitive to serotonin availability in the brain. Because serotonin participates in a heat-generating system in the body,[100] if REM-deprived animals have a serotonin deficit they should be less capable of sustaining body temperature in response to cold. In fact this proved to be the case in young rats. REM-deprived animals did not restore body temperature as rapidly as normal animals after exposure to cold. Then we determined whether biogenic amine reuptake inhibitors that were specific for serotonin (e.g., fluoxetine) or NE (desipramine) would rectify the thermoregulatory deficit. The answer was clear cut. As summarized in Figure 7.4, the serotonin reuptake inhibitor alleviated the deficit, while the NE inhibitor did not.[101] Of course, it should be emphasized that a serotonin-specific measure was selected, and it might be the case that the opposite result would have been obtained if an NE-specific measure, like selective attention, had been used. In fact, considering that both neuronal systems cease firing during REM (see the "Afterthought" of this chapter), it seems likely that both would have an excellent opportunity to be rejuvenated. In any event, both of these hypotheses face the same dilemma: Why would REM deprivation produce antidepressant effects?

More to the point, the restorative effects of sleep may be even broader, permitting restoration and rebalancing of many neurochemical systems in the brain. Future research should consider the possibility that SWS is a special period when behavioral excitatory processes in the brain are restored, while REM sleep is a period when inhibitory processes are restored (see Figure 7.3). Through the gradual reciprocity of these states, the brain may be brought back to a balance point of optimal functioning. Sleep is a phenomenon full of paradoxes. Let me address one final one that has been alluded to several times in this chapter.

If one of the major functions of REM sleep is to facilitate information processing, it is remarkable that

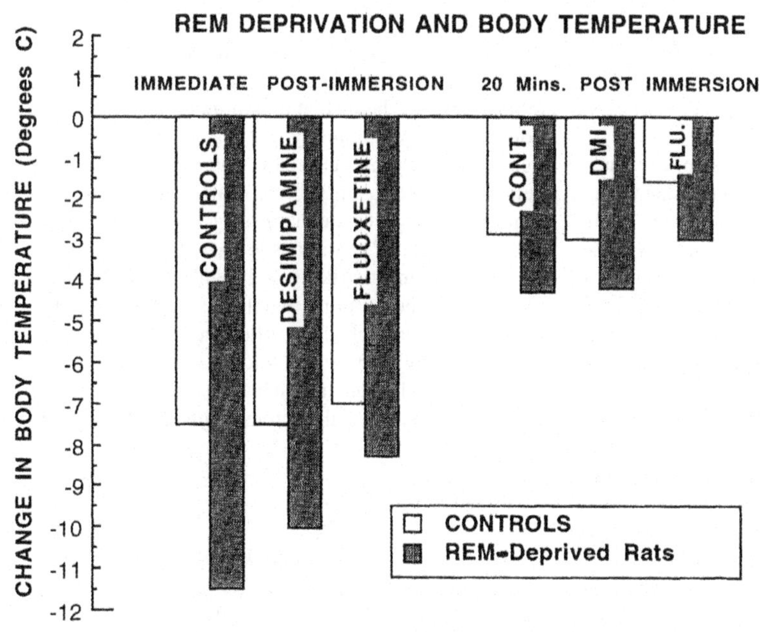

Figure 7.4. Changes in body temperature in REM-deprived animals as a function of treatment with a selective norepinephrine reuptake inhibitor (desipramine) and a serotonin reuptake inhibitor (fluoxetine/Prozac®). REM-deprived rats lose more body heat than control animals to the same cold-water challenge. The smaller reduction and faster restoration of normal body temperature recovery following fluoxetine, which selec-tively enhances serotonin activity, suggest that, in addition to many other brain effects, REM sleep may promote restoration of serotonin functions in the brain. (According to unpublished data, Bishop & Panksepp, 1980.)

humans have such great difficulty remembering the content of their dreams. The vast majority of dream material is never recalled, and many scientists believe that the consolidation mechanisms of the brain are shut down during REM. It is almost as if humans experience an amnesic syndrome similar to that which follows hippocampal damage. A famous neurological patient known as H. M. had such a syndrome—of living in the perpetual present—following bilateral temporal lobe surgery.[102] He, like many similar patients since then, was unable to transfer short-term memories to long-term stores. During the transition of dreaming to waking, we are all like H. M. The memory of the dream dries up like a shallow pool of water in the desert. Postdreaming amnesia may be due in part to the cessation of NE activity during the dream. It is known that facilitation of brain NE activity can promote memory consolidation,[103] and the dreaming brain has very little NE activity.

How then can the brain be actively processing information in REM, when subsequent conscious retrieval of this processing is so drastically compromised? Perhaps it is a consolidation of a subtle type. Perhaps consolidation during REM involves material destined to become so habitual that it no longer needs to be accessed by conscious awareness. Perhaps REM helps solidify the many unconscious habits that are the very foundations of our personality. In the final accounting, dreams may construct the powerful subconscious or preconscious affective psychological patterns that help make us the passionately creative, frustratingly average, or tediously boring people that we are. It may help construct the many emotional myths and beliefs around which our individual lives revolve. But, as usual in this nebulous area of "knowledge," the critical experiments to support such views remain to be done.

AFTERTHOUGHT: Activities of Neurochemically Characterized Neurons and Hallucinations

In Chapter 6, I discussed the geographies of the major biogenic amine systems of the brain: norepinephrine, dopamine, and serotonin. Since such biogenic amine neurons are tightly clustered in the brains of rats, it has been possible to characterize the neuronal activities of each of these systems during the various vigilance states. The results have been clear and striking.

Brain NE and 5-HT systems exhibit their highest levels of activity during waking. They slow down substantially during SWS, and a few moments prior to REM they cease firing and remain inhibited throughout the ensuing REM period.[104] In short, they are inactive during dreaming. By comparison, DA cells show comparatively little change from one vigilance state to the next, even though they begin to exhibit bursts of firing when animals seek rewards. Otherwise, they fire at a steady rate throughout waking, SWS, and REM, suggesting that they are prepared to perform their function at any time of day or night.[105]

The lack of firing in 5-HT systems during REM is especially intriguing, since this helps explain the hallucinatory activity of dreaming. On the surface, dreaming resembles an LSD-like state, and LSD is an excellent serotonin receptor blocker. As mentioned earlier, we can also generate REM-typical PGO storms in the waking brain by reducing brain serotonin activity, whether by administering LSD or giving serotonin synthesis inhibitors (e.g., PCPA) in combination with biogenic amine depletors (such as reserpine).[106] Indeed, drugs that reduce the availability of serotonin and other biogenic amines at synapses (e.g., reserpine) also tend to intensify LSD-induced hallucinatory states in humans and animals.[107] Conversely, drugs that promote brain serotonin activity usually attenuate LSD-induced hallucinations as well as REM sleep.[108] In general, it seems that one higher cerebral function of brain serotonin is to sustain stability in perceptual and cognitive channels. When this constraint is loosened by a global reduction of 5-HT activity, the probability of information from one channel crossing into another channel is increased. Thus a mild reduction in brain serotonin activity may be an important ingredient for the generation of new insights and ideas in the brain, while a sustained reduction of serotonin might lead to chaotic feelings and perceptions, contributing to feelings of discoherence and mania.

In sum, perhaps it is this loosening of sensory-perceptual barriers between different brain systems that characterizes dreams, hallucinations, and the florid phases of schizophrenia, as well as normal creativity. Maybe this loosening of information flow between various sensory and perceptual channels is one way in which REM sleep helps initiate the integration and consolidation of information that animals have faced during their waking states. It may also generate totally new permutations of associations. Only more research can shed further light on such intriguing possibilities. But in line with our theme that dreaming is related to emotionality, it is worth noting that just as low brain serotonin characterizes the dream state, it also promotes heightened emotionality, both positive and negative. It is a neurochemical state that leads to impulsive behaviors in humans,[109] even ones as extreme as suicide.[110] Probably the most striking and highly replicable neurochemical finding in the whole psychiatric literature is that individuals who have killed themselves typically have abnormally low brain serotonin activity. Was Freud right that there is a death wish hidden in the human soul? If so, it must be especially active during dreaming sleep.

Suggested Readings

Binkley, S. (1990). *The clockwork sparrow: Time, clocks, and calenders in biological organisms.* Englewood Cliffs, N.J.: Prentice-Hall.

Dement, W. C. (1974). *Some must watch while some must sleep*. San Francisco: Freeman.

Fishbein, W. (ed.) (1981). *Sleep, dreams, and memory: Advances in sleep research*, vol. 6. New York: SP Medical and Scientific Books.

Horn, J. (1988). *Why we sleep: The functions of sleep in humans and other animals*. Oxford: Oxford Univ. Press.

Hobson, J. A. (1988). *The dreaming brain*. New York: Basic Books.

Kryger, M. H., Roth, T., & Dement, W. C. (eds.) (1989). *Principles and practice of sleep medicine*. Philadelphia: Saunders.

Mendelson, W. (1987). *Human sleep: Research and clinical care*. New York: Plenum Press.

Miles, A., Philbrick, D. R. S., & Thompson, C. (eds.) (1989). *Melatonin: Clinical perspectives*. Oxford: Oxford Univ. Press.

Thorpy, M. (ed.) (1990). *Handbook of sleep disorders*. New York: Marcel Dekker.

Williams, R., & Karacan, I. (eds.) (1976). *Pharmacology of sleep*. New York: Wiley.

8

SEEKING Systems and Anticipatory States of the Nervous System

"I feel saved," he would say, "resurrected, reborn. I feel a sense of health amounting to Grace. . . . I feel like a man in love. I have broken through the barriers which cut me off from love." The predominant feelings at this time were feelings of freedom, openness and exchange with the world; of a lyrical appreciation of a real world, undistorted by fantasy, and suddenly revealed; of delight and satiety with self and the world.

Leonard L. in Oliver Sacks, *Awakenings* (1973)

CENTRAL THEME

The desires and aspirations of the human heart are endless. It is foolish to attribute them all to a single brain system. But they all come to a standstill if certain brain systems, such as the dopamine (DA) circuits arising from midbrain nuclei, are destroyed. Such was the tragedy that overtook Leonard L. in his childhood, and it was not until he was a grown man that he was able to partake again of worldly delights. What allowed him to achieve the feelings of success described by Sacks was L-DOPA, the precursor of DA. This medicine had already alleviated the psychomotor problems of ordinary parkinsonian patients, who had weaker forms of deterioration in their ascending DA systems. In such individuals L-DOPA can dramatically alleviate the inability to initiate movements, allowing them to enjoy everyday pleasures. Now we know that ascending DA tracts lie at the heart of powerful, affectively valenced neural systems that allow people and animals to operate smoothly and efficiently in all of their day-to-day pursuits. These circuits appear to be major contributors to our feelings of engagement and excitement as we seek the material resources needed for bodily survival, and also when we pursue the cognitive interests that bring positive existential meanings into our lives. Higher areas of the motor cortex are also energized into action by the presence of DA. Without the synaptic "energy" of DA, these potentials remain dormant and still. Without DA, human aspirations remain frozen, as it were, in an endless winter of discontent. DA synapses resemble gatekeepers rather than couriers that convey detailed messages. When they are not active at their posts, many potentials of the brain cannot readily be manifested in thought or action. Without DA, only the strongest emotional messages instigate behavior. When DA synapses are active in abundance, a person feels as if he or she can do anything. Is it any wonder that humans and animals eagerly work to artificially activate this system whether via electrical or chemical means? Cocaine and amphetamines are psychologically addicting because they facilitate activity in brain DA systems. When the activities of these synapses are excessive, however, in ways that we do not fully understand, people may be in the florid early phases of schizophrenia, seeking spiritual heights and philosophical insights that may not even exist. Many schizophrenics eventually become consumed by an emotional chaos that the rest of us can only imagine. Are we justified in labeling the functions and dysfunctions of brain DA systems in unitary psychological terms? I think so, if we wish to communicate effectively. But what word or phrase shall we use? Here I will call this emotional circuitry the SEEKING system of the brain, as opposed to the expectancy or behavioral activation system as originally proposed.[1]

The Appetitive Motivational or SEEKING System of the Brain: A Goad without a Goal

It may be hard for us to accept that human strivings are ultimately driven by the welling up of ancient neurochemicals in primitive parts of the brain. This view does not easily fit our conception of ourselves as moral and spiritual beings. Although the details of human hopes are surely beyond the imagination of other creatures, the evidence now clearly indicates that certain intrinsic aspirations of all mammalian minds, those of mice as well as men, are driven by the same ancient neurochemistries. These chemistries lead our companion creatures to set out energetically to investigate and explore their worlds, to seek available resources and make sense of the contingencies in their environments. These same systems give us the impulse to become actively engaged with the world and to extract meaning from our various circumstances. When these systems become overactive, our imagination outstrips the constraints of reality. We begin to see causality where there are only correlations.

In previous times, such individuals probably found places in society as soothsayers, seers, shamans, or sacred clowns. But if such a person's vision was limited or excessively bizarre, he or she was probably considered simply odd. Today we call many of the more seriously afflicted individuals schizophrenic or manic (or one of the other subvarieties of psychosis). Milder cases may pass as the creative inspiration of artists, some of them geniuses.[2] How shall we understand the neural systems that underlie such imaginative excess? Perhaps we can approximate the truth with theoretical leaps of the imagination, which help guide the conduct of one experimental step at a time!

To make mechanistic sense of certain brain systems in humans, we must imagine how the simplicity of certain animal behaviors relates to the vast complexity of human experience, and vice versa. This is surely a hazardous undertaking, but in this chapter I will pursue the idea that the mammalian brain contains a "foraging/exploration/investigation/curiosity/interest/expectancy/SEEKING" system that leads organisms to eagerly pursue the fruits of their environment—from nuts to knowledge, so to speak. Like other emotional systems, arousal of the SEEKING system has a characteristic feeling tone—a psychic energization that is difficult to describe but is akin to that invigorated feeling of anticipation we experience when we actively seek thrills and other rewards. Clearly this type of feeling contributes to many distinct aspects of our active engagement with the world.

The critical circuits for this intrinsic brain function are concentrated in the extended lateral hypothalamic (LH) corridor. This system responds unconditionally to homeostatic imbalances (i.e., bodily need states) and environmental incentives. It spontaneously learns about environmental events that predict resources via poorly understood reinforcement processes (Figure 8.1). I believe that these transhypothalamic circuits lie at the very heart of the SEEKING system. The LH continuum, running from the ventral tegmental area (VTA) to the nucleus accumbens, is the area of the brain where local application of electrical stimulation will promptly evoke the most energized exploratory and search behaviors an animal is capable of exhibiting. For instance, stimulated rats move about excitedly, sniffing vigorously, pausing at times to investigate various nooks and crannies of their environment. If one presents the animal with a manipulandum, a lever that controls the onset of brain stimulation, it will readily learn to press the lever and will eagerly continue to "self-stimulate" for extended periods, until physical exhaustion and collapse set in. The outward behavior of the animal commonly appears as if it is trying to get something behind the lever. In other words, an invigorated exploratory attitude is sustained throughout. This is not the type of behavior one sees when animals are either pressing levers to obtain conventional rewards or when they are actually engaged in *consuming* them. Thus, this system is unlikely to be a simple "reward" system that tells us a certain food is tasty.

On Labeling the Appetitive Motivational/SEEKING System

There is growing acceptance that this emotional function of the brain—the basic impulse to search, investigate, and make sense of the environment—emerges from the circuits that course through the LH. The anatomy of brain DA circuits (see Figure 3.6) corresponds to the general trajectory of this psychobehavioral system, and brain DA itself is an essential ingredient in allowing the circuitry to operate efficiently, although many other brain chemistries are involved in the overall construction of the SEEKING response. Investigators have generated diverse names for this system. Originally I called it the *foraging/expectancy* system, while Jeffrey Gray called it the *behavioral activation system*;[3] more recently, Richard Depue chose to call it the *behavioral facilitation system*,[4] and most investigators now working in the field are beginning to agree that it is a general "incentive or appetitive motivational system" that mediates "wanting" as opposed to "liking."[5]

Competition among terminologies can promote confusion, especially for students just being exposed to the relevant information, so I hesitate to contribute more variability to that trend. However, since there are problems with all of these terminologies,[6] SEEKING seems to be a more suitable term for psychology because it implies a distinct psychological dimension as opposed to a mere behavioral process. This harmoniously operating neuroemotional system *drives* and *energizes* many mental complexities that humans experience as persistent feelings of interest, curiosity, sensation seeking, and, in the presence of a sufficiently complex cortex, the search for higher meaning. Although this brain state, like all other basic emotional states, is initially without intrinsic cognitive content, it gradually helps cement the perception of causal connections in the world and thereby creates ideas. As we will see, it appears to translate correlations in environmental events into perceptions of causality, and it may be a major source of "confirmation bias," the tendency to selectively seek evidence for our hypotheses. The mental effects of psychostimu-

SEEKING SYSTEM

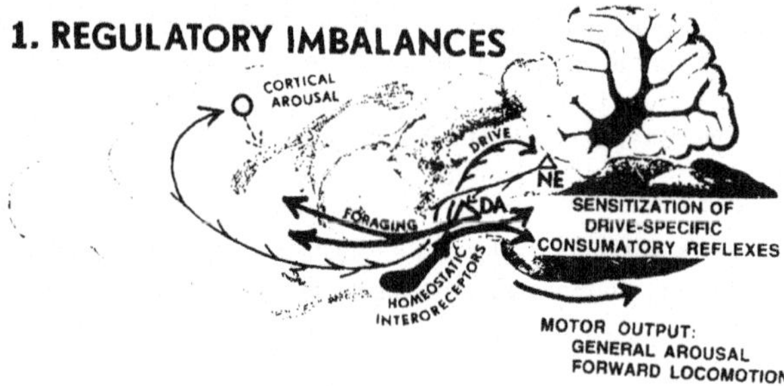

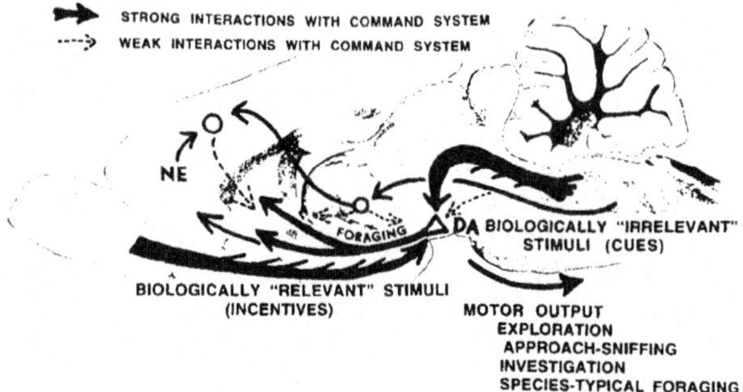

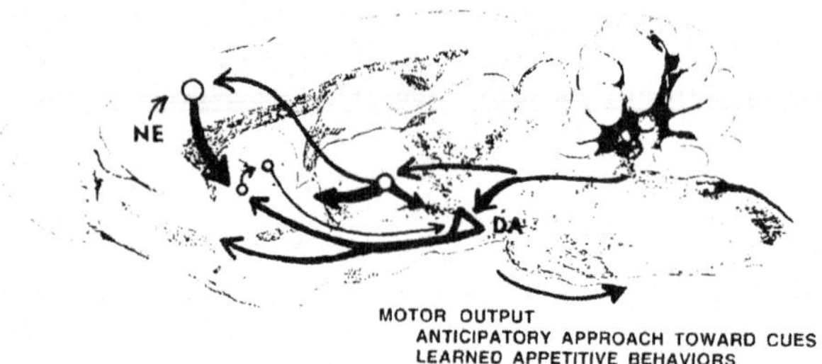

Figure 8.1. The SEEKING system is sensitized by (1) regulatory imbalances to yield general arousal and persistent forward locomotion and (2) external stimuli that can either have strong or weak interactions with this emotional system, and (3) it helps mediate appetitive learning so that animals will become eager and exhibit expectancies in response to cues that have been previously associated with arousal and disarousal of this system. Stimuli that have innate strong interactions with the SEEKING system are unconditional incentives (i.e., they are intrinsically relevant for survival), while those that have weak interactions are potential cues (and hence are designated as "biologically irrelevant" because their stimulus properties are not intrinsically associated with environmental events than can unconditionally promote survival). Fluctuations in the activity of this circuitry presumably mediate one form of "reinforcement." A general way this may be achieved is via the conversion of "weak interactions" in the system into "strong interactions" when reward-induced reductions in SEEKING arousal are registered as relevant events (which may solidify access routes from correlated stimuli into the SEEKING system). (Adapted from Panksepp, 1986; see n. 1.)

lants such as cocaine and amphetamines that arouse the DA system provide a direct porthole into the feelings evoked by this emotional system. The affective state does not resemble the pleasurable feelings we normally experience when we indulge in various consummatory behaviors. Instead, it resembles the energization organisms apparently feel when they are anticipating rewards.

Traditionally, all motivated behaviors have been divided into *appetitive* and *consummatory* components. This distinction is premised on the recognition that one must not only seek out and approach the material resources needed for survival (except for oxygen, of course) but also interact with them in specific ways once they have been found: One must eat, drink, copulate, or carry the desired items home. The SEEKING system appears to control appetitive activation—the search, foraging, and investigatory activities—that all animals must exhibit before they are in a position to emit consummatory behaviors.

Because of the type of evidence summarized in this chapter, there are reasons to believe that the trunk of this emotional system courses through the ventrolateral regions of the diencephalon—areas of the brain called the medial forebrain bundle (MFB) of the lateral hypothalamus (LH), which contains many neurochemically specific tracts. One major set of pathways, the ascending DA circuits, outlines the sites from which this psychobehavioral state can be most easily evoked with localized brain stimulation (see figures 3.6 and 8.1).[7]

Where Is the "Reinforcement" in Self-Stimulation Systems?

When given the opportunity, animals fitted with electrodes in most LH locations voluntarily self-administer electricity into this system. In short, they *self-stimulate*.

In the behaviorist lexicon, this system was called the brain "reinforcement" or "reward" system; some of the more courageous investigators even dared to call it the "pleasure" system. All of these labels now seem to be misleading because they suggest a close relationship between arousal of this brain system and the consummatory phase of behavior. As already mentioned, the emotive tendencies aroused by this type of brain stimulation most clearly resemble the normal appetitive phase of behavior that precedes consummatory acts. As we will see, the pleasures and reinforcements of consummatory processes appear to be more closely linked to a reduction of arousal in this brain system. It makes sense that the many reward objects that naturally satiate appetitive behaviors—such as food, water, and sex—should be closely linked to internal processes that signal encounters with objects of clear biological relevance. Indeed, consummatory behavior causes a transient inhibition of appetitive arousal. As the animal encounters a need-relevant reward object and shifts into the consummatory mode, the appetitive urge to move forward ceases temporarily. It is hypothesized that this rapid shift in the patterns of neural activity may establish the neural conditions that engage reinforcement processes in the brain (Figure 8.1).[8]

The transient external cues associated with life-sustaining events may be the ones that gradually develop conditioned neural routes back to the appetitive system. In other words, the SEEKING system is initially activated by the unconditional distal incentive *cues* of rewards, such as smells and sights; eventually, through learning, neutral cues can come to arouse and channel activity in this system through a reinforcement process that is linked to the inhibition of approach in some presently unknown manner (as schematized in Figure 8.1). In other words, the search system automatically evaluates the importance of environmental events and stores that knowledge for future use, perhaps through some type of "reinforced" memory process. Although we now know where the unconditional brain systems for foraging behavior are situated, we do not yet know precisely how they work. Nor do we know precisely how neutral cues gain conditional access to this system, although the best current hypothesis would be that they achieve such control through glutamate circuits from the cortex, hippocampus, and several subcortical areas such as thalamic nuclei that descend onto the SEEKING system. We can be certain that the SEEKING system does interact with higher brain circuits that mediate each animal's ability to anticipate rewards.[9] Later in this chapter, I will discuss one type of learning ("autoshaping") that appears to be an intrinsic function of this system.

Historically, it was all too easy to believe that the onset of brain stimulation contained all of the emotional/affective goodies, so to speak. Actually, both the onset and offset may have affectively desirable components, but they differ from each other: The onset may be desirable because of the energized anticipatory excitement that is induced, while certain types of offset may be desirable because they help signal that important events, perhaps even pleasurable ones, have occurred. In fact, it is quite possible that termination of "rewarding" brain stimulation is more intimately linked to the arousal of associative "reinforcement" processes than is the onset of stimulation.[10] This is a diametric reversal of traditional behaviorist thinking concerning the underlying nature of self-stimulation (SS). There is substantial evidence to support such an alternative view, although these lines of evidence have often been ignored because they do not fit into traditional modes of thinking.

Consider some relevant empirical findings. In one of the first studies to measure neuronal action potentials within the trajectory of the SEEKING system, it was found that neurons were typically aroused in the LH when animals were searching for food and shut down promptly when the food was found and feeding began.[11] In other words, the appetitive phase of behavior corresponds to high arousal of the LH system, while consummatory pleasures are more closely related to offset of neuronal activity in this system. This type of finding has been affirmed by a great deal of subsequent research. In monkeys, the system is more active in response to cues that predict reward than in response to the reward itself,[12] even though some neurons in the LH do respond during the actual experience of the reward.[13] This goes to show that no single psychological concept fully describes the functions of any given brain area or circuit. There are no unambiguous "centers" or loci for discrete emotions in the brain that do not massively interdigitate with other functions, even though certain key circuits are essential for certain emotions to be elaborated. Everything ultimately emerges from the interaction of many systems. For this reason, modern neuroscientists talk about interacting "circuits," "networks," and "cell assemblies" rather than "centers." Still, specific circuits do have psychological spheres of influence, and it is now evident that the LH behavioral arousal SEEKING system is much more devoted to anticipatory-appetitive arousal rather than simply to consummatory reward processes, which are even more ancient functions of the brain.

Historically, it has been of some interest to determine which aspect of brain stimulation—its onset or offset—is more attractive to an animal.[14] Consider an animal in a chamber with only two objects in sight. During training, "rewarding" stimulation is always turned on when the animal touches one object and off when it touches the other. During testing, when no more brain stimulation is available, where would the animal prefer to spend more time—at the site where the brain "reward" always came on or where it went off? If stimulus onset truly produces most of the reward, as traditionally assumed, one would predict animals would seek out the "onset object." This experiment has been done only in cats, and the answer was clear.[15] When tested in such an arena without any brain stimulation, cats spent significantly more time investigating the area where the stimulation had gone *off* rather than the area where it had come on! These results suggest that the offset signaled psychological relevance or positive reward value more than the onset. At the very least, the "off location" ranked higher in the animal's internal interest hierarchy than the "on location." Perhaps a type of reinforcement or relevance mechanism, distinct from the exploratory arousal induced by the onset of brain stimulation, had been repeatedly engaged at the off site, and hence the animal was most attracted to that location when it had nothing else to do.

From the present theoretical perspective, this paradoxical result makes good sense, for items in the world that can normally terminate foraging are typically goal objects that reduce the specific physiological deficits an animal is experiencing. Although LH brain stimulation may not evoke the neural representation of any specific deficit, it does evoke an aroused investigatory state characteristic of animals experiencing bodily need states, such as hunger. Behavior induced by LH stimulation most clearly resembles the type of arousal that animals exhibit in the presence of cues predicting the availability of appropriate rewards, such as a dog expressing eagerness at the sight of the leash that signals a walk or the sound of a can opener that signals forthcoming food. It is reasonable to suppose that termination of artificially induced arousal in this system may resemble the brain state that normally signals biological relevance. Of course, every scientific observation has several potential explanations. Perhaps the cats in the aforementioned experiment did not go to the "on location" simply because brain stimulation had induced a brief period of amnesia in which they forgot the importance of that location,[16] or because the stimulation had evoked aversive feelings, and relief from those feelings at the point of stimulus termination made the offset location an attractive place to be.[17] Obviously, more work needs to be done on this interesting issue.

In any event, all of the aforementioned processes must be conceived in dynamic terms, and mere words are certainly not sufficient to capture the real-life flow of the underlying brain systems in action. In fact, when animals eat, drink, or have sex there appears to be a chaotic, dancelike tension between the consummatory and appetitive phases of behavior. As the animal momentarily settles down to eat, each swallow is followed by the urge to reach out for more. Just picture yourself eating potato chips or some other favorite snack: Your hand repeatedly reaches out with an apparent mind of its own. In the present view, such cyclic urges to reach out and seek rewards constitute the basic adaptive function of the underlying SS circuits. Of course, this does not exclude the possibility that this system is also important in an organism's attempt to seek escape from negative events.

The Extent of the Self-Stimulation/ SEEKING System in the Brain

Besides the difficulties involved in delimiting the psychobehavioral function of this system, there are also problems in specifying its complete anatomical trajectory. SS can now be obtained from a great number of brain sites (for a visualization of the extended zones, see Figures 3.6 and 5.3), and it can bc accompanied by several distinct behavioral characteristics. From major SS sites within the LH, behavior tends to be frantically energized, while from other sites, such as the medial septal area and locus coeruleus, it is slow and methodical. Clearly, all brain sites that sustain SS need not be considered part of the same psychobehavioral system. Accordingly, we must refer to other behavioral criteria than the mere act of SS in designating the location of the SEEKING system. One useful criterion is whether the brain stimulation can motivate complex investigatory behaviors, or even provoke more simple manifestations of such behavioral tendencies when animals are anesthetized.

One such simple behavior in rats is sniffing. This behavior is present whenever a rat is searching, investigating, or expecting positive rewards. As will be discussed later, sniffing can be evoked by electrical brain stimulation (ESB) within the LH, as well as from more rostral frontal cortical areas and downstream mesencephalic ones to which LH circuits are interconnected.[18] Pharmacological activation of DA systems with psychostimulants such as cocaine and amphetamines also increases spontaneous sniffing. DA blocking agents (i.e., the antipsychotics), on the other hand, decrease the spontaneous behavior but have very little effect on electrically evoked sniffing behavior, suggesting that ESB-induced sniffing is provoked more by the activation of descending rather than ascending neural components such as DA axons. At present, we consider the whole trajectory of the sniffing system (both ascending and descending components) to constitute a coherently operating SEEKING system that helps place the animal in a distinct waking state characterized by exploration, investigation, and foraging—accompanied, presumably, by internal feelings of anticipatory eagerness.

It should be emphasized that even though the system is nicely outlined by the trajectory of DA circuits (see Figure 3.6), especially the mesolimbic and mesocortical ones from the VTA, the SEEKING system is not simply the DA system. There are powerful descending components, probably glutamatergic in part, that remain to be functionally characterized,[19] but they may be just as important for the generation of appetitive and SS behaviors as the DA systems whose participation is now well documented. When those descending systems are fully characterized, they may have powerful implications for understanding such psychiatric disorders as schizophrenia, which reflect, in part, some yet unfathomed derangement of this emotional system.[20]

To highlight an example of a powerful SS site that does not appear to be a major component of the SEEKING system, consider the case of the medial septal area. Animals will respond persistently to stimulation of that brain site, with no outward agitation. Indeed, these animals outwardly appear to be relishing a highly satisfying pleasure. They periodically shiver, as if their experience is remarkably intense. In fact, humans who have been stimulated at such locations report pleasurable sexual feelings, suggesting the location of a "sexual pleasure" system in the brain.[21] Although this system anatomically connects up with the SEEKING system, it appears more likely to be part of a separate pleasure-type response. Of course, SEEKING systems and pleasure systems must be intimately intertwined in the brain. As already mentioned, the present analysis suggests that pleasure emerges from the neural conditions that normally inhibit seeking—namely, from the many consummatory acts that are the terminal components of successful bouts of foraging.

The SEEKING System and Human Affective Experience

Before summarizing additional intriguing facts concerning the SEEKING system, let us briefly consider how its activation modifies subjective experience. This is especially important since many investigators who discuss human emotions have had difficulty agreeing what emotional state this system is supposed to mediate. I would suggest that "intense interest," "engaged curiosity," and "eager anticipation" are the types of feelings that reflect arousal of this system in humans. Obviously, in humans such a neural system has a vast reservoir of cortical potentials to interact with, yielding a menagerie of specific cognitive changes. However, at a more basic level of analysis, two issues concerning the nature of such psychobehavioral states are pertinent.

The first and more confusing issue is whether we should even consider an appetitive engagement or "interest" type of mental state to be an emotion. Although the affective expression of interest is quite clear and evident in young infants,[22] typically there is no intense outward expression of this state in adults. Of course, we should remember how socially important it is for humans to give the appearance of being "cool and collected" on the outside, even though they may be jumping up and down with childish excitement in their minds. The cultivated appearance of detachment may in fact be a learned human convention, used to promote a sense of power, control, and even useful deception in the practice of everyday social politics If you want to succeed, it is often best to keep a "poker face" rather than reveal the intense excitement or interest you may have.

Second, curiosity and interest seem to be relatively stable personality traits as opposed to passing emotional states. In fact, contrary to most other emotional responses, the SEEKING system is commonly tonically engaged rather than phasically active. As noted in the last chapter, DA neurons remain active throughout the various vigilance states. The level of sustained neural firing in this system may have clear psychological effects, as revealed by pencil-and-paper tests designed to evaluate relevant affective dimensions in humans. For instance, the level of activity in this system may be related to the personality dimensions of *positive emotionality*,[23] *sensation seeking*,[24] and other measures of appetitive engagement with the world.

Spielberger's State Trait Personality Inventory (STPI) is a well-standardized emotional test that aims to evaluate present levels (states) of anxiety, curiosity, and anger, as well as overall personality tendencies (traits) on those same dimensions. It asks 60 simple questions, 10 for each of the three emotional "states" and 10 for each of the "traits" (i.e., anxiety, curiosity, and anger). In analyzing all the intercorrelations among the six resulting scores, one finds only one stable relationship. "State curiosity" and "trait curiosity" exhibit high positive relationships across diverse subject populations.[25] In other words, the person who is likely to be engaged with curiosity "here and now" is likely to view him- or herself as highly "curious." This stability between *state* and *trait* variables does not hold clearly for anger or anxiety, or for the various other possible interrelationships. In other words, the neural substrates for the other emotions are not as chronically active.

Of course, the best way to gauge the feelings mediated by lateral hypothalamic SS circuits would be to monitor subjective feelings in humans while the system is being stimulated. This has been done, with a perplexing pattern of results. One aspect, however, is highly revealing from the present theoretical perspective. People typically have not reported simple sensory pleasures from the LH stimulation, but, rather, invigorated feelings that are difficult to describe. They commonly report a feeling that something very interesting and exciting is going on.[26] This contrasts with electrical stimulation of the septal area, where, as already mentioned, feelings of sexual pleasure have been evoked.

Finally, as mentioned earlier, the analysis of subjective responses to psychostimulants such as cocaine and amphetamines suggests that an energized psychic state accompanies arousal of the SEEKING system, while a sluggish depressive state accompanies blockade of the system with antipsychotics.[27]

Why Should We Consider SEEKING to Be an Emotional System?

In Chapter 3, neurobehavioral criteria were provided for considering certain brain systems as emotional ones.

The SEEKING system highlights the utility of neural criteria in defining basic emotional systems. Not only does this LH circuitry mediate a positive affective state, but it fulfills the other criteria outlined in Chapter 3. Let me summarize evidence for each of those criteria.[28]

1. *The underlying circuits are genetically prewired and designed to respond unconditionally to stimuli arising from major life-challenging circumstances:* That this system is innate is indicated by the ability to obtain SS in neonatal rats. The system is not dependent on higher brain functions, for it continues to operate effectively in adult animals even though most of their higher cognitive mechanisms have been surgically removed. The survival value of this system is indicated by the fact that damage along its trajectory at an early age reduces the probability of survival much more than damage at older ages.

2. *The circuits organize behavior by activating or inhibiting motor subroutines (and concurrent autonomic-hormonal changes) that have proved adaptive in the face of life-challenging circumstances during the evolutionary history of the species:* The mesolimbic/cortical DA circuits, which are deemed to lie at the heart of this system, allow animals to perform a large number of motivated goal-seeking behaviors. If the system is damaged, a generalized behavioral inertia results; if the system is stimulated, either pharmacologically or electrically, a large number of motivated behaviors and a variety of physiological changes are invigorated.

3. *Emotive circuits change the sensitivities of sensory systems relevant for the behavior sequences that have been aroused:* Electrically induced arousal of this system leads to more effective cortical processing, and the effect is restricted to the ipsilateral cerebral hemisphere. Such stimulation also metabolically arouses widespread sites on the ipsilateral side of the brain, including certain cortical areas.

4. *Neural activity of emotive systems outlasts the precipitating circumstances:* It has long been known that behavioral arousal induced by rewarding brain stimulation outlasts the stimulation. The original drive-decay theory of SS and the priming effects (behavioral excitation) that are commonly induced by activating this circuit are premised on the fact that the neural system sustains activity for some time beyond the point of stimulation offset.

5. *Emotive circuits can come under the conditional control of emotionally neutral environmental stimuli:* The SEEKING substrates of the brain exhibit spontaneous learning, as reflected by single-cell activity during simple forms of appetitive conditioning, as well as in the spontaneous anticipatory shaping of unconditional response systems, such as sniffing, during systematically administered brain stimulation (as will be detailed later). Recent evidence also indicates that ventral tegmental DA cells exhibit anticipatory learning during appetitive conditioning, and the mesolimbic DA system exhibits vigorous release of DA especially during the anticipatory phase of behavior during various forms of appetitive conditioning. Whether the system also responds to the anticipation of aversive events has yet to be resolved. My view predicts this will not be the case, at least not to the extent as in appetitive conditioning.

6. *Emotive circuits have reciprocal interactions with brain mechanisms that elaborate higher decision-making processes and consciousness:* When this system is mildly aroused, one would expect people's subjective experience to be filled with a pleasant energy that leads them to eagerly pursue various interests and life-sustaining activities. Vivid documentation of such effects is found in the life stories of the parkinsonian patients described by Oliver Sacks in *Awakenings*.[29] These men and women were placed on L-DOPA to facilitate activity in their impaired brain DA systems. Prior to medication, they were living a life of "suspended animation," in which time progressed with a dull monotony. As highlighted by Leonard L.'s description of his own awakening in the epigraph to this chapter, L-DOPA restored life's vibrancy in individuals whose DA systems had been damaged by disease. Although tragic tribulations eventually followed, as excessive psychomotor arousal and schizophrenic symptoms were induced by the L-DOPA therapy, the power of DA to "fire" a positive, interest-filled engagement with the world was apparent in all individuals who received the medication. The psychic attractions of cocaine and other psychostimulants emerge largely from the ability of these drugs to arouse this fundamental emotional system of the brain. The precise biochemical effect has been delimited to the dopamine transporter sites that mediate the reuptake of synaptically released dopamine back into presynaptic endings.[30] The affective state these drugs induce is not simply "pleasure" but a highly energized state of psychic power and engagement with the world during which one is eager to pursue a variety of goal-directed activities.

A Historical Overview of the Self-Stimulation System

It is remarkable how long it has taken psychobiologists to begin to properly conceptualize the function of the SS system in the governance of behavior. The history of this field highlights how an environmental-behavioral bias, with no conception of internal brain functions, has impeded the development of compelling psychobehavioral conceptions of SS—one of the most fascinating phenomena ever discovered in biopsychology and one that is still largely ignored by mainstream psychology.[31]

Still, it is historically understandable why the SS system of the brain was initially characterized as one that mediates reward, pleasure, or reinforcement. But ever since James Olds and Peter Milner of McGill University first stumbled upon the phenomenon in 1954, there has been an abundance of dilemmas and paradoxes. These remain unresolved from the theoretical perspective that the underlying brain system mediates reinforcement or pleasure. Perhaps the most puzzling feature of the behavior pattern during these bouts of SS was the fact that the animals simply did not have the behaviorally settled outward appearance of animals consuming conventional rewards. Self-stimulating animals look excessively excited, even crazed, when they worked for this kind of stimulation. When a normal animal begins to eat, it tends to calm down rather than get more and more excited (even though it does get highly excited between rewards if only very small portions of food are provided intermittently, especially when it is very hungry). A generation of behaviorally oriented investigators (who refused to deal in psychological concepts) may have been misled when they allowed their animals to self-stimulate. Perhaps the *arousal* of the system did not activate an internal experience of reward but instead excited the animal into an appetitive search strategy, and the SS was more reflective of an animal caught in a "do-loop" (i.e., a repetition of the same instruction), where each stimulation evoked a reinvigorated search strategy. Few investigators chose to emphasize that self-stimulating animals did not appear to behave as if they were experiencing anything akin to the pleasure of eating or being touched.

Investigators seemed loathe to suggest the obvious—that self-stimulating animals appeared to be in a state of anticipatory eagerness. It was not clearly recognized that such a state might have positive incentive properties of its own. To better appreciate this issue, perhaps an apt analogy would be male sexual behavior, which consists of at least three phases: the initial appetitive behavior (some have called it "cruising and courting"), the actual copulatory behavior (which is a proximal appetitive behavior), and ejaculation/orgasm, the climactic terminal component, which may contain the most pleasurable aspects of the behavior sequence. In feeding there is a comparable trichotomy, with the generalized approach pattern being the initial component, the biting, chewing, and tasting reflecting the proximal appetitive component, and swallowing the terminal component. In any event, lateral hypothalamic SS did not provoke behavior resembling the terminal components, when the body becomes quiescent. Indeed, that was the component that seemed to be largely missing from SS, even though there were some sites where males would eventually ejaculate in the midst of their excitement. This, of course, was "spontaneous," since the animals had no partner in the cage, nor had they physically stimulated their own genitalia. However, the animals did not typically cease behaving when this happened. They continued self-stimulating in an apparent anticipatory frenzy.

In any event, when "rewarding" brain stimulation is applied unconditionally into the LH, without requiring animals to work for it, one always observes a sustained exploratory-investigatory pattern. It would have been straightforward to postulate that this reflects the action of a basic neural system for exploration, but the prevailing modes of behavioristic thinking led investigators to infer that they had discovered the brain's fundamental reward or reinforcement system. Instead of suggesting that the evoked search behaviors actually reflected the most evident function of the underlying brain circuit, they proceeded to suppose that those behaviors were secondary consequences of animals having been given the neural essence of reward, which they then proceeded to seek avidly within their immediate environments. By a strange quirk of logic, the searching was presumed to be secondary to an unobserved internal event ("reinforcement" or a feeling of reward) as opposed to the primary reflection of an exploratory urge!

Why was there no clear conception that animals needed a brain system to seek rewards? Because behavioral psychologists were loathe to discuss any "inner causes." Obviously, rewards in the world are meaningless unless animals can search them out. All organisms need powerfully ingrained emotive systems to make sure they get to the available resources in a timely fashion. Now, almost half a century after the discovery of SS, investigators are still assimilating the possibility that "rewarding" brain stimulation actually evokes search strategies, not the intrinsic neural representation of specific reward or pleasure processes.

Just as the sea hare *Aplysia* described in Chapter 2 goes into a search mode to find a stable footing when it is suspended in a tank of water, all mammals go into a search mode when their bodies are hungry, thirsty, cold, or desirous of social/sexual companionship. Indeed, it is hard to imagine that an organism could survive if such an appetitive function was not well ingrained within its basic neural infrastructure. Since nature did not always provide the necessary resources for survival immediately at hand, each animal has a spontaneous tendency to explore and learn about its environment. When an animal has established a knowledge of its local terrain (probably through the development of cognitive maps),[32] it can move about flexibly and efficiently to find the things it needs. It also begins to spontaneously anticipate occurrences that are important in its quest for survival by using informative temporal or environmental cues.

Of course, animals pursue most of these behavioral endeavors mechanically, presumably without much forethought, but there are now many reasons to believe that forethoughts (e.g., positive expectancies/anticipatory states) do in fact emerge from the interactions of the SEEKING system with higher brain mechanisms, such as the frontal cortex and hippocampus, that generate plans by mediating higher-order temporal and spatial information processing. Indeed, circuits coursing through the LH can trigger a hippocampal theta rhythm, which, as noted in the previous chapter, is an elemental signal of information processing in that structure.[33] At the peak of each theta wave, there is a glutamate-induced strengthening of the hippocampal marker of learning known as *long-term potentiation.* The hippocampus also has strong downward connections with the hypothalamus via the descending fiber bundle of the fornix (and these connections may convey cues from spatial maps to foraging impulses).[34] Other projection zones of this system, such as those in the basal ganglia, also have strong downward influences onto the hypothalamic sources of the SEEKING system.[35]

The Many Paradoxes in the Study of This Emotional System

Ever since the discovery of SS, a variety of oddities and paradoxes have been evident in conceptualizing this system as one that simply encodes the positive reinforcing properties of external reward. Let us first consider one behavior that frequently disrupts ongoing SS—namely, grooming.[36] To the chagrin of early investigators, highly excited self-stimulating animals often would run away from the lever and stop responding. Instead of returning promptly, they would go into a prolonged grooming sequence of the type that is common after animals finish their meals or complete their sexual activities. Such animals would not readily resume SS, especially early in training. However, it was noted that giving the animal a few free *priming* stimulations would often reevoke the appetitive mood. This was often necessary to induce animals to behave at the beginning of the test session as well. No such priming was necessary for hungry and thirsty animals working for conventional rewards.

The comparatively weak motivation for the stimulation suggested to some investigators that there was something motivationally unusual about brain-stimulation "reward." An intriguing early suggestion was that the stimulation had two distinct effects: It evoked a drive (an internal feeling of being in a state of homeostatic imbalance, sort of like a hunger) and the concurrent appropriate "reward" or satisfaction of that drive. Since the artificially induced drive decayed after the offset of stimulation, the animal would gradually exhibit a diminishing level of motivation.[37] This drive-decay or "dual-process" theory sought to explain several odd properties of SS, including phenomena such as rapid acquisition, overresponding, and extinction without reward, but two factors were really not needed.

Subsequent investigators demonstrated that these unusual behaviors could be more simply explained by a single factor—an "incentive" process independent of normal homeostatic imbalances (i.e., the drive state) that normally tend to sensitize responsivity to potential sources of external rewards.[38] Thus, the same odd properties of SS could be obtained with conventional rewards in nondeprived animals if one sustained behavior using similar response contingencies by administering high-incentive rewards, such as chocolate milk, directly into the mouths of rats when they pressed levers.[39] The trouble with the early "incentive" concept of brain-stimulation reward was that it was defined with respect to properties of objects in the world as opposed to circuit functions in the brain. At present, it is essential to conceptualize an *incentive process*—a fundamental appetitive motivation process—as an intrinsic brain function.

Let us examine this issue in greater detail. From the behaviorist perspective, the incentive properties of a reward were traditionally defined in terms of attributes such as the *quality*, *quantity*, and *delay of reward* rather than in terms of any conception of what the nervous system experiences or undergoes when it is confronted by highly desirable objects. In fact, the high incentive state, from the nervous system perspective, may be the arousal of an emotive process that invigorates search and foraging behaviors. In other words, the unconditional incentive state within the brain may largely consist of the arousal of a psychobehavioral integrative system (e.g., SEEKING) of the brain. An increasing number of studies measuring DA cellular activity, as well as dopamine release in the pathways emanating from the VTA, now indicate that this system is especially highly tuned to stimuli that predict rewards, rather than to rewards themselves.[40]

LH Self-Stimulation as a Unitary Process

In the 1970s and 1980s, most investigators focused their attentions on the anatomical and neurochemical details of the LH-SS system.[41] Because of its rich microanatomy, and the many goal-directed behaviors that could be elicited during LH stimulation, it was widely doubted that a single psychobehavioral process could really be the foundation of the LH-SS phenomenon. Although a few attempted to conceptualize the DA system as a pleasure or hedonic system,[42] their efforts eventually faltered as many experimental inconsistencies with the pleasure interpretation were revealed.[43]

Clearly, the LH contains many ascending and descending neural systems with many interconnections to other brain areas. It seemed overly simplistic to assume that a homogeneous motivational system coursed through this brain area. Indeed, many other basic emotional and homeostatic sytems are represented in nearby zones of the hypothalamus, but these facts do not preclude the possibility that the main trajectory of the LH-SS system was functionally homogeneous. Obviously, many distinct neural subcomponents may operate in a coordinated and harmonious fashion to generate a single psychobehavioral response. Activation of that LH-SS trajectory has long been known to evoke a singular neuropsychological process. One line of evidence was derived from animals' ability or lack of ability to discriminate the internal brain states evoked by activation of two SS electrodes at distant locations within the trajectory of this system. Another line emerged from the analysis of the many specific consummatory behaviors that can be evoked by activation of the LH.

First, the discrimination studies indicated that stimulation at many distinct SS sites evoked a single type of internal experience. This conclusion was based on the fact that if one evaluates the discriminative cue properties of electrical current applied to two distant electrodes within the trajectory of this system—with one electrode signaling the availability of a conventional reward (CS+) and the other indicating that reward is not available (CS–)—animals exhibited great difficulty acquiring the discrimination.[44] For instance, hungry rats require only a few dozen trials to discriminate lights from tones in this type of situation when food is used as a reward, but it takes them several hundred trials to discriminate between the activation of two separate electrodes placed at distinct sites along the LH.

The fact that discrimination is eventually obtained in such experiments does not argue against a single type of process being activated, since there must always be several distinct neural components to every emotive process, and also because other emotive systems, such as those that mediate fear, rage, and various social processes, overlap massively in the LH. In any event, discrimination learning, which is one of the few experimental ways to get at the internal states of an animal, progresses much more rapidly when one of the electrodes is outside the bounds of the SEEKING system. For instance, rats readily make the discrimination if one electrode is in the LH and the other is in the septum. As discussed previously, there are good reasons to believe that septal SS electrodes evoke a psychic process that is more akin to feelings of pleasure.

On the Nature of Consummatory Behaviors Evoked from the SEEKING System

The other powerful line of evidence for the existence of a unitary emotive system within the SS zone of LH circuitry comes from the study of the many distinct types of consummatory behavior patterns that can be evoked by stimulation in this part of the brain. Throughout the 1960s it was demonstrated that a diversity of specific "stimulus-bound" behaviors could be triggered from the LH by electrical stimulation of the brain (ESB)—for instance, feeding, drinking, wood gnawing, sexual behavior, pup carrying, and even tail preening. There was considerable hope that the close study of the underlying circuitry would yield an understanding of how specific instinctual behaviors were mechanistically coded within specific neural circuits of the brain.

Then Elliot Valenstein and his colleagues did a series of experiments with "stimulus-bound" feeding, drinking, and gnawing that startled the behavioral neuroscience community.[45] These results laid to rest the simpleminded mechanistic hope that distinct circuits would be found in the LH for all the observed consummatory behaviors. The experiments indicated that the hypothalamic motivational system that was activated when animals exhibited distinct behaviors was *nonspecific*. The LH apparently mediated some process other than the specific behaviors that were being observed! However, because of existing preconceptions in the field, Valenstein's finding sent both research and thinking in the area into a nosedive from which it is only recently recovering, largely because of the development of new analytical neuroscience tools that can tell us precisely what is happening in this system at neurophysiological and neurochemical levels. A few insightful behavioral experiments are also again appearing. For instance, through a detailed analysis of taste-induced facial response patterns in rats (i.e., lip-licking responses), it is clear that ESB-induced feeding is not accompanied by a pleasurable state resembling gustatory pleasure.[46]

Why specifically were the findings of Valenstein and colleagues so devastating for traditional thinking in the field? What these researchers did, quite simply, was to study "stimulus-bound" eaters, drinkers, and gnawers *after* they took away each animal's preferred goal objects, while leaving the other two goal objects available throughout prolonged overnight periods of intermittent ESB. By morning, most of the animals had shifted to another behavior. And this was not just a modest shift in preference, for when the originally preferred goal object was returned, the newly acquired consummatory behaviors competed effectively with the original behaviors. Many additional observations further undermined the notion of motivational "specificity." For example, the stronger the initial "stimulus-bound" behavior (vigorous eating, etc.), the more rapidly the animal would shift to a new consummatory behavior (e.g., it would become a vigorous drinker). Along the way it also became clear that the initially exhibited consummatory behaviors were not really motivationally specific. Even the most vigorous stimulus-bound eaters were not really highly focused on getting food; if one replaced an animal's initially preferred food with another type, the probability of remaining a "stimulus-bound" eater was no higher than the probability of shifting to another behavior such as drinking. For animals that were drinkers, one could remove the water from a bottle and place it in a dish; some of the animals became stimulus-bound eaters, while others continued licking the now empty tube.[47] Normal thirsty rats simply are not so foolish as to begin eating just because their water is moved to a nearby dish.

These researchers made many other perplexing observations, all suggesting that "stimulus-bound" consummatory behaviors evoked with LH stimulation were deceiving us about the actual motivational process that was being artificially aroused. Valenstein sided with the idea that the underlying neural substrates, presumed to be evenly distributed throughout the hypothalamus, exhibited considerable motivational "plasticity." He chose not to advocate a clear theoretical position as to what psychobehavioral process was actually being activated by the brain stimulation. Rather, he simply emphasized the broad possibility that the underlying hypothalamic substrates were motivationally nonspecific, and that learning was the critical process determining which specific behaviors an animal would exhibit. Unfortunately, Valenstein failed to clearly indicate that a variety of other behaviors, such as fear and ragelike aggression, which can also be obtained from many nearby sites in the hypothalamus, could never be modified into the types of consummatory behaviors that he was studying.

Instead, the whole explanatory burden was placed on learning, perhaps because that jibed with traditional behavioristic (and humanistic) conceptions of how the nervous system was organized. In fact, Valenstein made an inaccurate statement when he suggested that all parts of the hypothalamus could learn to generate consummatory behavior. That would certainly have indicated a remarkable degree of plasticity for the underlying tissues activated by the ESB. Actually, when one statistically computes the locations of Valenstein's own effective electrode sites, one finds the heaviest density situated within the dorsolateral quadrant of the hypothalamus, where most of the ascending DA fibers are concentrated (Figure 8.2). This distribution of electrode sites corresponds to the circuits that are here conceptualized as the SEEKING system.

Although investigators who promoted motivational specificity suggested some clever counterinterpretations of Valenstein's observations (e.g., that many overlapping fiber systems for specific consummatory behaviors were being stimulated), their own experiments finally proved that this was not the case. For instance, if there were many systems coursing through the LH, one would have predicted that a movable electrode could be repositioned into different sites to yield different motivated behaviors as it passed through different neural systems. In fact, a single animal tended to show a single behavior in such experiments,[48] and animals also tended to show essentially the same behavior pattern when the two sides of the brain were stimulated with different electrodes at substantially different locations.[49] Furthermore, it was demonstrated that the animal's emotional temperament could predict what type of stimulus-bound behavior it would exhibit. Rats would exhibit "stimulus-bound" predatory behavior, such as attacking mice, only if they already had a natural tendency to indulge in it. Animals that appeared especially likely to exhibit what ethologists call "displacement activities" (motivational spillover between emotive systems) were most likely to exhibit strong appetitive behaviors.[50]

The conclusion seemed inescapable: The LH-SS system activates a unitary motivational process. However, the prevailing intellectual zeitgeist was not conducive to conceptualizing this single process in psychological terms. This would have required a discussion of the inner neurodynamic aspects of the animal's "mind"—including perhaps a discussion of the nature of intentionality and subjective experience in animals—rather than simply focusing on how behavior was controlled by external events. That was, and still *is*, considered anathema in behavioral neuroscience. Accordingly, most investigators decided to remain in a theoretical limbo that is now only slowly dissipating.[51]

On the Unity Underlying the Behavioral Diversity That Emerges from the SEEKING System

The preceding results are highly consistent with the idea that a unitary neuropsychological process is evoked by LH stimulation. Even though animals are prone to ex-

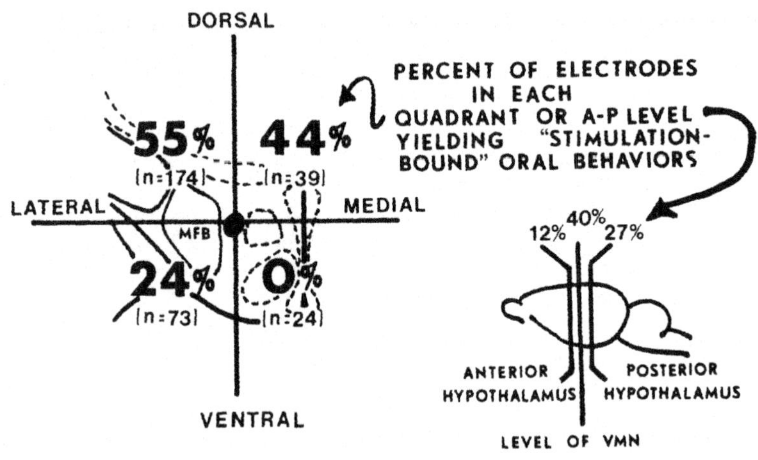

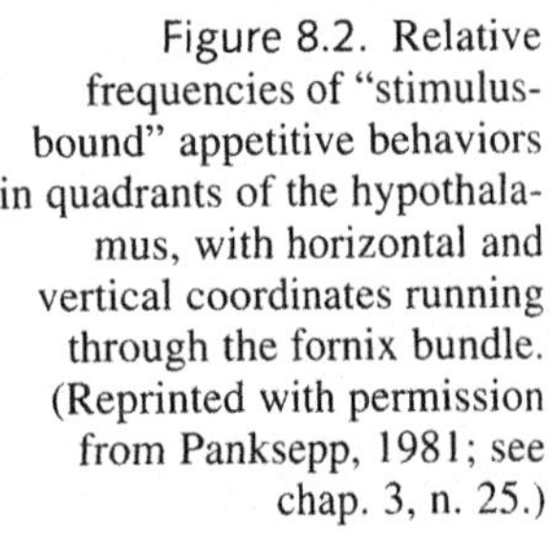
Figure 8.2. Relative frequencies of "stimulus-bound" appetitive behaviors in quadrants of the hypothalamus, with horizontal and vertical coordinates running through the fornix bundle. (Reprinted with permission from Panksepp, 1981; see chap. 3, n. 25.)

hibit many distinct consummatory behaviors when this system is activated, depending on their "personality" tendencies and bodily needs, there is one behavior that is exhibited by all. All animals move forward in an energetic search pattern, sniffing vigorously and investigating, mouthing, and manipulating prominent objects in the environment. Every rat stimulated in the LH exhibits this behavior pattern, even though they go in many different consummatory directions if provided a variety of interesting objects with which to interact. Indeed, one might expect that with the right choice of an environment, all animals might, in fact, exhibit a single type of "stimulus-bound" appetitive behavior, and that is precisely what happens.

Several investigators configured experimental situations in such a way that ESB was applied only when the animal was on one side of a test chamber, the side that had been provisioned with a variety of "junk" objects, while the other side, where stimulation went off, was empty. After some experience with this situation, most animals begin to systematically carry the objects from the stimulation side to the no-stimulation side.[52] The end result was that the pile of junk was transferred from one side of the chamber to the other. One way to understand this is to surmise that LH stimulation arouses a brain state that normally occurs when animals forage for worldly goods outside of their home burrow, and that animals tend to drop objects when this type of neural activity ceases: The foraging impulse naturally declines when they reach home. Although this procedure yielded consistent behavioral results, object-carrying behavior is still rather complex and perhaps not the ideal choice for a mechanistic analysis of the underlying functional process.

What, then, is the best single behavioral measure to focus upon when one is interested in analyzing the basic nature of this brain system? In my estimation, the best way to study the unconditional behavioral properties of the SEEKING system in rats is via the analysis of "stimulus-bound" sniffing. All animals exhibit this response during the arousal of the circuitry. The response can be readily quantified, and it can even be studied in the anesthetized animal. Indeed, the presence of ESB-induced sniffing at an electrode site during surgery is an excellent indicator that the site will subsequently support SS. Also, the level of electrical current needed to provoke sniffing is almost perfectly related to the threshold for SS at various points in the trajectory of the system (the correlations are above .90).[53] It is noteworthy that the number of microamperes (i.e., electrical current threshold) for evocation of sniffing is never higher than that for SS. This suggests that the sniffing response may be a more primal indicator of the function of the system than is the SS response.

However, the ESB-evoked sniffing response is probably elaborated by both ascending and descending connections in the brain and is not controlled directly by ascending DA systems. It is not diminished markedly by DA receptor blocking agents (a manipulation that markedly reduces SS from the same electrodes).[54] On the other hand, it is clear from a great deal of research that natural exploratory sniffing does require DA activity. Injections of DA blocking agents that have no effect on ESB-induced sniffing markedly reduce exploratory sniffing.[55] This suggests that electrical stimulation evokes sniffing at a point in the neural circuitry that is beyond the DA control point, perhaps via descending glutamatergic circuits that provide regulatory control over bursting activity within the DA system.[56] As highlighted later in this chapter, by measuring sniffing, one can begin to untangle how animals spontaneously learn about the resources in their environments.

It was not until recently that one could put some of these ideas to a direct test via the analysis of DA release in behaving animals. Now it has been demonstrated that DA is released from the ventral striatum (i.e., nucleus accumbens) of rats quite vigorously during the anticipatory phase of behavior but not during the consummatory phase.[57] Comparable DA release is not evident in the dorsal striatum (caudate nucleus), which receives DA projections mainly from the more lateral nigrostriatal system arising from A9 DA neurons. In a typical experimental situation, a male rat is exposed to a sexually receptive female, but physical access is prevented by a wire mesh cage placed over the female. Brain DA is released selectively in the ventral striatum while the male eagerly investigates the situation and searches for a way to get into the cage. DA release diminishes when a route of entry is provided and copulation occurs.

A similar pattern of DA release is seen when animals are anticipating other rewards, such as food.[58] In sum, data from in vivo neurochemical analyses have confirmed that the activation of DA systems is related more closely to the appetitive than to the consummatory phase of motivated behavior. However, the possibility that this system also responds to stressors and the anticipation of aversive events has received provisional support, suggesting that it responds not simply to positive incentives but also to many other emotional challenges where animals must *seek* solutions.[59]

Although a great deal of detailed work remains to be done on this system, the idea that the LH contains a variety of distinct consummatory behavior circuits is no longer tenable.[60] Many investigators now accept the simple alternative that a great deal of behavioral learning can emerge from the intrinsic flexibility of broad-reaching emotional systems in the brain. Behavioral variety is further promoted by the motivationally generalized SEEKING system because it can be modulated by a variety of specific homeostatic detectors within medial strata of the hypothalamus. As will be summarized in the next chapter, many need-specific regulatory systems in the hypothalamus can modulate the arousability of the SEEKING system. Interoreceptive neurons, which detect water, energy, thermal, and other imbalances, energize the search for vital resources in part by promoting the arousability of the SEEKING system.

The Neurodynamics of the Self-Stimulation System: Single-Unit and Neurochemical Studies

Although the SEEKING system is certainly more extensive than the brain DA system, the best electrophysiological evidence of how the system operates can be obtained from a study of how DA neurons fire in response to environmental contingencies. Studies of this sort in awake animals have been made possible by the identification of an electrophysiological "fingerprint" for the activity of these cells. DA neurons typically fire in a fairly rhythmic pattern, with two or three spikes at a time, diminishing spike amplitudes, and longer than normal durations of the action potentials.[61] It is worth noting again that DA neurons have endogenous pacemaker activities. They continue firing at a fairly stable rate throughout the day, including during REM sleep, when other biogenic amine neurons are "sleeping." This may suggest that the system is ready to mediate behavioral arousal at a moment's notice. Also, it may be a way for the brain to keep abreast of the passing of time. It is almost like the second hand of a watch. When the system is aroused and begins to actively mediate behavior, the neurons assume a *bursting* pattern—whereby a series of action potentials are generated in a row—that more effectively promotes dopamine release in the synaptic fields.[62] Also, this type of bursting may help speed up the internally sensed passage of time, thereby leading to the elevation of anticipatory behaviors, as is seen in the scalloped response patterns animals exhibit when working for rewards on fixed-interval schedules (see Figures 1.4 and 8.4).

There is also now a great deal of evidence that VTA-DA neurons are exquisitely responsive to "incentive stimuli"—namely, stimuli that predict the occurrence of rewards in the environment. In one of the most compelling initial studies, investigators analyzed the activity of mesencephalic DA neurons in primates as a function of "go" and "no-go" stimuli predicting the availability and nonavailability of reward, respectively, and how the activity of these neurons related to the animal's reward-seeking arm movements.[63] To facilitate the discrimination of sensory-perceptual and motor responses, arm movements had to be inhibited until the door to the reward boxes was opened. Essentially, the researchers found that "go" stimuli were especially effective in arousing DA neurons (i.e., during a time when no explicit motor response was evident), while similar "no-go" stimuli were not. The "door-opening" stimulus also provoked a comparable response in DA cells, but this was accompanied by motor movements.

Extensive analyses of neurophysiological responses of neurons in the DA terminal fields in the amygdala and basal ganglia have also been conducted.[64] It has been observed that many neurons there are especially responsive to learned contingencies, suggesting that instinctual tendencies and acquired behaviors blend in those areas. Several investigators have also identified putative areas of the brain where reward registration occurs. Temporal and frontal cortices contain an abundance of neurons that fire only in response to stimuli that have acquired meaning by being predictably associated with rewards.[65]

The Neurochemistry of Self-Stimulation

And so the core of the SEEKING system is remarkably well highlighted by the trajectory of brain DA systems, especially the mesolimbic and mesocortical components which ascend from the A10 DA neurons of the VTA to the shell of the nucleus accumbens, and areas of the frontal cortex and amygdala (see Figure 3.6). Manipulation of this system by any of a variety of means yields highly consistent effects on SS: Reductions in DA activity reduce SS, and increases facilitate it. Moreover, SS clearly promotes the release of DA in the brain.[66] However, many other systems are also involved, and there is good evidence that ascending norepinephrine (NE) and epinephrine systems play a modest facilitatory role, while serotonin generally inhibits SS. However, at some sites near the mesencephalic central gray, serotonin promotes a form of SS.[67]

At present, it is widely believed that ascending DA systems are only one link within the complex chains of electrophysiological and neurochemical events that mediate SS, and it is certain that the system also has important descending components that can promote sniffing behaviors, perhaps via glutamate release.[68] Acetylcoline fibers, apparently acting on muscarinic receptors on DA neurons, may constitute an important stage within the system, since muscarinic blockers placed into the VTA can reduce SS.[69] In addition, many neuropeptide systems converge on VTA neurons, including strong neurotensin, opioid, and substance P systems, all of which can promote SS to some extent.[70] Also, cholinergic and GABAergic influences are prominent in the system, and animals will self-inject cholinergic agonists and GABA antagonists into the VTA.[71]

One key task is to determine how these various chemistries control normal appetitive behavior. The most comprehensive analysis of various points along the extended SEEKING system indicates that appetitive approach is affected more substantially than consummatory behaviors following local neurochemical manipulations.[72] In general, the manipulations that selectively decrease appetitive approach behavior to a sucrose reward are DA and cholinergic receptor blockade, and facilitation of GABA activity, which match results observed with SS. It should be an intriguing future chapter of psychobiology when investigators unravel the distinct types of information that modulate the SEEKING system through these and other chemistries. Do different categories of cognitive, classically conditioned, and unconditioned (olfactory, gustatory, and homeostatic) sources of information access DA cells via different neurochemical inputs?

Sometimes it seems that most of the important facts about SS are already known, but then we find, once more, how much remains to be discovered. There are bound to be many more surprises in our analysis of these systems. As mentioned earlier, it is clear that sniffing, the superlative indicator of arousal of this system in rats, operates through neurochemistries other than DA. Why does haloperidol, a potent antipsychotic DA receptor blocker that severely impairs SS, have practically no effect on "stimulus-bound" sniffing, while the same doses can essentially eliminate spontaneous exploratory sniffing?[73] Presumably, the sniffing evoked by ESB is aroused by activation of a descending neural system beyond the DA synapse. No one has yet identified the neurochemistry that mediates this output pathway, but since glutamate is the most prolific excitatory transmitter in both cognitive and emotional systems of the brain, there are good reasons to suspect that glutamate is essential for the sniffing response.

Further, since the sniffing response is at the very heart of the SEEKING system in rats, we can expect to achieve a new and deeper understanding of SS when the neurochemistries of the descending components are identified. Indeed, because of the relationships of SS to learning processes, as well as to schizophrenia (see later discussion), it is possible that such knowledge may yield novel ways of controlling certain spontaneous forms of learning that elaborate delusional thinking.[74]

Role of the SEEKING System in Learning and Memory

It is widely believed that the SS system exerts a key role in learning. James Olds, who along with Peter Milner discovered SS in 1954, spent the last 15 years of his life trying to identify precisely how the brain constructs a fundamental form of knowledge—the knowledge that one is about to be rewarded. Olds and his colleagues recorded action potentials from neurons in SS systems, as well as many other areas of the brain, while rats were learning a very simple classically conditioned appetitive task—namely, anticipatory behavior during a state of hunger.[75] When a one-second tone was sounded, the hungry rat learned to anticipate the delivery of a small pellet of food (for summary see Figure 8.3). The rats typically exhibited no behavioral signs of learning during the first 20 trials, but neuronal indications of learning were evident in the LH and anatomically related areas (midbrain, preoptic area, pons, and amygdala) during trials 10 to 20. Learned behaviors, although poorly executed, were apparent from trials 20 to 30, and during this period various thalamic and hippocampal areas indicated learning. From trials 30 to 40, clear purposive behavior became evident, and the basal ganglia (caudate and globus pallidus) began to exhibit learned responses. By trials 40 to 50, behavior typically became skilled, and the animal seemed to know what was happening. Only at this late stage did the medial geniculate of the thalamus, which decodes auditory stimuli, and the cortical projection areas for auditory processing exhibit learning.

Olds and his colleagues not only identified how learning was prioritized in the brain but also sought to identify the neurons that first exhibited learned changes in individual trials with well-trained animals. To answer the latter question, the investigators sought to identify the neurons that first responded to the onset of the tone signaling food. Again, neurons within the LH exhibited primacy, responding within the first 20 thousandths of a second following onset of the tone. However, other parts of the brain that had taken longer to exhibit initial learning, such as the cortex and posterior nuclei of the thalamus, also exhibited such early responses. Relatively late players in this knowledge game were the frontal cortex, the hippocampus, and the basal ganglia, suggesting that they represented other aspects of the knowledge, perhaps conscious perception of the reward contingencies.

This pattern of results suggests that the LH-SS or SEEKING system is one of the first brain areas to learn an appetitive task, and in well-trained animals it is among the first to express its learning. These results suggest that a fundamental appetitive learning mechanism, which generates positive expectancies, resides within the lateral hypothalamic tissue. Other investigators have affirmed the importance of neurons along the trajectory of this circuit for appetitive learning.[76] Indeed, an animal's ability to exhibit anticipatory excitement is severely compromised by LH damage.[77] However, investigators have hesitated to exploit these findings theoretically, since LH lesioned animals are globally debilitated: It is entirely possible that generalized motor incompetence rather than learning capacity prevents these animals from exhibiting anticipatory behaviors. In any event, these results do affirm the importance of the SEEKING system in the appetitive competence of animals.

If this brain area contributes to animals' intrinsic ability to generate appetitive learning, the mere application of electrical stimulation to this circuitry on a predictable schedule should spontaneously generate anticipatory learning. Indeed, one would predict that the pattern of responding on fixed-interval (FI) schedules may reflect the natural operations of this brain system. Specifically, on a FI schedule, where the possibility of obtaining reinforcement occurs only at set times, animals tend to withhold their responses during the first half of each postreward interval, and operant behavior

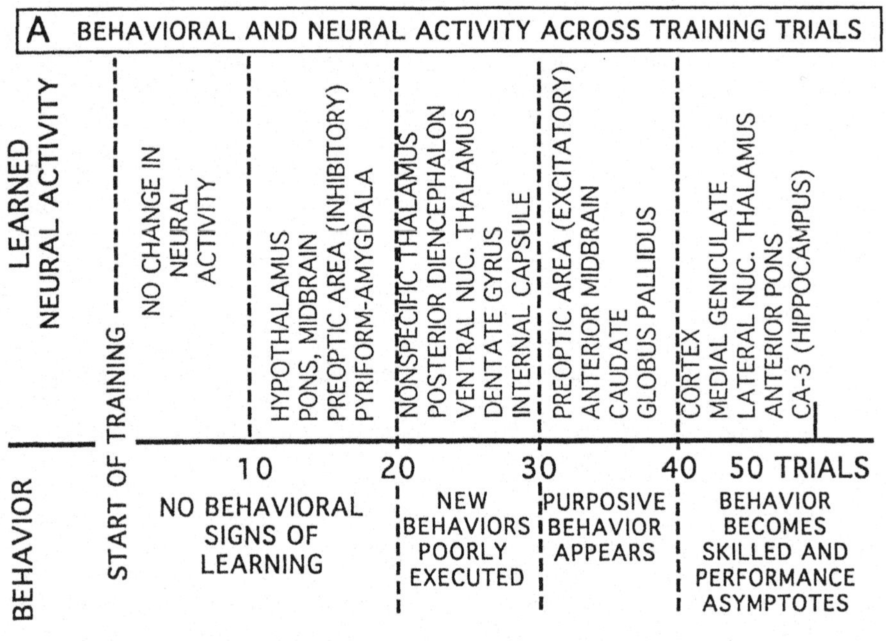

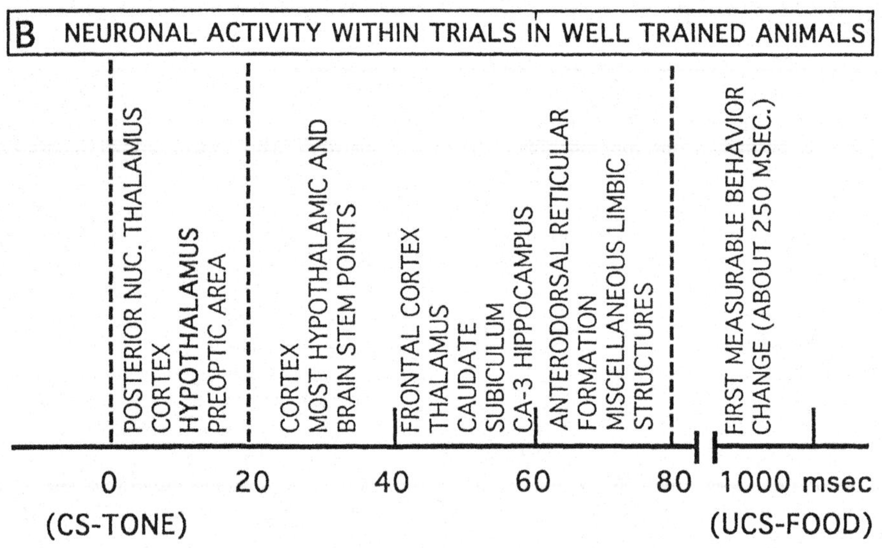

Figure 8.3. Changes in neuronal activity during simple appetitive learning consisting of a tone followed by food one second later. (A) summarizes behavioral changes and learned neuronal changes during acquisition of the task. (B) summarizes the temporal sequence with which brain areas start to exhibit neuronal changes in the well-trained animal. (Adapted from Panksepp, 1981; see chap. 3, n. 25.)

increases gradually during the second half of the interval, before there is any realistic opportunity to obtain rewards. Thus, animals appear to be natural "optimists," invariably underestimating the amount of time they need to wait. After their first response of each FI segment, they begin to respond at ever-increasing rates as the time for reward approaches, yielding a "scalloped" response pattern (see Figure 1.4). Although behaviorists are loath to use terminologies such as expectancies,[78] it seems as if animals working on FI schedules exhibit a gradual intensification of behavioral excitement, or anticipation, as each interval draws to a close.

In fact, rats *spontaneously* exhibit learned behavioral changes resembling the "scalloped" response pattern of FI schedules when they are given free "rewarding" brain stimulation at set intervals: The natural instinctive behavior that exhibits this form of spontaneous learning is exploratory sniffing, the same response that can be evoked by rewarding brain stimulation.[79] Specifically, when free stimulation is administered into rewarding LH sites for 1 second every 20 seconds, anticipatory eagerness develops. During the initial trials, the animals go into a sustained exploratory pattern, with intense sniffing, throughout the interstimulation interval (see Figure 8.4). Gradually, the sniffing begins to diminish following each stimulation but systematically increases as the interval progresses. At the end of training, animals exhibit scalloped sniffing patterns during the interstimulation intervals. This pattern closely resembles the operant behavior animals normally exhibit on such schedules of reinforcement. The difference is that, in this situation, animals *did not need to*

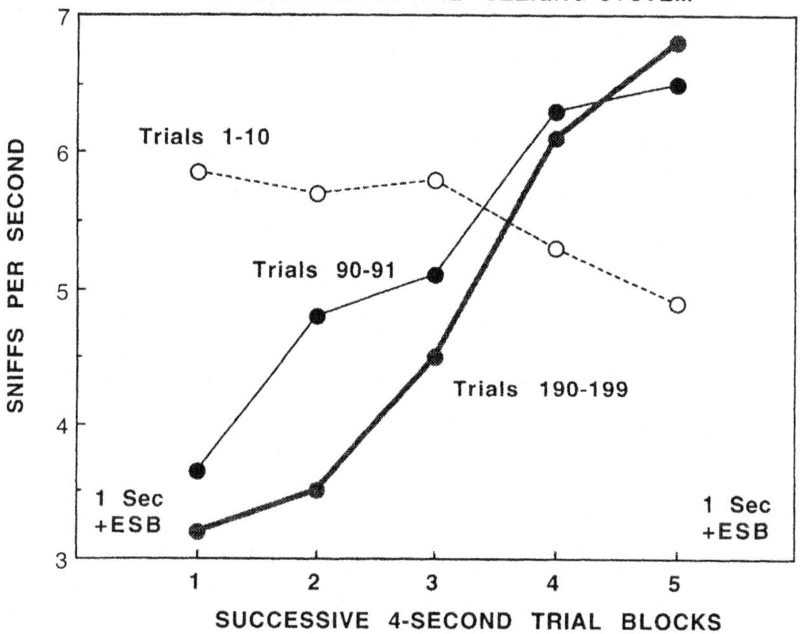

Figure 8.4. Elaboration of sniffing during free fixed-interval 20-second administration of rewarding LH stimulation. During the beginning of training (first 10 trials), animals exhibited only generalized overall energization of sniffing throughout the interstimulation interval. By the end of training (trials 190–199), animals were exhibiting a scalloped pattern, which is reminiscent of animals working for conventional rewards on a fixed-interval schedule (see Figure 1.4). An important point to note is that all of these stimulations were free, and the animals did not have to change their behavior patterns to obtain all "rewards." However, the system spontaneously developed an instrumental pattern of behavioral output. This can explain how patterns of behavior emerge on the schedules of reinforcement that have long been described in the behavioral literature. (Adapted from Panksepp, 1981; see chap. 3, n. 25.)

do anything systematic to obtain rewards. The underlying neural system spontaneously exhibited a scalloped response pattern. Thus, since this acquired behavior served no formal instrumental function, it could be deemed delusional.[80] Of course, it could be assumed that the behavior helps animals prepare for receiving available rewards efficiently. Indeed, that is why I originally called this the "expectancy system."

To determine whether this spontaneous form of anticipatory conditioning has primacy over scalloped operant responding, the spontaneous sniffing of rats was monitored while they were working for sugar water on an FI schedule.[81] It was of special interest to determine what happened during the moment just prior to the first "voluntary" lever press within each FI response segment. In fact, the rats exhibited an invigoration of sniffing just before they made their first lever press. Sniffing continued to increase further after this initial "optimistic" but invariably ineffective response (Figure 8.5). Thus, the brain system that generates sniffing became engaged a moment before the animal emitted its first operant responses. This suggests that the spontaneous arousal of the SEEKING system helped arouse the instrumental behavior. If we understood the mechanisms that allow the SEEKING system to spontaneously generate scalloped sniffing patterns, we would gain a profound understanding of how the brain spontaneously mediates anticipatory states. Presumably this occurs through the ability of LH circuits to generate theta rhythms that sensitize both the associative abilities of the hippocampus and DA-mediated timing functions of the striatum. A neurophysiological understanding of these brain systems can explain how animals spontaneously generate solutions to the various environmental contingencies they encounter in their lives. Presumably, these same systems allow us to develop a sense of causality from the perception of correlated environmental events. This type of spontaneous associative ability characterizes normal human thinking, as well as the delusional excesses of schizophrenic thinking. Indeed, as highlighted in the "Afterthought" of

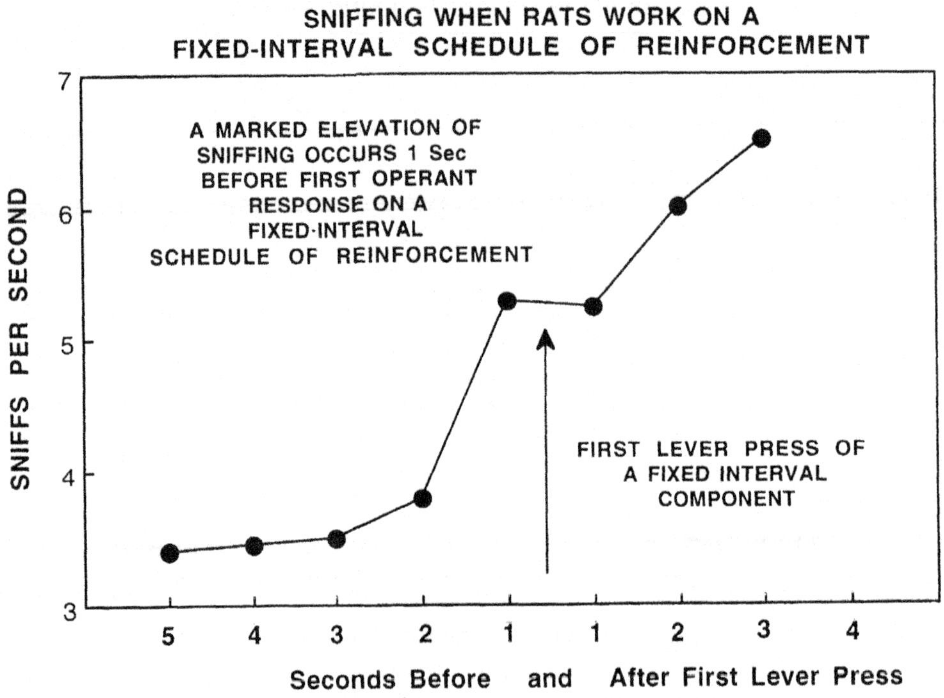

Figure 8.5. Elaboration of sniffing in rats working for rewarding brain stimulation on a fixed-interval schedule of reinforcement. It is noteworthy that spontaneous sniffing increased markedly one second prior to the first lever press within each response segment. This suggests that the brain substrates that arouse sniffing, namely, the circuits of the SEEKING system, mediate appetitive behavior patterns seen when animals are required to exhibit operant responses in order to obtain food. It should be noted that the theta rhythm, which invades the hippocampus when it is integrating information, is of the same frequency as sniffing, and the neuronal systems that activate theta arise from the brain stem and course through the lateral hypothalamus. (Reprinted with permission from Panksepp, 1981; see chap. 3, n. 25.)

this chapter, profound relationships exist between the neural underpinnings of SS in rats and schizophrenia in humans.[82]

The SEEKING System and Sources of Delusional Behaviors in Animals

Arousal of the SEEKING system spontaneously constructs causal "insights" from the perception of correlated events. Some of the relationships may be true, but others are delusional. Indeed, all forms of inductive thought, including that which energizes scientific pursuits, proceed by this type of logically flawed thinking (see Figure 2.3). An intrinsic tendency for "confirmation bias" appears to be a natural function of both human and rat minds.[83] Indeed, the classically conditioned confirmation bias that characterizes many brain learning systems, including the SEEKING system, perplexed investigators when it was first discovered.

An example of this type of spontaneous learning is called "autoshaping," which reflects an animal's tendency to spontaneously behave as if correlated cue-reward contingencies reflect causal relationships. In the classic demonstration of this phenomenon, pigeons were exposed to an illuminated key just prior to the delivery of food.[84] With repeated exposure to this contingency, pigeons exhibited anticipatory pecking at the illuminated key, even though there was no formal connection between anything the animal did and the appearance of food. It was as if the animal believed its behavior was instrumental in procuring the food, although, in fact, it was not. Of course, this is a very effective way to train animals to do various things, even though at a formal level such behaviors reflect delusional thinking. Comparable phenomena have now been observed in all mammalian species that have been studied. The "rain dances" of Indian shamans and the prayers of the devout may reflect such processes in humans. If performed long enough, such rituals are bound to "work," even though there may be no causal relationships between the dances or prayers and events in the world. Nonetheless, we should note that it is possible that the dust kicked up during hours of rain dancing may help seed colloidal suspensions of moisture that can promote precipitation. Also, prayer may put individuals in a frame of mind to behave in ways that may change the social world. However, to the best of our current knowledge, most of such autoshaped behaviors simply reflect a form of classical conditioning within the SEEKING system of the brain. The role of DA in the generation of this type of behavior is affirmed by the ability of DA blocking agents to reduce autoshaping.[85]

Another bizarre behavior generated by the SEEKING system is schedule-induced polydipsia (SIP). This is the excessive drinking that can be produced in hungry rats by giving them small portions of food on an FI schedule; using about two-minute intervals between food delivery produces the maximal response.[86] If water is not available, the animal will exhibit other behaviors such as compulsive shredding of available objects or schedule-induced wheel running. One can even obtain aggression if another animal is nearby. Animals appear to vent the frustration of neuroemotional energy emerging from unfulfilled expectations on any available target.

As a group, these behaviors are called "adjunctive" or "displacement" behaviors, and they resemble the "superstitious" behaviors that Skinner described in his pigeons when they worked on FI schedules of reinforcement.[87] During the interreinforcement intervals, some would strut around the cage and flap their wings in predictable patterns, as if their dance had some meaningful consequence for world events. These behaviors were explained by "adventitious reinforcement"—the chance pairing of randomly emitted behaviors with the delivery of rewards. A deeper cause may be overarousal of the brain's SEEKING system. Adjunctive behaviors probably emerge from the same neural substrates as the "stimulus-bound" behaviors evoked by electrical stimulation of the LH: Animals can dissipate their appetitive "energies" on any of a number of goal-directed behaviors. Indeed, rats that exhibit the most intense SIP behavior are also the most likely to develop intense "stimulus-bound" behaviors.[88] In other words, hungry animals may experience sustained foraging arousal, and if they cannot satisfy this urge by homeostatically appropriate consummatory behavior, they will start to exhibit alternative consummatory behaviors that can partially alleviate feelings of excessive appetitive arousal. The fact that LH lesions as well as DA receptor blockade can markedly reduce schedule-induced behaviors affirms such a conclusion.[89]

Such adjunctive behaviors may resemble the obsessive-compulsive (OC) behavior patterns that humans exhibit under stressful circumstances. However, one of the cardinal attributes of OC psychopathology in humans is the conscious desire to avoid the compulsions. Since we cannot measure the thoughts of animals, the obsessive component of OC disorders may never be properly evaluated in animal models, although adjunctive behaviors may help highlight the nature of impulse control disorders: compulsive acts that are not accompanied by the internally experienced need to withhold behavior.[90]

Another remarkable finding in this area is that most of the behaviors evoked by LH stimulation in rats can also be evoked by applying mild pressure to their tails.[91] Behaviors induced by tail pressure include feeding, drinking, and gnawing, all of which can be diminished by DA receptor blocking agents. This suggests that the phenomenon also arises from excessive activity of the SEEKING system.

Thus, the SEEKING system can promote many distinct motivated behaviors, and the underlying neural system is prepared to jump to the conclusion that correlated environmental events reflect causal relationships. It is easy to appreciate how this may yield a consensual understanding of the world when the underlying memory reinforcement processes are operating normally (i.e., yielding a "reality" that most of the social group accepts). It is also easy to understand how it might yield delusional conclusions about the world. If the system is chronically overactive, it may be less constrained by rational modes of reality testing. The fact that the mesolimbic DA system is especially responsive to stress could explain why paranoid thinking emerges more easily during stressful periods, and why stress may promote schizophrenic thinking patterns.

One critical task for better understanding how this system operates is to identify which neural change actually constitutes reinforcement within the dynamic operation of such brain circuits. In line with the suggestion that positive reinforcement may be linked to reductions in firing within the SEEKING system, we might anticipate that in schizophrenics bursting patterns and internally generated cessations of such patterns may occur with abnormal frequency in response to internal cues rather than to real-life events.[92] Perhaps neurons of the VTA-DA system exhibit excessive bursting, leading to many cessations of bursting for internal as opposed to external reasons. If the spontaneous, internally generated relationships between certain persistent thoughts and the modulation of neuronal bursting are sufficiently systematic, then we can envision how schizophrenics might develop delusional insights from poor regulation of neuronal firing in the SEEKING system.

Relationships of the SEEKING System to Schizophrenia

Some psychobiologists believe that SS of the LH circuitry is an excellent model for type I, or paranoid, schizophrenia, as opposed to type II schizophrenia, which is characterized by demonstrable brain damage (CAT technology reveals ventricular enlargement, suggesting deterioration of surrounding brain tissues).[93] There is general agreement that paranoid schizophrenia is characterized by excessive brain DA activity. The most commonly observed biochemical correlate is an increase of DA receptors (the D_2 variety), especially in the ventral striatum,[94] with occasionally reported abnormalities such as elevated DA levels in the amygdala of the left hemisphere.[95] All antipsychotic drugs reduce DA activity at D_2 receptors, and here is where the parallel between schizophrenia and SS circuitry becomes striking: Virtually all drugs that reduce schizophrenic symptoms also reduce SS along the SEEKING system. Conversely, drugs that worsen schizophrenic symptoms generally increase SS behavior.[96] For instance, psychostimulants facilitate SS and, when administered repeatedly, eventually precipitate symptoms of paranoid schizophrenia that are psychiatrically indistinguishable from the spontaneously occurring variety.[97]

Since schizophrenic breaks can also be precipitated by stress, it is especially noteworthy that the mesolimbic DA system (A10) is highly stress-responsive, more so than the other brain DA systems.[98] During stress, certain ascending DA systems become rapidly depleted of DA, with consequent development of hypersensitivity in the receptors to the little that is left, causing increases in psychological symptoms resembling schizophrenia. Functionally, this may reflect an adaptive process: One should exhibit increased amounts of seeking behaviors when one is under stress in order to ferret out resources to alleviate the stressful situation.

Similar long-term brain changes can be induced by chronic administration of psychostimulants such as cocaine and amphetamine, reflecting a permanent elevation in the sensitivity of the underlying brain systems.[99] This "sensitization" may reflect a long-term brain adjustment that is important for understanding not only schizophrenia but also such phenomena as drug craving and other obsessions, as well as overall reductions in the ability to tolerate stress. It is now clear that a number of neurochemical influences can facilitate such sensitization, including opiates and other drugs of abuse, while drugs that reduce memory consolidation, such as glutamate receptor antagonists, tend to block sensitization. A different syndrome is precipitated by chronic treatment of animals with the direct DA receptor agonist apomorphine, which can influence both postsynaptic and presynaptic DA receptors (i.e., ones situated on DA neurons). Rats that have received such drugs eventually begin to exhibit a high spontaneous level of fearlike emotionality as well as aggression.[100] Many investigators believe such findings are of considerable importance for understanding such psychiatric disorders as mania, but the precise relations have not been determined.

The ideas and facts that presently predominate in biological psychiatry are quite astounding. We can finally make some sense of schizophrenic symptoms by conceptualizing SS circuitry as an appetitive emotional system that can become unstable. If the normal function of this system is to mobilize the organism for seeking out resources in the world, then we begin to appreciate how the SEEKING system might also generate delusional thoughts. Apparently when this emotional system is overtaxed and becomes free-running, it can generate arbitrary and unrealistic ideas about how world events relate to internal events. Is delusional thinking truly related to the unconstrained operation of spontaneously active associative networks that are uncoupled from the reality testing that is created by the brain's normal ability to compute relationships among events? If so, we may have a great deal more to learn about schizophrenia from a study of the SEEKING circuits that mediate SS behavior in animals. Through a study of this system, we can also begin to understand the natural eagerness that makes us the emotionally vibrant creatures that we are. This emotion is harder to visualize than the others, but we have tried to capture the essence of this pervasive emotional process in Figure 8.6.

AFTERTHOUGHT: Self-Stimulation and Dreaming

In the previous chapter, I focused on possible relationships between schizophrenia and dreaming. As we have now seen, there is also a credible linkage between schizophrenia and SS. Accordingly, one might predict that there is an intimate relationship between SS and dreaming. Indeed, interesting connections between the two have been found in REM-deprived animals. REM deprivation in rats leads to an increased sensitivity of the LH-SS system: Animals work at higher rates for lower current levels, as if REM deprivation sensitized the substrates of the SS system.[101] Conversely, it has also been found that allowing animals to self-stimulate for a few hours during the course of ongoing REM deprivation eliminates the need for subsequent REM recovery sleep. In other words, the drive for increased levels of REM following REM deprivation is apparently discharged by allowing animals to self-stimulate during the deprivation period.

It is noteworthy that schizophrenics also fail to exhibit compensatory elevations of REM sleep following imposed periods of REM deprivation.[102] Thus, there appears to be a fundamental relationship between the schizophrenic process and the neuropsychological (emotional?) discharge that occurs during both REM sleep and SS. These findings suggest that there may yet be considerable substance to psychodynamic theories that relate dreaming mechanisms to symbol- and reality-creating mechanisms of the brain.[103]

Such findings also bring to mind old theories of the function of REM sleep, for example, that it provides a time for the discharge of excessive "bottled-up" psychic energies.[104] If we add to these observations the common speculation that there may be a fundamental relationship between REM sleep and schizophrenia, one is led to wonder whether the type of psychic discharge that occurs during SS might also help alleviate schizophrenic symptoms. Could one dissipate the excess energies of this system through various life activities? Could the symptoms of schizophrenia be alleviated simply by providing more outlets for the foraging tendencies of individuals? Can one dissipate SEEKING urges simply through new types of emotional exercises? Of course, speculative ideas such as these—provocative products of brain SEEKING systems—will remain without substance until they are evaluated through rigorous empirical studies.

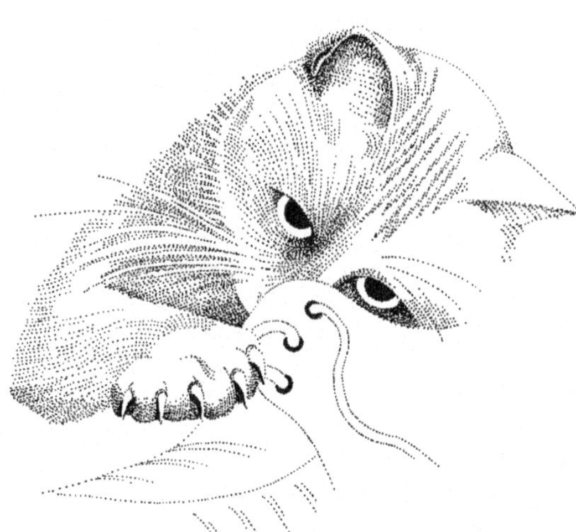

Figure 8.6. The SEEKING system in action. (Adapted from photograph in Panksepp, 1989; see chap. 11, n. 5.)

Suggested Readings

Le Moal, M., & Simon, H. (1991). Mesocorticolimbic dopaminergic network: Functional and regulatory roles. *Physiol. Revs.* 71:155–234.

Liebman, J. M., & Cooper, S. J. (eds.) (1989). *The neuropharmacological basis of reward.* Oxford: Clarendon Press.

Olds, J. (1977). *Drives and reinforcements: Behavioral studies of hypothalamic function.* New York: Raven Press.

Panksepp, J. (1981). Hypothalamic integration of behavior: Rewards, punishments, and related psychological processes. In *Handbook of the hypothalamus.* Vol. 3, Part B, *Behavioral studies of the hypothalamus* (P. J. Morgane & J. Panksepp, eds.), pp. 289–431. New York: Marcel Dekker.

Plutchik, R., & Kellerman, H. (eds.) (1986). *Emotion: Theory, research, and experience.* Vol. 3, *Biological foundations of emotion.* New York: Academic Press.

Rolls, E. T. (1975). *The brain and reward.* Oxford: Pergamon Press.

Routtenberg, A. (ed.) (1980). *Biology of reinforcement: Facets of brain stimulation reward.* New York: Academic Press.

Schultz, S. C., & Tamminga, C. A. (eds.) (1989). *Schizophrenia: Scientific progress.* New York: Oxford Univ. Press.

Valenstein, E. S. (ed.) (1973). *Brain stimulation and motivation.* Glenview, Ill.: Scott, Foresman.

Wauquier, A., & Rolls, E. T. (eds.) (1976). *Brain-stimulation reward.* Amsterdam: North-Holland.

9

Energy Is Delight

The Pleasures and Pains of Brain Regulatory Systems

> As the human understanding surpasses that of the ape, and that of the ape surpasses that of the fishes, so in almost as extreme a degree the vertebrate brain surpasses the nervous organs of the invertebrates. A reason for this difference, one thinks, is to be found in history, and in a very elementary biological fact. All animals are dependent on either plants or animals for food, and from its beginnings the evolution of the animal kingdom has in the main presented a pageant of predator and prey—eat or be eaten!
>
> H. W. Smith, *From Fish to Philosopher* (1953)

CENTRAL THEME

Mammals can survive only if they maintain relative constancy of various bodily processes, including oxygen and carbon dioxide content in blood, body water levels, salt and energy balance, and body temperature. Complex brain and body systems sustain these constancies, and the overall concept used to describe this ability is *homeostasis*. Some people prefer the word *heterostasis*, since the level of regulation sometimes changes as a function of environmental conditions as well as internal bodily cycles (e.g., 24-hour rhythms). Homeostasis is sustained by a diversity of mechanisms ranging from rapid physiological changes, such as reflexive modification of breathing rate as a function of oxygen need (which is actually signaled to the brain by carbon dioxide buildup in the bloodstream), to instinctual behavioral tendencies, such as an animal's urge to seek resources needed for longer-term survival, including food, water, warmth, and micronutrients such as vitamins and minerals. Bodily needs instigate distinct forms of bodily arousal and psychological feelings of distress such as hunger, thirst, and coldness. Animals have exquisite sensory systems to identify the most important items they need—for example, the ability to taste sweetness identifies foods laden with sugar, and saltiness identifies sources of sodium. It is commonly believed that color vision evolved, in part, to help primates identify the ripest fruit. The needed items that cannot be identified by taste—for instance, many vitamins and other micronutrients—can usually be regulated via learned selection of foodstuffs, based on their postingestive consequences. Most interesting from the affective point of view are the intrinsic brain mechanisms that mediate pleasure and displeasure to provide an intrinsic guide for food selection. The pleasures of sensation arise from the interactions of many sensory systems with poorly understood hedonic mechanisms of the brain. Sensations generate pleasure or displeasure in direct relation to their influence on the homeostatic equilibrium of the body. For instance, if one is depleted of energy resources, foods taste better than when the body is already replete with energy. Although it is difficult to study internally experienced pleasures and displeasures in animals, for an accurate description of certain brain functions it will be essential to conceptualize how such processes are elaborated by specific neural circuits. A variety of distinct pleasures may arise from essentially the same types of neurochemical systems, such as the release of endogenous opioids. Likewise, regulation requires some type of set-point mechanisms, resembling the thermostats that control furnaces in our homes, which help specify deviations from physiological equilibrium and thereby promote SEEKING behaviors. To highlight general principles of how regulatory processes operate, in the present chapter I will focus largely on the physiological, behavioral, and psychological mechanisms that help sustain body energy balance. In more than a poetic sense, energy is delight.

Feeling States Related to Homeostasis

For those who have never been extremely hungry or thirsty, it is hard to imagine the distress that such bodily imbalances create within the brain. Consider this archetypal situation: the Black Hole of Calcutta, the horror of 146 survivors of the British garrison that lost Fort William to a Bengali attack on a summer evening in the middle of the 18th century. The prisoners were crammed into a room 18 feet square, and only a few survived that sultry Indian night. The description, by the officer in command, tells of the agony of thirst and the manner in which powerful motivations funnel mental energies to one single goal—survival:

> We had been but a few minutes confined before every one fell into a perspiration so profuse, you can form no idea of it. This brought on a raging thirst. . . . Water! water! became the general cry. . . . [A little was brought by the guards]. . . . There ensued such violent struggles and frequent contests to get it. . . . These supplies, like sprinkling water on fire, only seemed to feed the flame. Oh! my, how shall I give you a just conception of what I felt at the cries and cravings of those in the remoter parts of the prison, who could not entertain a probable hope of obtaining a drop, yet could not divest themselves of expectations, however unavailing, calling on me by the tender considerations of affection and friendship. The confusion now became general and horrid. . . . Many, forcing their way from the further part of the room, pressed down those in their passage who had less strength, and trampled them to death. . . . My thirst now grew insupportable. . . . I kept my mouth moist from time to time by sucking the perspiration out of my shirt-sleeves, and catching the drops as they fell like heavy rain from my head and face; you can hardly imagine how unhappy I was if any of them escaped my mouth. . . . I was observed by one of my companions on the right in the expedient of allaying my thirst by sucking my shirt-sleeve. He took the hint, and robbed me from time to time of a considerable part of my store, though, after I detected him, I had the address to begin on that sleeve first when I thought my reservoirs were sufficiently replenished, and our mouths and noses often met in contact. This man was one of the few who escaped death, and he has since paid me the compliment of assuring me he believed he owed his life to the many comfortable draughts he had from my sleeves. No Bristol water could be more soft or pleasant than what arose from perspiration. . . . At six in the morning the door was opened, when only three and-twenty out of the hundred and forty-six still breathed.[1]

Clearly, a broad range of subjective feelings are associated with intense regulatory imbalances and the many specific sensations that accompany the satisfaction of bodily needs—the hungers, thirsts, cravings, and the various sensory delights that arise from interacting with needed resources. These types of feelings have posed troublesome issues for investigators devoted to a scientific analysis of motivations. It has been difficult to conceptualize mechanistically how such feelings might actually participate in the causal control of animal behavior, but here we recognize that they are the brain's value-coding devices, which can be studied through the analysis of various behavioral indicators, ranging from food choices to facial gestures.

Although the preceding topics may seem somewhat remote from our main goal of clarifying emotional processes, they do highlight the types of neuropsychological analyses of animal feelings that will be required in order for us to make sense of energy-balance regulation. We will eventually need to understand the affective nature of hunger, as well as the more nebulous feeling of metabolic well-being. At the end of this chapter, I will also tackle the important issue of gustatory pleasures. In general, I trust the reader appreciates that we will have to understand the various regulatory mechanisms of the brain and body in order to really understand the nature of the many affective experiences that surround our eating habits and other regulatory behaviors. To achieve such knowledge, we must be willing to use measures of behavioral events as indices of mental events. The logic is the same as the use of cloud chambers to track the movements of subatomic particles in physics.

Many other related feelings are impossible to study in animal models. For instance, the problems people develop with their self-image when they are anorexic or obese cannot be addressed in animal models, probably because they emerge from the higher reaches of the human brain, which can generate thoughts beyond the imagination of other creatures. However, the simpler feelings that are more directly related to primitive homeostatic processes shared by all animals can be indirectly (i.e., inferentially) studied in animals by carefully observing their behaviors. Let us consider one example that has received virtually no experimental attention.

One of the most powerful and rapidly acting regulatory urges is our continual need for oxygen. Of course, breathing regulation is very different from the other motivations, since the needed resource, under most circumstances, is readily available. Most other motivations, such as the need for food or sex, can be fulfilled only by active exploratory and search behaviors generated by the SEEKING system. Breathing does not require such assistance. When breathing proceeds normally, the controls remain totally at a subconscious level. Obviously, evolution has automated and eliminated choice in the most important aspects of homeostasis. Indeed, our bodies do not actually detect oxygen need directly. Our brain only monitors correlated variables such as the buildup of carbon dioxide in the body and changes in the acid-base balance of the bloodstream.

An increase in systemic carbon dioxide elevates the

rate and depth of breathing, without being accompanied by major psychological distress. What causes respiratory distress is impairment of our rhythmic breathing—for instance, by airway obstruction, suffocation, or strangulation. When such events occur, a very powerful emotional state arises—a paniclike condition that reflects the existence of a primitive brain stem response system, called the "suffocation alarm" reflex. When this happens, one's mind is rapidly filled with a precipitous anxiety, and one begins to flail about in anguish. Indeed, human "panic attacks" may emerge, in part, from activation of this powerful emotional response system.[2] This example exquisitely indicates how rapidly feeling states and behaviors can change in response to a regulatory crises. Although the spontaneous activation of such an emotional state leads to a large number of cognitive evaluations, there is no reason to believe that the suffocation-alarm response itself is normally activated by any higher appraisal mechanism. This highlights the normal flow of motivational events in the brain—emotions and regulatory feelings have stronger effects on cognitions than the other way around.

Obviously, several types of cognitive and emotional arousal occur in any strong motivational situation. Consider the simple cases of excessive bladder or rectal distention. The concern these sensations often cause derives from the type of social inhibitions that do not seem to worry other animals. Still such feelings of distention can become incredibly insistent, filling our minds with nothing but the urge for relief. The feelings are so insistent that it is difficult to sustain other thoughts in one's mind. Unfortunately, we know little about the neural systems that subserve such feelings, but it is possible that they are organized quite low in the neuroaxis, perhaps at the brain stem level. If we could specify the exact neural systems that create such feelings, we would probably understand more about consciousness than can presently be found in most of the learned texts on the topic (see Chapter 16).

Regulatory urges rarely become as intense as in the examples described earlier because we can anticipate their coming and their consequences. To some extent, our cognitive abilities allow us to anticipate such events and relieve ourselves of potential embarrassments. The higher cognitive processes can also promote, at least in humans, many other subtle emotional concerns that are not directly related to aroused needs. For instance, during one's search for resources, anxiety can easily arise from contemplations such as "Will I find what I need? Will there be enough? And what if someone gets there before me?" Frustration and anger may be engendered if a competitor is successful in snatching away a valued resource. If the needed resources are rare or consistently lost in competitive encounters, one may develop such chronic behavioral tendencies as hoarding or learned affective habits such as greediness. Indeed, these tendencies also appear to be part of the instinctive potential of the mammalian nervous system, even though they are typically expressed only if resources are perceived to be scarce for prolonged periods.[3]

Conversely, it should be noted that virtually all emotional states affect the intensity of our motivations. Most animals, even humans, are unlikely to eat much or exhibit any inclination for play or sex when they are very scared or angry. One long-term emotion that is especially incompatible with normal appetite is separation distress. When young animals are socially isolated, they typically lose weight even if they have free access to lots of food. When the young are reunited with their kin, and a mood of apparent contentment is reestablished, appetite returns. From this vantage, it is not surprising that one's appetite is best in the presence of social companionship and social facilitation of feeding is such a robust phenomenon in nature.[4]

Because of the lack of relevant brain data, we will rarely address the cross-modal influences among emotional and motivational systems, but the available behavioral data indicate that such interactions are pervasive—which makes it difficult to study regulatory influences, such as satiety factors, without also considering a host of other affective changes in the organism.

As a heuristic exercise into the nature of regulatory feelings associated with bodily need states, I will provide a fairly detailed brain overview of one major motivational system—the one that mediates body energy regulation. I will also seek to illuminate the nature of the affective feelings that accompany energy need states—the distress engendered by hunger, as well as the pleasures arising from consummatory acts.

Regulatory Behaviors and the SEEKING System

As we saw in Chapter 8, the SEEKING system can motivate animals to pursue a diversity of distinct rewards in the environment. The nervous system does most of this automatically, with no obvious deliberation. Many bodily needs access the SEEKING system and thereby arouse appetitive search tendencies that motivate animals to approach and learn about available resources. It would have been wasteful for evolution to have constructed separate search and approach systems for each bodily need. The most efficient course was for each need-detection system to control two distinct functions: a generalized, nonspecific form of appetitive arousal and various need-specific resource-detection systems. In addition, learning would increase the efficiency with which the SEEKING system could guide animals to appropriate goal objects. This is, in fact, what transpires in the mammalian brain.

Thus, resource depletions within the body can lead to a generalized arousal of seeking behaviors regardless of the specific regulatory imbalances that exist, and specific need states that sensitize distinct consummatory reflex tendencies (e.g., licking, biting, chewing, and swallowing) and key support mechanisms, such as sensory, perceptual, and memory fields relevant for the specific needs. By the interplay of these processes, a generalized search system can efficiently guide animals to relevant environmental goal objects. In other words, the nonspecific SEEKING system, under the guidance of various regulatory imbalances, external incentive cues, and past learning, helps take thirsty animals to water, cold animals to warmth, hungry animals to food, and sexually aroused animals toward opportunities for orgasmic gratification (Figure 9.1).

Existing evidence suggests that the SEEKING system is under the control of internal *homeostatic* receptor systems that detect various bodily imbalances. This is suggested by the fact that many imbalances can modify the rate at which animals self-stimulate lateral hypothalamic (LH) electrode sites.[5] For instance, hunger reduces the current threshold needed to sustain LH self-stimulation while also increasing the rate at which animals behave. Similar effects can be evoked by thirst, cold, and various sex hormones, even though these have not been studied as thoroughly as the effects of food deprivation. The exact manner in which the various interoreceptive systems interface with the foraging system remains to be worked out in detail, but there are many candidate neurons with the right anatomical and physiological characteristics throughout the LH and adjacent zones of the medial hypothalamus.

The axons of many medial hypothalamic neurons make synaptic contact with the ventral tegmental area (VTA). Their dendrites extend radially across the ascending and descending axons of the SEEKING system, providing feedback loops that can regulate the vigor of foraging.[6] Many of these neurons are sensitive to circulating nutrients such as amino acids, fatty acids, and blood sugar, or glucose.[7] Other nearby interoreceptive neurons, known as *osmoreceptors*, are sensitive to the osmotic concentrations of solutes in the blood. Various others, known as *thermoreceptors*, are sensitive to bodily (core) and peripheral temperature fluctuations.[8] There are also specialized neurons that are sensitive to the various hormones that control sexual tendencies (e.g., steroid-receptive neurons for testosterone, dihydrotestosterone, estrogen, and progesterone).[9] There are bound to be other detectors (e.g., sodium and perhaps other micronutrient detectors), but our knowledge about their locations and properties remains more rudimentary.

It is important to note that electrode locations that readily yield self-stimulation in rats typically yield predatory aggression in cats.[10] Obviously, this is a reasonable species-typical SEEKING behavior for a carnivorous animal that subsists at the top of the food chain. Outward behavior can sometimes mislead us about the functions of an underlying brain system. The failure to recognize this appears to have been another instance in which the variety of behaviors evoked by LH stimulation has deceived investigators about the generalized emotive functions of a brain circuit. As we will see in the next chapter, a great deal of evidence suggests that predatory aggression is a result of arousal of the SEEKING system, as opposed to activation of a distinct emotional system. As discussed in the previous chapter, a comparable mistake was the idea that activation of the LH self-stimulation system evoked consummatory pleasure or reward responses in animals.[11]

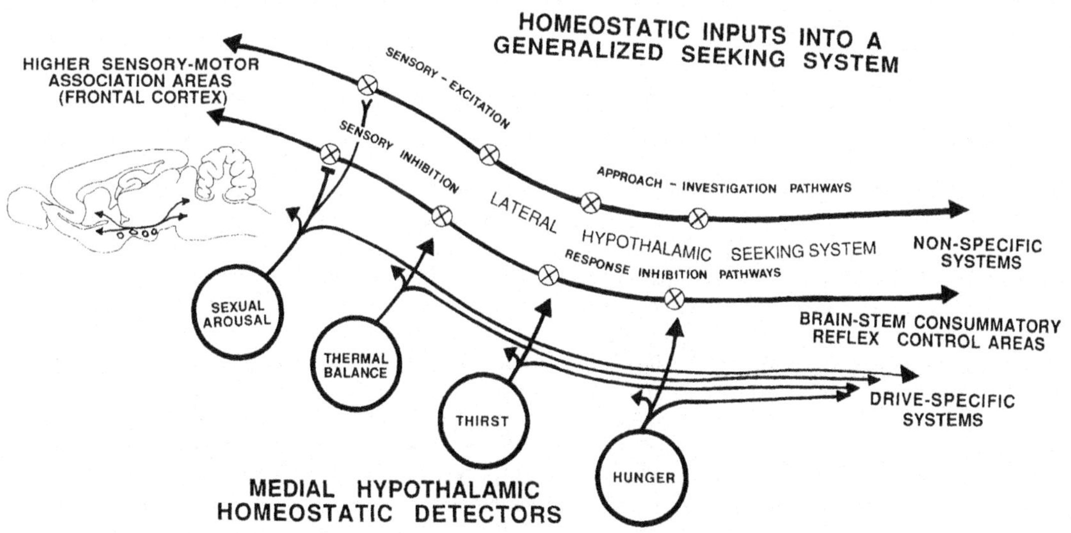

Figure 9.1. A conceptual schematic of how specific regulatory detector systems in the medial hypothalamus access a shared SEEKING system in the lateral hypothalamus. (Adapted from Panksepp, 1981; see n. 5.)

Drives, Incentives, and Appetitive Arousal in the Brain

In the old psychological terminology, the bodily need detection systems of the brain were thought to generate "drives," but the use of that concept has diminished as we have come to realize that such a broad abstract *intervening variable* cannot be credibly linked to unitary brain processes. Indeed, it has been recognized that at a logical level, the notion of drive may be redundant for a coherent explanation of behavior. *Incentive* concepts may suffice, especially since specific deprivation states primarily facilitate an animal's response to specific external incentive stimuli.[12] Here, we will use the concept of a bodily *need state* as opposed to *drive* to indicate the presence of regulatory imbalances. For instance, need states such as energy depletion lead to dramatic increases in motor arousal only when animals are in the presence of incentive stimuli—namely, those stimuli that predict the availability and characteristics of relevant primary rewards such as food. At a physiological level, increased arousal can be measured by the intensification of reflexes as well as neural changes.[13]

It should also be noted that there are problems with the traditional concept of incentive, as defined by the attributes of quantity, quality, and delay of reward. If the incentive process is defined only with respect to the external qualities of rewards, we may tend to overlook important properties of brain systems that evolved to respond to these attributes. In other words, the incentive process, as instantiated by specific properties of neural circuits, may respond to certain properties of external rewards so as to integrate an affective/motivational state within the brain. Once the incentive stimuli have interacted with such circuits, the aroused psychological response is only indirectly related to the outward properties of rewards.

As summarized in the previous chapter, a major type of incentive-related process in the brain is arousal of the SEEKING system. It is reasonable to consider this an incentive system because it establishes an appetitive arousal bias within animals so they can seek and eventually come to anticipate the diversity of rewards the environment has to offer. As an animal learns about the rewards in its world, the degree of conditioned arousal of the SEEKING system appears to be systematically related to external incentive properties of reward objects—namely, the quantity, quality, and delay of reward. The SEEKING system presumably integrates this information spontaneously through its exposure to previous reward experiences. However, the arousability of this emotive system is more than the sum of those experiences. In other words, the brain's intrinsic, evolutionarily derived mechanisms add a new dimension to those inputs—namely, the incentive-directed psychobehavioral "energy" of the animal. The system sensitizes animals to respond vigorously when there are predictable rewards. Presumably this activation optimizes the likelihood that an animal will "be first in line" to obtain available resources. Evolution has provided a special psychic "energy" to the arousal of this system. Of course, this can easily lead to a behavioral free-for-all if the brains of several animals, each seeking to be first in line, are aroused in the same way at the same time.

Although the SEEKING system is well situated to be influenced by an array of bodily need states (Figure 9.1), the extent to which those sources of arousal produce direct or indirect effects on the SEEKING system remains unanswered experimentally. There are many possibilities. For instance, do homeostatic interoreceptors directly modulate SEEKING by sending synapses to VTA-dopamine neurons, or do they merely gate various sensory inputs into the system? As with any set of scientific alternatives, the truth often lies somewhere in between. Thus, it is to be expected that energy balance detectors may promote searching, both directly and indirectly, via the amplification of relevant sensory inputs that can also energize the search process.

However, the key question for this chapter remains: How do specific neurons know that the body has too little or an overabundance of available energy? This appears to be achieved in large part through specialized cells in medial and lateral zones of the hypothalamus that interact with various bodily factors. Indeed, this serves as one specific example for the general principle of how homeostatic imbalances operate through the auspices of the SEEKING system. However, before exploring those details, I will first focus on the diversity of behavior patterns that animals exhibit in harvesting energy from their environments. Obviously, there is great variability in the feeding patterns of different species. After all, each is adapted to its own ecological niche.

Meal-Taking Behavior and Energy Homeostasis

There are as many unique feeding strategies in the wild as there are nutritional environments in which different species subsist. No two diets or feeding methods are exactly alike. Seed-eating birds often cache supplies of food far and wide and use remarkable spatial memories in retrieving their hidden tidbits. Indeed, birds that actively hide seeds for later use have larger hippocampi, the brain areas that specializes in processing spatial information, than those that do not. Omnivores such as rats also show energized exploratory behaviors for scattered food items and often exhibit hoarding; they typically consume many small meals each day. Herbivores, on the other hand, spend much time grazing on more readily available, energy-dilute resources. Hence, their foraging systems are designed to progress methodically across a field as the animals consume large meals. Carnivores, on the other hand, must stalk, chase down, pounce upon, and kill their quarry before they have an opportunity to gorge on energy-rich meals. Parenthetically, it is more difficult to obtain consistent self-stimulation from the LH of cats than of rats, perhaps because of the predatory foraging style of carnivores. The high degree of behavioral inhibition necessary for stalking followed by rapid pursuit may be incompatible with vigorous self-stimulation behavior.

Although the goal of energy balance regulation can be achieved by a variety of easily observed behavior patterns—from the consumption of one meal a day to continual nibbling—the nature of the regulated process is not as evident. The essence of energy regulation is well hidden from scientific view, apparently in the deep metabolic recesses of the hypothalamus. Because of the difficulty of studying such hidden processes, investigators have generally focused on the clear and measurable characteristics of feeding patterns, rather than on the intrinsic nature of internal processes that can only be inferred from outward behavioral signs. Indeed, for a long time it was assumed that if we carefully study the relationships between meals and intermeal intervals, special insights would emerge concerning the underlying regulatory processes. This hope has been fulfilled only marginally, since the balancing of energy intake is typically only accurate in the long term, with many inaccuracies in the short term. One reason that individual meals tell us rather little about the regulatory mechanisms of the brain is because regulatory patterns change during the animal's circadian metabolic cycles. In addition, many other psychological processes, from fear to pleasure mechanisms, can easily subvert the brain's regulatory actions for extended periods. For instance, fearful animals eat little. On the other hand, animals take large meals if their food is especially tasty but become finicky nibblers if it is not. They also take large meals if food is hard to find but tend to make many small meals if food is abundant.[14]

Let us consider in some detail one example of why a single meal may tell us little about regulation. Omnivores, such as rats and humans, are opportunists. If given sudden access to rich and appealing food, they typically gorge like carnivores, with little heed for their immediate energy needs. This "dessert effect" makes the analysis of overall energy regulatory processes problematic unless one uses constant dietary conditions, which obviously makes human research especially difficult. Humans actively seek culinary variety, which can temporarily override regulatory signals. The variability in short-term regulation also appears to be greatest among individuals who have a constitutional tendency toward obesity and those who follow sedentary lifestyles. Likewise, if rats living in small cages are given continuous access to a variety of tasty foods, comparable to a typical human diet (the so-called supermarket diet), they generally become poorer regulators and plateau at substantially higher body weights than they would normally sustain.[15] In other words, constant access to tasty junk food (cookies, chocolates, etc.) promotes overeating and fat deposition in both rats and humans. On the other hand, if maintenance food is not tasty, animals tend to sustain chronically lower body weights. Thus, to study the underlying principles of body energy regulation, one has to minimize the influence of such external variables. It is best to test the feeding behavior of animals kept on maintenance diets to which they have been well habituated. It is also well established that animals regulate their body weight more effectively when they have access to abundant exercise.[16] Thus, it is now accepted that long-term energy homeostasis in all mammalian species is accomplished only across many discrete eating episodes. One meal does not suffice.

When one does control all of the many factors that can affect spontaneous meal taking, one can obtain a clear understanding of what normally regulates feeding. It is the energy content of food. It does not matter whether the calories come from fats, proteins, or carbohydrates; animals seek enough to maintain a certain level of available bodily energy. This can be demonstrated in a large variety of ways, the most common of which has been to modify the caloric density of food. Animals rapidly adjust intake downward or upward depending on whether their diet is concentrated or diluted. Animals also correctly adjust feeding if part of their daily energy intake is infused directly into their stomachs (Figure 9.2).[17]

This type of overall energy intake adjustment, now observed in hundreds of studies, suggests that regulation is linked to the body's energy extraction processes, namely, intracellular metabolism. For instance, all macronutrients converge on the Krebs cycle, where more than 80% of the energy content of food is extracted into a metabolically usable form. Also, it appears that the brain can indirectly monitor the amount of energy that is retained in long-term storage pools such as adipose tissue. It seems that the long-term results of these processes of energy extraction and disposition are eventually sensed by specialized areas of the hypothalamus, and certain forms of obesity arise from disruptions of these mechanisms. Thus, the brain's regulatory mechanisms resemble centers of gravity around which relevant psychobehavioral processes revolve. For instance, these systems control the intensity of the desire to eat, the pleasure reactions elicited by foods, the amount eaten during each meal, and the length of time animals wait before taking subsequent meals. Clearly, our understanding of regulatory processes, as well as many related behavioral changes, hinges on our ability to fathom the details of long-term homeostatic mechanisms. At present, we are only partway there, but the last few years have seen dramatic advances.

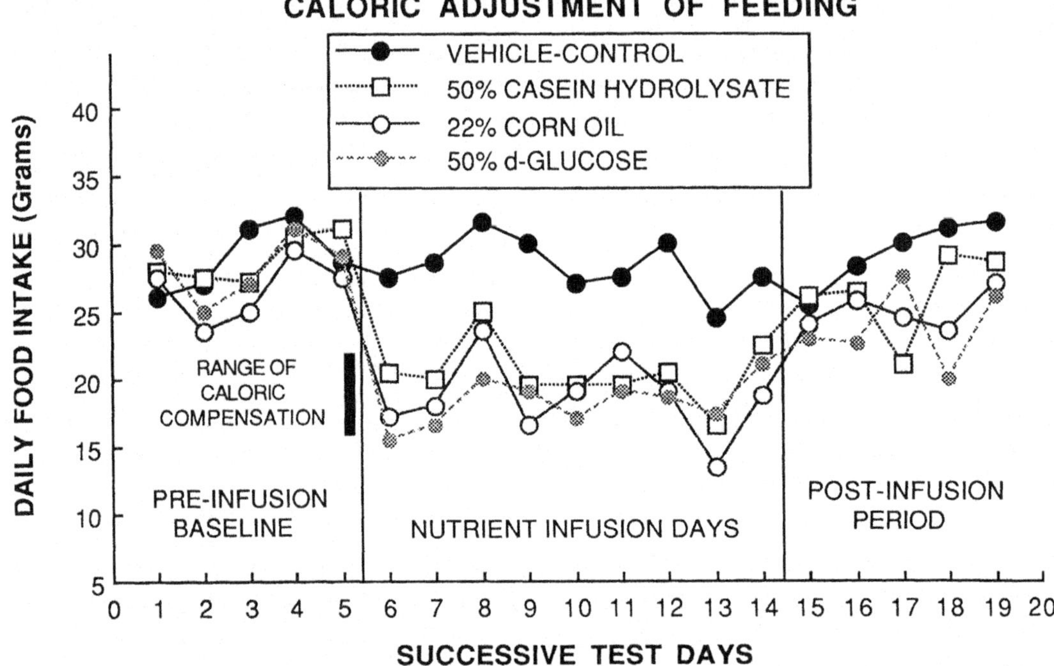

Figure 9.2. Daily food intake of rats during a nine-day period when animals receive approximately a quarter of their daily caloric intake directly into the stomach, but all of the nutrients infused are fats, proteins, or carbohydrates. (Adapted from Panksepp, 1971; see n. 17.)

Methodological Difficulties in Sifting Important Regulatory Energy Balance Effects from Trivial Feeding Ones

Before discussing what we do know about long-term energy regulation, let us not underestimate the complexity of short-term feeding control mechanisms. The signals include (1) many oral factors; (2) a large array of stomach and gastrointestinal factors that act upon various brain mechanisms; (3) a diversity of metabolic factors from various body compartments, especially the liver, which are reflected in circulating nutrients, some of which can affect the brain; (4) a great many neurochemical factors; and (5) a vast array of nonspecific influences that have little to do with energy regulation, such as feelings of sickness and malaise, as well as emotional and mood changes that can dramatically affect feeding behaviors. Indeed, an enormous number of short-term factors have been shown to control feeding—from rattling an animal's cage to giving drugs that make them ill—but most tell us little about the mechanisms that normally mediate long-term body-energy regulation. On the other hand, various short-term controls, such as rapid distention, and also metabolic signals from the gastrointestinal system, which ascend into the brain via the vagus nerve, are essential for the normal short-term patterning of food intake.[18] Obviously, we must always be concerned about the behavioral specificity of our manipulations and must utilize various experimental means to distinguish nonregulatory affective influences from those that normally control appetite. Since so many factors can reduce feeding in the short term without having much to do with the physiology of normal regulatory mechanisms, how shall we discriminate the important physiological factors that normally reduce feeding from those that decrease intake for trivial and temporary reasons?

This is no simple matter. Obviously, such issues are especially problematic in studies that analyze feeding for short periods after experimental manipulations, especially when psychoactive drugs are used. We must seriously consider the feeling states of animals in order to avoid misleading ourselves about the types of effects that are reducing appetite. Accordingly, manipulations that increase feeding generally provide more insight into the nature of the underlying physiological controls than manipulations that reduce feeding. However, ongoing research is still strongly biased toward the study of agents that inhibit feeding, because the discovery of a truly effective long-term appetite control agent would be financially lucrative. In any event, careful investigators agree: To interpret appetite-inhibition effects correctly, one must conduct a variety of controls to evaluate whether the effects are behaviorally specific. Unfortunately, the recognition of such interpretive problems is more widespread than are empirical solutions.

The most common way to evaluate behavioral specificity is by determining whether agents that reduce food intake also produce *conditioned taste aversions* (CTAs).[19] This procedure relies on the fact that animals will typically not eat foods that have been followed by illness. All drugs that make animals sick will provoke learned rejections of novel foodstuffs with which the feelings of malaise have been associated. A single incidence of sickness is usually sufficient to establish a specific food aversion, and the illness can even occur many hours after exposure to a new food source. Thus, if appetite-reducing drugs also produce conditioned food aversions, investigators typically infer that the agent reduces food intake by nonregulatory means. For instance, one widely touted "satiety agent" called cholecystokinin (CCK), a neuropeptide, has been found, upon close analysis, to reduce food intake by causing gastrointestinal distress, transmitted up to the brain via the vagus nerve, rather than a natural feeling of satiety.[20] It has also recently become apparent that CCK fragments may precipitate panic attacks in humans.[21] Many other putative "satiety agents" may be comparably flawed.

One potential shortcoming of the CTA criterion is that animals can also learn "conditioned satieties." Thus, the reduced intake of a novel foodstuff that has been associated with an experimental treatment may simply indicate that the animal is treating it as a very high-energy food source. Of course, this could be evaluated by testing the animal under conditions of hunger. If the aversion persists, it is unlikely to have been a "conditioned satiety," but investigators rarely implement such control maneuvers.[22] Another shortcoming is that many substances produce CTAs, including presumably pleasurable items such as amphetamines and opiates, so it remains possible that the CTA measure also detects agents that simply produce new and powerful feelings other than malaise.

Another suggested control procedure has been to monitor the behavior patterns of animals after a normal, satisfying meal. This typically consists of a sequence of grooming, exploration, and then a nap.[23] However, this is a fairly diffuse behavioral criterion of satiety, since an animal behaves in this way even if a meal is prematurely terminated or following other satisfying activities such as sex. Thus, it would be useful to have more specific behavioral assays that leave less room for ambiguity.

One measure that has not received the attention it deserves is the tendency of animals to rapidly eat massive amounts of tasty food they receive only occasionally, even when they are not hungry. Indeed, well-fed rats will eat as much of foods they greatly prefer, such as raw ground meat, as very hungry rats. By comparison, starved animals eat much more of their normal maintenance chow than nondeprived animals (see Figure 9.3). This "pig-out" phenomenon, whereby animals become quite insensitive to the cues of long-term energy balance because of the overwhelming effect of taste, could be used as a credible measure of normal satiety. For instance, if one has a drug that is presumed to evoke a normal feeling of satiety, the drug should selectively reduce intake of a maintenance food to which an ani-

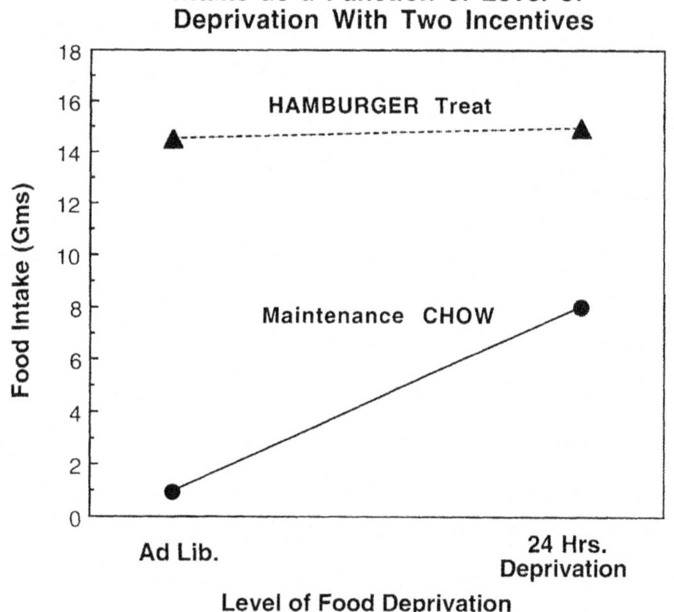

Figure 9.3. A summary of the effects of high-incentive (raw hamburger) and much lower-incentive food (the animals' normal maintenance chow) on intake as a function of degree of prior food deprivation. (According to unpublished data, Panksepp, 1974.)

mal is habituated but have little effect on the intake of a very tasty food that is provided infrequently. A feeling of sickness should reduce the intake of both types of food. Unfortunately, this test has rarely been employed in feeding research.[24]

An even better way to evaluate this troublesome issue might be to identify an active behavior that is markedly increased by normal satiety. We have identified one such behavior: rough-and-tumble social play in young rats.[25] Hunger produces a dramatic reduction in their play behaviors, as do other aversive states (see Figure 1.1), but a single meal brings play right back to normal. One could argue that the ability of a substance to restore play could be used to determine that a normal "satiety process" has been activated. Thus, not only should an agent reduce feeding; if it produces normal satiety it also should increase play. In our attempt to evaluate several agents in this way, we have found that opiate antagonists, which are quite effective in reducing eating, have no ability to increase play in hungry animals. Similar problems have been observed with CCK. However, some increase in play was observed following treatment with bombesin, another potential satiety peptide that is released into the circulation from the stomach following eating. More recently, I evaluated the ability of another new "satiety agent," named glucagon-like peptide-1 (GLP-1),[26] to reverse play inhibition caused by hunger; if anything this "satiety factor" reduced play even further, suggesting it was provoking anxiety rather than satiety.[27]

Much more work needs to be done on the many postulated "satiety agents." Until adequate work along these lines is conducted, we simply will not know whether the ability of specific agents to reduce feeding should be deemed important for clarifying the underlying physiological issues. For this reason, the exceedingly long list of substances that have been found to reduce short-term food intake will not be discussed in this chapter. There are many reasons to believe that short-term satiety processes and long-term regulatory processes, which surely interact, can also be distinguished in the brain.[28]

The Underlying Nature of Energy Regulation

We have already seen that feeding controls are subservient to the body's energy-regulating processes (Figure 9.2). To understand how animals maintain their body energy at stable levels, we must examine the nature of the specific nutrient detector systems that monitor bodily energy transactions, especially in the long term, and we must clarify their interconnections to behavioral control networks such as the SEEKING system (Figure 9.1). In other words, to fathom the underlying regulatory processes, we need to know as much about what food does to the animal's body as we know about what animals do to food.

To maintain a stable level of energy and hence stable body weight, animals must consume as much food as

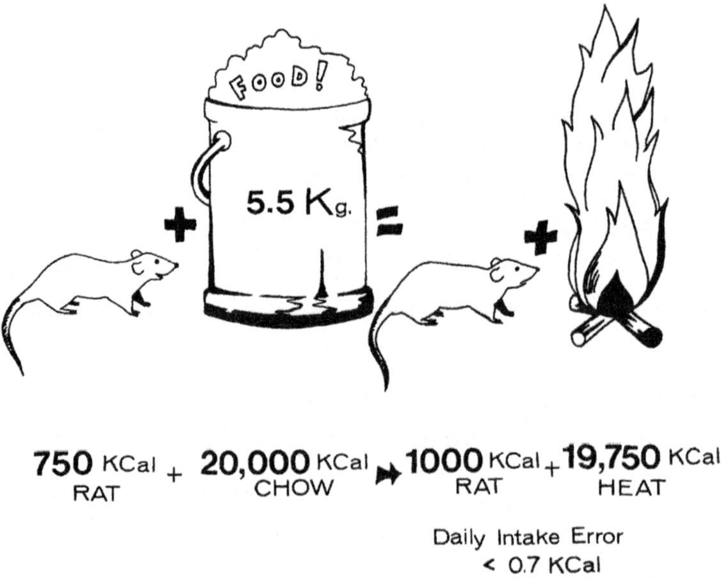

Figure 9.4. A female rat's approximate yearly energy balance equation. A great deal is eaten without much change in body weight. With the small increase in body weight, the daily intake error was less than a kilocalorie. The remaining energy was dissipated as heat, most of it in the conduct of essential metabolic transactions. (Adapted from Panksepp, 1978; see n. 32.)

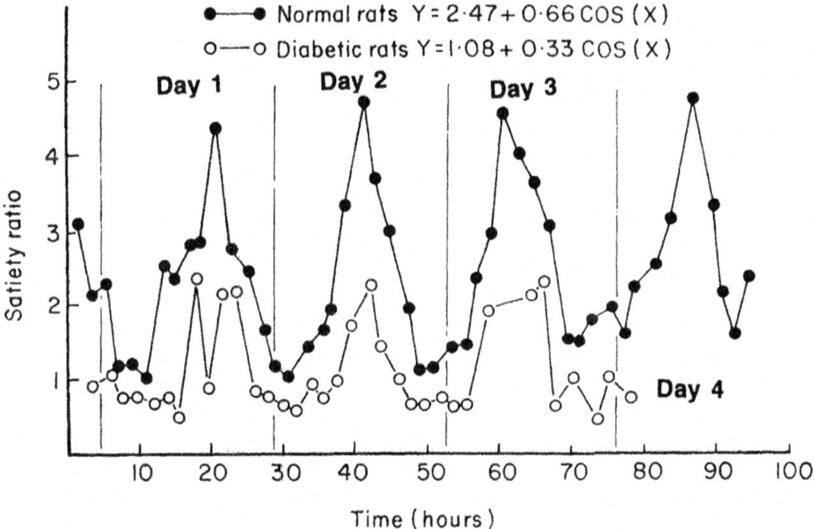

Figure 9.5. Average daily feeding cycle across three to four days in a group of 10 normal rats and 10 diabetic rats given free access to food. The satiety ratios (postmeal interval/meal size) reflect the duration of feeding inhibition for each unit of food eaten. The low points indicate where the animal is eating many meals that do not quell its appetite for a long period, while the peaks reflect periods during the day when the animal eats fewer meals and the meals are much more satiating. The equations reflect the best-fitting cosine function for these results. (Adapted from Panksepp, 1978; see n. 32.)

they dissipate in metabolic activity (Figure 9.4). In animals maintained under routine laboratory conditions, the daily difference or error in input and output is minuscule. This is also generally the case in most humans across long spans of time, even though inactivity and free access to many tasty foods promote instabilities in the regulatory system.[29]

Unlike energy utilization, depicted on the right side of the equation in Figure 9.4, the process of energy acquisition (i.e., meal taking) is discontinuous. Feeding is a periodic series of discrete events, and a great deal of effort has been devoted to analyzing the temporal structure of these events in the laboratory rat. One finding stands out: Animals can maintain stable body energy patterns through a variety of behavioral strategies.[30] Even under conditions where animals are allowed to eat a single large meal a day, they tend to maintain a weight only slightly below normal. Also, this is the type of regulation animals exhibit when they are given distasteful food or when they must expend a great deal of effort to get meals. In other words, when rats must work on very high fixed-ratio schedules (see the "Afterthought" of Chapter 1 for a description of schedules of reinforcement) to gain access to a feeding dish, they typically take infrequent, large meals. On less demanding schedules of reinforcement, they take smaller and much more frequent meals. Thus, under various economic conditions, animals regulate their energy balance equally well. However, the behavioral details differ,[31] indicating that regulation can be achieved through several distinct behavior patterns.

Overall, one of the strongest influences on the patterning of feeding when there is plenty to eat is the influence of circadian variables (see Chapter 7). Humans and animals alike eat quite differently at different times of day. A key to understanding the nature of energy regulation is that circadian differences are also evident in the way our bodies process food.

Meals and the intervals between them have different effects depending on the time of day. The satiating capacity of food and the hunger-inducing capacity of time without eating vary across the day.[32] Units of food are more satiating during the half day when animals normally sleep. Similarly, long intervals between meals are less likely to evoke hunger during those times of day (Figure 9.5). Conversely, during the half day or so when animals are typically active, food is relatively less satiating, and time without eating is more liable to provoke hunger. The overall result is that during half of the day, animals typically consume more energy than their bodies need, whereas during the other half, they eat less than they need. Of course, nocturnal animals such as rats and light-loving animals such as humans exhibit these phases at different times. The two distinct phases of the daily feeding cycle correspond to high energy storage (i.e., the *anabolic* phase when fat is deposited) and high energy utilization (the *catabolic* phase when lipids are extracted from stores) of the daily energy cycle.[33] This cycling is distally due to the internal 24-hour clock of the suprachiasmatic nucleus (see Chapter 7). It is proximally linked to the cyclic hormonal tides that control the dispersion of energy throughout the body (e.g., Figure 7.3).

The body's daily energy cycle is largely regulated by the pancreatic secretion of insulin,[34] the primary energy storage (anabolic) hormone. Insulin allows glucose to enter cells in most tissues, especially in adipose tissue. The brain is the only organ that extracts glucose from the bloodstream completely without assistance from insulin, except for the small groups of neurons at the base of the hypothalamus that regulate long-term energy balance. This insulin insensitivity allows animal brains to continue to function efficiently when energy resources are low so they can continue to seek food. Indeed, when animals are starved, their insulin levels drop to very low levels.

Insulin secretion normally occurs promptly at the outset of eating as a conditioned response to the taste of food; this is called the *cephalic phase* of insulin secretion.[35] This anticipatory surge of insulin reduces glucose output by the liver and allows increased absorption of blood glucose into muscles and adipose tissue. These rapid changes probably contribute to the "appetizer effect" that small units of tasty food exert when given just prior to a larger meal. It is known that in rats a small reduction of blood sugar begins to occur a few minutes before the initiation of meals, suggesting that such a reduction either triggers meal initation or is a conditioned "appetizer" response when animals begin to "think" about eating.[36]

After the meal is consumed, there is a larger surge of insulin secretion in the *metabolic phase*, which is proportional to the food consumed. This serves to distribute the incoming energy to long-term storage pools of adipose tissue.[37] There is no reason to believe that the energy deposited in these peripheral fat stores has any direct effect on the brain's feeding-control mechanisms, since surgical removal of body fat has relatively little effect on appetite.[38] However, as will be discussed later, molecules signaling satiety do appear to emanate from the fat. Fat stores may also affect feeding metabolically when the energy currency is slowly withdrawn during the course of each day. During the half day when these stores are being utilized, appetite remains low for long periods, and eating tends to be light and infrequent. One can easily imagine the weight problems that could emerge if the normal mechanisms that control this energy withdrawal process were compromised. If one stored energy effectively but could not retrieve the stores, one would get hungry easily, overeat, and soon become obese. Indeed, many feeding and body weight disorders arise because certain organisms tend to persist in the storage phase of their daily energy cycle. In short, the normal balancing of the daily energy account has gone awry in certain forms of obesity. Some of the problems arise from peripheral dysfunctions, while others, as we will see, reflect disorders in several brain mechanisms that monitor energy flow within the body.[39]

These issues cannot be overstated. To really understand the manner in which the brain regulates long-term energy balance, we will need to know as much about the details of energy metabolism, and correlated neurochemical events, as about feeding behavior. It will probably be in the area of long-term metabolic and regulatory feedback processes that truly effective medical maneuvers for the control of eating disorders will eventually be found. Indeed, results obtained in the last few years are true breakthroughs.

Recently it has been found that genetically obese rodents (i.e., *ob/ob* mice) lack certain fat-derived plasma proteins, called *leptins* (after the Greek *leptos* for "thin"), that are abundant in their lean counterparts. When leptins have been restored by injections, the obese mice begin to sustain normal body weight.[40] Although we do not yet understand what these proteins normally do within the metabolic system, the lure of profits has led biotech firms to spend fortunes to purchase the patent rights to develop and market such gene products as potential weight-control agents. Obviously, an effective medicine to control obesity will reap great profits, but it presently seems unlikely that much money will be made directly from leptin. There is no evidence that obese humans typically have a deficit of this protein.[41] As I will describe in detail later, some forms of human obesity may be due to a lack of the receptor for this peptide signal rather than to a deficit in the amount of leptin released from the adipose tissue.

Brain Mechanisms of Energy Balance Regulation

The promise of substantive biomedical help for long-term body-weight problems remains on the horizon. Most of the pertinent work has been conducted on the omnivorous laboratory rat, which, fortunately, appears to have an energy regulatory system closely resembling that of humans. Adult rats exhibit a remarkable ability to balance their body energy equation (Figure 9.4), and this is accomplished partly by metabolic changes on the output side of this equation. For instance, the regulation of energy output can be achieved by changes in muscular activity in addition to spontaneous changes in metabolism. However, a great deal is also accomplished on the input side, through changes in feeding behavior. Variations in nutrient absorption from the gastrointestinal tract do not appear to be a major factor in either input or output regulation, since all available metabolic energy is absorbed by a healthy digestive system. The fact that energy balance is typically sustained over time suggests that the brain is sensitive to the overall flow of energy, and modifying factors on one side of the equation are balanced by compensatory changes on the other side.

Although most investigators assume that an energy-regulatory mechanism exists somewhere in the hypothalamus, our knowledge about its precise nature remains incomplete. A key question that needed to be answered before one could actually study the regulatory mechanisms in the brain was: What is regulated? There have been many proposals concerning the major signals that may mediate the homeostatic control of feeding, including *glucostatic*, *aminostatic*, *lipostatic*, and *thermostatic* theories of regulation. These perspectives viewed blood sugar, blood amino acids, some aspect of adipose tissue metabolism, or the overall ability of the body to maintain a consistent temperature to be the regulated variables.[42]

Although all of these factors surely participate in feeding control, the common denominator for long-term regulation appears to be the overall ability of the body to sustain energy metabolism. Hence an *energostatic* theory has been proposed by several investigators as the "center of gravity" around which feeding behavior and bodily energy balance are regulated.[43] The basic evidence for this theory is that animals adjust their daily food intake quite well when a proportion of their daily energy need is administered directly into their stomach, regardless of the energy source. If animals are given a sufficient amount of time to adjust, the compensation is quite precise and comparable for all the major macronutrients—fats, proteins, and carbohydrates (Figure 9.2). However, this does not really tell us much about the exact mechanisms by which the regulation is achieved.

In general, how might the brain's energy balancing mechanism work? Conceptually there are two possibilities: (1) that the brain merely senses circulating nutrients or correlated substances in the blood and adjusts feeding accordingly, and (2) that the brain itself sustains an ongoing energy-dependent integrative process that parallels bodily processes and adjusts feeding in response to its own local energy transaction mechanisms or highly correlated processes. It presently seems likely that both types of mechanisms are operative, and it seems clear that the key to overall body-energy balance resides in some type of longer-term regulatory process that operates throughout the day rather than among the short-term signals that arise from individual meals. Two intriguing findings highlight the need for a clear distinction between short-term feeding control and long-term energy-regulatory factors.

First, many years ago investigators joined two rats together in parabiotic union ("Siamese twins," who shared each other's blood circulation via a surgically produced skin-flap connection).[44] Each of these normal animals gradually ate less, and eventually each contained only half the body fat that a normal rat contains. This peculiar result suggests that each animal's brain was perceiving their joined metabolic dynamic as if two bodies constituted a single fat mass (Figure 9.6). This suggests that the circulating metabolic signals were integrated as if each animal was contributing one half of a critical signal to the other's brain. The critical area of the brain that probably receives this signal is the ventromedial hypothalamus (VMH). VMH lesions have long been known to produce overeating and eventual obesity, and when a VMH-lesioned animal was joined to a normal nonlesioned partner, the results were striking. The VMH-lesioned animals were not affected by the signal emerging from the neurologically normal "Siamese twins." On the other hand, the normal partners detected too much of a repletion signal from the VMH-lesioned animals. While the VMH-lesioned animals still overate and became obese, their partners lost their appetite completely and became emaciated.

We still do not know exactly what the fat-repletion signal is in this situation, although it might arise from the leptin protein mentioned earlier, since normal animals parabiosed to an *ob/ob* animal also lose weight. However, such weight patterns may also reflect metabolic energy from the excessive eating of the VMH animal as it is monitored by the long-term energy integrator in the VMH of the normal animal. In other words, if the brain's integrative systems sense more meals coming into the body than are actually consumed, feeding behavior may be reduced.

The second finding was related to the long-standing assumption that the VMH senses some type of "satiety signal" that normally terminates bouts of feeding (Figure 9.7). This part of the brain clearly contains glucoreceptive neurons, but, surprisingly, direct administration of glucose into this brain area does not reduce the size of subsequent meals. Animals without this brain area fail to exhibit normal responsivity to food deprivation. These paradoxes led to a simple modification of the notion of a "satiety center": The VMH does not elaborate a short-term satiety signal but rather a longer-term signal of body-energy integration.[45] Accordingly, the prediction would be that direct administration of glucose into this brain area would reduce daily food intake, but not necessarily the size of the meal that followed. In fact, this is the case,[46] and many of the paradoxes in our knowledge of brain feeding control systems were resolved by this shift of theoretical perspective. Of course, such facts concerning regulatory signals form only a small, albeit central, part of the feeding story.

Considering the essential role of energy intake in sustaining survival and reproductive fitness, it is not surprising that feeding-control systems are located in several areas in the brain, from frontal cortical and temporal areas that register the value of specific foods to brain stem levels that govern chewing, swallowing, and simple gustatory acceptance.[47] However, the most important findings in the field have been made at the hypothalamic level (Figure 9.7). Damage to the LH was found to produce severe feeding deficits, and for a while that area of the brain was thought to contain a "feeding

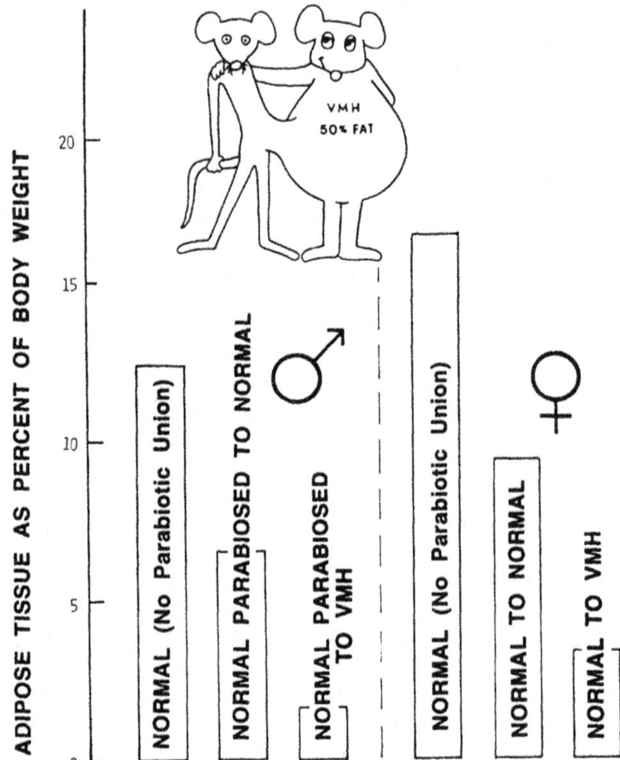

Figure 9.6. Changes in body fat content as a function of parabiotic union of two normal rats, as well as that between normal rats and those with ventromedial hypothalamic lesions that cause obesity. (Adapted from Panksepp, 1975; see n. 44.)

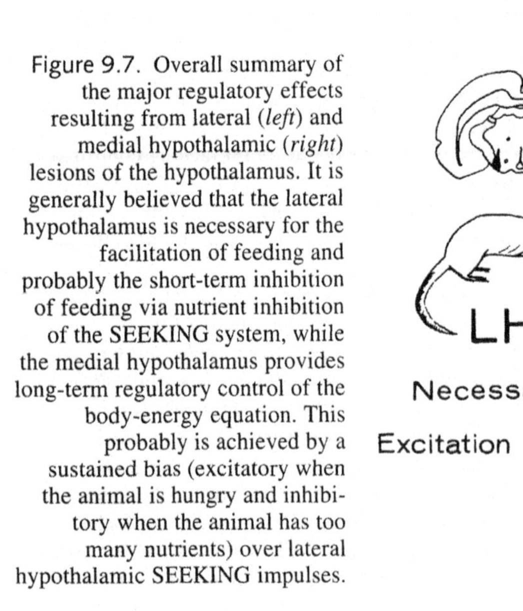

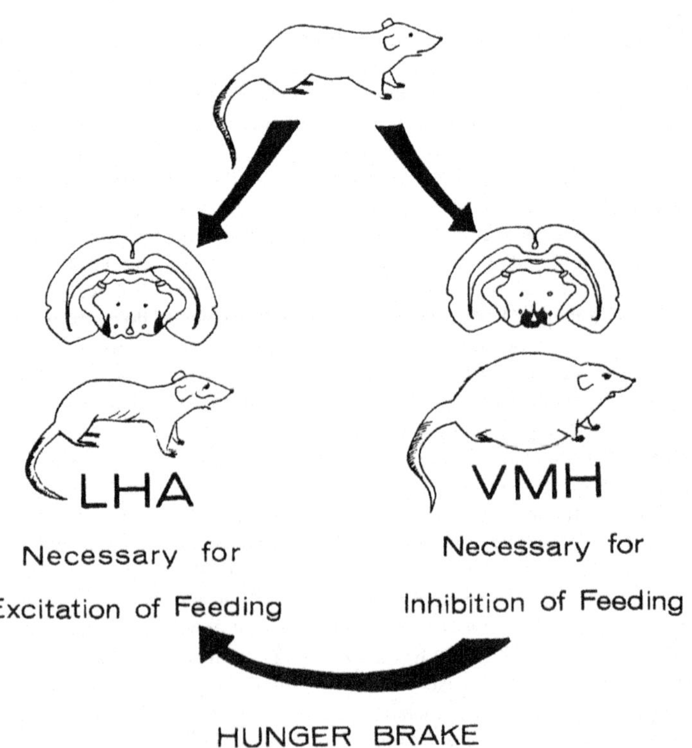

Figure 9.7. Overall summary of the major regulatory effects resulting from lateral (*left*) and medial hypothalamic (*right*) lesions of the hypothalamus. It is generally believed that the lateral hypothalamus is necessary for the facilitation of feeding and probably the short-term inhibition of feeding via nutrient inhibition of the SEEKING system, while the medial hypothalamus provides long-term regulatory control of the body-energy equation. This probably is achieved by a sustained bias (excitatory when the animal is hungry and inhibitory when the animal has too many nutrients) over lateral hypothalamic SEEKING impulses.

system." In fact, as we have already seen, the circuits of the LH elaborate seeking strategies, which require a great deal of sensory and motor integration. Many of these psychobehavioral routines are governed by interactions with the basal ganglia, especially ventral striatal areas such as the nucleus accumbens, as well as ventromedial zones of the caudate nucleus (i.e., of the dorsal striatum). With massive lesions in the LH, animals are essentially parkinsonian and have difficulty doing anything. They typically have an abnormally high metabolic rate and proceed on a downhill course toward death unless they are given extended nursing care.[48]

With smaller LH lesions, animals gradually recover, but they always remain sluggish in both regulatory and behavioral situations that require them to respond to metabolic and environmental stressors.[49] With quite small lesions, the behavioral deficits are minimal, and the animals simply sustain a lower than normal body weight. This lower level of body weight continues to be actively defended, so enforced weight reductions lead to increased feeding and experimentally induced weight increases lead to appetite reduction. Accordingly, some have suggested that the LH contains a body-weight set-point mechanism.[50] This conclusion remains controversial, since merely giving a rat a relatively unpalatable diet has the same effect. Obviously, it would be incorrect to suggest that a palatability manipulation can modify a physiological set-point mechanism. Since the LH probably contains not only SEEKING circuits but also ones that contribute to the pleasure of eating,[51] it remains possible that LH lesions may simply be making the available food less palatable or attractive. Such deficits, in addition to impairments of sensory-motor and foraging abilities, seem to be sufficient to explain the feeding deficits of these animals with no involvement of a long-term energy regulatory mechanism.

There is substantial evidence that the VMH actually contains the metabolic information integrators of the long-term energy balance system, even though the function of this area was originally misconceptualized as a meal-terminating "satiety center." Early investigators thought that the VMH harvested incoming information by which individual meals were brought to an end. In fact, short-term satiety stimuli may operate directly on the LH SEEKING system to inhibit foraging activities.[52] The medial hypothalamus, rather than containing a short-term satiety mechanism, appears to contain a long-term metabolic detector by which overall energy balance is regulated. In short, it is not a lack of sensitivity to *short-term* internal factors that causes VMH-lesioned animals to overeat. Their gluttony reflects the fact that they are perpetually stuck in the lipogenic phase of the daily energy regulatory cycle (i.e., the phase of the day when they eat more than their bodies need) and hence they become imprecise regulators because they cannot accurately detect body energy repletion or depletion. Their failure to detect hunger is indicated by reduced motivation when they have to work for their food, the fact that they only become obese when given reasonably palatable foods, and their willingness to exhibit severe anorexia if given unpalatable diets. In general, they still appear able to integrate short-term signals that normally terminate meals.[53]

Metabolically, VMH-lesioned rats remain permanently in the nighttime, lipogenic phase of their energy dispersion cycle. Is this due simply to changes in bodily metabolic control mechanisms or to their brain's inability to sense their *long-term* internal energy stores? Both mechanisms probably are impaired. VMH-lesioned animals do oversecrete insulin, which automatically leads to increased storage of body fat in peripheral adipose depots (after all, insulin injections are the most effective way to induce obesity in normal animals),[54] and they may also overeat because their brain can no longer gauge the metabolic output of those energy stores. In any event, there is compelling evidence that the integrated signal of body energy depletion and repletion enters the brain via the medial hypothalamic gateway. However, the exact location and anatomical dispersion of the mechanisms may be more extensive than originally envisioned, extending to dorsomedial zones of the anterior hypothalamus such as the paraventricular nucleus, since lesions there can also elevate food intake.[55]

Behavioral evidence suggests that detectors along this neural corridor to the pituitary gland detect an animal's overall energy storage status. In other words, this system integrates daily energy flow and provides a signal of body energy depletion and repletion to the nearby SEEKING system of the LH. It monitors longer-term deviations from optimal body energy conditions rather than the short-term signals that terminate meals. In order to understand the puzzle of overall energy balance regulation, we have to understand the metabolic and neurochemical properties of these medial hypothalamic cells. Parenthetically, it is noteworthy that the brain location of this long-term energy regulatory mechanism is very appropriate. It sits astride the pituitary stalk, in an ideal position to orchestrate the many hormonal changes that control body energy transactions (including the control of thyroxine, growth hormone, and cortisol secretion).

We will find that this same area of the brain also controls female sexual receptivity (see Chapter 12), and it is important to note that reproduction is generally reduced by starvation conditions (it is not wise to have children when food is scarce!). The onset of female puberty is also triggered to some extent by weight (if one has abundant food, one should begin to reproduce earlier), which indicates how closely energy detectors and female sexual receptivity systems are coupled in the brain.

Being situated just adjacent to the SEEKING system in the LH, the VMH is in an ideal position to regulate appetitive eagerness. How, then, is this achieved?

It is due in part to the ability of cells to detect peripheral adipose tissue metabolism through signals such as those provided by the leptin peptide discussed earlier,[56] but part of the job is probably achieved metabolically. Let us first consider recent evidence suggesting that special signaling molecules from adipose tissue influence the long-term regulatory mechanisms of the VMH. I will then discuss the less well appreciated possibility that the VMH may *directly* integrate long-term metabolic information.

Direct Long-Term Signals from the Adipose Tissue

In addition to metabolic information, it now seems likely that the VMH also detects the status of peripheral energy stores directly through information molecules such as leptin. Animals that do not properly manufacture this protein, such as the genetically mutant *ob/ob* mice, become grossly obese.[57] However, other genetic variants, such as the *db/db* mouse and *Fatty* rat, which also become obese, appear to be missing the hypothalamic receptor for this protein. If a similar deficit occurs in many human obesities, it is unlikely that administration of leptin will be of much help in controlling excess body weight, and presently it is hard to genetically restore leptin receptors to individuals who do not express them normally.

It is evident that the *db/db* type of deficit prevails over the *ob/ob* deficit. Parabiotic union of *db/db* mice with normal controls as well as *ob/ob* mice has yielded clear results (Figure 9.8). Both normals and *ob/ob* animals lose weight as a result of this union. There is a clear asymmetry in the effect of the two animals when the two types of obese mice are joined. The *ob/ob* animal is affected much more by the *db/db* animal than vice versa, presumably because the *db/db* animals are restoring a substantial amount of the leptin protein that the *ob/ob* animal is missing.[58] However, from the perspective that this is the only signaling pathway for body fat control, the reduction of weight by the *db/db* animals is perplexing because they are presumably simply missing the leptin receptor. The fact that their weight is still affected by being connected to *ob/ob* animals suggests an alternate control factor, such as the local metabolic pathways in the VMH discussed in the next section. Indeed, there are already several manipulations that paradoxically reduce circulating leptin level and reduce food intake,[59] and others that increase leptin levels and increase food intake.[60]

In addition to the newly discovered leptin system, several less well understood body-weight information systems in the hypothalamus may eventually provide

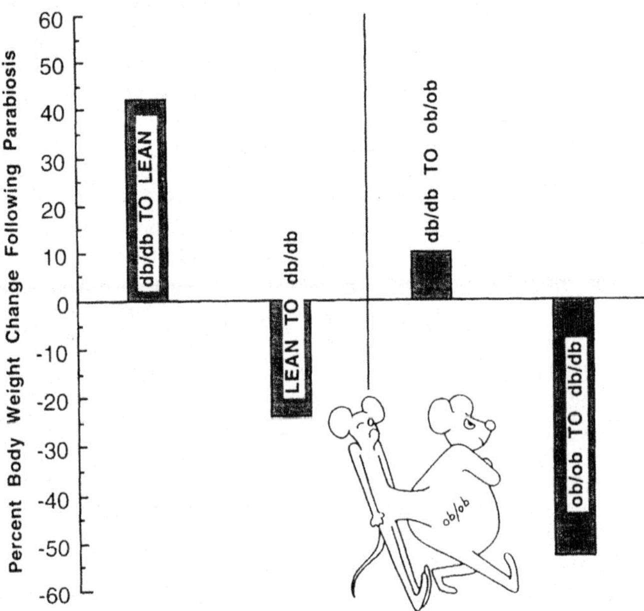

Figure 9.8. Body weight changes of different types of genetically obese mice (*db/db* and *ob/ob*) parabiosed to each other as well as lean controls. (Adapted from Panksepp, 1975; see n. 44.)

additional ways to control body weight. A variety of endogenous molecules, most of them neuropeptides, have now been found that can dramatically reduce appetite and body weight in normal animals. Among the most exciting recently discovered ones are items such as GLP-1, fibroblast growth factor, and urocortin.[61] Of course, as already discussed, it will be critical to determine which of these is actually producing a normal type of satiety as opposed to illness or some other emotional effect. Good control experiments of the type described earlier remain to be done, and they will be needed to resolve such issues.

It should also be remembered that most of these molecules, which are fairly large peptides, do not cross the blood-brain barrier readily. Chemists would have to develop new variants of regulatory molecules that could get into the right areas of the brain before we could ever use them as magic bullets to curb appetite. Also, in the regulation of bodily functions such as energy balance, everything is multiply determined. Thus, it may be essential to use several strategies concurrently, including ones that take advantage of metabolic mechanisms to help balance the body's energy equation. Recent work with mutant mice, where one enzyme that is important for fat metabolism has been changed, leads to chronic leanness, even when animals are challenged with high-fat diets.[62] Clearly, better ways to control metabolic information transactions may be essential for long-term control of appetite and body-weight problems.

What Type of Metabolic Information Does the VMH Integrate?

The VMH has metabolic properties that distinguish it from the rest of the brain. For instance, as mentioned, it contains cells that are insulin-sensitive. Thus, it is likely that the VMH elaborates a long-term signal of body energy status partly via the local storage of nutrients. Local VMH energy stores may help generate a neural signal that dampens feeding during repletion states and facilitates food seeking during depletion states. For instance, local oxygen consumption of this brain area is more responsive to starvation than are other brain areas, and the VMH also retains radioactivity for a longer time following isotopically labeled glucose loads than do other brain areas. These VMH nutrient stores may reflect an energy integration process that provides a long-term metabolic signal by which feeding behavior is regulated. This local energy storage mechanism is probably insulin-sensitive (unlike the rest of the brain, which requires no insulin for glucose utilization). Local glucose infusions into the VMH can decrease daily food intake without having any discernible effect on the size of the meal that immediately follows. In other words, the infusions have small cumulative effects across many meals, and with continuous, around-the-clock infusion, the effect is sustained for many days. The selective retention of nutrients in the medial hypothalamus is partly due to a selective increase in lipid pools; the degree of retention is related to the feeding behavior of the animal—the more energy that is retained, the larger the suppression in feeding. If retention is selectively diminished, feeding is increased.[63] More recently it has been observed that nearby regions of the brain behave in a manner similar to the liver,[64] which is an intermediate-duration energy storage depot of the body. This suggests that several distinct types of energy storage processes may be reflected within hypothalamic subareas.

The selective insulin sensitivity of the VMH can help explain various paradoxical feeding effects that have been observed in the past. Although peripherally administered insulin can dramatically increase food intake (because it diverts nutrients to body fat stores), when this hormone is administered directly into the brain, feeding is reduced.[65] This may be explained by direct receptor-mediated effects or the tendency of central insulin to increase brain energy storage. The metabolic insulin sensitivity of the VMH may also explain why it is more sensitive to the neurotoxic effects of gold-thio-glucose (GTG), a man-made research molecule that can selectively destroy the VMH, and thereby produce overeating and obesity.[66] Although the whole brain takes up this molecule, selective VMH damage may well arise from local weakness in the blood-brain barrier and from insulin sensitivity that allows GTG to selectively accumulate to neurotoxic levels.

VMH Metabolism and the Neurochemical Control of Feeding

How is metabolic information from the VMH interfaced with feeding control circuits? The most obvious way would be for neuroactive information to be extracted directly from intracellular metabolic processes of the VMH. The major metabolic cycle of the body that extracts energy from food is the Krebs, or tricarboxylic acid, cycle. It is noteworthy that several neuroactive amino acids are produced via the metabolic reactions of this cycle; one of them, gamma-aminobutyric acid (GABA), is unique to the brain. In many neurons, the Krebs cycle has a "GABA shunt" whereby this major inhibitory transmitter is constructed as a by-product of energy production. This provides a very attractive way for brain energy stores to be interfaced with a modulation of neural activity in foraging circuits.

Several laboratories have now tested this proposition, and it seems to be a promising approach for controlling feeding. Various manipulations that increase GABA levels strongly inhibit feeding, especially when administered to the specific areas of the VMH where glucose can also reduce feeding. Conversely, manipulations that reduce the influence of GABA in this area can increase feeding.[67] Perhaps the most powerful manipulations are GABA-transaminase inhibitors such as amino-oxyacetic acid and ethanolamine-O-sulfate (EOS), both of which increase GABA by preventing its breakdown. By administering such GABA-breakdown inhibitors into the ventricular system of the rat, one can inhibit feeding to the point where the animal will starve itself to death (Figure 9.9).[68] It is unlikely that GABA exerts its effect just on the VMH. Rather, it could provide control over arousal tendencies that accompany hunger throughout the brain. These may be relatively short-term influences, compared with the regulatory signal that emanates from the VMH. In this scheme, one metabolite of GABA, gamma-hydroxybutyrate, is a powerful inhibitor of dopamine neuron firing, providing yet another avenue for controlling foraging tendencies. There are bound to be others.

In sum, there is a great deal of evidence that at least part of energy regulation is affected by local metabolic mechanisms within the VMH itself. Although the details remain to be worked out, it seems that specialized medial hypothalamic cells (perhaps the same ones that contain leptin receptors) can integrate the flow of metabolic energy that has passed its insulin-sensitive gates. This flow of energy may be translated into various neuroactive signals, especially through a variety of amino acids that arise from the Krebs cycle, especially the GABA shunt.

So which signaling routes are most deficient in human body-weight regulation problems? We have already noted that peripheral leptins that provide regulatory feedback concerning the status of adipose tissue stores seem to be normal in human obesities. Very recent work also suggests that most human obesities may not be due to deficits in leptin receptors, since recent work indicates that the brains of seven lean individuals, who weighed 151 pounds on average, did not differ from those of eight obese individuals, who weighed 264 pounds on average.[69] It remains possible that the main deficit is in the signaling pathways that convey information within the brain *following* leptin's interactions with its receptors.

On the Multiplicity of Feeding Controls

Although the preceding description leaves out many details of the puzzle, it represents a general view of how overall body energy regulation is achieved. However, we should recognize how much work is left to be done before we truly understand the multiplicity of brain systems that contribute to regulation. The number of relevant variables is vast. Important controls that have not been emphasized here are amino acids and brain biogenic amines. Placement of many amino acids di-

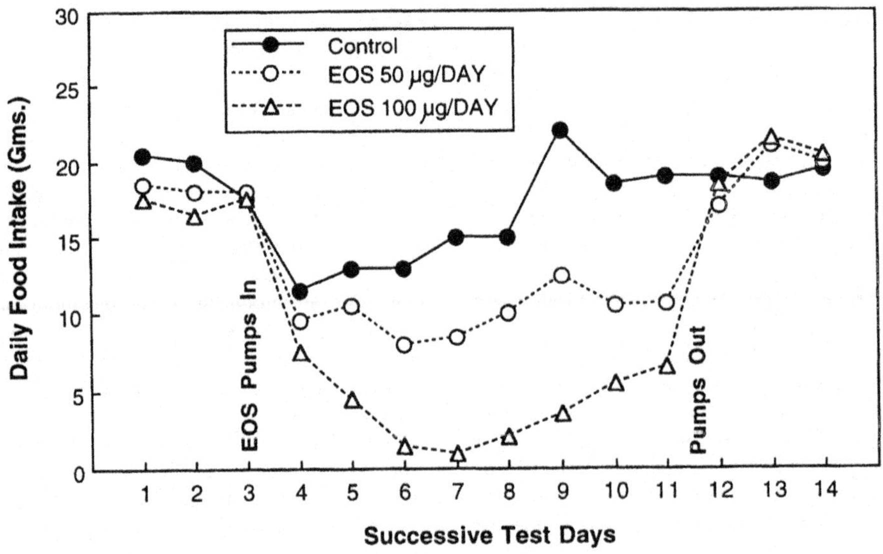

Figure 9.9. Daily food intake of animals infused with two doses of ethanolamine-O-sulfate, an inhibitor of GABA breakdown, into the third ventricle region of the medial hypothalamus. The inhibition of feeding was dramatic and dose-dependent. (Results according to unpublished data, Panksepp & Bishop, 1980.). At twice the higher dose (data not shown), animals stopped eating completely, and most starved themselves to death during the infusion.

rectly into the hypothalamus can reduce food intake. Likewise, facilitation of brain serotonin activity and depletion of norepinephrine activity decrease feeding. Also, various neuropeptides reduce feeding, including cholecystokinin, oxytocin, corticotrophin releasing factor, and bombesin.[70] Some of these probably do so because they participate in the normal brain control of feeding, while others do so because of other emotional or motivational effects. We simply do not yet have good answers to such questions.

Also, we have not focused on the several neurochemical systems that can increase feeding, including increases in brain opioid and benzodiazepine activities.[71] Among the most powerful is neuropeptide Y (NPY), which can dramatically increase feeding, to the point of inducing obesity with repeated injections.[72] Indeed, bulimic humans have been found to have excess levels of NPY circulating in their cerebrospinal fluid.[73] Likewise, dynorphins can increase feeding,[74] and recently it has been found that galanin can selectively increase fat appetite.[75] Development of pharmacological agents to reduce the arousal of these systems has the potential to provide new medications for the control of appetite. For instance, it might be expected that an NPY antagonist would be an excellent appetite-control agent, although this is contradicted by the recent development of a "knockout" mouse missing NPY, which seems to exhibit normal appetite and energy balance regulation.[76] Still NPY remains a top candidate to be a major hunger neuromodulator of the brain.

All these factors, and many more, deserve attention in our attempt to understand the controls that can modify feeding. These lines of research, most conducted on laboratory rodents, have direct relevance for understanding energy regulatory systems in humans. Although the energy regulatory systems of the brain are ultracomplex, they are probably remarkably similar in all omnivorous mammals. Once new orally effective drugs are developed that can interact with the receptors for these neuropeptide systems, we should have some truly powerful medicines to control appetite in clinical disorders characterized by body energy imbalances. Eventually we may also be able to directly control the energy dynamics of the VMH in useful ways.

In addition to the intrinsic elements of the homeostatic systems of the body, learning has a major role in maintaining regulation of bodily states. Many items, such as individual vitamins, are needed for health, but the body does not have separate detectors for them. Rather, when animals are missing certain micronutrients, they feel unwell; when they encounter foods that restore those needed items, they feel healthier. Apparently animals are able to utilize restoration of health as a signal for the types of dietary choices they should make.[77]

The many feelings that accompany energy balance regulation and the other homeostatic systems of the brain are not yet widely recognized by scientists. However, it remains likely that bodily constancies are behaviorally sustained, at least in part, through the ability of specific brain systems to create feelings—various forms of regulatory distress when systems are out of balance, and various forms of satisfaction when systems are returning to balance. Most of these feelings will be difficult to decode using animal models because there are no clear external indicators of an animal's feelings, except for a few measures such as the facial taste responsivity patterns of rats. Although scientists have been loathe to accept the possibility that certain regulatory urges are mediated by internal feeling states, the probability seems high that such states do participate in body weight regulation. By working out the biochemical details of the regulatory underpinnings in the animal brain, we may eventually develop enough knowledge about the working of these systems to provide clues about the more subtle neurodynamics that, at present, can be evaluated only through the subjective verbal reports of humans.[78] We will not reach a complete understanding of the underlying brain processes until we consider the varieties of motivational- and taste-induced feelings that can be generated in the brain. Let us now tackle this most difficult issue.

The Pleasures of Regulatory Systems

Many primitive feeling states are associated with feeding and other consummatory behaviors, but since such feelings cannot be directly measured, most remain to be addressed by modern brain research. By comparison, the measurement of consummatory behaviors is uncontroversial, and most investigators have been satisfied to simply monitor these behaviors without indulging in any speculations concerning the accompanying affective states. Like the smile of the Cheshire cat, we can only glimpse feelings indirectly, for they are not tangible entities, and neuroscientists are prone to ignore neurodynamic processes that must be inferred. Of course, physics would be in a sorry state if physicists had ignored the internal dynamics of atoms. Although it is understandable why neuroscientists might be prone to ignore feelings, it is remarkable that psychologists and emotion researchers have also tended to ignore the feelings associated with regulatory behavior patterns.

The brain's ability to generate a variety of subjective feelings during homeostatic imbalances may be nature's way of providing a simple general-purpose coding device for discriminating the relevance of both external objects and internal states, thereby providing a powerful intrinsic motivational mechanism for guiding behavioral choices. It is generally accepted that pleasurable taste probably indicates that a foodstuff is likely to contain nutritionally useful materials, while bitter or disgusting taste indicates that a foodstuff may contain harmful poisons or be unwholesome.

Indeed, one can readily predict the affective consequences of various external stimuli in humans from a knowledge of bodily imbalances. It has been experimentally affirmed that pleasant and unpleasant feelings provoked by external stimuli arise from their ability to predict the alleviation of bodily imbalances. Stimuli that promote a return to homeostasis are routinely experienced as pleasurable, while those that would impair homeostasis are unpleasant or even distressing. Thus one and the same stimulus can be pleasurable under certain circumstances while being unpleasant under others.[79] For instance, if one is moderately thirsty, the first few gulps of water are more pleasant than the last. If one is cold, a hot temperature that might be deemed unbearable on a warm day is considered pleasant.

Such findings also allow us to rigorously define "pleasure." For science, it does not suffice to say that pleasure is something "that feels good," for such circular word juggling cannot lead us to a new understanding of a phenomenon. A general scientific definition of the ineffable concept we call pleasure can start with the supposition that pleasure indicates something is biologically *useful*. This takes us in the right direction, for we can provide a credible description of what it means for something to be biologically useful. Useful stimuli are those that inform the brain of their potential to restore the body toward homeostatic equilibrium when it has deviated from its biologically dictated "set-point" level. Indeed, this has turned out to be a powerful concept. The same temperature can be pleasant or unpleasant depending on whether we are warmer or colder than our ideal temperature of 37°C. The same goes for body energy and water balance, and perhaps the levels of micronutrients such as sodium. In short, since we must interact with the world on a periodic basis to sustain bodily equilibrium, we have brain mechanisms to generate various forms of distress (hunger pangs, thirst, coldness, etc.) when body resources deviate from equilibrium, and we feel pleasure and relief when we undertake acts that alleviate disequilibrium. Clearly, affective processes cannot be ignored if we wish to understand how bodily constancies are regulated by the brain.

Thus, in addition to focusing on food intake, we can probably evaluate regulatory pressures in the brain by looking at how animals respond to various pleasant stimuli. Rats appear to exhibit pleasure-related adjustments in their gustatory choices depending on the homeostatic consequences of their behaviors. For instance, if one gives rats free access to two bottles of sugar water, one much more concentrated and sweet than the other, they will initially consume much more of the sweeter source.[80] Across days, however, the animal will gradually forsake its initial preference and will drink more and more of the dilute source (Figure 9.10), almost as if the organism's natural hedonism gives way to an attitude of compromise. The sweeter substance simply provides too many calories too rapidly. In order to maximize pleasure, animals learn to exhibit behavior patterns that balance their intrinsic desire for sweets with the metabolic consequences of excessive indulgence. Further, the rate at which animals make such adjustments is dependent on their metabolic states (Figure 9.10).[81]

Genetically obese animals, as well as those induced to become obese with hypothalamic lesions or chronic insulin treatment, do not show such shifts. However, experimental diabetic animals that have very high resting blood glucose levels, and those recovering from induced obesity, shift to the dilute sugar source more rapidly than normal animals. Thus, the speed of this shift in gustatory preference is dependent on the energy regulatory status of the animal. It is unlikely that these are deliberate choices. Rather, they are probably related to changes in the animal's affective pleasure experiences. In sum, pleasure is not simply a response to a specific environmental event but one that is guided by the internal status of relevant physiological systems. We are finally beginning to understand the nature of these homeostatic systems and the pleasure responses they evoke within the brain. A sweet taste that is deemed to be pleasant when one is hungry is not as pleasant if one has already eaten more than one's fill. The same goes for sex and other forms of bodily touch (see Chapters 12 and 13). All these experiments point to one overwhelming conclusion: Pleasure is nature's way of telling the brain that it is experiencing stimuli that are useful—events that support the organism's survival by helping to rectify biological imbalances.

There are other regulated systems within the body, many of which do not require immediate interaction with the outside world. When they are out of kilter, we tend to feel ill, a neurochemical response that is partly mediated by the neural effects of immune system chemicals called *cytokines* such as the interleukins (as mentioned in the "Afterthought" of Chapter 3). Thus, rather than generating pleasure and displeasure, other internal regulatory systems can generate affective consequences that are commonly labeled as feelings of sickness or well-being. We do not yet understand the neural circuits that mediate these reactions. Indeed, they may arise from quite diffuse effects on the brain. However, conditioned taste aversions—for example, those induced by illness—are known to be mediated in part by specific areas of the brain that have weaknesses in the blood-brain barrier, such as the *area postrema* in the brain stem just below the cerebellum, as well as the medial zones of the temporal lobes.[82]

Although the issue of using animal models to investigate feelings remains controversial, we should remember that states of pleasure and displeasure are no more difficult to study in animals than in young babies, as long as we are willing to trust certain behavioral indicator variables (e.g., Figure 2.3). Even newborn babies react distinctly to the four intrinsic gustatory qualities. They pucker their lips and squint their eyes in response to sour flavors. They exhibit a concerned look and pull away from the taste of salt. They express an open-

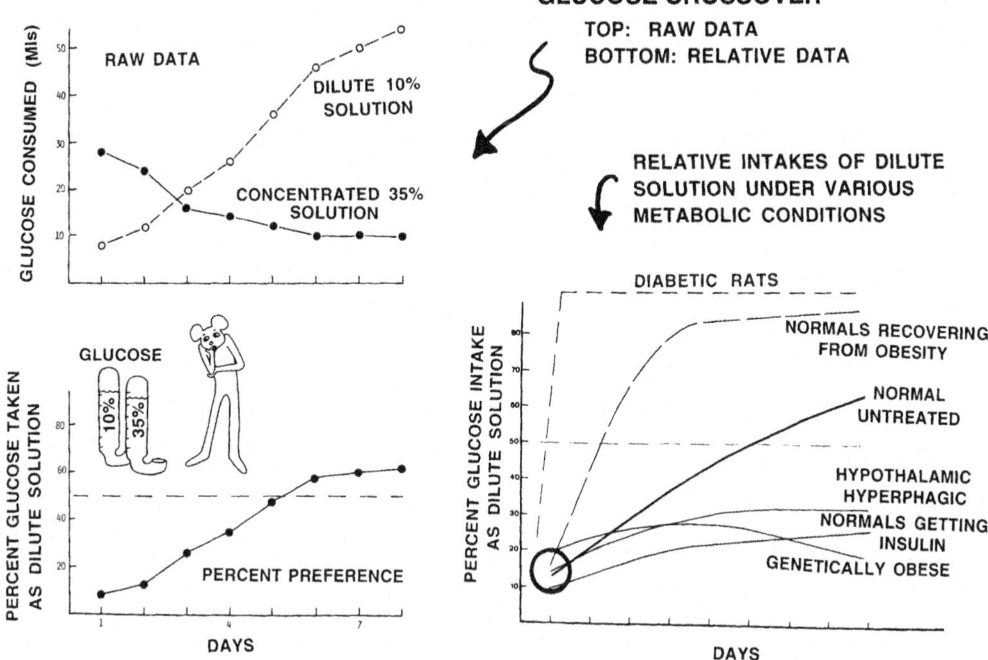

Figure 9.10. Summary of the patterns of sugar water consumption in animals given continuous daily access to two solutions of different concentrations. Animals initially take most of their sugar from the concentrated solution but gradually shift over to the less sweet dilute source. The right-hand graph summarizes the glucose crossover patterns of various animals having different regulatory problems. (Adapted from Panksepp & Meeker, 1977; see n. 81.)

mouthed, revulsive disgust, furrowed brow, and lateral head shaking to bitterness. And they exhibit a relaxed savoring and lip-smacking response to sweetness. All these behavioral responses are distinct and clear, and comparable measures have been developed in animals. For instance, rats "lick their chops" in response to sweet solutions; in response to a bitter taste, they shake their heads laterally (in a "no"-type gesture) and wipe their chins on the floor.[83]

Such affective responses are subcortically organized, and they are presently being used to analyze the neurochemical basis of gustatory pleasure. It is already clear that brain opioids and benzodiazepine systems are important for generating these affective states.[84] As mentioned in the previous chapter, the facial pleasure response of rats is not intensified by "rewarding" lateral hypothalamic stimulation. This implies that so-called brain reward does not resemble gustatory pleasure, even though it is clear that gustatory inputs are important for governing the arousal of the SEEKING system.[85] In addition to using taste preference tests and reflexive facial action responses to monitor affect, we can also utilize a variety of choice tasks to infer the internal affective states of animals. For instance, animals consistently seek locations in their environments where they have previously found palatable food.[86]

The preceding examples, simple as they may be, highlight a profound principle of brain organization. Although people use many different adjectives to describe the states of satisfaction they experience, most of our feelings of sensory pleasure arise from the various stimuli that signal the return of bodily imbalances toward an optimal level of functioning. This type of analysis suggests that an understanding of subjective experience may be an especially important key to the deep neural nature of many homeostatic functions. Feeling states may have been a neurosymbolic way for the brain to encode, in relatively simple fashion, intrinsic values for the various behavioral options that are open to an organism in a specific situation. Those that help reestablish homeostasis are experienced as good, while those that do not are felt to be either neutral or bad, depending on whether they have no effect on homeostasis or actually increase homeostatic disequilibrium.

It is more reasonable to assume that sensory pleasure is an ancient brain coding system for some of the most crucial biological values that all mammals share rather than to believe it is unique to humans, or even to assume, as did the behaviorists, that pleasure is a figment of the human imagination. We will need to understand the pleasurable nature of certain tastes and the distressful nature of hunger to fully grasp the overall pattern of energy regulatory processes in the brain. Once the neural basis of such processes has been credibly characterized in animals, the knowledge will probably also apply to humans. At present, we do not know where gustatory pleasure is mediated in the brain. It could take place in higher brain areas such as the septal area, where other pleasures (e.g., sexual) are elaborated; in the amygdala, where certain conditioned taste aversions are generated; or even the taste input areas of the brain stem.[87] As with other emotional functions, the processes are probably widely distributed throughout the brain.

At present, we do not even know whether there are several distinct pleasure systems in the brain or whether the affective differences we experience under different motivational conditions are simply due to the distinct sensory correlates that accompany different consummatory behaviors. Perhaps many stimuli can converge on a single pleasure system. Just as the SEEKING system can control many types of behaviors, a single pleasure system may provide affective import for many different gustatory sensations. In other words, the large number of sensations we can discriminate may delude us into believing that there is a greater variety of pleasant gustatory feelings than can be distinguished on a neurological basis. Of course, there may be distinct pleasure circuits for food, warmth, and sex. However, they may still arise from similar neurochemical effects, perhaps opioid actions, in slightly different parts of the brain.

On the Neurochemistry of Pleasure

What are the neurochemical messages that weave together the magical experience of pleasure? Many believe pleasure ultimately reflects the action of opioid systems in the brain; others believe that dopamine systems are at the heart of the experience.[88] There are bound to be many neurochemical surprises, especially among the neuropeptide systems that are just beginning to be studied in earnest. However, if one contrasts data on the opioid and dopamine systems, it is clear that a role for opioid components presently has the most empirical support.[89]

The evidence for brain opioid participation in the elaboration of consummatory pleasure is quite compelling. Animals that are given nonnutritive sweet solutions such as saccharin initially consume a great amount but gradually diminish their intake if they also do not have access to nutritive food. This suggests that the pleasure of taste is not sufficient to sustain consumption if it is not followed by beneficial metabolic consequences. Hedonism diminishes even faster if the saccharin is given in the presence of opiate receptor antagonists such as naltrexone. Presumably, the opiate receptor blockade diminishes the pleasurable aspects of sweet taste even further. Recent work also suggests that clinical disorders such as bulimia nervosa can be inhibited by the same drugs.[90] Indeed, sweet substances have been found to promote opioid release in the brain, and young animals (as well as human babies) become analgesic and cry less after the administration of sugar water into their mouths. Again, these effects are partly reversed by opiate receptor antagonists.[91] These experiments demonstrate that sweet substances promote opioid release in the brain.[92] Although many other neurochemical systems are likely to participate in these hedonic functions, an analysis of brain opioids has provided a robust beginning to the search for the neurochemical underpinnings of gustatory pleasure.

It seems likely that food preferences are largely mediated by two factors—taste pleasure and postingestive consequences. If opioids control taste pleasure (which is not to exclude them from also playing a role in metabolic consequences), one should be able to shift taste preferences by artificially stimulating and blocking opioid receptors as animals consume various foodstuffs. This is supported by one of our unpublished experiments summarized in Figure 9.11. Animals were give access to two saccharin solutions of the same sweetness, one that was made distinct with vanilla flavoring and the other with lemon. If either of these flavors was given following mild morphine activation of the opiate receptor system, and the other solution was given following naloxone blockade of this same system, when given a choice between the two, animals overwhelmingly preferred the flavor they had consumed under the opiate state. As is evident in Figure 9.11, this effect can be seen in two-bottle preference as well as single-bottle intake tests. When the drug pairing was stopped, the preference gradually extinguished; it could also be counterconditioned by reversing the drug-solution pairings. Such results suggest that brain opioids are important in governing gustatory choices. We seem to be addicted to foods that naturally activate our opioid systems.[93]

It also seems likely that opioid-mediated pleasure is a key ingredient in many other rewards. For instance, sexual reward has a strong opioid component. Male rats exhibit a place preference for locations in which they have copulated, but opiate receptor blocking agents decrease this preference, without reducing copulatory acts (see Chapter 12). There is evidence that opioids participate in the good feelings generated by maternal behavior and other social interactions involving touch (see Chapters 13 and 14). Indeed, brain opioids may participate in every pleasure, serving as a general neurochemical signal that the body is returning to homeostasis.[94]

In this context, it is a bit surprising that low doses of opiates activate feeding, but this may be due to the fact that mild opiate stimulation can arouse the SEEKING system.[95] At high doses, opiates dramatically reduce the desire for food but also for practically all other rewards. At present, it does not appear likely that

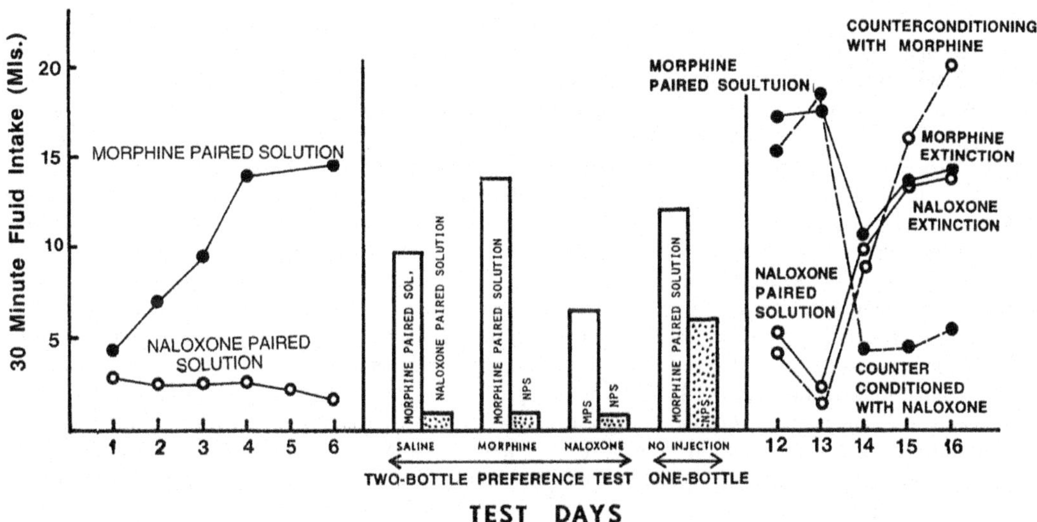

Figure 9.11. Changes in saccharine solution intake in animals in which one solution odorized with lemon or vanilla was paired with 1 mg/kg of morphine, while the other was paired with 1 mg/kg of the opiate antagonist naloxone. Clearly, animals preferred the morphine-paired solution under a variety of testing conditions, and these preferences could be extinguished and counterconditioned readily. (According to unpublished data, Panksepp & Jalowiec, 1982.)

pharmacological modulation of opioid systems will ever be able to be molded into a generally effective therapy for appetite disorders. It may be more important to target the actual brain mechanisms that mediate regulation rather than the many affective manifestations that are normally controlled by the regulatory processes.

The key question that must now be answered to provide useful treatments for energy balance disorders is the precise molecular nature of the regulatory system in the brain that determines how body energy homeostasis is sustained. Once we unravel the details of those processes, we should be in an excellent position to devise ways to help people control their body weight with the aid of biomedical interventions At the present time, available appetite-control drugs are simply not adequate for the task, and very little has been introduced to the market in the past 20 years. Fenfluramine, which has recently been marketed as a weight-control agent, reduces appetite, more than anything, by slowing gastric passage.[96] The greatest stumbling block is that most of the substances that reduce feeding do not do so by simulating normal long-term satiety—an internal feeling that body energy levels have been restored. Rather, they operate on a variety of short-term mechanisms that can inhibit appetite only briefly. It is possible that congeners of leptin will help normal people to better control their appetites in the long term, but for most obese individuals, one may need to amplify the normal functioning of leptin receptors or the postsynaptic chemical messages that leptin controls. Alternatively, we may need to fool the energy detectors in the hypothalamus that the body is processing more energy than is actually being consumed.

In sum, the analysis of food-intake regulation has proved to be a remarkable puzzle. Although there is an abundance of relevant facts, the precise nature of the regulatory system still eludes us.

AFTERTHOUGHT: Comments on Some Other Motivational Systems

Our understanding of such processes as thermoregulation and water balance, as highlighted in the following, is substantially more complete than energy balance regulation largely because it is easier to understand the regulation of these comparatively simple commodities. Unfortunately, our understanding of the accompanying affective states—the intense feelings of thirst described at the beginning of this chapter—are less well understood. In any event, drinking (or body water regulation) is controlled by two distinct systems, one for osmotic thirst and another for volumetric thirst.[97] The former is designed to monitor bodily dehydration (or intracellular salt concentration) in the blood via osmoreceptors situated in the anterior hypothalamus in an area called the *organum vasculosum of the lamina terminalis* (OVLT), while the latter is responsive to the loss of extracellular body fluids (largely reflected in blood volume); its major receptive elements appear to be in a specialized area at the juncture of the lateral and third ventricles called the *subfornical organ*. The need for increased water intake when the vascular volume goes down is especially important in emergency situations such as loss of blood following injuries. The brain system that induces *hypovolemic* (low-blood-volume) thirst does so largely by activation of a peptide in the lung called *angiotensin*. This circulating peptide is activated during blood volume loss (as detected by the kidney) and is also manufactured within the thirst circuits of the brain. Minute quantities of this peptide placed into the brain produce voluminous drinking.[98]

Our understanding of other receptive systems, such as that for sodium, is less thorough. However, it should be recognized that sodium chloride is such an essential bodily constituent that there are distinct mechanisms to assure that this commodity does not fall in short supply within the body. Aldosterone is a specialized adrenal hormone that facilitates sodium reabsorption from the blood passing through the kidney. A powerful brain mechanism also facilitates salt craving when plasma levels of sodium diminish.[99] Sodium is a relatively rare commodity in the real world, especially in inland regions. Certain herding animals will travel hundreds of kilometers to salt licks to replenish their sodium stores. The mammalian brain is designed with special-purpose mechanisms to assure that animals will remember sodium sources in their environment even when they do not need sodium. This intrinsic memory capacity was strikingly demonstrated many years ago by investigators who exposed sodium-replete animals to salt either in certain locations in their environment or within water supplies which they were required to work for while thirsty.[100] When these animals were first confronted by rapidly induced sodium depletion, they immediately sought out the locations at which sodium had previously been encountered, and they worked more vigorously for water sources that had contained the salt (even though they were now on an extinction schedule on which no salt reward was forthcoming). In other words, the memory of salt had been firmly recorded in their brains at a time when salt was not needed. This memory was retrieved at a future time when sodium was desperately needed. This remarkable feat suggests that the brain is evolutionarily prepared to remember sodium sources because that rare and precious commodity may be needed at unforeseen times. Indeed, the value of salt is recorded within our language in the word *salary*, which comes from the Latin *salarium*, meaning "salt money," which was provided for Roman soldiers as part of their compensation.

Our brains contain many types of subconscious metabolic memories. Our bodies can automatically judge the energy and micronutrient (i.e., vitamin and mineral) contents of foods and base future dietary choices on such knowledge. Likewise, we can learn to avoid substances that are bad for us from the postingestive consequences of the things we eat.[101] For instance, young rats can learn to make the correct dietary choices by observing the dietary behavior of their parents.[102] Even human infants make sophisticated dietary choices. In one experiment, they were given equal experience with two food sources that are essentially identical except for color and energy content (e.g., red versus green jello, where one contained sugar and the other was made to taste equally pleasant with noncaloric sweeteners). When given subsequent choices between these two food sources, infants selected the one that contained carbohydrate energy over the one that did not.[103] We still know little about the neural nature of metabolic memories that permit organisms to make such appraisals, but they show us, once again, that the intrinsic abilities of the brain are remarkable indeed.

Suggested Readings

Bolles, R. C. (1975). *Theory of motivation* (2d ed.). New York: Harper and Row.

Booth, D. A. (ed.) (1978). *Hunger models: Computable theory of feeding control.* London: Academic Press.

Brownell, K. D., & Foreyt, J. P. (eds.) (1986). *Physiology, psychology, and treatment of the eating disorders.* New York: Basic Books.

Katsuki, Y., Sato, M., Taklagi, S. F., & Oomura, Y. (eds.) (1977). *Food intake and chemical senses.* Tokyo: Univ. of Tokyo Press.

Kleiber, M. (1975). *The fire of life.* New York: Krieger.

LeMagnen, J. (1992). *Neurobiology of feeding and nutrition.* San Diego: Academic Press.

Novin, D., Wyrwicka, W., & Bray, G. A. (eds.) (1976). *Hunger: Basic mechanisms and clinical implications.* New York: Raven Press.

Panksepp, J. (1974). Hypothalamic regulation of energy balance and feeding behavior. *Fed. Proc.* 33:1150–1165.

Stunkard, A. J., & Stellar, E. (eds.) (1984). *Eating and its disorders.* New York: Raven Press.

Young, P. T. (1961). *Motivation and emotion.* New York: Wiley.

10

Nature Red in Tooth and Claw

The Neurobiological Sources of Rage and Anger

> Our ferocity is blind, and can only be explained from below. Could we trace it back through our line of descent, we should see it taking more and more the form of a fatal reflex response. . . . In childhood it takes this form. The boys who pull out grasshoppers' legs and butterflies' wings, and disembowel every frog they catch, have no thought at all about the matter. The creatures tempt their hands to a fascinating occupation, to which they have to yield . . . and . . . we, the lineal representatives of the successful enactors of one scene of slaughter after another, must, whatever more pacific virtues we may also possess, still carry about with us, ready at any moment to burst into flame, the smoldering and sinister traits of character by means of which they lived through so many massacres.
>
> William James, *Essays on Faith and Morals* (1910)

CENTRAL THEME

Although aggression has multiple causes, in psychiatric practice the most problematic forms arise from anger. Many stimuli can provoke anger, but the most common are the irritations and frustrations that arise from events that restrict freedom of action or access to resources. Although psychologists have documented numerous environmental precipitants of anger and aggression, they have yet to clarify the difficult question: What is anger? One reason this topic has been avoided is that anger is a primitive state of the nervous system that cannot be explained by mere words or environmental events. It must be clarified through a study of the underlying neuroevolutionary processes. As most observers have agreed throughout history, the emotion of anger is a human birthright, arising from our ancestral heritage. During this century, we have finally come to understand, at least in part, the nature of brain circuits that generate these powerful and often dangerous feelings, which yield behaviors that moral philosophers of the previous century said "deserved reprehension" and which emerge from our potential for "evil." Modern evidence suggests that anger emerges from the neurodynamics of subcortical circuits we share homologously with other mammals. The general locations of these circuits have been identified by localized electrical stimulation of the brain. The RAGE circuits run from medial areas of the amygdala, through discrete zones of the hypothalamus and down into the periaqueductal gray of the midbrain. These areas are hierarchically arranged so that higher functions are dependent on the integrity of lower ones. The more we understand about these circuits, the more we will understand the fundamental nature of anger itself. A knowledge of the brain areas where rage is evoked now allows us to work out the neurochemistries of this basic emotion. Such knowledge should eventually permit development of new medications to control pathological rage, as well as other impulse-control disorders that promote aggression. Unfortunately, most forms of human aggression may be instrumental or predatory in nature, and an understanding of anger will not help us solve the prevalent social problems that arise from such sociopathological motivations. In sum, aggression is a broader phenomenon than anger itself. Aggression is not always accompanied by anger, and anger does not necessarily lead to aggression, especially in mature humans who can control such base impulses. Because the two do not always go together, a tradition has evolved in animal brain research of overlooking the concept of anger, which cannot be observed directly. Thus, we rarely find terms such as *rage* and *anger* in the modern brain research literature. Indeed, students are commonly discouraged from using such concepts in relation to animal behavior. Even though we have abundant data on the deep neurobiological nature of ragelike aggression (or "affective attack," as it is called by behavioral neuroscientists), few bridges have been built between this database and the nature of anger and rage in human experience. These connections will be cultivated in this chapter. Of course, the primitive neural circuits of RAGE also interact with higher cognitive processes. However, before we can understand how appraisals and other acquired symbolic processes can trigger or inhibit anger, we must first fathom the lower reaches of RAGE circuits and the affective experiences that emerge therefrom. In sum, to understand anger, we must come to terms with that powerful brain force we experience as an internal pressure to reach out and strike someone.

On Aggression

At times animals threaten, bite, and kill each other.[1] Such behavior is known as aggression. Its manifestations range from a threatening baring of teeth to the tearing of flesh, from the graceful dive of a hunting hawk to the spitting spectacle of a cornered cat, from the display of pompous sexual plumage to the catastrophes of well-oiled guns and hidden bombs. Aggression is neither a universal nor a unidimensional phenomenon. Many invertebrates, like mollusks, exhibit no apparent aggression during their life cycles. However, nearly all vertebrates exhibit aggression from time to time, and such behavior can have several distinct environmental and brain causes.

Three distinct aggressive circuits have been provisionally identified in the mammalian brain: predatory, intermale, and affective attack or RAGE circuits. Only the last one provokes enraged behaviors, and presumably the experience of anger. For instance, males that fight each other for access to sexual resources do not appear to be enraged but instead present themselves as potential champions on the field of competition. Of course, they may eventually become angry at each other as they lock horns. Likewise, predators kill other animals not out of anger but because they need food to live. We must assume that the hunt and the kill is as positive a psychological experience for the predator as it is a fearful one for the prey. Predatory attack is a distinct type of aggression that arises from different circuits than anger or the seasonal competition for dominance among males of "tournament species." However, as we will see, it is not fully distinct from the SEEKING circuits discussed in Chapter 8.

Are there other aggression circuits? Perhaps, but we do not have sufficient evidence to discuss them as distinct entities. For instance, killing and injury of the young (infanticide and child abuse) are common behaviors in nature and human societies, but these tendencies may emerge from some combination of the three brain systems already mentioned, as well as others. Also, does defensive aggression arise from a distinct system in the brain? We simply do not know, but here we will assume it emerges largely from a dynamic intermixture of RAGE and FEAR systems.

In addition to distinctions we can make among different forms of aggression, all forms share certain features, such as the potential for bodily injury and individual concerns about the distribution of resources. In humans, such resources may even be psychological ones. Because aggression entails many destructive potentials, intrinsic biological restrictions are placed upon it within all species (i.e., few animals, besides humans, kill other adult members of their own kind), and there are numerous societal sanctions against it in most human cultures. In general, there is much less aggression when animals have known each other for a long time than when they are strangers.

Animals in stable societies usually develop an acceptance of their social status, and hence their "rightful" priority in the line for resources, yielding dominance hierarchies.[2] Among those that know each other, competition is often resolved by glances and gestures rather than blows. However, when organisms do not know each other, they are more likely to take the path toward physical confrontation and, if neither side backs down, bloodshed. At the cultural level, our laws attempt to ensure that humans do not impose their will on others; those who fail to comply with societal expectations are commonly recipients of various forms of societal retribution, which, with a modest stretch of the imagination, may also be defined as aggression.

At the outset, I wish to make one disclaimer: The most broadly destructive kinds of human aggression—wars between nations and competing cultural groups, as well as many violent crimes—do not arise directly from brain circuits of the type discussed here. These are instrumental acts that arise as willful activities of humans. Only weak precedents have been described in our kindred species, the chimpanzees, who occasionally exhibit group aggressive activities that resemble human tribal skirmishes, or miniwars, against others of their kind.[3] Very little of what we have to say here can highlight the causes of similar instrumental political phenomena in human societies, except that aggression may seem like a reasonable strategy among those who have little to lose or much to gain.[4] Of course, warlike tendencies in humans are ultimately accompanied by many hateful emotions, including avarice, spite, and triumph, but to the best of our meager knowledge, most of these complex feelings are not instinctual potentials of the old mammalian brain. They probably arise from higher brain areas through social learning. Without the neocortical sophistication that we humans possess, other animals simply are not able to have the complex thoughts and feelings about such matters that humans have. Still, elemental emotions like fear and anger occur on every battlefield, and the subcortical nature of these brain states can be understood through animal brain research.

Evolutionary Sources of Aggression and Rage

Some individuals are more prone to aggression than others, partly because of the quality of their neural circuits and partly because of the constrictive, irritating, and impoverished environments in which they live. As James continued in the passage from *Essays on Faith and Morals*: "Our ancestors have bred pugnacity into our bone and marrow, and thousands of years of peace won't breed it out of us." Perhaps the proper kind of education may. In any event, genetic selection experiments in both male and female rodents indicate that one can markedly potentiate aggressiveness through selective breeding within a half dozen generations, and that breeding for aggression is as effective in females as in males.[5]

Tendencies for sociopathy also appear to be genetically transmitted in humans,[6] and certain families with very high levels of aggression have been found to be characterized by neurochemical traits such as high plasma monoamine oxidase-A (MAO-A) activity,[7] the enzyme that breaks down several biogenic amines, including serotonin, within the brain. Likewise, animals and humans that have constitutionally low brain serotonin activity are more prone to aggression and the impulsive acting out of other emotions than those with higher levels.[8] In addition, males are generally more aggressive than females partly because of fetal organizational and adolescent activational effects of testosterone on their brains (see Chapter 12).[9] However, when it comes to defending their young, females of most species develop a propensity to become more defensive and assertive soon after giving birth. This may be partly due to a shift in brain chemistries within certain aggression circuits toward patterns that are more typical of males (see Chapter 13 for more on this topic).

In many species, males are disproportionately larger than females (e.g., "tournament species," such as elk and walruses, which seek to captivate many females in "harems"); especially high levels of intermale aggression are evident among such creatures. However, the fighting is typically restricted to the breeding season, when testosterone levels are particularly high. In species where males and females are closer in size, pair-bonding is more common, and sex differences in aggression are less evident; but often, as in wolf packs, only a single dominant female in a group reproduces. In a few avian species, females are bigger and more pugnacious than males, and similar patterns are evident in some mammals, most notably the spotted hyena.[10]

Female hyenas have unusually high levels of circulating testosterone, and, quite remarkably, the appearance of their external genitalia resembles that of males; one cannot tell the sexes apart with a casual peek, for the female's enlarged clitoris is as large as a male penis, and as capable of erectile activity. Female hyenas are also more aggressive than males, and it is suspected that they exhibit increased development of the underlying emotional systems that are typically more robust in the males of most species. Newborn hyenas, commonly twins, begin life with rather aggressive temperaments and remarkably high levels of circulating testosterone. They seem to be born in a fighting mood, and because of their sharp teeth, one of the two commonly dies before they enter the gentler phase of youth that is characterized by friendly play-fighting (see Chapter 15). However, there is no reason to believe that this form of aggression emerges from anger, although it might. It is more likely to reflect an early expression of dominance urges. This is not to say that anger cannot occur during such vigorous antagonistic interactions.

Although anger appears to have several obvious precipitating stimuli in the environment, the emotion is not created out of environmental events but represents the ability of certain types of stimuli to access the neural circuitry of RAGE within the brain. For instance, a human baby typically becomes enraged if its freedom of action is restricted simply by holding its arms to its sides.[11] This highlights a general and lifelong principle. Anything that restricts our freedom will be viewed as an irritant deserving our anger, contempt, and revolutionary intent. Of course, restriction of freedom is not the only precipitant of our anger and scorn. The same response emerges when one's body surface is repeatedly irritated or when one does not receive expected rewards, namely, when one is frustrated. To take a trivial example: Who has not experienced a brief flash of frustration-induced anger when a vending machine takes one's money without dispensing any goods? Most can shrug off the feeling rapidly with cognitive intervention, especially if one is not too hungry and still has sufficient coins available to try again elsewhere. This simple observation suggests that unfulfilled expectancies within the SEEKING system activate the neural patterns of frustration, probably in frontal cortical areas, which compute reward contingencies. As will be explained in detail later, reward and expectation mismatches may promote anger by downward neural influences that arouse RAGE circuits.

Such cognitive precipitants of anger would, of course, require prior learning. By contrast, a young baby who becomes enraged because it is prevented from moving may not initially conceptualize the external source of its anger, but with social development and insights into the nature of social dynamics, it rapidly learns to appraise the sources of the irritations and frustrations in its world. And then the neural paths have been prepared for retributions.

Indeed, human brains are evolutionarily "prepared" to externalize the causes of anger and to "blame" others for the evoked feelings rather than the evolutionary heritage that created the potential for anger in the first place. Of course, this makes adaptive sense. The aim of anger is to increase the probability of success in the pursuit of one's ongoing desires and competition for resources. But this is also the dilemma that therapists commonly highlight when they exhort their clients "to take responsibility for their feelings."[12] Other people do not cause our anger; they merely trigger certain emotional circuits into action. Ultimately, our feelings come from within, and perhaps only humans have a substantive opportunity, through emotional education or willpower, to choose which stimuli they allow to trigger their emotional circuits into full-blown arousal.[13] Animals, because of their limited ability to conceptualize the nature of emotions and intentions, do not appear to have such options.

Although we cannot go back in evolution to explore the origins of anger circuitry (since the brain does not fossilize well), we can at least provide reasonable scenarios concerning those sources. Perhaps one of the earliest evolutionary vectors was the adaptive advantage of having invigorated psychobehavioral responses to physical constraint, as commonly occurs in predator-prey encounters. Once a predator has captured its prey, there are two behavioral strategies that might benefit the diminishing behavioral options of the prey. The "victim" may become totally still, feigning death, which might fool the predator into releasing its grip. Indeed, this type of "tonic immobility" is a common response of several prey species (e.g., rabbits, guinea pigs, and chickens), and it is referred to by the rather sensational label "animal hypnosis."[14] The other strategy is for the animal's behavior to become vigorous very rapidly, which might startle or otherwise dissuade the predator from pursuing its course of action, thereby giving the prey a chance to flee and escape. I assume it was this latter response, initially an adaptive reflex of invigorated movement, that guided the evolution of the full-fledged emotional system that now mediates anger.

That a complex form of psychological constraint such as frustration would eventually provoke the same type of psychobehavioral activity highlights the evolution of emotional systems. New controls, including layers of learning, have been gradually added to ancient emotional integrative systems, thereby enhancing and expanding the range of behavioral control. In other words, circuit openness (see Figure 4.2) has been promoted in emotional systems by the addition of hierarchical layers of new control (see Figure 2.2). With multiple inputs and control functions, the degree to which animals can exhibit emotional regulation has been expanded. However, the more recently evolved controls continue to depend critically on the nature of preexisting emotional circuit functions. In adult humans, higher cortical controls can be refined to the point that we can, to some extent, choose to be angry or not. But also, because of such higher cognitive functions, we can become angry merely in response to symbolic gestures (reflecting how past learning and current appraisals can come to arouse emotional systems).

Appraisals, Higher Cognitive Functions, and Aggression

Since the study of violence and aggression has become a sensitive societal and academic topic (see note 4), many investigators hesitate to discuss the potential insights that a psychobiological analysis of aggression circuits could provide. It is not generally accepted that the potentials for aggression are inborn. Rather, the prevailing view is that most impulses for aggression emerge from the appraisal of events. Here I will advocate the idea that the subcortical neural systems that generate anger are inborn, although it cannot be emphasized enough that a great deal of learning comes to modulate these underlying emotional forces, perhaps in all mammalian species,[15] but most certainly in humans. Conversely, it is also likely that the neuropsychic force we call anger promotes certain types of cognitive activities in humans, such as thoughts of vengeance and the pursuit of retribution.[16] Higher cerebral abilities must be taken into account in any comprehensive explanation of angry behavior, and it is incorrect to believe that a study of animals will fully explain why humans exhibit and inhibit aggression. Many cognitive aspects of anger are undoubtedly unique to the human species. What animal research can provide is lasting insight into the fundamental sources of primal feelings of rage within the brain.

Even limited claims such as this are not especially popular in the present intellectual zeitgeist, where ideas are commonly constructed and deconstructed without recourse to the evidence. Nonetheless, there are abundant reasons to believe that the subcortical anatomies and major neurochemistries for the feeling of anger are remarkably similar in all mammals. For instance, one can evoke angry behaviors and feelings by electrically stimulating the same brain areas in humans as in other species. Angry behaviors can also be modulated by manipulating the same neurochemistries in all mammalian species that have been studied.[17] Thus, the major differences between species probably lie in the cognitive subtleties that incite and channel the internal emotional force we commonly call anger. The material values upon which cognitive appraisals are premised are bound to differ substantially among species, depending on the resources they value and how much competition is needed to obtain them.

Although the cognitive activities that accompany anger will be harder to analyze across species, it remains possible that some cross-species analyses will be informative. For instance, anger may provoke certain types of primitive thoughts and perceptual changes in all animals. During anger, rapid movement on the part of other animals may be viewed as provocations, as opposed to irrelevant pieces of information. Certain cues from other animals that have been repeatedly associated with the provocation of anger may also develop the ability to sustain angry moods for extended periods through classical conditioning. This type of learning, once it becomes cognitively represented, may be called "hatred." Is the feeling of hatred, then, little more than the emotion of anger, conditioned to specific cues, that has been cognitively extended in time? This may well be the case, and it would explain why hatred should not be called a basic emotion, even though it has certain features that differentiate it from anger. Hatred is obviously more calculated, behaviorally constrained, and affectively "colder" than the passionate "heat" of rage.

In fact, anger does not always provoke explicit threat or aggression in humans. Mature humans can voluntarily inhibit the expression of their primitive impulses and, with a great deal of social learning, can express their anger with the cool detachment of barbed words. However, when we humans experience anger, even at times when we are unwilling to express the underlying urges to others, our mental dialogues overflow with statements of blame and scorn for the individual(s) or institution(s) that provoked (or seemed to provoke) the anger. These internal dialogues deserve more study by psychologists, but there are other aspects of anger that cannot be studied through the analysis of words or human actions. To be angry is to have a specific kind of internal pressure or force controlling one's actions and views of the world. This affective "force" within the human brain can be reasonably well understood, if one is willing to consider that it emerges from the neuropsychic energies aroused by RAGE circuits shared by all mammalian brains. A similar analysis can be done for brain systems that can reduce anger.

Both psychologically and behaviorally, certain attitudes and gestures are especially efficacious in reducing anger.[18] Among many types of animals, appeasement signals—for instance, lying on one's back, exposing vulnerable parts like the belly and neck—commonly reduce aggression by others of the same species. Defeated rats often emit long 22 Khz vocalizations. Do these submissive gestures release specific neurochemicals that counteract angry urges, or is the reaction purely cognitive? Although it is next to impossible to probe the thoughts of emotional animals, we will here assume that there are certain neurochemical profiles that can promote peaceful relations among animals, including chemistries that emerge from circuits mediating sexuality (see Chapter 12), nurturance (see Chapter 13), and social bonding (see Chapter 14). But before we can understand the influence of these factors, we will first have to understand the nature of anger within the mammalian brain.

The General Neurocognitive Substrates of Anger and the Frustration-Aggression Hypothesis

In the body, anger is accompanied by an invigoration of the musculature, with corresponding increases in autonomic indices such as heart rate, blood pressure, and muscular blood flow. As is so well conveyed by idiomatic descriptions of anger (e.g., "getting hot under the collar"), body temperature also increases during anger. In the brain, there emerges an intense and well-focused tendency to strike out at the offending agent. The emotional state aroused in the brain is a fiery mental storm, capable of being defined in neurophysiological and neurochemical terms, that rapidly persuades us that the offending agent is below contempt and deserves harm. Previous memories related to the anger episode are easily remembered and potential plans for vengeance are automatically promoted.[19] This indicates powerful interactions of RAGE systems with memory encoding systems of the brain, although, as already indicated, we know little neurophysiologically about such matters.

The study of such internal experiences of humans could provide some testable hypotheses concerning the properties of anger systems. Since anger is most easily aroused when the availability of desired resources diminishes, it should have close anatomical and neurophysiological linkages to the SEEKING system. Indeed, arousal of the self-stimulation system entails an increased possibility of frustration, since this system establishes neural conditions for an affective state of high expectations and hence their failure to be met (Figure 10.1).

To the best of our knowledge, positive expectations, and the possibility of frustration, arise from neurodynamic activities of higher brain areas that compute reward contingencies—psychological processes that are linked intimately to the cognitive functions of the frontal cortex.[20] A rapid suppression of activity within the SEEKING system, in the absence of homeostatic pleasures, which would normally index that a reward has been obtained, should unconditionally promote the arousal of anger circuitry. Indeed, such effects have been observed in animals' elevated tendency to bite when rewarding brain stimulation is terminated.[21] In comparable circumstances, humans tend to to clench their jaws and swear epithets. In other words, the RAGE and SEEKING circuits may normally have mutually inhibitory interactions (see Figure 3.5), even though both may be comparably sensitized by other processes such as the feelings of hunger aroused by the body's energy needs. This makes psychological sense, since such need states would heighten the value of positive expectations, and hence the feelings associated with those expectations not being met.

The frustration-aggression hypothesis has been one of the most well-developed theories in the psychological literature (as highlighted in the famous book by Dollard and colleagues, cited in the Suggested Readings). Frustrating experiences have traditionally been linked to anger through the hypothesis that if a goal response is interrupted, aggression follows. A basic postulate of this view is that aggression will increase in proportion to the level of frustration—namely, in

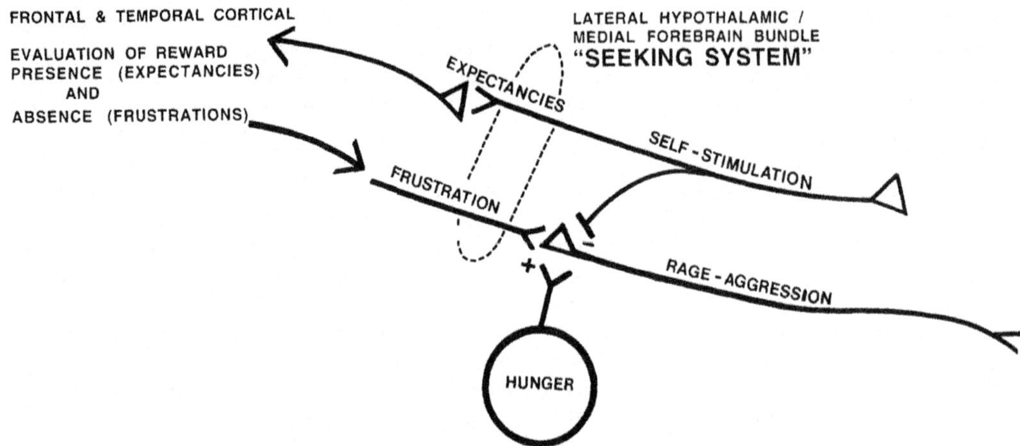

Figure 10.1. Schematic suggestion of likely interactions between neural systems that mediate the anticipatory behaviors of SEEKING and arousal of the RAGE system. (Adapted from Panksepp, 1981; see chap. 3, n. 25.)

direct relation to the intensity of the desire that is thwarted and the number of times the thwarting occurs. Such predictions are supported by a large amount of human data. For instance, children who have not been allowed to participate in a favorite activity will subsequently tend to exhibit higher levels of aggression, and such frustrations bring other dark thoughts to the surface such as prejudice toward minority groups.[22]

From both neural and affective perspectives, we must also ask some deeper questions. Is the feeling of frustration really substantially different than that of anger? Psychobiological evidence certainly allows us to conclude that they are intimately linked, since manipulations that reduce the effects of frustration, such as antianxiety agents and temporal lobe damage or more restricted amygdaloid lesions, also tend to reduce emotional aggression.[23] Thus, the emotional feeling of frustration may largely reflect the mild arousal of RAGE circuitry, in the same way that anxiety may reflect weak arousal of the FEAR circuitry (see Chapter 11). In other words, the outputs of cognitive brain systems that evaluate reward contingencies may simply have special access to RAGE circuitry. Even though there is little evidence on this, it also remains possible that feelings of frustration arise directly from higher brain activities, such as of the frontal cortex, that evaluate reward contingencies. Certainly, the fact that patients with frontal cortical damage can become angry rapidly, but can also lose their anger rapidly,[24] suggests that frontal cortical influences are important in sustaining instinctual anger responses that are elaborated by lower regions of the brain.

Although it remains to be empirically demonstrated which brain systems are essential for generating *feelings* of frustration, such feelings may very well arise from mild arousal of RAGE circuitry. Since the frontal cortex elaborates reward expectancies, presumably a neural representation of those perceptions feeds back onto the subcortical components of the anger system. However, in this context it is important to remember that there are many other facilitators of aggression beside frustration—including hunger, pain, and perhaps some of the neural effects of testosterone. Conversely, it is also worth considering that such intense feelings may also sensitize the higher neural substrates that instigate frustration through the computation of positive expectancies. How this might operate for specific commodities that alleviate hunger and pain is more straightforward than it is for testosterone, unless we consider that the hormone may generate greater expectations by promoting feelings of social strength and dominance. Such strong feelings may help set the stage for stronger feelings of frustration when things do not go as well as anticipated, especially during intermale competition. Because of the likelihood of multiple layers of neural interactions among the various aggression systems, as well as the other basic emotions, it is important to consider all the various forms of aggression that have been documented by animal behaviorists.

Taxonomies: Environmentally Induced Varieties of Aggression

Although the frustration-aggression hypothesis has been of great value in promoting coherent psychological analysis of aggression, we must remember that behavioral manifestations of aggression are quite diverse. There are several distinct brain systems that can precipitate aggressive acts and an even greater number of external stimuli that can trigger such systems into action. As we saw in Chapters 2 and 8, all emotional circuits appear to be designed to permit a great deal of behavioral flexibility, which helps explain the variability of behavior patterns seen during a single emotional state, within as well as between species. Thus, it is understandable why there would still be considerable confusion about how aggression should be subcategorized and studied. Taxonomies of aggression can be based on (1) the possible psychological causes of aggression (as in the previous section), (2) the varieties of behavioral expressions, as well as (3) the basis of the types of underlying neural systems. Let us now move to the second level of analysis.

The types of aggression that have been distinguished on the basis of eliciting conditions are more numerous than those based on the behavioral manifestations and the types of aggression-organizing systems that have been discovered in the brain. Even though many distinct circumstances lead to aggression, several forms, distinguished on the basis of eliciting conditions, probably do emerge from the same neural operating systems. For instance, the aggression that a mother exhibits to defend her offspring may not be fundamentally different from the aggression a male exhibits when an intruder infringes on his territorial "rights." In both situations, aggression may be evoked by essentially one and the same brain circuit, even though the two can be distinguished taxonomically by the different psychosocial/cognitive precipitating conditions. Thus, a single brain process can be activated by several different inputs.

The most widely cited behavioral taxonomy based on the eliciting conditions for aggression was developed by Kenneth Moyer.[25] His list includes seven distinct forms of aggression: (1) *Fear-induced aggression* occurs when an animal cannot escape from an aversive situation; (2) a female often displays *maternal aggression* when an intruder is perceived to threaten the safety of her offspring; (3) *irritable aggression* results from annoying occurrences in the environment that are not strong enough to provoke flight; (4) *sex-related aggression* occurs in the presence of sexual stimuli; (5) *territorial aggression* occurs when a strange animal enters the living space claimed by a resident animal; (6) *intermale aggression* reflects the fact that two males placed together are much more likely to begin fighting than two females placed together; and (7) *predatory aggression* is a food-seeking mechanism in certain omnivorous and carnivorous species. One could even suggest others, such as *play-fighting*, *defensive aggression*, and perhaps even *lovers' spats*, but these types of distinctions are presently not very useful at the neuroscience level of analysis.

As will be highlighted later, all these forms of aggression are certainly not distinct at the subcortical level. Environmentally based taxonomies such as Moyer's do not reflect the distinct types of brain operating systems that can mediate aggression. Several items in his taxonomy share underlying controls, while others do not. For example, most investigators consider predatory aggression to be motivationally and neurologically distinct from other forms. Indeed, William James, in his famous *Essays on Faith and Morals*, may have been conflating distinct forms, such as predatory aggression (little boys' pulling of butterfly wings) and those aggressive passions that can lead to intermale conflict and warfare. Unlike most of the other forms, predatory aggression is largely endogenously generated and accompanied by positive affect (even though the concurrent energizing contributions of hunger may be aversive), and I will argue, contrary to traditional wisdom, that hunting largely emerges from the SEEKING system discussed in the previous chapter. Of course, this does not mean that the whole predatory attack sequence or any other real-life emotional pattern ever remains under the control of a single emotional system. A predator surely experiences irritability or frustration if the prey struggles so vigorously that it seems liable to escape. Thus, in real life, there are sudden shifts in emotions depending upon the success or failure of specific behavioral acts, as well as in the changing cognitive expectations and appraisals of each situation.

Let us now shift to the third level of analysis and focus on the distinct circuitries for aggression that actually exist in the brain. The final word on this is not in, but it is certain that there are fewer aggression systems than are highlighted in Moyer's taxonomy. How might we empirically winnow the list and then empirically distinguish among them? One problem is that many environmental, neuroanatomical, and neurochemical influences act similarly on each and every type of aggression listed. For instance, prolonged social isolation or hunger may increase all forms of aggression, while high brain serotonin activity may reduce them all.[26] Such important shared variables do not allow us to make useful distinctions. At present, the most effective way to distinguish among the various neural systems is via the analysis of "stimulus-bound" aggressive tendencies evoked by localized electrical stimulation of specific circuits in the brain, and via the analysis of which variables modify the sensitivities of these circuits.

Varieties of ESB-Induced Aggression and Their Affective Consequences

Distinctions among neural pathways for aggression have been effectively made by the careful psychobehavioral analysis of aggressive sequences evoked by direct electrical stimulation of the brain (ESB). The fact that coherent patterns of aggression can be produced in this way is remarkable in itself. If, as many scientists used to believe, aggression is largely a learned response rather than an intrinsic potential of the nervous system (e.g., see the contribution by John Paul Scott in the Suggested Readings), it would be unlikely that localized ESB could evoke attack behaviors. However, since Walter Hess's work in the 1930s (see "Afterthought," Chapter 4), it has been clear that rage can be precipitously provoked by ESB administered to specific brain areas.

My own initial experience with this technique was revealing. When I first applied ESB to a cat that had been surgically prepared with an indwelling electrode in the medial hypothalamus, within the first few seconds of ESB the peaceful animal was emotionally transformed. It leaped viciously toward me with claws unsheathed, fangs bared, hissing and spitting.[27] It could have pounced in many different directions, but its arousal was directed right at my head. Fortunately, a Plexiglas wall separated me from the enraged beast. Within a fraction of a minute after terminating the stimulation, the cat was again relaxed and peaceful, and could be petted without further retribution.

As mentioned at the outset of this chapter, at present three distinct kinds of aggression can be aroused by applying ESB to slightly different brain zones: predatory aggression, angry, ragelike aggression, and perhaps intermale aggression, even though the last may also have strong components of the other two. It is the second of these systems that will be the center of attention in the remainder of this chapter, even though I will summarize selected issues related to the other two.[28]

Several early investigators called aggressive displays induced by ESB "sham rage," based on the assumption that the animals were not experiencing true affect. This seemed plausible because some of the subjects could be petted even while they were hissing and snarling.[29] However, such sites appear to be quite low in the brain stem and in the minority. Now it seems more likely that most electrode placements above the mesencephalon do evoke a central state indistinguishable from normal anger (except perhaps for the fact that stimulation-induced rage is not sustained for a long time after ESB offset, perhaps because of the sudden release of an opponent neural process). Perhaps the most compelling evidence that the ESB evokes a true affective feeling is that humans stimulated at such brain sites have reported experiencing a feeling of intense rage.[30]

At a logical level, it is by no means clear whether the experience of anger should be deemed an unambiguously aversive emotion. It could easily become positive if it succeeds in changing the world in desired ways. However, we can conclude that most animals do have unpleasant affective experiences during such stimulation, since they readily learn to turn off ESB that generates affective attack.[31] Although some electrode sites, especially those low in the brain stem, may only activate motor-pattern generators with no accompanying affective experience, most animals are truly enraged by the ESB. They readily direct their anger to the most salient potential threat in their environment. However, other forms of aggression evoked by ESB do not appear to be accompanied by anger.

The early distinction between *affective* or *defensive attack* and *quiet-biting* or *predatory attack* has been most extensively analyzed. During affective attack (see Figure 10.2), animals exhibit piloerection, autonomic arousal, hissing, and growling during their attack pattern, while during quiet-biting attack they exhibit only methodical stalking and well-directed pouncing.[32] Subsequent studies in rats established a similar taxonomy.[33] Additional work with rats has provided evidence for a third form: intermale aggression.[34]

The fact that only these three forms can be provoked with ESB suggests that the many environmental influences outlined by Moyer probably converge on a limited set of aggressive operating systems in the brain. For instance, maternal and fear-induced aggression may reflect a convergence of inputs onto an affective attack or RAGE system. On the other hand, intermale, territorial, and sex-related aggression may have some common influence on the system that elaborates *intermale fighting*, whereas instrumental and predatory aggression may largely arise from the quiet-biting attack systems. Of course, as already mentioned, it must be emphasized that in real-world encounters, several emotive systems are bound to be recruited concurrently or successively in the excitement of ongoing events.

Although the so-called quiet-biting attack or predatory attack system described in cats is surely distinct from the one that mediates rage, the notion that it is separate from the SEEKING system is probably a misinterpretation. A great deal of evidence suggests that both emerge from a homologous brain system on the basis of anatomical, neurochemical, and functional grounds. The two behaviors are obtained from essentially the same brain areas, and in rats the most effective quiet-biting attack electrodes always evoke self-stimulation.[35] Self-stimulation is facilitated by antianxiety agents,[36] as is ESB-induced quiet-biting attack,[37] and both behaviors are reduced by dopamine-blocking agents.[38] It is evident that the segregation of these two lines of research (i.e., work on the lateral hypothalamic self-stimulation system in rats and the quiet-biting attack system in cats) has overlooked this remarkable commonality in the underlying brain substrates. To the best of our knowledge, the two response patterns are simply two distinct behavioral expressions of SEEKING tendencies that arise from homologous systems in the brains of different species. The species-typical expressions of this system lead to foraging in some species and predatory stalking in others.

But how about the distinction between affective attack and quiet-biting attack systems? Can that distinction be defended on the basis of hard empirical evidence, as opposed to mere differences in outward appearance? Might it not be that these seemingly distinct forms of aggression emerge from a single system, and the apparent differences are due to activation of extraneous influences, such as other emotional systems located nearby—for example, those that elaborate FEAR or PANIC? The answer appears to be no. A substantial amount of evidence now shows that affective attack and quiet-biting attack systems are quite distinct

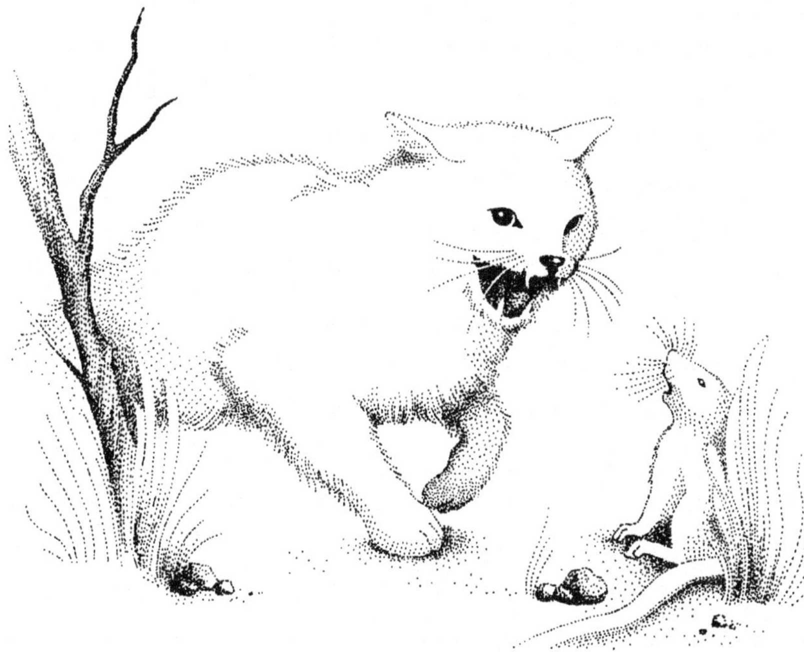

Figure 10.2. Artist's rendition of a cat in the midst of a stimulus-bound affective attack episode (electrodes to cat not depicted). Although the behavior of the animal is well directed and apparently intentional, there is substantial autonomic arousal and an anger type of behavioral presentation. (Adapted from a photograph by John Flynn, 1967; see n. 28.)

in the brain. In addition to the observable behavioral differences and neuroanatomical divergencies to be discussed in the next section, quiet-biting attack is typically evoked during ESB of the dorsolateral hypothalamus, while affective attack sites are more concentrated in the ventrolateral and medial hypothalamus.[39] The approximate neuroanatomy of the RAGE system is summarized in Figure 10.3.

The two forms of aggression can also be distinguished in rats by several other criteria. First, with respect to affective correlates, brain sites that yield quiet-biting attack invariably also support self-stimulation, while affective attack sites yield escape behaviors.[40] This same trend is apparent in the periaqueductal gray (PAG), where affective attack and aversive responses can generally be aroused from the dorsal half of the PAG, while quiet-biting attack and self-stimulation are more readily obtained from the ventral half.[41] This does not mean that anger must necessarily be considered a wholly negative emotion. As mentioned, if the ener-

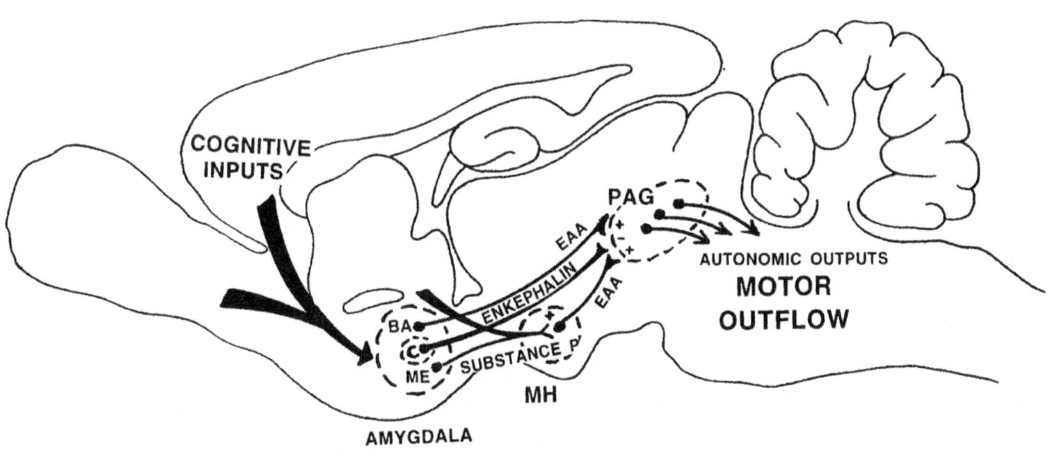

RAGE CIRCUITS

Figure 10.3. Summary of the localization of RAGE circuitry in the brain. (Adapted from data in Siegel & Brutus, 1990; see n. 39; and Siegel & Schubert, 1995; see n. 81.)

gized behavior of rage produces the desired changes in the environment, then it is rapidly mixed or associated with positive emotional feelings.

The differentiation of predatory and affective attack can also be made in terms of the higher brain areas that control these tendencies, as can be evaluated by stimulating two brain areas concurrently. For instance, stimulation of the bed nucleus of the stria terminalis facilitates affective attack while suppressing quiet-biting attack.[42]

The two types of attack can also be distinguished with respect to eliciting conditions. Rats exhibiting quiet-biting attack will, in addition to attacking live prey, also bite dead mice, while stimulation of affective attack sites does not support the latter behavior. On the other hand, when confronted by conspecifics (members of the same species), no attack is generated from quiet-biting attack sites, while intense attack is still evoked from affective attack sites. Apparently, during anger, the type of available target is not as important as the fact that there is a living target upon which to vent one's rage. Yet as one does these types of ESB manipulations in more complex creatures such as monkeys, the aroused animals tend to vent their rage on more submissive animals and avoid confronting more dominant ones. With repeated stimulation within a colony-living situation, however, it has been found that animals can actually ascend in rank within their dominance hierarchies.[43]

Affective and predatory attack sites can also be distinguished pharmacologically. While minor tranquilizers such as chlordiazepoxide (Librium®) reduce affective attack and increase quiet-biting attack, psychostimulants such as amphetamine can increase affective attack without clearly affecting quiet-biting attack.[44] In sum, quiet-biting and affective attack circuits are clearly distinct. Also, as mentioned earlier, there is preliminary evidence that one can activate aggressive intermale fighting independently of these two systems. Let us now focus on the details of each of these "aggression" systems.

Brain Circuits for Affective Attack (RAGE)

It seems highly probable that the emotion we commonly call *anger* or *rage* derives much of its motivating energy and affective impact from the neural circuits that orchestrate affective attack. The most compelling evidence, of course, comes from subjective reports that have been obtained from humans. The core of the RAGE system runs from medial amygdaloid areas downward, largely via the stria terminalis to the medial hypothalamus, and from there to specific locations within the PAG of the midbrain. This system is organized hierarchically (Figure 10.4), meaning that aggression evoked from the highest areas in the amygdala is critically dependent on the lower regions, while aggression from lower sites does not depend critically on the integrity of the higher areas.[45] In other words, lesions of both medial hypothalamic and PAG zones dramatically diminish rage evoked from the amygdala, but not vice versa. Thus, from diencephalic zones, around the medial hypothalamus, the aggressive tendency is critically dependent on the integrity of the PAG but not of the medial amygdala. This probably indicates that the higher areas provide

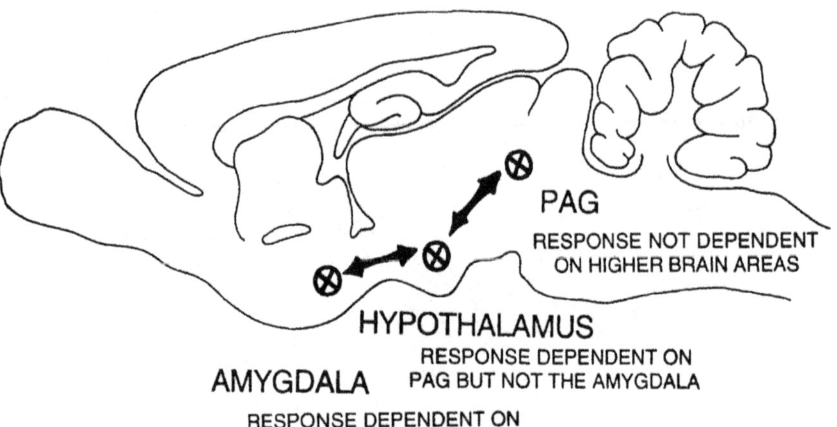

Figure 10.4. Hierarchical control of RAGE in the brain. Lesions of higher areas do not diminish responses from lower areas, while damage of lower areas compromises the functions of higher ones.

subtle refinements to the orchestration that is elaborated in the PAG of the mesencephalon. For instance, various irritating perceptions probably get transmitted into the system via thalamic and cortical inputs to the medial amygdala, while more basic physiological "irritations," such as hunger and basic hormonal/sexual influences, enter the system via medial preoptic and hypothalamic inputs.

Since the primary evolved function of anger is to motivate individuals to compete effectively for environmental resources, we would anticipate that reciprocal relations would exist between the SEEKING and RAGE systems (see Figures 3.5 and 10.1). Indeed, as mentioned earlier, animals are less likely to bite during "rewarding" lateral hypothalamic stimulation, but they tend to bite more at the offset of such stimulation. In addition, frustration, a major precipitant of anger, seems to be elaborated largely within frontal cortical areas, where neurons register conditional stimuli that predict forthcoming rewards.[46] These neurons can track reward-relevant stimuli, so that when CS+ and CS– (i.e., the conditional stimuli predicting reward presence or absence) are reversed, the neurons reverse their firing patterns to follow the new reward relationships. Neurons within the temporal lobes, which also exhibit similar initial discrimination of conditional reward associations, do not readily exhibit response patterning reversals when the valences of the conditional stimuli are reversed.[47] It is not clear which type of brain tissue is more important for the generation of frustration, but presumably frustration emerges from the ability of such cognitive systems to monitor the probability of forthcoming rewards. If an expected reward is not registered, the higher cell assemblies send out *opponent process* messages that invigorate activity within the RAGE system. Does the relevant neuroanatomy support such a scenario?

Detailed maps have now been constructed of the brain interconnectivites of the executive system for RAGE which ultimately terminate in the PAG. Both the retrograde and anterograde maps of these brain sites yield a provocative set of connections.[48] PAG sites that support rage behaviors receive inputs primarily from six areas of the brain (Figure 10.5), including several areas of the cortex, the medial hypothalamus, and several zones of the lower brain stem. The six major areas, with their potential psychobehavioral functions are as follows: (1) The highest brain areas sending direct information to the PAG emerge from the frontal cortex—primarily from medial areas that contain reward-relevance neurons, as well as from a more lateral area called the frontal eye fields, which help direct eye movements to especially prominent objects in the environment. It seems appropriate that the basic anger circuits receive information from brain systems that regulate these important integrative areas. (2) Another set of inputs comes from the orbitoinsular cortex, especially the insular area, where a multitude of senses converge, especially ones related to pain and perhaps hearing. These areas presumably code the affective content of certain irritations, including vocalizations, and may give specific sounds direct access to RAGE circuitry. For instance, it is not an uncommon human experience that an angry tone of voice directed at you activates your own anger in return. (3) Powerful inputs emerge from the medial hypothalamus. Not only is this brain area part of the trajectory of the anger system itself, but it also elaborates energy homeostasis (see

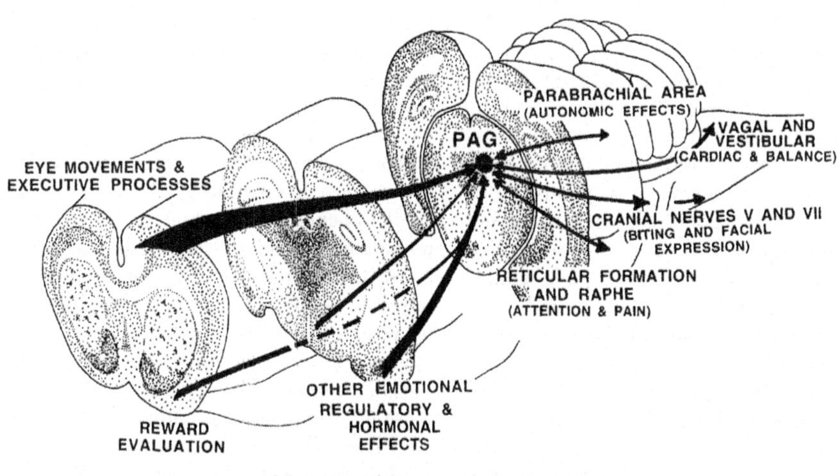

Figure 10.5. The anterograde and retrograde connectivities of mesencephalic RAGE sites in the cat brain. (Adapted from Bandler, 1988; see n. 41.)

Chapter 9) and sexual matters (see Chapter 12); thus it is an ideal area where those influences come to modify anger. For instance, both hunger and testosterone are capable of sensitizing the anger circuit, while satiety and estrogen are able to quell activity within this system. Inputs from lower areas include (4) the vestibular complex, which may help enrage animals when their bodily orientation is disrupted; (5) amine cell groups such as the locus coeruleus and raphe, which are known to exert nonspecific modulatory control over all behaviors (see Chapter 6); and (6) the nucleus of the solitary tract, which collects visceral information via the vagus nerve and probably is important for apprising the anger systems of the tone of peripheral autonomic processes such as heart rate and blood pressure. It is important to emphasize that most of these connections are reciprocating two-way avenues of interdependent control (i.e., they reflect reciprocating feedback mechanisms).

Indeed, it is known that some peripheral inputs can control the sensitivity of rage systems. For instance, increased activity in *baroreceptors* of the carotid arteries monitors levels of blood pressure and can facilitate the sensitivity of RAGE circuitry. When blood pressure goes up, the sensitivity of RAGE systems does, too.[49] Probably the most important brain area for the actual integration of the overall anger response is in the PAG, an area that also sends reciprocal efferent feedback to most of the systems mentioned previously. This reciprocity indicates that the RAGE system remains informed of its activities at all of the hierarchical levels of the basic control circuitry. This, of course, makes considerable adaptive sense.

Quiet-Biting Attack

As already indicated, the major brain areas that yield predatory aggression during ESB overlap remarkably with brain areas where self-stimulation is obtained, although quiet-biting attack has typically been studied in cats, while rats have been the species of choice for self-stimulation studies. If both self-stimulation and predatory attack actually emerge from a homologous basic brain function, it is understandable why cats are so rarely used in self-stimulation research. Cats do not acquire self-stimulation behavior as readily as rats, and when they do, they do not behave in a rapid, agitated way like rats. Presumably, this is because a cat's typical food-aquisition strategy is stealthy hunting that requires considerable motor inhibition. Rats, on the other hand, acquire the behavior rapidly and behave energetically, probably because their natural foraging style, which is accompanied by vigorous activity and object manipulation, fits nicely with vigorous lever pressing.

Conversely, it is much easier to obtain quiet-biting attack from cats than from rats, probably because rats normally harvest energy by searching and scavenging for their food rather than hunting. In one of the first studies to map out aggression circuits in the rat brain, it proved remarkably difficult to demonstrate quiet-biting attack until subjects were preselected for the tendency to exhibit predatory intent.[50] In other words, predatory attack could be obtained easily only in those individual animals that had a preexisting strong tendency to approach and vigorously investigate potential prey objects such as mice. In these animals, brain stimulation at lateral hypothalamic sites would eventually induce systematic pursuit and attack of available mice.[51] However, if mice were not available, the same animals would readily exhibit one of the other stimulus-bound behaviors, such as eating or drinking, that is typically evoked from the lateral hypothalamus (see Chapter 8). There was no reason to suppose that quiet-biting attack was aroused from different circuits than those alternative behaviors (even though the terminal behavioral component obviously requires some different circuitry in the brain stem and spinal cord for the differential patterning of the final behavioral output). In short, ESB-induced quiet-biting attack could be obtained readily only from those animals that already exhibited some predisposition to attack. Accordingly, it seems that quiet-biting attack is simply one behavioral product of the SEEKING system. Even though this behavior has been extensively studied within the context of aggression, from the animal's point of view, there is no apparent anger involved in this food-seeking response. Indeed, it has always been more reasonable to assume that the emotive pattern was, in fact, accompanied by positive affect, since cats, just like rats, readily exhibit feeding during low-intensity stimulation of those lateral hypothalamic sites where higher levels of stimulation provoke predatory attack.[52]

Moreover, it should be noted that many of the perceptual sensitivity changes that have been obtained in stimulus-bound aggression studies on felines are restricted to quiet-biting attack rather than affective attack circuitry. For instance, during application of this kind of brain stimulation, the perioral regions of cats are sensitized, so that light touch along the lip line is more likely to evoke orientation and biting than it is without the brain stimulation (Figure 10.6).[53] The stronger the current, the broader the area of sensitization. A similar phenomenon is obtained in rats with lateral hypothalamic stimulation that sustains stimulus-bound appetitive behavior,[54] which further affirms the commonality of these systems in the two species. In a similar way, this type of stimulation sensitizes the skin of the cat's paws, so that mild touch is more likely to provoke a vigorous striking reflex.[55] Again, the more intense the stimulation, the broader the area of sensitivity. In neurological terms, the more intense stimulation recruits more *dermatomes* along the forearm (i.e., dermatomes are skin zones served by the individual spinal sensory nerves).

Another fascinating aspect of brain stimulation is that it provokes a predatory temperament only on the

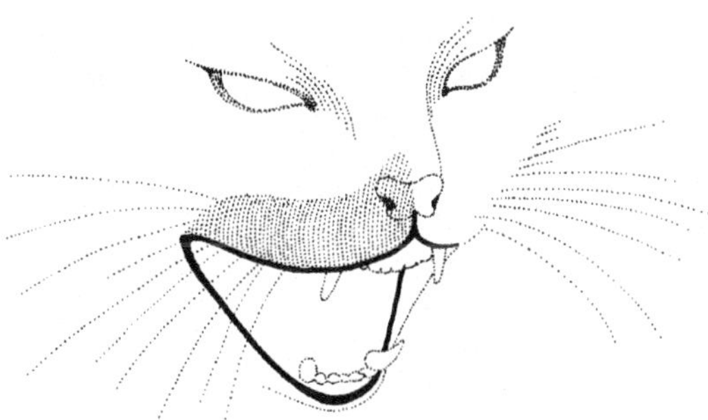

Figure 10.6. Animals stimulated in quiet-biting attack areas exhibit a clear sensitization of various sensory fields, especially that around the lip line and around the muzzle. The area of sensitization increases with increasing stimulation intensity. Similar changes may occur at brain sites that produce affective attack, but that is not clear from the available literature.

side of the brain that is stimulated directly, and this is reflected in the sensitization of the corresponding visual fields. Specifically, ESB applied to the right side of the brain makes an animal exhibit predatory aggression in its left visual field but not in the right (please note that information from the right visual field is transmitted to the left cerebral hemisphere because of the way the optic nerves cross in the optic chiasm). Conversely, stimulation of the left side of the brain leads to attack directed at target animals in the right visual field. In other words, lateral hypothalamic stimulation sensitizes sensory processing within the ipsilateral cerebral hemisphere, which sensitizes the animal's response to information coming in through the contralateral sensory fields.[56] Accordingly, a prey moving across one half of a subject animal's visual field will provoke attack, but when it reaches the opposite visual field, attack behavior ceases.[57] A similar unilateral sensitization of higher areas has been demonstrated for self-stimulation circuitry in rats,[58] again reinforcing the relationship of that circuitry to predatory aggression. Comparable types of brain effects have yet to be demonstrated with electrode placements that generate affective rage, but they may well exist once studies are done.

Intermale Aggression and Dominance

In nearly all mammalian species, males fight more than females. In neural terms, this is the case because males possess more active aggression circuits, at least those types of aggression circuits that were evolutionarily designed to assure reproductive success. Females possess the more precious reproductive resource (the egg and gestational abilities), so it has been left for males to compete for the sexual favors of females. Some have even speculated that male assertiveness is a selection process driven by the female, whereby the most vigorous males within a breeding population are allowed preferential access to reproductive opportunities.[59] To put it bluntly, from the female's point of view, a male that can trounce his rivals is more likely to be carrying competitive, winning genes.

In virtually all mammals, male sexuality requires an assertive attitude, so that male sexuality and aggressiveness normally go together. Indeed, these tendencies are intertwined throughout the neuroaxis, and to the best of our limited knowledge, the circuitry for this type of aggression is located near, and probably interacts strongly with, both RAGE and SEEKING circuitries. Our knowledge about the intermale aggression system remains preliminary, but the general neurogeography of the system is highlighted by the high density of testosterone receptors running from the medial amygdala, through the preoptic, anterior hypothalamic area, and down into the PAG of the brain stem (which is really quite distinct from the trajectory of the RAGE system). One can dissociate intermale social aggression from the other types in various ways, including the types of brain damage that affect them. For instance, many forms of brain damage (including lateral septum, nucleus accumbens, medial hypothalamus, and raphe) intensify aggressive responses directed toward experimenters and prey objects but tend to reduce fighting between males.[60] Thus, brain manipulations that appear to intensify anger and predatory aggression, such as ventromedial hypothalamic damage, do not necessarily intensify social aggression, suggesting that they are independently controlled in the brain.

An especially critical question from both philosophical and empirical points of view is to what extent neurons "irritated" by testosterone in the service of sexual arousal (see Chapter 12) also participate in aggressive arousal. Are these extensively or only mildly overlapping systems? This question is actually more philosophical than practical because testosterone emanating from the testes would affect both systems simultaneously. It would be of practical interest, however, to discover whether the systems are extensively independent and capable of independent modulation. If they are essentially a single system in the human brain, then the only hope for tempering the negative aspects of this neural dilemma would be through education—namely, cognitive specification as to what is acceptable and unacceptable behavior. Although we do not have an answer for humans, the question is partly answered for hamsters. Using *cfos* visualization of neural activity, it is known that many neurons in the amygdala that are aroused by aggressive encounters are also aroused by sexual activity.[61]

Although there is no longer much dispute that, in most natural circumstances, males are more aggressive than females (with a few exceptions, such as spotted hyenas), the brain mechanisms for this difference have only recently been revealed. Testosterone has powerful effects on the expression of several brain neurochemical systems. The most extensively studied is the neuropeptide arginine-vasopressin (AVP). There are extensive AVP-based systems in the brain; major nuclei are situated in the anterior hypothalamus, with projections to the hippocampus, septal areas, and downward through the diencephalon, to the midbrain PAG (see Figure 6.7).[62]

Testosterone sustains the genetic expression of AVP in a large number of these circuits. Accordingly, males have more extensive vasopressinergic circuits than females.[63] When male rats are castrated, AVP is markedly reduced in approximately half of their vasopressinergic circuits. This is paralleled by a decline in both sexuality and aggressiveness.[64] If one replaces testosterone directly into the brain via microinjections into the appropriate hypothalamic tissues, these behavioral tendencies return. Several experiments have now directly manipulated the AVP systems, revealing that elevating AVP levels by direct central administration increases intermale aggression in rats.[65] In hamsters, centrally administered AVP markedly increases territorial marking behavior, even in the absence of other males.[66] If one places an AVP receptor antagonist into the brain, both of these behavioral tendencies are markedly reduced.[67] Thus, it would seem that AVP is certainly one factor that promotes intermale aggression; as we will see in Chapter 12, it is also a powerful factor in promoting male sexuality and the formation of social memories. Thus, we can speculate that a molecule such as AVP that can facilitate intermale aggression may only do so because it increases a more generalized male tendency such as behavioral persistence—the relentless and single-minded pursuit of a goal. Clearly, we have much more to learn about this aggressive system in the brain that plays a key role in the elaboration of social dominance. At an affective level, we might expect that the initial motivation for intermale aggression is positive, since both combatants readily enter the fray; it is only later, when frustration occurs and defeat is imminent, that more negative emotions begin to intervene. There is a distinct possibility that brain systems that mediate social play (see Chapter 15) are highly interrelated with intermale aggression systems, which would be another reason for seeking linkages to positive affect within intermale aggression circuits.

Although testosterone can clearly increase intermale aggression, we should also briefly consider how those processes relate to RAGE circuits. Although evidence is sparse, the present supposition is that they are largely independent but highly interactive systems. It is possible that testosterone modulates activity in the RAGE system in a way quite comparable to its effects on the intermale aggression systems,[68] but the evidence is not definitive. There is little reason to believe that testosterone promotes anger independently of its effects on male assertiveness and the potential conflicts and problems that can lead to. Intermale aggression is an ideal behavioral circumstance where anger could be evoked. Because of such interactions, we cannot be certain that testosterone is directly sensitizing RAGE circuits. For instance, human studies have not provided unambiguous evidence that testosterone increases feelings of irritability. Indeed, some recent human work indicates that testosterone administration does not facilitate such feelings, and human males given supplementary testosterone typically tend to feel better than those who received placebos.[69]

Learning and Aggression

As with any emotional system, a great deal of aggressive behavior is learned. Animals can be trained to be more aggressive or more passive. They can be trained to be winners or losers.[70] However, it is remarkable how the hormones that promote intermale aggression also provide feedback and reinforce the learning of status. One series of recent findings has shown that victory in a variety of forms leads to increased secretion of testosterone in male animals as well as humans. In humans, such victories as the completion of law or medical school or military training increase plasma testosterone levels.[71] Victory on the tennis court can have the same effect.[72] To what extent these hormone changes help reinforce future assertive behavior remains to be evaluated, but it would come as no surprise if the neurophysiological solidification of assertiveness was the end result.

Of course, many antiaggressive factors also influence the brain. The "female hormones" estrogen and progesterone have been found to exert antiaggressive effects,[73] and it is known that the pleasures of touch and sexuality can inhibit certain types of aggressive tendencies.[74] Perhaps the most striking example of inhibition has been found with infanticide, a form of sex-related aggression.[75] Males of many species will harm young animals already present in a new territory to which they wish to lay claim. This is an evolutionarily adaptive strategy. By eliminating lactation-induced infertility, infanticide increases the probability that new males will be able to rapidly fertilize available females, producing offspring of their own. At the same time, males should have natural evolutionarily derived inhibitions against harming their own offspring.

To evaluate this possibility, investigators monitored the pup-killing habits of male rats as a function of copulatory experiences.[76] It was reasoned that if males were given a chance to mate, they might reveal an inborn system that diminishes the likelihood that they will kill their own offspring at some future point in time. Considering that female rats have a three-week gestational period, it was anticipated that the pup-killing tendencies of males might diminish approximately three weeks after mating, at about the time their own offspring might be born. That, in fact, was what happened (Figure 10.7). While males exhibited about 80% infanticide at the

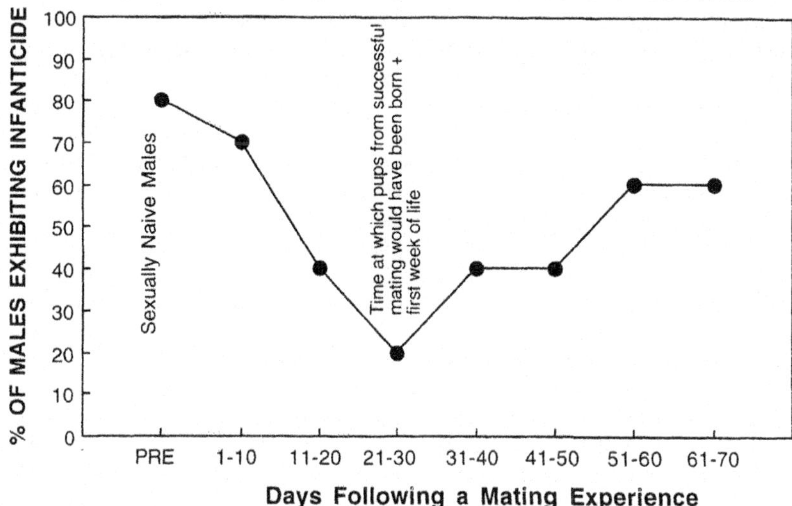

Figure 10.7. The percentage of male rats exhibiting infanticide on a weekly basis following one sexual encounter. (Adapted from Mennella & Holtz, 1988; see n. 76.)

beginning of testing, they gradually diminished to 20% at the three-week time point and then gradually returned to original levels. This points to a specific form of sociosexual memory: Male rats seem to "recognize," on the basis of their own prior sexual activity, which pups are likely to be their own offspring.

Although it has not been demonstrated which brain changes register this type of memory that promotes peaceful coexistence, a reasonable candidate is the gradual induction of oxytocin in the brain. This hormone, which is more prevalent in females than males (see Chapter 12), promotes nurturant behavior (see Chapter 13). Not only is it known to be an effective antiaggressive agent,[77] but it can be increased in the brains of male rodents by preceding sexual activity (see Chapter 12). If similar mechanisms exist in humans, the knowledge might have important implications for the discussion of sociosexual policies and politics.

Although females generally exhibit less infanticidal behavior than males, it is certainly not absent, but it often serves a different function. A mother may kill and consume some of her own offspring if food is scarce, even though such killing can also occur for more subtle "political" reasons. Perhaps the most famous perpetrators of such acts were the cruel female chimpanzees, Passion and her daughter Pom, who killed off at least three and probably more of the young infants of other females in the group that Jane Goodal studied for many years.[78]

Although learning controls many forms of aggression, is it important in the mediation of rage? Unfortunately, there is practically no work on the issue since animal models of angry behavior remain poorly developed—partly because most investigators are not willing to study angry animals and partly because it is somewhat difficult to bring anger under systematic laboratory control. Perhaps the best approach has been to analyze the biting tendencies of organisms that are confronted by frustration induced by reward reductions.[79]

In lieu of critical data, we can only speculate. I would suggest that the classical conditioning of anger should proceed readily. If one pairs certain neutral stimuli with the unconditional response of anger, one would expect that conditioned anger responses would emerge rapidly. Perhaps one of the best ways to do this would be using electrical stimulation of the relevant brain circuits, but to my knowledge, no work along these lines has yet been done. If it were to work, it would be a useful model to analyze how trigger points for anger develop in the nervous system. This would allow us to understand, both pharmacologically and behaviorally, how to reverse or minimize the development of such excessive sensitivities.

Pharmacology and the Neurochemistry of Aggression

One of the most difficult psychiatric problems is aggression. Before the era of psychotropic drugs, it was not unusual for newly admitted patients to arrive at psychiatric hospitals in straitjackets or other restraints to prevent them from hurting themselves and others. Antipsychotic drugs discovered in the early 1950s, such as chlorpromazine, were rapidly found to be quite effective antiaggressive agents, but only at high doses. The effects were largely due to sedation arising from global reduction of brain catecholamine activity. Although a variety of newer and more specific antipsychotic drugs can now be used to reduce violent behaviors, they are still little more than chemical straitjackets. To this day there is no highly specific way to treat pathological anger pharmacologically.[80]

However, there are now many drugs that can reduce various forms of aggression in animal models,[81] and some of them may be effective against pathological anger. Most prominent among the current generation of antiaggressive drugs are those that promote the activity of the serotonin, gamma-aminobutyric acid (GABA), opioid, and oxytocin systems of the brain. The opiate receptor stimulants exert an especially powerful inhibitory effect on various forms of aggression, which may be partly due to their ability to promote pleasurable feelings of satisfaction and general well-being (see Chapter 9), but it is unlikely that this system can be harnessed for useful medical purposes because of the addictiveness of opiates.

Indeed, opiate addiction gradually strengthens a variety of physiological "opponent processes," which tend to counteract the high levels of opiates in the body. Because of the release of these opponent processes during opiate withdrawal, irritability and impulsive aggression can be dramatically increased. This is one reason that opiate addicts undergoing withdrawal have a heightened tendency to initiate violent acts. Of course, as long as they have opiates in their systems, the tendency to exhibit aggression remains very low. Should society recognized this "Catch-22" when it wages various wars against drug abuse? Whose fault is it if an opiate addict in withdrawal has no legal source of drugs to reduce irritability and becomes aggressive in an effort to obtain such agents? The answer is not obvious.

It is not yet clear which brain neurochemistries promote anger, but one neuropeptide, substance P, may be a key modulator in the RAGE system. Angry displays elicited by brain stimulation can be increased by brain infusions of substance P and they can be reduced with substance P antagonists.[82] Perhaps an orally administered substance P antagonist, or some other peptide receptor antagonist, can one day be used as an antiaggressive agent in clinical practice. If so, it will be because human anger has been studied through the analysis of RAGE systems in the animal brain.

Which system is most likely to provide a medically useful antiaggressive drug at the present time? Among the biogenic amines, both norepinephrine (NE) and serotonin (5-HT) control anger, the first tending to increase it because of general arousal effects and the second reducing it, just as it controls every other emotional response. Clinically, it has been found that drugs that block the ß-NE receptors, such as propranolol, are clinically useful antiaggressive agents. Unfortunately, the overall efficacy of such ß-blockers has not been as uniform as desired, and serotonin has been the focus of the most intense efforts to yield better agents that are desperately needed.

Eltoprazine, a serotonin receptor agonist that acts specifically on the 5-HT-1A receptor, has emerged during the past decade as a very specific antiaggressive agent. It is one of a number of drugs called *serenics*. Eltoprazine and related drugs are effective in reducing virtually every form of aggression that has been studied in the laboratory, but it is no longer on the fast track for general medical use.[83] Not only does eltoprazine decrease aggression without any sedation, but it actually increases other friendly and social exploratory behaviors (Figure 10.8). Dissection of the precise mode of action of this drug has indicated that the antiaggressive effects are due to *postsynaptic* 5-HT receptor activity, while the pro-social effects are due to *presynaptic* inhibition of serotonin cell bodies, both being mediated by the same type of 5-HT-1A receptor.[84] In other words, eltoprazine reduces aggression by facilitating brain serotonin receptor activity in higher limbic circuits, but increases social interactions by reducing serotonin neuronal activity throughout the brain.

However, the increase in social interaction resulting from decreased serotonin is found only in well-socialized animals. Across different strains of rodents, aggressiveness produced by prolonged social isolation is highly correlated to isolation-induced decreases in brain serotonin activity,[85] and serotonin supplementation can decrease aggression in animals that have become irritable because of long-term social isolation.[86] In general, reduced brain serotonin activity also tends to increase impulsive and acting-out forms of behavior in humans.[87] A higher tendency toward delinquency has been observed in human males who have low serotonin activity (as indexed by low cerebrospinal fluid levels of the serotonin metabolite 5-HIAA).[88] Such evidence suggests that the same neurochemical dynamics known to control animal aggression may also control human criminality and social assertiveness.

Conversely, socially dominant animals, who can control aggression with a glance, have been found to have high brain serotonin activity. Indeed, monkeys tend to climb higher in their dominance hierarchies following long-term treatment with drugs such as the selective serotonin reuptake inhibitors (SSRIs), which increase serotonin availability in the brain.[89] In sum, many serotonin-promoting drugs, as well as other agents, can provide inhibitory control of aggression.[90] But specific antianger agents will have to emerge from our understanding of the specific brain modulators that promote RAGE in the brain, in the way that AVP seems to promote intermale aggression.

The neurochemical systems that have been found to promote aggression are less numerous than those that reduce it. In addition to the work on substance P mentioned earlier, the two best candidates for specifically promoting the impulse of anger are glutamate and acetylcholine. One can provoke defensive hissing by ad-

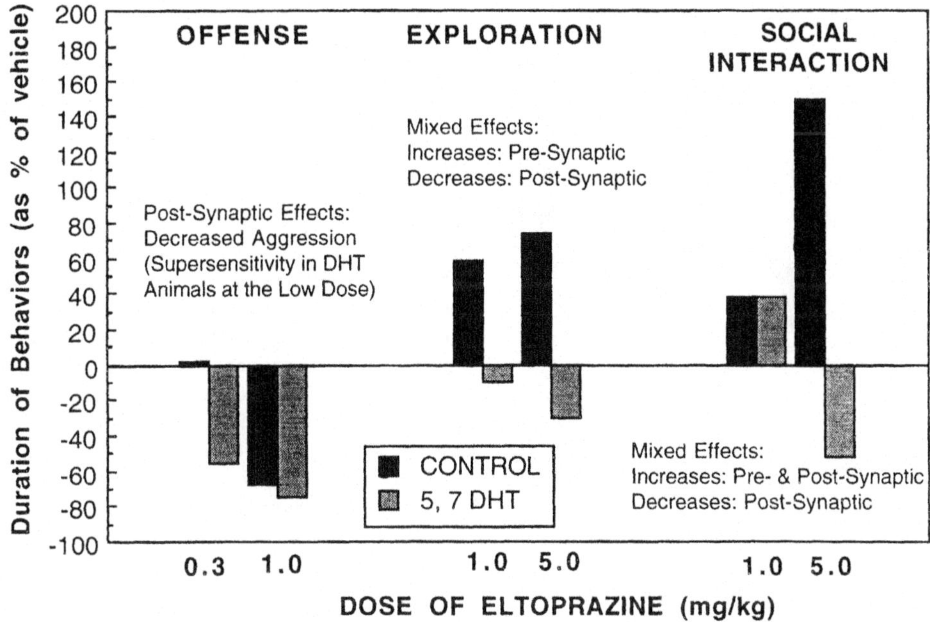

Figure 10.8. Dose-response effects of eltoprazine on offense, exploration, and social interest in normal rats and those whose midbrain serotonin neurons had been destroyed with the selective 5-HT neurotoxin 5,7-dihydroxytryptamine (5,7-DHT). (Adapted from Olivier et al., 1991; see n. 83.)

ministering cholinergic agonists into those regions of the brain where ESB has been found to provoke rage,[91] but it is possible that this hissing response is merely an alarm-fear response rather than an angry one.[92] A somewhat clearer effect is obtained following localized glutamate administration into specific areas of the brain.[93] From this one might conclude that glutamate antagonists or acetylcholine antagonists will prove to be excellent antiaggressive agents. Unfortunately, because of the participation of these transmitters in so many brain processes, there is little hope that their manipulation will ever provide clinically useful antianger/antiaggression agents.[94] Clearly, the most important neuromodulators for the instigation of rage have not yet been definitively identified.

In any event, existing evidence suggests that mammalian anger emerges from a homologous RAGE circuit that has been remarkably conserved during mammalian brain evolution. Accordingly, a cross-species comparison has a greater potential to reveal neurobiological sources of human anger than any other strategy that is presently available. Of course, this will tell us little about the cognitive sources of anger in humans. It will only tell us how the feeling of anger emerges from specific brain activities. Also, because aggression is such a multidimensional phenomenon, considerable insight will be needed to develop models of anger and aggression that are reasonably pure and distinct from the multifaceted mixtures of aggression and fear that one normally sees in nature.

In conjunction with data summarized in the next chapter, we now know that circuits for aggression and fear overlap in many areas of the brain, including areas extending from the anterior hypothalamus to the PAG. Thus, one of the easiest aggressive responses that can be elicited with brain stimulation in cats is a hissing-defensive response with no attack (see Figure 10.9). Although this type of response could be interpreted as supporting the existence of a distinct "defense system" within the brain,[95] at present the most parsimonious conclusion is that such defense responses arise from the concurrent stimulation of two distinct but highly overlapping and interactive emotional systems, namely, those of RAGE and FEAR. This second emotional system will be the focus of the next chapter.

AFTERTHOUGHT: Autonomic and Cerebellar Control of Rage

The outdated James-Lange theory (see "Afterthought," Chapter 3) suggested that peripheral autonomic effects that feed back onto the thinking brain create our experience of emotions. Although the modern view is that emotional circuits within the visceral brain coordinate affective processes, there are certainly many feedback

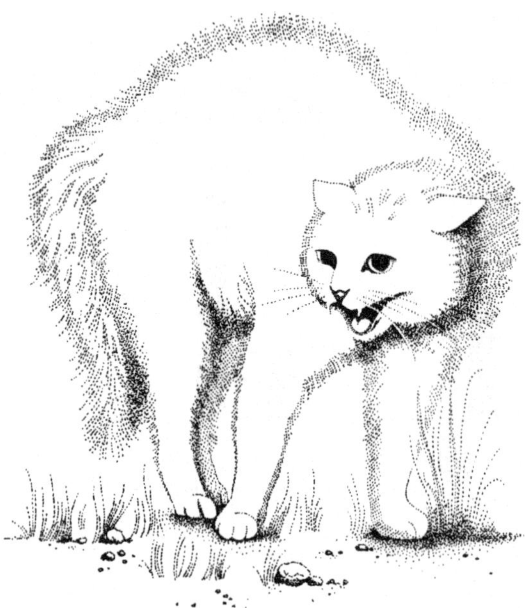

Figure 10.9. Brain stimulation–induced defensive behavior, which may reflect a mixture of simultaneous activation of ANGER and FEAR systems. (Adapted from a photograph by Walter Hess.)

relationships between the relevant peripheral and central processes. For instance, while centrally induced anger increases blood pressure, the arterial detectors for blood pressure changes (i.e., the baroreceptors in the carotid arteries) can modify the sensitivity of the RAGE circuit. As mentioned earlier, if we artificially increase blood pressure, it is easier to evoke angry behavior in cats by hypothalamic stimulation. Thus, we must remember that the actual brain mechanisms that control anger are complex, are under multiple physiological, neuroanatomical, and neurochemical controls, and are only roughly understood. Many details of this emotional system remain to be revealed, and many surprises are bound to emerge from future research.

For instance, one of the most intriguing recent findings is that knockout mice, which are lacking the gene for nitric oxide synthetase (NOS), exhibit high levels of violent behavior and hypersexuality.[96] However, this psychopathic tendency, presumably caused by reduced brain levels of the gaseous transmitter nitric oxide (NO), is evident only in male rats, and the finding was totally serendipitous. Because of past data implicating NO in learning, the experiment was being conducted to evaluate the role of genetic deletion of the enzymatic machinery needed for NO synthesis on memory. As it turned out, these animals, missing one form of NOS, exhibited normal learning. The tendency of such NOS-deficient animals to be aggressive was discovered only because animal caretakers noted that many of the animals were dying with injuries on their bodies. It turned out that only the males were killers; they were also hypersexual, with an apparent reduced ability to understand the meaning of "NO."

Will such knowledge help us deal better with human violence, a most serious social problem? Most think it is unlikely that our society can implement biological interventions for such matters of personal conduct, but new possibilities for biological control are bound to emerge. They will pose enormous ethical problems for future generations, unless we can teach individuals who have aggressive "hair triggers" to voluntarily utilize pharmacological or other aids to control their negativistic urges. Indeed, there are also bound to be nonpharmacological interventions to control aggression, ranging from meditation to the well-established effects of castration and new forms of brain stimulation. Let me focus on the last of these options.

One of the most unusual ways that violent tendencies have ever been controlled in the annals of medicine is by cerebellar stimulation. Although the cerebellum was long believed to simply control motor coordination, it is now known to contribute to attentional and emotional processes as well. This emerging knowledge was utilized by one daring and controversial neurosurgeon, Robert Heath, to control violent pathological aggression. Electrical stimulation was applied to the cerebellum via a plate electrode implanted at the back of the head (over the cerebellum), and the whole contraption was given the provocative name "cerebellar pacemaker."[97] Of course, this radical maneuver was attempted only in seriously ill individuals whose aggressive outbursts could not be controlled by any other means, including high doses of heavily sedating antipsychotic drugs.

Heath reported remarkable success in reducing the irritability of such individuals with his "cerebellar pacemaker." Folks who had been totally incapacitated by their persistent violent thoughts and impulses, could now lead peaceful lives. How this strange therapy works is still unknown, but there are sites in the most ancient part of the cerebellum (in the deep cerebellar nuclei, such as the *fastigial* and *interpositus*) where one can elicit aggressive tendencies with ESB.[98] Maybe just like the cerebral cortex, which tends to provide chronic inhibition over subcortical processes, the neocerebellar cortex exerts a similar effect on its deep nuclei, and Heath's "cerebellar pacemaker" facilitates that effect.

Now that new procedures have been developed to activate the brain through the application of intense magnetic fields several inches outside the head (i.e., via rapid transcranial magnetic stimulation [rTMS]; see Chapters 5 and 16), the day may soon arrive when such procedures will become an accepted part of psychiatric practice.[99] Already, several investigators have had considerable success using this noninvasive rTMS approach to alleviate drug-resistant depressions.[100] It is widely believed that this fairly gentle form of brain stimulation will eventually replace electroconvulsive therapy (ECT) as a treatment for those depressed individuals who do not respond to the many new medications that have recently become available during this "Age of SSRIs."[101] Will someone eventually construct an antiaggression chair, where the back of the headrest contains a magnetic stimulator that is able to change underlying cerebellar activity to such an extent that one's impulsive urges melt away as if by magic? If such a useful device is constructed, it should be used only with a clear recognition that anger, at a cognitive level, may be not only a destructive but a useful force in society.

Although affective neuroscience research can provide us with a substantive knowledge of the experience of anger, it cannot explicate the cultural, environmental, and cognitive causes of aggression. In humans, it is usually the appraisal of events that triggers anger; obviously, many values upon which appraisals are premised are culturally learned in humans. For instance, presently many humans are angry at others for the views they hold about abortion, capital punishment, and innumerable other sociopolitical issues. With sufficient depth of personality, the psychic energy of human anger can be diverted into outrageously creative or constructive efforts. Where would we be today if our ancestors had not had the passion to say: "Give me liberty or give me death." Psychobiology presently has little of importance to say about the many cognitive components of human anger, especially the firey human energies that help change societies.

Suggested Readings

Averill, J. R., (1982). *Anger and aggression: An essay on emotion.* New York: Springer-Verlag.

Dollard, J., Miller, N. E., Doob, L. W., Mowrer, O. H., & Sears, R. R. (1939). *Frustration and aggression.* New Haven, Conn.: Yale Univ. Press.

Johnson, R. N. (1972). *Aggression in man and animals.* Philadelphia: Saunders.

Miczek, K. A. (ed.) (1981). *The psychopharmacology of aggression and social behavior.* Special issue of *Pharmacology Biochemistry and Behavior* 14 (suppl. 1). Fayettesville, N.Y.: ANKHO International.

Moyer, K. E. (1976). *The psychobiology of aggression.* New York: Harper and Row.

Olivier, B., Mos, J., & Brain, P. F. (eds.) (1987). *Ethopharmacology of agonistic behaviour in animals and humans.* Dordrecht: Martinus Nijhoff.

Scott, J. P. (1958). *Aggression.* Chicago: Univ. of Chicago Press.

Svare, B. B. (ed.) (1983). *Hormones and aggressive behavior.* New York: Plenum Press.

Valzelli, L. (1981). *Psychobiology of aggression and violence.* New York: Raven Press.

Valzelli, L., & Morgese, I. (eds.) (1981). *Aggression and violence: A psychobiological and clinical approach.* Milan: Edizioni Centro Culturale E. Congressi Saint Vincent.

11

The Sources of Fear and Anxiety in the Brain

Fear produces an agony and anxiety about the heart not to be described; and it may be said to paralyze the soul in such a manner, that it becomes insensible to every thing but to its own misery. . . . When the effects of fear operate powerfully, without any mixture of hope, these passive impressions are predominant but where there is a possibility of escape, the mind re-acts with wonderful energy . . . enabling the sufferer to precipitate his flight, by exertions that would have been impracticable in a more composed state of mind.

T. Cogan, *On the Passions* (1802)

CENTRAL THEME

Contrary to traditional thinking on the topic, which taught that fears simply reflect *learned anticipation* of harmful events, it now appears that the potential for fear is a genetically ingrained function of the nervous system. This should come as no surprise. An organism's ability to perceive and anticipate dangers was of such obvious importance during evolution that it was not simply left to the vagaries of individual learning. Even though learning is essential for animals to utilize their fear systems effectively in the real world, learning does not create fear by pasting together a variety of external experiences. Evolution created several coherently operating neural systems that help orchestrate and coordinate perceptual, behavioral, and physiological changes that promote survival in the face of danger. The emotional experience of fear appears to arise from a conjunction of neural processes that prompt animals to hide (freeze) if danger is distant or inescapable, or to flee when danger is close but can be avoided. To understand the deep experiential nature of fear in humans, we must probe the genetically ingrained neural components that mediate homologous fearful states in other mammals. Our understanding of the neurobiology of human fears has emerged largely from basic research on the brains of "lower" animals. These investigations indicate that the capacity to experience fear, along with fear-typical patterns of autonomic and behavioral arousal, emerges primarily from a FEAR circuit that courses between the central amygdala and the periaqueductal gray of the midbrain. Fear behaviors can be evoked by artificially activating this circuit, and conditioned fears can be developed by pairing neutral stimuli with unconditional stimuli, such as electric shock, that can arouse this emotional system. In other words, conditioned fears emerge by neutral stimuli gaining access to this system via learning. Higher cortical processes are not necessary for the activation of learned fears, although those processes refine the types of perceptions that can instigate fear. The neurochemistries that control this emotional system include excitatory amino acids such as glutamate and a variety of neuropeptides (e.g., CRF, α-MSH, ACTH, CCK, and DBI), each of which may eventually be found to instigate slightly different anxieties—for instance, fear of pain, fear of heights, fear of predators. Minor tranquilizers of the benzodiazepine (BZ) class act by partially dampening activity in this emotional system, through GABA-mediated neural inhibition. Other antianxiety drugs such as buspirone are able to attenuate anxiety in totally different ways, such as by modifying serotonin sensitivity in the brain. New agents—for instance, those that inhibit cholecystokinin (CCK) and other neuropeptide receptor systems (especially CRF) as well as those that stimulate neuropeptide Y and oxytocin systems—show considerable promise of yielding a new generation of antianxiety agents. Others are bound to follow as our knowledge of the FEAR system becomes complete.

On the Characteristics of Fear

One of the most horrible experiences of life is to be stricken by sudden terror. Another is to be continually consumed by the persistent feelings of anxiety that gnaw away at you, destroying your sense of security in the world. It is likely that the affective impact of both experiences emerges ultimately from the differential arousal of one and the same brain system—a coherently operating FEAR circuit that produces terror when precipitously aroused and chronic anxiety during milder, more sustained arousal. The FEAR system can be activated by various world events, as well as by internal ones. External stimuli that have consistently threatened the survival of a species during evolutionary history often develop the ability to unconditionally arouse brain fear systems. For instance, laboratory rats exhibit fear responses (increased freezing and inhibition of other motivated behaviors) to the smell of cats and other predators (see Figure 1.1), even though they have never encountered such creatures in their lives, having grown up in the safety of a controlled laboratory setting (for more on the underlying neural mechanisms, see the "Afterthought" of this chapter).

In addition to such inborn tendencies, a variety of specific anxieties can be acquired during the life span of each individual. These are usually triggered by specific external events that have been paired with pain or other threatening stimuli, but it is important to recall that feelings of fear can also emerge simply from the internal dynamics of the brain (so-called free-floating anxieties). Internal stimuli that can arouse the FEAR system range from irritative epileptic foci in the limbic system to conscious as well as unconscious memories of past occurrences. Although a neural circuit coursing between the central amygdala and the periaqueductal gray (PAG) of the midbrain has now been well established as a major FEAR circuit, it remains possible, even likely, that there are multiple neural systems that can make us afraid. We do not yet have an accepted neural taxonomy of various fears, but I will address some possibilities.

Although feelings of fear are as hard to define as they are to measure directly, most people have a natural understanding of what it means to be afraid. For those who do not, imagine an archetypal situation. You are alone in the woods, in the darkness of night, lost and with little confidence in your ability to find the way out. The moon filters through racing clouds on the heels of a chilly wind. The branches above sway menacingly. Your imagination runs wild with the archetypal monsters and demons that populated the fantasy landscape of your childhood imagination. Suddenly, a branch cracks and falls behind you. You exhibit a reflexive startle much larger than you would have made to the same sound in the safety of your backyard; this is due to the potentiating effect of the background fear. After this intense reaction, you hold very still for a moment, frozen in one position, as your mind fills with dread, all your senses riveted on the perceived source of the noise. Your cognitive processes are rapidly analyzing sundry imagined and real possibilities. If this analysis attributes the sound to a mythical werewolf or a real mountain lion, you may explode into a vigorous flight pattern, running faster than you thought your legs could ever carry you. If you are fortunate enough to find a momentary place of perceived safety (perhaps an abandoned cabin in the woods), you will hide, tremble, with heart throbbing (not just from your physical exertions); you remain alert for a long time in a cold sweat as you vigilantly evaluate each new environmental stimulus. You may have wet your pants, or worse, along the way.

Fortunately, at daybreak you find your way out. On future occasions you will be more careful not to get lost again. You may dream about the episode for several nights. Had you encountered truly frightful events such as sustained wartime battles, then mixtures of fear and anger would incubate in the neural substrates of your psyche for years to come, until you might develop what is called a post-traumatic stress disorder. Even though many higher cortical perceptions sustained and exacerbated your fears, to the best of our knowledge, the resulting chronic hyperemotional state is created by deep subcortical networks that can become sensitized and can operate independently of your higher cognitive faculties. For this reason, long-lasting fears and anxieties can lead to chronic psychological distress that does not always respond well to standard cognitive therapies.

Experientially, fear is an aversive state of the nervous system, characterized by apprehensive worry, general nervousness, and tension, which tells creatures that their safety is threatened. It is accompanied by specific forms of autonomic and behavioral arousal. The most common clinical symptom of fear is generalized anxiety. The current *Diagnostic and Statistical Manual* (*DSM-IV*) of the American Psychiatric Association offers standard criteria for generalized anxiety that include a variety of psychological symptoms, such as uncontrollable apprehensive expectations, with jumpiness and a tendency for excessive vigilance and fidgeting. The various autonomic symptoms include frequent tendencies for gastrointestinal disturbances, including upset stomach, diarrhea, and frequent urination, as well as other visceral symptoms like tachycardia, chronic dryness of the mouth, and increased but shallow respiration.[1] Some individuals who have anxiety problems complain more about physical symptoms, while for others psychological anguish is the prevailing concern.

Where in the brain is the array of fear responses organized? Obviously, the overall neural control is complex, including many cognitive analyzers as well as autonomic and somatic-motor circuits. Most of the brain is involved. However, there are distinct sites in the brain where electrical stimulation will provoke a full fear response in all mammalian species, and these are locations where the executive system for FEAR is concentrated.[2] These are in the lateral and central zones of the amygdala, the anterior and medial hypothalamus, and, most clearly (and at the lowest current levels), within specific PAG areas of the midbrain. Of course, this highly interconnected network interacts with the many other emotional systems discussed in this book, especially RAGE circuits (which contribute to the balance between fight and flight reactions), as well as the behaviorally nonspecific chemistries of the brain such as norepinephrine and serotonin. My aim is not to assess all the components of a global fear response but rather to summarize information on what we know of the central FEAR system.[3]

At present, the precise manner in which fears and anxieties are created by brain tissue remains a matter of intense debate and inquiry. But the original idea that captivated psychology—that fear is simply a conditioned response to the cues that predict pain—is no longer tenable. Although pain is an especially effective stimulus for creating fear and generating learned fears, it does not constitute fear itself. To the best of our present knowledge, fear—the subjective experience of dread, along with the characteristic set of bodily changes—emerges from the aforementioned circuit, which interdigitates extensively with the RAGE circuit. In the amygdala, however, the two systems are fairly clearly segregated, with FEAR being more lateral and RAGE more medial. As mentioned, the FEAR circuit courses from the lateral and central nuclei of the amygdala, through the ventral-anterior and medial hypothalamic areas, down to the mesencephalic PAG (Figure 11.1). Freezing, as well as flight behavior and the autonomic indices of fear (e.g., increased heart rate and eliminative behavior), can be evoked along the whole trajectory of this system.[4]

It makes good evolutionary sense for FEAR and RAGE circuits to be intimately related, for one of the functions of anger is to provoke fear in competitors, and one of the functions of fear is to reduce the impact of angry behaviors from threatening opponents. Although it has not been empirically demonstrated, it is reasonable to suppose that at low levels of arousal, the two systems are mutually inhibitory (see Figure 3.5). At very sudden or intense levels of arousal, however, both the fear response and the rage response may be concurrently aroused. Of course, the existence of a major FEAR system does not preclude the existence of other systems that may mediate other forms of alarm and trepidation. Indeed, as we will see in Chapter 14, separation anxiety emerges largely from brain systems other than the FEAR circuit. For clinical reasons detailed there, I have chosen to call it a PANIC system.

Since mild fear is characterized largely by behavioral inhibition components, while intense fear is commonly characterized by active flight, it is important to consider how these diametrically different response tendencies might be elaborated by the FEAR system. By carefully following the behavioral responses evoked by different intensities of stimulation, it has become clear that one can promote freezing during mild arousal of this system and flight at higher stimulation intensities (Figure 11.2). Whether the shift in response tenden-

Trajectory of a Trans-hypothalamic FEAR System

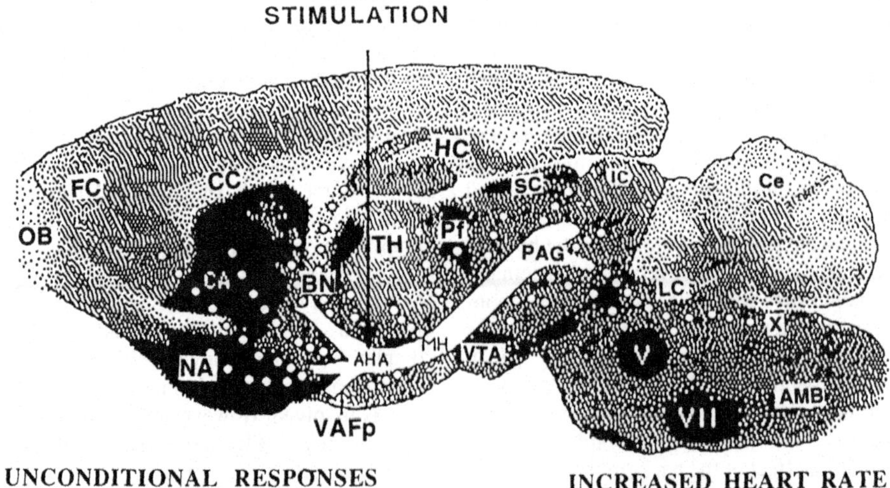

Figure 11.1. Schematic summary of the trajectory of the FEAR system and the various symptoms induced by stimulation of the system. (Adapted from Panksepp, 1990; see n. 2.)

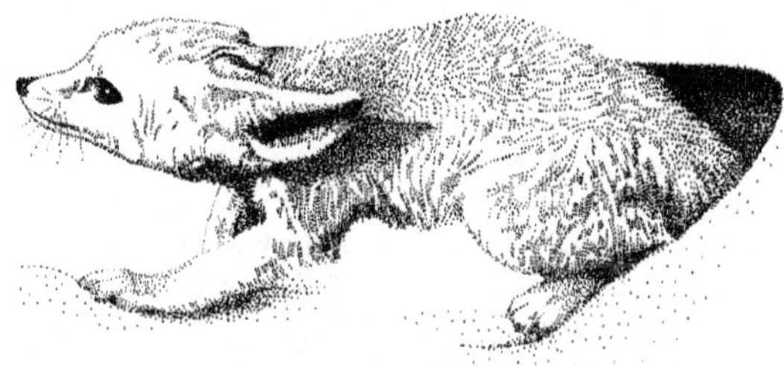

Figure 11.2. Artist's rendition of the type of freezing behavior that can be generated by mild stimulation of the FEAR system. (Adapted from a photograph in Panksepp, 1989; see n. 5.)

cies is organized by different subcomponents of the FEAR system at the stimulation electrode site or the different response characteristics are generated by differential outputs at the aroused synaptic fields downstream from the stimulation is presently unresolved. However, it does seem possible that both of these fear responses are governed by the same basic emotional system within the brain.

Before proceeding with a discussion of the major amygdalo-hypothalamo-mesencephalic FEAR circuit, it will be helpful to present an overview of the vast number of animal models of anxiety that have been developed by behaviorists over the past few decades. Most of the preclinical pharmacological work aimed at identifying and developing new antianxiety agents is emerging from the systematic analysis of such animal models. It is not yet clear how each of these models relates to arousal of the FEAR system versus other negative emotional systems of the brain. The many inconsistencies in the literature may eventually be resolved by an appropriate taxonomy of brain circuits that mediate anxiety. Since this has not yet been achieved, and since most of the available animal models remain to be linked to specific neural circuits, the existing literature may give an impression of chaos and incoherence. But we can at least summarize the diversity of models in a systematic way, and thereby focus on the most promising lines of future inquiry.

Preclinical Models for the Study of Fear

In contrast to the paucity of natural animal models for anger, there is an overabundance of models for fear. This probably reflects the widespread recognition that fear responses are learned readily and that they have distressing consequences for the lives of many people. The various preclinical laboratory models for the study of anxiety can be conveniently broken down into those that use painful stimuli to produce symptoms of anxiety (i.e., via use of punishment procedures) and those that use no explicit punishment. In addition, each of these categories includes several models to analyze changes in learned fears and others to measure unconditional, or instinctual, fear behaviors, yielding four types of models, as summarized in Table 11.1.

Although most of these models are quite sensitive to the effects of minor tranquilizers (which are typically called antianxiety agents), suggesting that they share common affective features, a conceptual problem runs through much of the literature on this topic. Antianxiety effects are generally *assumed* to exist when previously punished behaviors are released from inhibition, but such effects can be explained in several ways: Animals may be less anxious, or they may simply be more impulsive and disinhibited. The second alternative was rarely considered in earlier discussions of how animal models can relate to our understanding of human anxiety.[5]

Another problem is that there are so many differences in formal procedures and drug sensitivities among the various experimental models that it is not yet possible to argue for a common anxiety process that underlies all of them. There are also no accepted guidelines regarding which models are the best predictors for which specific anxiety-related disorders in humans and why. Accordingly, the literature may actually be describing many different types of fears or different ways in which the brain handles one type of fear. Although I

Table 11.1. A Taxonomy of Animal Models of Fear

	With Punishment	No Punishment
Learned	Active avoidance tasks Conditioned emotional responses Punished behavior tasks Passive avoidance tasks	Partial reinforcement extinction effect
Spontaneous	Freezing to shock Defensive burying Stimulation of fear circuits Responses to loud sounds (startle)	Open-field exploration Avoidance of bright lights Social-interaction tests Plus-maze test Predatory odors

will not attempt to contrast and compare these models, I will provide a systematic organizational scheme that may help us visualize how the various models interrelate (Table 11.1). The models will be divided into those that use punishment and those that do not, and also according to those that require learning and those that do not.

Quadrant 1 (learned tasks with imposed punishments): The first models that were used to study fear simply measured an animal's tendency to learn new responses to escape and avoid aversive stimuli such as foot shock (which is usually administered through metal rods that constituted the cage flooring). Many of these models were widely implemented by pharmaceutical firms for evaluating the potential antianxiety effects of new drugs. It turned out that these specific models were not especially sensitive to antianxiety agents, probably because, by the time investigators tested their drugs, the learned behavior had become so efficient that test animals no longer experienced much fear. Subsequent models tried to circumvent such problems by establishing stable baselines of learned approach behaviors, on which fears could be imposed via classical conditioning principles (the so-called conditioned emotional response [CER] procedures).[6] Such designs turned out to be much more sensitive to the effects of minor tranquilizers.

Models of this type first conditioned anxiety in experimental animals by systematically pairing environmental cues with aversive events, after which investigators evaluated the effectiveness of those cues in suppressing various appetitive behaviors. For example, the readiness of hungry rats to press levers for food would be measured during baseline periods, as well as during presentation of the fear stimuli. When the danger cue was presented, an internal state of anxiety presumably was produced, and the degree of behavioral inhibition was used as an operational measure of the anxiety. Such CER tasks were most effective when the cue-shock pairings were administered directly upon the appetitive baselines. Eventually such behavioral inhibition tasks were further simplified by using spontaneous consummatory baselines, such as voluntary feeding and drinking, which were periodically accompanied by cue-contingent or even uncontingent administration of foot shock, yielding a very direct measure of the amount of behavior an animal was willing to emit while expecting and receiving mild punishment. If the shock was contingent on an animal making a specific consummatory response, it was considered to be a punishment task. Of course, in this last model the only learning consisted of the animal's presumed realization that it would be punished if it exhibited consummatory behavior.

A variant of this model involved placing animals in well-lit arenas, with immediate administration of shock when they entered an accessible dark hole or, alternatively, when they stepped down from a safe perch. In such circumstances, animals typically exhibit much longer latencies for their spontaneous avoidance behaviors on the second trial if they have already been punished for their efforts on the first trial, yielding "passive avoidance" measures that presumably reflect the behavior-inhibiting effects of anxiety. In other words, a smart animal that has received a shock when stepping to the floor has "second thoughts" about taking such a step the next time. Of course, these models do not readily distinguish between the effects of pharmacological and physiological manipulations on memory processes as opposed to emotional ones. For instance, drugs may evoke amnesia in the animals. A variety of additional controls are needed to evaluate those issues.

Perhaps the most effective model of this type, one that has now been extensively exploited, employs what is called a "potentiated startle." Animals and humans show a characteristic startle response to sudden loud sounds. The vigor of the startle reflex (whose neural details have been worked out and will be discussed later) is increased markedly by concurrent exposure to a classically conditioned fear stimulus (i.e., a light that previously had been paired with electric foot shock). Indeed, the potentiation of the startle response in this manner appears to be elaborated by the FEAR system, which runs from the amygdala to the PAG,[7] and this experimental model can readily be implemented in humans.[8]

Quadrant 1 models were especially prevalent during the initial era of preclinical psychopharmacology in the 1950s to 1970s, but, as mentioned, they were often flawed by their failure to distinguish between antianxiety effects and simple behavioral disinhibition. This noncritical approach produced a long-lived, but questionable, serotonin theory of anxiety.[9] The first neurochemical theory of anxiety ever proposed, was based largely on the observation that serotonin receptor antagonists could increase punished behaviors. However, it is now clear that a reduction of brain serotonin makes animals more manic and impulsive in general, with a very broad pattern of behavioral disinhibition in situations that entail anxiety as well as those that do not. Accordingly, increased behavior in the face of punishment could have simply reflected a generalized release of active behavioral tendencies, not a reduction of anxious feelings. Although some recent data do suggest that certain serotonin receptor subtypes may in fact promote anxiety (especially 5-HT_2 and 5-HT_3), while other receptors for this same amine decrease anxiety,[10] there is presently little empirical reason to believe that serotonin neuronal activity is a major player in producing the actual experience of fear within the brain. Rather, it is clear that the serotonin system modulates the intensity of fear, but to no greater extent than it modulates other negative emotions. In fact, most of the available data is still consistent with the alternative conclusion that an overall increase of serotonin activity decreases anxiety and produces feelings of relaxation. Of course, the vast proliferation of serotonin receptor subtypes discovered over the past few years (15 are presently known) reveals a level of complexity that is still not well integrated into a solid base of accepted knowledge.

Quadrant 2 (learned tasks with no explicit punishment contingencies): Only one model of anxiety has attempted to utilize a learning task without any explicit punishment. This task is the partial reinforcement extinction effect (PREE), whereby animals exhibit high response rates during extinction because they have presumably become accustomed to frustrative nonreward, which is proposed to resemble a central state of anxiety.[11] Although this model is sensitive to benzodiazepines (BZs) and other antianxiety agents, such as barbiturates, that also block the PREE, it remains more probable that frustration and fear emerge from separate brain mechanisms, in which case these results may not be valid antianxiety effects. Rather, the data may simply indicate that minor tranquilizers diminish the effects of frustration and anger, which is consistent with data presented in the previous chapter and, of course, quite interesting in itself.

Quadrant 3 (instinctual fear behaviors with no explicit punishment): The prototypical model of this type is the "open-field" task in which an animal is placed into an unfamiliar chamber. One then measures exploratory activity (which increases as a function of repeated test sessions), the amount of defecation (which initially is high and diminishes as a function of sessions), and a variety of autonomic indicators of stress and fear, such as elevated heart rate and adrenal glucocorticoid secretion.[12] Perhaps because of the new regulations imposed on animal research in many countries around the world, with restrictions on the use of procedures that may produce distress in experimental animals, a large variety of fear models that do not use punishment have now been developed. All of them rely on the fact that each species has specific sensory and perceptual access routes to fear circuitry. For instance, rodents do not require explicit physical punishment to motivate them to avoid events. They naturally prefer to enter dark holes,[13] yielding *the latency to enter a dark hole task.* When forced to remain under bright light, rats also exhibit reduced social activity, yielding the *diminished social-interaction test*, an anxiety that is effectively counteracted by BZs.[14] They also tend to avoid leaving the security of well-protected (i.e., high-walled) areas for the insecurity of wide-open areas, yielding the *plus-maze test* in which two arms have high walls and two have no walls.[15]

We now also know that rats exhibit an intrinsic fear of the smell of potential predators such as cats and ferrets, yielding various fear-smell tests in which one can measure behavioral disruptions of any of a variety of behavioral baselines (for rough-and-tumble play in juveniles, see Figure 1.1). Most of the preceding measures of fear are diminished by BZs, but it is noteworthy that the plus-maze test and the cat-smell test in rats are not especially sensitive to such drugs.[16] Morphine, which is only moderately effective in these models, strongly counteracts the disruption of play behavior produced by cat smell, suggesting that these models arouse distinct types of trepidation that may need to be differentiated from each other.[17]

Quadrant 4 (instinctual fear behaviors resulting from explicit punishment): The analysis of unconditional (instinctual) responses to punishment is likely to provide the clearest view of the unlearned brain mechanisms mediating fear, since punishment can presumably directly activate instinctual fear behaviors that arise most directly from underlying FEAR circuitries. There are now many such models, including simple ones, such as measuring how long animals "freeze" (show behavioral immobility) in response to "contextual cues" that have been paired with shocks (Figure 11.1),[18] as well as those that measure more complex behaviors, such as rats' tendency to cover up shock prods placed in their living quarters;[19] both of these behaviors can be reduced with BZs. The most compelling model of this type, probably the one that evokes fear most directly, is direct electrical stimulation to specific subcortical locations (including central amygdala, anterior hypothalamus, and PAG) to evoke a central aversive state accompanied by powerful fearlike response patterns.[20] Such brain stimulation induces freezing at low currents and flight at higher current levels, accompanied by intense autonomic indicators of fear such as increases in defecation, urination, heart rate, blood pressure, and adrenal stress responses. This approach provides a direct estimate of the localization of the major unconditional FEAR circuit in the mammalian brain (Figure 11.1) and also permits the dynamics of the underlying circuits to be studied effectively in the fully anesthetized subject.[21] Since some of these fear responses can be evoked under anesthesia, one can presumably study the sources of anxiety without imposing powerful (and no doubt unpleasant) emotional experiences on the experimental animal, but such approaches have not yet become fashionable.

The many models that exist for the analysis of fear suggest that a variety of processes may elaborate anxiety within the brain. Fearful states can be evoked by painful stimuli, cues that have become associated with aversive stimuli, various nonpainful stimuli that have indicated danger in the evolutionary history of a species, and perhaps even certain frustrations. These models are often differentially sensitive to pharmacological manipulations that may reflect the variety of distinct cognitive and motivational controls that interact with a limited set of unconditional anxiety processes that exist in the brain.

Thus, many of the distinct stimuli and situations that can evoke fearful states may derive their motivational impact from shared neural circuits. Indeed, this is how most emotional systems usually appear to operate—by responding to a multiplicity of inputs and controlling a multiplicity of outputs, all of which can be modulated by ongoing learning processes. It is unlikely that a single FEAR system of the brain can explain how all of the preceding models derive their affective force, but we anticipate that this system will account for a substantial part of the variance. Thus, before discussing the FEAR system in greater detail, let us first summarize some evidence for multiple anxiety systems based on the pharmacological treatment of anxiety disorders in humans.

On the Varieties of Anxiety Systems in the Brain

The abundance of animal models, and the overall clinical complexity of anxiety indicate that we should be cautious in simplifying the issues that confront us as we seek a definitive understanding of anxiety within the mammalian brain. Let me briefly consider some other neuroemotional systems that contribute to aversive brain states related to anxiety. One of these is the system that functions primarily to elaborate separation distress (i.e., the PANIC system discussed in Chapter 14) as indexed by measures of separation calls in species as diverse as primates, rodents, and birds. This circuit is clearly distinct from FEAR and runs from the preoptic area and bed nucleus of the stria terminalis, down through the dorsomedial thalamus to the vicinity of the PAG.[22] This system presumably mediates such negative feelings as loneliness and grief, and may also contribute substantially to the precipitous forms of acute distress known as panic attacks.

Clinically, a distinction between brain mechanisms that control panic attacks and those that control everyday anticipatory anxiety first became apparent when it was found that the best available antianxiety agents (e.g., BZs such as chlordiazepoxide and diazepam) did not quell either panic attacks in humans or separation anxiety in animals. However, tricyclic antidepressants such as imipramine and chlorimipramine, which had no clear effect on simple generalized anxieties, were found to exert clear antipanic effects in humans and to also reduce separation distress in animals.[23] Quite remarkably, people whose panic attacks had been effectively attenuated with tricyclics still feared that the attacks might recur; hence they often did not consciously appreciate the therapeutic effects of the drugs, although they objectively experienced far fewer attacks. In other words, anticipatory anxiety and panic were modulated by different neurochemical systems.

Other symptomatic distinctions can also be made between fearful anxiety and separation anxiety. The former is characterized by generalized apprehensive tension, with a tendency toward various autonomic symptoms such as tachycardia, sweating, gastrointestinal symptoms, and increased muscle tension. The latter, especially in intense forms such as grief, is accompanied by feelings of weakness and depressive lassitude, with autonomic symptoms of a parasympathetic nature, such as strong urges to cry, often accompanied by tightness in the chest and the feeling of having a lump in the throat. While the former emotional state beckons one to escape situations that intensify the anxiety, the latter tends to motivate thoughts about the lost object of affection and impels one to seek the company of special loved ones.[24]

Recently, a strong case has been put forward claiming that panic attacks emerge from primitive suffocation-alarm systems of the brain, which may be closely coupled with separation-distress systems.[25] Thus, although PANIC and FEAR systems can be distinguished in the brain (also see Chapter 14), it is to be expected that they can also operate synergistically: Chronic anxiety can increase the incidence of panic attacks, and panic attacks can lead to chronic anxiety. The effectiveness of some new antianxiety agents, such as alprazolam, in reducing panic[26] may also indicate that the two emotional systems share some common neurochemical influences, perhaps because of shared nonspecific influences such as increased serotonin and reduced norepinephrine (NE) activity.

Another anxious state that may result from distinct neural activity is post-traumatic stress disorder (PTSD), which is characterized by chronic negative feelings, including mixtures of anger and anxiety. The severity of PTSD can be diminished with antiseizure medications, such as carbamazepine, an agent that is not consistently effective in the control of either panic attacks or anticipatory anxiety.[27] In addition to facilitating GABA activity, carbamazepine has a spectrum of other neurochemical effects. This drug also blocks "kindling," which is the experimental induction of chronic epileptic potentials in the brain via the periodic application of brief electrical stimulation to seizure-prone areas of the temporal lobe such as the amygdala (see "Afterthought," Chapter 5). It is not unusual for kindled animals to exhibit chronic emotional changes (increases in irritability as well as heightened sexuality), further suggesting that similarities may exist between this type of evoked brain change and PTSD.[28] Kindled animals also startle more easily than controls.[29]

A variety of other psychiatric disorders are commonly accompanied by anxiety. For instance, obsessive-compulsive behaviors and rituals often reflect an attempt to ward off encroaching anxieties. We do not know whether such incipient anxieties are mediated by any of the systems discussed earlier. It is noteworthy, however, that the serotonin-reuptake inhibitors such as chlorimipramine, which are effective antipanic agents, are also highly effective in controlling obsessive-compulsive behaviors,[30] suggesting a shared neurochemical substrate for both. Selective serotonin reuptake inhibitors (SSRIs) are also effective in reducing separation distress in animals, although their efficacy in generalized anxiety disorders is more modest.[31] However, since serotonin modulates all emotional systems (see Chapter 6), such lines of investigation are not going to be especially useful for distinguishing emotional processes.

It seems likely that brain systems that mediate anticipatory and chronic generalized anxiety can be differentiated from those that mediate panic attacks, separation anxiety, and PTSDs in terms of the specific brain mechanisms involved, even though they also share many neural components. For instance, all may share a hypersensitized "alarm" component, reflecting an initial alerting response when threatening stimuli first appear on the psychological horizon; this response may arise, in part, from generalized cerebral arousal/attentional systems such as cholinergic and noradrenergic alerting circuits of the brain stem (see Figure 6.5). Many anxieties may also share arousal of the pituitary-adrenal stress responses,[32] although, surprisingly, this response system is not vigorously engaged during panic attacks.[33]

During the past few decades, several brain systems have been proposed as basic substrates for anxiety, including noradrenergic arousal from the locus coeruleus,[34] serotonergic arousal from midbrain raphe cell groups,[35] and a hippocampal-septal behavioral inhibition system.[36] Each of these theories remains controversial, with considerable contradictory data. Perhaps the most serious problem is the simple fact that animals still appear able to experience a great deal of fear after these systems have been experimentally damaged. Animals with damage to the brain areas mentioned above can learn to avoid foot shock and continue to exhibit anxious behaviors in many of the models discussed here. Accordingly, these systems probably contribute to fear in nonspecific ways. Indeed, they contribute substantially to practically every behavior an animal exhibits.

The Basic FEAR System

Brain-stimulation studies have long suggested that a coherently operating FEAR system exists in the brain. As mentioned previously, it extends from the temporal lobe (from central and lateral areas of the amygdala) through the anterior and medial hypothalamus to the lower brain stem (through the periventricular gray substance of the diencephalon and mesencephalon) and then down to specific autonomic and behavioral output components of the lower brain stem and spinal cord, which control the physiological symptoms of fear (including increases in heart rate, blood pressure, the startle response, elimination, and perspiration; for a summary see Figure 11.1). A growing consensus is emerging that this neural system mediates a fundamental form of unconditional fear.[37] Minor tranquilizers exert part of their antianxiety effect by reducing arousal of this brain system.[38]

When this system is activated by electrical stimulation of the brain (ESB), animals exhibit a variety of fearlike behaviors, ranging from an initial freezing response at low current levels to an increasingly precipitous flight response at higher current intensities. These, of course, reflect the types of fear responses animals normally exhibit when dangers are either far or close. In other words, the responses evoked artificially by ESB look very similar to the behavior of animals that have either noticed a predator at a distance or are being pursued by one. Likewise, the behaviors resemble those of animals that either have received foot shock recently or are in the midst of being shocked. Even though such animals appear to be severely distressed, it seems unlikely that the brain stimulation is activating a pain pathway, since the stimulated animals normally do not squeal or exhibit other apparent symptoms associated with pain. For some time, investigators believed that this kind of brain stimulation did not evoke a subjective state of fear. They were wrong.

As in the case of rage described in the previous chapter, the fearlike behaviors evoked with brain stimulation have commonly been considered to simply reflect motor control mechanisms for flight. The failure to more fully consider the possible role of this emotional response system in affective experience arose from a single peculiar fact: Even though animals exhibit flight when this system is stimulated, they do not readily learn to avoid the brain stimulation that evoked the fearful behaviors. In other words, a neutral cue predicting the onset of ESB in the FEAR system does not readily become a conditional source of fear that is sufficient to motivate the learning of discrete avoidance responses. By comparison, peripheral pain (e.g., foot shock) does so readily. Accordingly, investigators concluded that only somatic and visceral motor output systems had been activated rather than the emotional integration system for fear itself. We now know that this conclusion is incorrect: Animals will exhibit conditioned fear to this kind of ESB, as long as sufficiently sensitive behavioral tests are used (Figure 11.3).[39] It is possible that animals did not avoid the centrally evoked fear state in earlier studies because ESB-induced emotions are simply too pervasive and cannot be effectively linked to discrete external cues. Also, it is possible that the fear outlasted the ESB to such an extent that normal reinforcement processes could not be properly engaged.

Although we cannot directly measure subjective experience, the behavioral evidence from all mammals that have been studied strongly suggests that a powerful internal state of dread is elaborated by the FEAR system. First, all animals readily learn to escape such stimulation, implying that this type of ESB is highly aversive. The more closely the requisite learned response resembles the ESB-induced flight, the more rapidly the animal learns. Thus, the act of running away is learned more rapidly than a lever-press response.

If given the opportunity, animals will avoid environments where they have received such stimulation in the past, and if no avenue of escape is provided, they

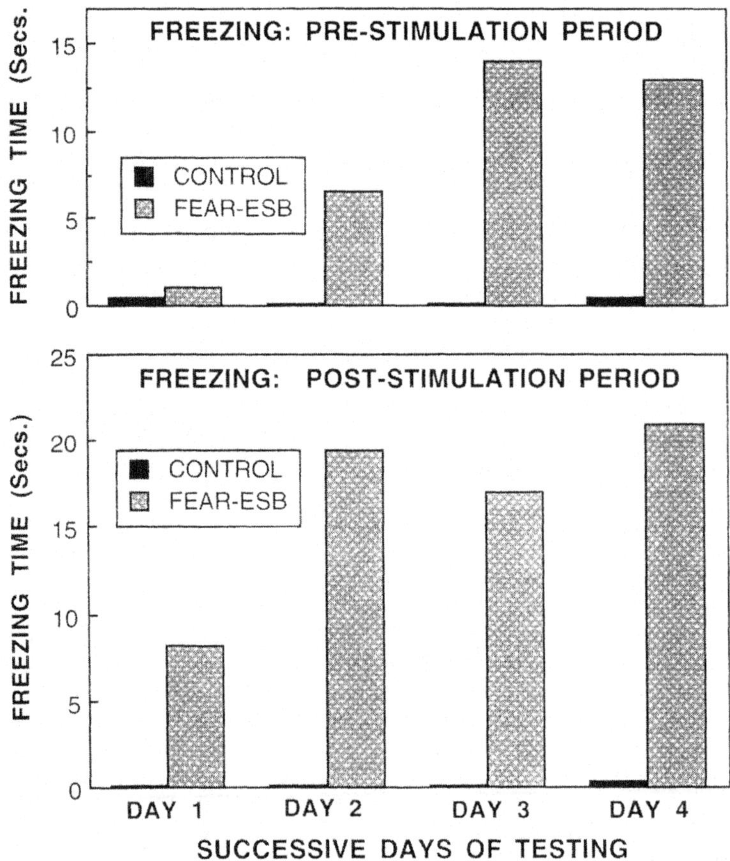

Figure 11.3. Freezing time during the minutes prior to and after electrical stimulation of the FEAR system on four successive days of testing. (Unpublished data, Sacks & Panksepp; adapted from Panksepp, 1996; see n. 40.)

will freeze as if in the presence of a predator.[40] Thus, although it is certainly difficult to train animals to avoid (i.e., anticipate) this kind of brain stimulation using traditional behavioral procedures (such as shuttle boxes and lever presses), animals do exhibit clear conditional responses if one utilizes simpler measures of learned behavior. Indeed, during stimulation of this system at very low current levels, the first response animals exhibit is an increase in freezing. Only when current levels increase does one begin to see a dramatic flight response. Perhaps most important, humans verbally report powerful feelings of foreboding during stimulation applied to these brain sites. The subjective fear responses are usually described in metaphoric terms.[41] For instance, one patient said, "Somebody is now chasing me, I am trying to escape from him." To another, onset of stimulation produced "an abrupt feeling of uncertainty just like entering into a long, dark tunnel." Another experienced a sense of being by the sea with "surf coming from all directions."

Whether the subjective experience of fear is mediated directly by this circuit or in conjunction with other brain areas will have to be addressed in further research. A modest amount of evidence favors the explanation that affective experience is an intrinsic subcortical function, since decorticate animals still exhibit escape and fear behaviors when these circuits are stimulated. To resolve how specific emotions are subjectively felt may require clarification of the primordial neural substrates elaborating affective experience, which may be organized at levels as low as the midbrain (see Chapter 16). At present, we do not have a detailed understanding of how affective experience is actually generated by such emotional circuits, but an understanding of the relevant behavioral substrates opens up a provocative avenue for determining how the conscious aspects of human and animal anxieties are created. Although precise neural evidence concerning the connectivities of the FEAR system remains modest, as will be summarized later, substantial progress is being made in defining how learned inputs enter the circuit in the amygdala and how unconditional ones such as pain come to enter the circuit in the PAG.[42]

Relationships between Pain and Fear

In addition to various forms of anxiety, there are many other types of aversive internal feelings—ranging from pain to hunger, thirst, and other bodily needs that may modulate the intensity of fear. It is especially important to consider the role of pain in the genesis of anxiety, since that has been the traditional way of producing fear conditioning in animal models. Animals readily learn to escape from and avoid places where they have been hurt. Current evidence suggests that pain and fear systems can be dissociated even though they interact strongly at various locations within the neuroaxis (including the lowest reaches in the PAG, as well as the highest reaches in the amygdala).[43]

Perhaps the clearest evidence for the dissociation is that fearlike behaviors in animals and fear states in humans are not readily produced by electrical stimulation of the classic spinothalamic pain systems. It is only at midbrain levels, where the classic pain systems diverge into reticular fields, that localized ESB begins to yield such fearful behaviors as freezing and flight. Further, humans who have been stimulated in these latter brain areas typically report fear rather than pain, and animals exhibit flight and escape with no vocal expressions of pain. Likewise, lesions in brain areas containing fear circuitry do not typically affect pain thresholds in animals.[44] Thus, even though pain systems do send inputs into areas of the brain that mediate fear (especially at the PAG of the mesencephalon), electrical activation of the FEAR system does not appear to readily evoke the sensation of pain in either humans or animals.

However, it is also clear that the FEAR system does control pain sensitivity. It is commonly observed that animals and humans do not focus on their bodily injuries when they are scared,[45] and fear-induced analgesia emerges, at least in part, from arousal of pain-inhibition pathways such as serotonin and endogenous opioids, near the PAG of the mesencephalon.[46]

Learning within Fear Systems

Learning mechanisms allow organisms to effectively channel their specific fears into environmentally appropriate responses. The FEAR system contains certain intrinsic sensitivities, in that it responds unconditionally to pain and the smell of predators and other intrinsically scary stimuli, but it can also establish new input components that function through learning to inform the organism about cues that predict threats. Some environmental circumstances lead to rapid conditioning, presumably because certain perceptions have ready access to the FEAR system, while neutral stimuli take longer to condition. For instance, it has been found that in humans autonomic fear responses condition more rapidly when a mild electric shock is paired with images of angry faces than when it is paired with smiling faces.[47] In other words, the brain is predisposed to associate fear with the potentially threatening configuration of anger more readily than with a pleasant face. Neural assemblies at the base of the temporal lobes decode the facial patterns of emotions, and from there they probably transmit information along evolutionarily prepared input channels to the FEAR system, as well as to other emotional circuits of the amygdala.[48]

There are bound to be several preferential input channels to the FEAR system, reflecting the different intrinsic fears of different species. Thus, humans readily exhibit fears of dark places, high places, approaching strangers (especially those with angry faces), and sudden sounds, as well as snakes and spiders.[49] Rats are especially apt to fear well-illuminated areas, open spaces, and the smell of cats and other potential predators. But completely neutral stimuli can also access the FEAR system of the brain. During the past few years, great progress has been made in unraveling the manner in which this system becomes classically conditioned when neutral cues are paired with shock.

One of the first breakthroughs in the field was the finding that conditioned fears access the FEAR system at the central nucleus of the amygdala.[50] When this area is lesioned on both sides of the brain, animals no longer exhibit increased heart rates to stimuli they had learned to fear.[51] It is now becoming clear that the central nucleus is one major brain area where conditional synaptic control of fear is created. This provides a precise neurogeographical end point for analyzing how neurotic behaviors might be generated through learning.

Several intensely focused research programs have now revealed the precise mechanisms that allow simple conditioned fears to access the unconditional FEAR system. Effective models have been derived from studies of fearful responses to lights and tones paired with the administration of electric shock. Consider a situation in which a tone is followed by shock: The sound enters the eighth cranial nerve, and after synapsing in the cochlear nucleus, the information moves on to the inferior colliculus of the midbrain, then to the medial geniculate of the thalamus, and then to the auditory cortex in the brain's temporal area (Figure 11.4). One can ask whether damage to any of these areas diminishes the conditioned fear response, and the answer is a clear yes for all auditory relay areas below the cortex.[52] This makes sense because the animal has been rendered deaf. However, the conditioned fear remains intact if only the auditory cortex is removed. In other words, the highest levels of auditory processing are not necessary for conditioned fears to be exhibited to simple sounds. This implies that a conditional linkage to the FEAR system has emerged at some subcortical location.

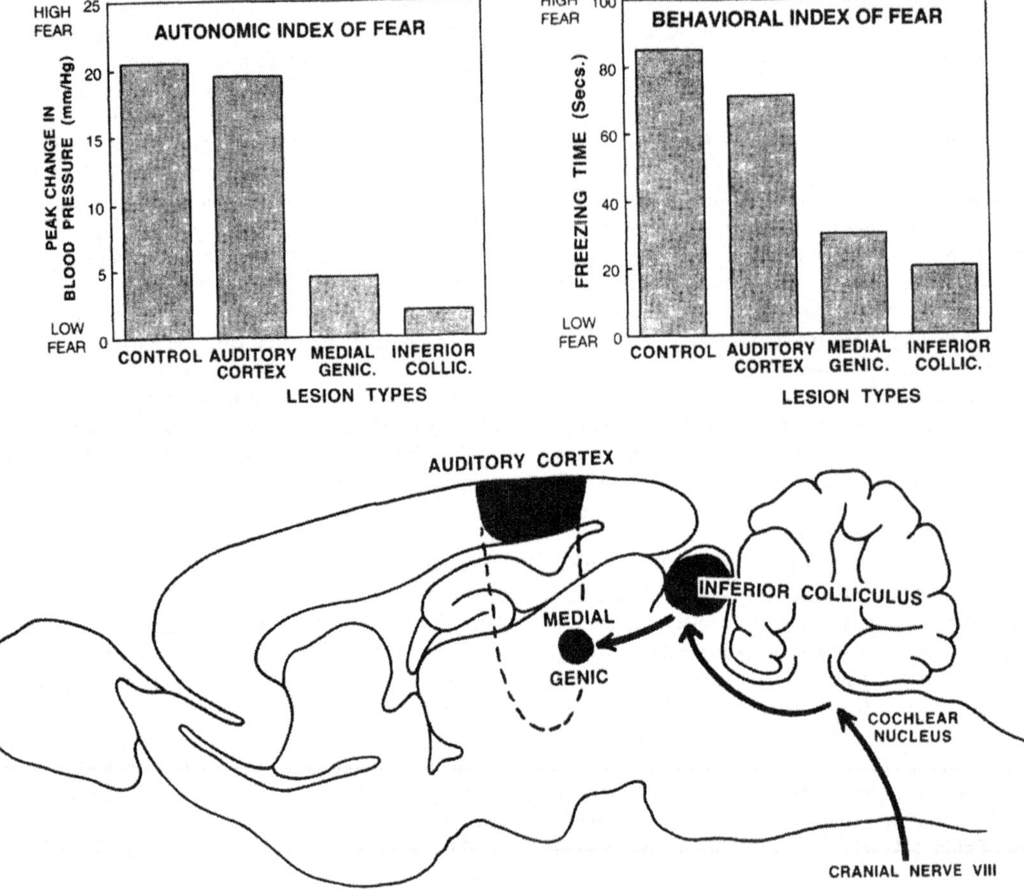

Figure 11.4. Lesions of subcortical but not cortical auditory processing areas disrupt conditioning of fear response to acoustic stimuli paired with foot shock. (Results adapted from Le Doux, 1993; see n. 53.) Behavioral data on top, and locations of lesions on bottom. The damage to the auditory cortex was on the lateral surface of the brain, depicted by dotted lines.

This important finding did not mean, of course, that cortical processing is irrelevant for fear learning. Complex fearful perceptions probably do require input from the cortex, but the finding did encourage investigators to search for a direct connection from thalamic auditory relays to the highest reaches of the FEAR circuit in the amygdala. Indeed, retrogradely labeled neurons were found in the thalamic auditory nucleus, the ventral part of the medial geniculate body, after placement of retrograde tracers into the headwaters of the FEAR system in the lateral amygdala.[53]

Although the analysis of amygdalopedal connections from the auditory thalamus did not yield powerful connections to the central amygdala as was initially expected, there were strong connections from the medial geniculate to the lateral and basolateral parts of the amygdala—areas which earlier ESB studies had implicated as FEAR circuits of the temporal lobes.[54] These lateral amygdaloid areas connect directly to the central amygdaloid nucleus, which then sends axons down to the lower reaches of the hypothalamus and midbrain, where the information is distributed to various, hormonal, autonomic, and somatic output channels that characterize the overall fear response.[55]

In other words, a direct thalamic-amygdaloid connection can convey low-level auditory information directly into the FEAR system without cortical participation.[56] However, additional work indicates that higher cortical processing is necessary for more complex auditory information to access the FEAR system.[57] By extrapolating these results to humans, we might hypothesize that the cortex decodes the affective lexical content of what is said as opposed to decoding the angry or fearful way something is said, but detailed evidence for this at the human level is nonexistent.

Much of the conditioning that occurs in the amygdala is mediated by glutamate synapses, since the conditioning process can be prevented by placement of antagonists to n-methyl-d-aspartate (NMDA) glutamate receptors directly into the lateral amygdala.[58] The acquisition of fear can also be modulated by ascending NE systems, since blockade of ß-adrenergic synapses concentrated within the amygdala tends to diminish consolidation and retention of fearful information.[59] It is to be expected that many other amines and neuropeptides localized in the amygdala will also prove to be influential in the overall integration of fear responses. It may well be that different peptides here help elaborate the various types of fearful sensations and perceptions.

In any event, the preceding results affirm that emotional learning can occur without the intervention of the highest reaches of the cognitive brain. There are direct anatomical entry points from the thalamus into the relevant amygdaloid circuits, but it is clear that the more indirect cortical and hippocampal connections also provide information about external threats. For instance, the hippocampus informs animals about threatening aspects of their spatial environments, but it does not process discrete fear stimuli as does the amygdala.[60] Conditioning, as well as affective experience, can probably also be elaborated at lower levels of the fear circuit (i.e., at hypothalamic and mesencephalic levels), but such important issues remain to be empirically evaluated.

Once all the details of the learning mechanisms have been worked out, it should be possible to specify how new pharmacological maneuvers might facilitate the deconditioning of long-lasting learned fears. Glutamate antagonists have already been evaluated and found to block not only the acquisition of conditioned fears but also their extinction.[61] Thus, since glutamate facilitates both learning and unlearning of fears, as well as most other forms of learning, such information is unlikely to yield any useful clinical interventions.

A vast number of cognitive studies have now demonstrated that glutamate participates in virtually every form of memory and cognitive information processing imaginable. All cortical information descends onto the basal ganglia via glutamate synapses (see Figure 4.9). As we will see in the next section, glutamate receptors control not only fear conditioning but also control unconditioned fear responses. Thus, drugs that modify glutamate receptors will be useful in the clinical control of anxiety only if we are fortunate enough to find variants of such receptors that will allow specific modulation of deconditioning processes. This presently seems improbable.

It is more likely that pharmacological modulation of a variety of neuropeptides, including CRF, α-MSH, ACTH, NPY, and others, will provide more specific neurochemical control of anxiety than does glutamate. These systems are constituents of the FEAR system[62] and afford excellent routes for new drug development. Indeed, our understanding of how minor tranquilizers (i.e., antianxiety agents) work in the brain by interacting with BZ receptors has so far provided the most abundant information for understanding how anxiety is produced and how it can be controlled.

The Neurochemistry and Pharmacology of FEAR

For medical purposes, the most useful knowledge about fear and anxiety will emerge from an understanding of the neurochemical systems that mediate fearful impulses. An extensive body of evidence has already been assembled on the brain systems that are sensitive to BZs.[63] BZ receptors are concentrated along the trajectory of the FEAR circuit, from the central amygdala, downward via the ventral amygdalofugal pathway, through the anterior and medial hypothalamus, and down across the substantia nigra to the PAG and the nucleus reticularis pontis caudalis (the RPC), where fear modulation of the startle reflex occurs.[64] BZ receptors are closely coupled to gamma-aminobutyric acid (GABA) function in the brain. Just as glutamate is the brain's most prolific excitatory transmitter, its metabolic product GABA, via one decarboxylation step, is the most pervasive inhibitory transmitter and is capable of suppressing fear as well as many other emotional and motivational processes.[65] In short, BZs reduce fear by facilitating GABA activity in many parts of the brain, including by directly inhibiting the FEAR circuit.

The discovery of this BZ-GABA receptor complex has been the single most important development for explaining how BZs and the older antianxiety agents (alcohol and barbiturates) inhibit fearfulness. The BZ receptors promote GABA binding, which then increases neuronal inhibition in the FEAR system by facilitating chloride influx into neurons.[66] In other words, anxiety is quelled by BZs through the hyperpolarization of the neuronal elements that pass anxiety messages through the neuroaxis. While agonists for the BZ receptor, such as the many variants of BZ-type minor tranquilizers, suppress activity in the FEAR circuit, they may also modulate higher cognitive processing of the relevant information (anxious thoughts and appraisals), perhaps via effects on the relatively abundant BZ receptors in the neocortex.

Antagonists for the BZ receptor (such as flumazenil) are usually behaviorally inactive by themselves,[67] suggesting that endogenous anxiety signals are not tonically present at BZ receptor sites. Of course, such BZ receptor antagonists can block the antianxiety effects of exogenously administered BZs, as well as the anxiety provoked by a class of drugs known as "inverse agonists" for BZ receptors, which *decrease* inhibition within the FEAR circuit and can produce chronic anxiety disorders.[68] This "inverse agonist" concept was first generated by the discovery of various ß-carboline drugs that produced effects opposite to those of BZs; they actively inhibited chloride entry into neurons via interaction with the BZ-GABA complex, thereby promoting anxiety in both humans and animals.[69]

One key task has been to discover what type of endogenous brain molecule normally acts on the BZ receptor. Even though definitive evidence is not available, and many natural brain metabolites have some effect on BZ receptors, a key candidate for some time has been an endogenous neuropeptide called diazepam binding inhibitor (DBI), which appears to promote anxiety when released onto BZ receptors, perhaps via an inverse-agonist effect.[70] As yet there is no conclusive evidence that DBI is in fact the major anxiety-generating transmitter of the brain, although most agree that if there is one that acts on the BZ receptor, it is likely to be an inverse agonist. In any event, existing data suggest that BZs promote serenity, in part, by promoting GABA-mediated inhibition within the FEAR system.

Which, then, are the neurotransmitters that directly convey the signal of fear through the neuroaxis? There are several possible candidates. Although NE and serotonin (5-HT) were once touted as specific anxiety transmitters, those early hypotheses have seemed improbable for some time, since biogenic amines operate as nonspecific control systems for all behavior.[71] Although increasing NE and 5-HT activity with drugs such as yohimbine and m-chlorophenylpiperazine (MCPP), respectively, can promote the experience of anxiety in humans,[72] such effects may be nonspecific. They may simply reflect general arousal effects that amplify whatever tendencies already exist in the nervous system, rather than reflecting any specific type of emotional arousal. Certainly, several other neuropeptides and amino acids modulate anxious behaviors more specifically and powerfully, at least in the animal models in which they have been studied. They will figure prominently in our future understanding of the neurochemical substrates of fear.

As indicated, one compelling option is that the simple amino acid neurotransmitter glutamate, which, as already noted, mediates the learning of fears, is also a key transmitter for generating the unconditioned response of fear.[73] A powerful fear syndrome can be evoked by administering the glutamate agonists kainic acid and also the specific agonist NMDA into the PAG or lower and higher areas near the ventricular system. Within minutes after placement of these agents into the brain, animals begin to exhibit spontaneous bouts of flight (often in a semicrouched posture) accompanied by an apparent psychic anguish. Visually oriented animals such as birds exhibit rapid head scanning, persistent vocalization, and bulging eyes suggestive of profound terror. These episodes can be inhibited by appropriate glutamate receptor antagonists (those that block kainate or NMDA receptors).[74] However, as already mentioned, such glutamate receptors are widespread in the brain, and only with remarkable luck (e.g., the discovery of unique emotion-specific variants of glutamate receptor antagonists or modulators) could we ever hope to develop antianxiety agents based on such knowledge. At present, the neuropeptides are more promising targets for pharmacological development in the ongoing search for new and useful ways to control anxiety.

In addition to DBI, several other anxiogenic neuropeptides have anatomical pathways along the trajectory of the FEAR system. Central administration of the neuropeptides CRF, α-MSH, ACTH, and CCK can promote an array of anxiety symptoms in animals.[75] CRF (see Figure 6.7), for example, causes agitated arousal and can reduce a variety of positively motivated behaviors, including feeding, sexual, and other positive social activities. Animals also tend to freeze in environments where they previously received CRF. Conversely, foot shock–induced freezing is diminished by CRF receptor antagonists.[76] Parenthetically, it should be reiterated that CRF arising from the paraventricular nucleus of the hypothalamus also controls the pituitary-adrenal stress response (see Figure 6.9) that accompanies virtually all emotions and many psychiatric disturbances, especially depression. Thus, it is generally believed that CRF receptor antagonists will eventually yield potent antianxiety and antistress agents. Nonpeptide CRF antagonists are already being developed for oral use.[77]

The neuropeptide α-MSH promotes camouflage-type pigmentary changes in many fish and reptiles. When such animals are scared, their skin tends to turn black. Although this peptide does not control skin pigmentation in higher vertebrates, a vigorous freezing/hiding pattern can be evoked in chicks by central administration of this peptide. ACTH, which comes from the same segment of the proopiomelanocortin (POMC) gene as α-MSH, has similar effects. Although there is little comparable information on mammalian behavior patterns, microinjections of high doses of ACTH into the PAG can precipitate vigorous flight, as well as freezing, in rats and other animals.[78] The affective effects of such treatments remain to be evaluated using conditioned freezing and place-avoidance paradigms, but it is anticipated that centrally effective antagonists of these neuropeptide receptor systems may reduce fearful behavioral inhibition.

An especially well-studied anxiogenic peptide is cholecystokinin (CCK). It, and various CCK fragments, can precipitate panic attacks in humans and a broad spectrum of anxiogenic symptoms in animals with the use of a variety of anxiety models described previously. Thus, from animal studies, it is to be expected that a CCK antagonist should have powerful antipanic and/or antianxiety effects, but preliminary clinical work has not been promising.[79]

A variety of other neuropeptides and neuropeptide antagonists appear to reduce anxiety symptoms following central administration. Centrally administered opioids (acting at *mu* sites), as well as oxytocin and somatostatin, are very effective agents for reducing separation distress vocalization (see Chapter 14). Recent work with putative neuropeptide Y (NPY) antagonists has suggested that they can evoke anxiety in animal models.[80] If such findings are supported by further research, it may eventually yield an especially useful category of drugs: In addition to reducing aspects of fear, an NPY agonist would be expected to markedly increase appetite, since this is the most powerful appetite-promoting peptide presently known.[81] Also, a number of steroids can modulate anxiety.[82] An especially important dimension of future research is to specify more precisely how these various neurochemical vectors mediate inputs and outputs of the FEAR system. Do certain neurochemistries convey specific fears, while others are indirect modulators (e.g., providing gain settings and duration controls) within the FEAR system? Future research should be able to tease apart the distinct functions of the many chemistries that control the diverse aspects of the anxiety/fear response and provide more precise avenues for the pharmacological control of various anxiety disorders.

Current Treatment of Anxiety in Clinical Practice

Progress in the treatment of anxiety was a matter of chance and exceptional good fortune during the early days of biological psychiatry. Until the development of benzodiazepine-type minor tranquilizers, the only drugs that could successfully control human anxiety were opioids, alcohol, barbiturates, and meprobamate.[83] Unfortunately, these drugs had many side effects, the worst of which was a poor safety margin, where the difference between the clinically effective dose and the lethal dose (ED/LD ratio) was rather small, increasing the probability of accidental death or suicide. The treatment of anxiety was revolutionized by the serendipitous discovery of the drug chlordiazepoxide (CDP). The efficacy of CDP was identified in 1960 during the final phase of research just prior to the scheduled termination of a relatively unfruitful research program on BZs at Hoffman-LaRoche labs. Almost as a last resort, it was found that one of the BZ molecules, CDP, was very effective in taming wild animals at a local zoo.[84] CDP rapidly became a great success in controlling various anxiety disorders, but for many years no one knew what it, and related BZs, did in the brain. As already summarized, now we do.

The entry of CDP into pharmaceutical practice, under the trade name Librium®, was rapid because of the drug's remarkable specificity and safety margin as compared with anything used previously. CDP could reduce anxiety at less than a hundredth of the lethal dose, which was a remarkable improvement over any other antianxiety agent, and soon many more potent BZs such as diazepam (Valium®) became available. The mild sedative effects commonly observed at the beginning of BZ therapy exhibit rapid tolerance, while antianxiety effects are sustained during long-term use. Initially, these drugs seemed to produce no apparent physical dependence during modest use. However, long-term use of high doses, which became a common practice, eventually was found to yield dependence and a withdrawal syndrome resembling the delirium tremens (DTs) of alcohol withdrawal.[85] This suggested that both agents work upon common substrates in the brain, and it is now well established that both promote GABA activity.

As BZs rapidly supplanted all other antianxiety medications on the market, several additional medical uses were discovered, including inhibition of muscular spasms and effective control of certain types of seizures, especially those that emanate from the limbic system.[86] BZs also found a receptive market as sleep-promoting agents and, because of their cross-tolerance (but relative lack of toxic effects), became effective medications for the alleviation of symptoms of alcohol withdrawal. In other words, subjects who were well habituated to taking high doses of alcohol could be placed on BZs without having to experience the harsh DT symptoms of alcohol withdrawal.[87] Of course, as long as people continued to take the BZs, the addictive state/process was sustained in their brains.

It was also anticipated that molecules of this class might be capable of being developed that would reverse some of the symptoms of drunkenness. Indeed, BZ receptor antagonists, such as flumazenil, can alleviate some of the symptoms of drunkenness, but not the toxic effects of alcohol. Such drugs will probably never be marketed because they do not reduce blood alcohol levels, and the manufacturers might be liable for accidents caused by people who have taken such drugs.[88]

A great variety of BZs eventually came on the market, but it was not until 1979 that the BZ receptor was finally identified in the brain; later, a different type of BZ receptor, which can control involuntary muscle spasms, was identified in the periphery. BZs are now tailor-made and marketed for specific disorders, even though the basic neuronal action is the same for all of them. The practice of using specific agents for each disorder is not based on any fundamental differences in their mode of action but rather on differences in potency and speed of entry into and exit from the brain. Thus, fast-acting BZs are used for sleep disorders, and longer-acting BZs are used for alcohol withdrawal and anxiety.[89]

Even though BZs turned out to be remarkably safe medicinal agents, the main shortcoming has been the previously mentioned dependence syndrome during long-term use. Other side effects include increased appetite, disorientation and memory loss (especially in the elderly), and the release of aggressive tendencies in passive-aggressive individuals.[90] Presumably this latter effect, which is somewhat paradoxical from the perspective that BZs can reduce affective attack (see Chapter 10), reflects release of an underlying irritability that has been kept in check by overriding anxieties or other social inhibitions. By reducing the impact of such concerns, the underlying aggressive impulses may be temporarily released. Because of the shortcomings of BZs, as well as the intense profit motives of pharmaceutical firms, there has been a concerted effort to develop additional antianxiety agents.

Many antianxiety candidates are now in the wings, but the only item that has reached the center stage of the pharmaceutical market is buspirone (Buspar®), which has a profile of action quite distinct from that of the BZs. The therapeutic effect of this agent appears to be based on anxiety modulation through the 5-HT system. Buspirone has the relatively selective effect of stimulating 5-HT-1A receptors, which are predominantly concentrated on serotonin cell bodies. At this site, buspirone reduces 5-HT neuronal activity in the brain and hence diminishes serotonin release in higher brain areas.[91] Although many investigators believe that buspirone alleviates anxiety by reducing 5-HT activity, it should be remembered that there are also postsynaptic 5-HT-1A receptors in the brain (see Figure 10.7), and it presently remains possible that the postsynaptic effects of buspirone, which act to facilitate 5-HT activity, are more important in the control of anxiety than the presynaptic ones, which reduce serotonin activity. Since the reduction of 5-HT release occurs promptly upon buspirone administration, while effective control of anxiety takes up to several weeks, it also remains likely that the effects of buspirone emerge from a long-term regulatory effect of the drug, perhaps upon the postsynaptic sensitivity of the 5-HT system. Thus, the antianxiety effects of buspirone could well be due to a long-term facilitation of 5-HT sensitivity in the brain.

Once therapeutic effects are obtained with buspirone, they tend to be milder than those obtained with BZs, but fewer side effects are encountered. Buspirone does not produce any sedative effects, does not produce any desirable short-term psychic effects (hence it is not subject to abuse), and does not produce dependence or withdrawal upon discontinuation. Unfortunately, buspirone provides little benefit to those individuals who have already used Bzs for a long time.[92] Thus, buspirone is now the best initial treatment option at the outset of any long-term pharmacotherapy for excessive anxiety. Unlike some of the newer BZs such as alprazolam, however, buspirone has exhibited no efficacy as an antipanic agent.[93]

For common physiological symptoms of anxiety, such as palpitations and sweating, ß-noradrenergic blockers, such as propranolol, still appear to be the drugs of choice. "ß-Blockers" are generally deemed to be useful medication for the symptomatic control of anxiety that accompanies certain activities such as public presentations and performances.[94] Finally, it is noteworthy that MAO inhibitors such as phenelzine have been found to be highly effective for the control of social phobias and other neurotic personality disorders.[95] On the other hand, tricyclic drugs that are effective in reducing the incidence of panic attacks are also useful for reducing childhood anxiety-related disorders such as school phobias and enuresis, which may arise from overactive separation distress systems of the brain (see Chapter 14).

An Overview of the Complexity of Fears and Anxieties in the Brain

There remains little doubt that there exists a highly coherent FEAR system in the brain that contributes substantially to the overall emotional response that we typically call anxiety, as well as to more intense forms of terror and dread. Although it is not yet known how the FEAR system helps create the phenomenological experience of anxiety,[96] we can be reasonably certain that it does, leading perhaps to the remarkably widespread manifestations of fear in the brain as revealed by Fos immunohistochemistry.[97] As mentioned earlier, the whole brain seems to be involved.

In addition to real-world threats and dangers, ESB along the FEAR circuit generates powerful fear responses and the corresponding negative affective states in experimental animals and humans. Pharmacological and surgical dampening of activity along this system can make both animals and humans placid. In short, many expressions of fear emerge directly from this neural system, and it is only a matter of time before the many subjective feelings of fears will be understood with the tools of modern neuroscience.

The definitive data concerning the sources of affective experiences must come from human subjective reports following various brain manipulations, as well as from scans of brain activity during emotional episodes. Although data from the available imaging technologies at times can be misleading[98] and also rather insensitive when it comes to deeper brain stem structures such as those we have focused on here, recent work does indicate that the amygdala is aroused when anxiety is precipitated in various ways.[99]

Also, during the past few years, a number of neuropsychological studies have demonstrated that damage to the amygdala can reduce fear conditioning in humans just as it does in animals, and that such brain-damaged individuals are no longer able to recognize the facial expressions of emotions.[100] In a recent single-case study, a young man with massive bilateral temporal lobe damage extending far beyond the amygdala has exhibited unconscious emotional conditioning, and still exhibits preferences for individuals who had treated him especially well.[101] Whether and how such preconscious affective information can influence consciousness remains an unstudied issue.

Although many believe that the conscious readout of affective experiences is mediated by fairly high regions of the brain such as the amygdala and frontal cortex, the position taken here is that the whole continuum of each emotional command system is important for contributing to the feeling of anxiety. To anyone who has studied decorticate animals, it is clear that they can still exhibit a great deal of fearful behavior,[102] and the affect of fear is probably a primitive state of consciousness that can be elaborated by ancient reaches of the brain stem such as the PAG (see Chapter 16). Even though the anxiety experiences of normal adults may be critically dependent on neural processing at the highest levels of the FEAR circuit,[103] the likelihood that young animals who have lost the higher reaches of the system can still experience fearful affect through the lower levels of the FEAR circuit remains a clear possibility that has not been adequately evaluated. If such low subcortical levels of affective processing do exist, we should be able to demonstrate some fear conditioning, especially changes in conditioned fears and place preference,[104] during stimulation of the lower reaches of the FEAR system in animals whose lateral and central amygdaloid nuclei have been completely destroyed at an early age (as in Figure 11.3). Clearly, much work remains to be done.

Just over a century ago, Freud bemoaned the fact that we knew practically nothing about the creation of anxiety in the brain. Now we have a mountain of important evidence that points to specific circuits in primitive parts of the brain that must have evolved long before organisms developed substantial cognitive abilities. This adds special meaning to that famous bit of wisdom from President Franklin D. Roosevelt during World War II, that "the only thing we have to fear is fear itself." In essence, the brain's capacity for fear is an evolved process that arises ultimately from internal neural causes rather than simply from the terrors of the environment.

The existence of this primitive state of fearfulness has been noted by many thoughtful observers down through the ages. My favorite is Jack London's description of how the instinct of fear begins to develop in his canine protagonist, White Fang,[105] The young wolf had never "encountered anything of which to be afraid. Yet fear was in him. It had come down to him from a remote ancestry through a thousand lives. It was a heritage he had received directly . . . through all the generations of wolves that had gone before. Fear!—that legacy of the Wild which no animal may escape." This fictional portrayal contains more than a grain of truth for humans as well. Because we share such ancestral emotions, animal brain research can finally clarify how we come to experience fear in our interactions with the world.[106]

AFTERTHOUGHT: Innate Fears—The Smell of Predators

Psychology has typically focused on how animals learn fearful behaviors, but now that we recognize that some fears represent the innate potentials of the brain, we can begin to ask how innate fears might be elaborated. Presumably, certain patterns of sensory stimulation have direct access to FEAR circuitry. This is affirmed to some extent by the patterns of fear development in human children. Children under 2 years typically exhibit the greatest fear in response to sudden noises, strange objects, pain, and loss of physical support, but all these fears decline steadily with age.[107] Other fears develop only as the child matures. For instance, only gradually do children become afraid of animals, strangers, the dark, and specific thoughts such as fears of drowning and death. Unfortunately, it is next to impossible to study the biological sources of these fears in the human brain.

By comparison, we can easily study some innate fears of animals. For instance, as exemplified in Figure 1.1, rats exhibit an innate fear of the smell of predators. When a very tiny sample of cat hair (a few milligrams will do) is placed in its cage, a rat exhibits dramatic changes in behavior—it plays less, eats less, and demonstrates an elevated level of wary attention. Such animals do not simply freeze (even though that behavior is elevated) but outwardly appear to be in a confused state, full of trepidation about something, although they do not appear to be afraid of the hair itself. Although most will eventually avoid the hair, individual animals will come very close, smelling and investigating it furtively. How does this olfactory stimulus actually enter the FEAR circuitry of the rat's brain?

Like all mammals, the rat has a *main olfactory system* (MOS) that transmits information from the olfactory epithelium to the olfactory bulb, which then distributes the information into various areas of the brain, including many circuits of the amygdala and hypothalamus. This system is designed primarily to sample odors from a distant source. The other olfactory system, called the *vomeronasal complex*, also known as the *accessory olfactory system* (*AOS*), tends to collect information from more nearby objects.[108] The animal actually has to be very close to the source to properly sample objects (indeed, when a snake flicks its forked tongue in and out of its mouth, it is sampling the air by depositing molecules directly into the accessory olfactory system at the roof of the reptilian mouth).

Which of these systems is the rat using when it exhibits trepidation in response to the smell of predators? This question has been answered by selectively damaging the MOS, by topical application of zinc sulfate, in one group of animals and eliminating the AOS input, by snipping the vomeronasal nerve as it enters the brain on the medial surface of the MOS, in another group.[109] We originally did these experiments anticipating that the smell of a cat was exerting its emotional effects via the distal olfactory system (i.e., input via the MOS). This would allow the rat to sense an approaching predator in order to effectively hide or flee. Quite surprisingly, the anxiety-provoking smell reached the brain via the AOS! This was measured by the ability of MOS and AOS destruction to reduce or eliminate the play-reducing effect of cat smell. Accordingly, the evidence indicated that the short-range rather than the long-range olfactory system was mediating the aversive effects of cat smell. This adaptation would mainly allow rats to avoid locations where predators have been, and presumably where they are likely to be again, since most predators are territorial. The olfactory fear of cats is apparently not an evolutionary design that allows rats to detect predators that are prowling at a distance.

Do humans have a similar dual olfactory system? For a long time, investigators thought these structures were vestigial, with only some children still having a functional system. But now it appears that most adults do, in fact, have a functional AOS.[110] There is an increasing amount of evidence that it might act upon our level of sexual arousal—the topic of the next chapter. This is also a pervasive function of the AOS in animals. Already companies are trying to develop new perfumes targeted for this primitive system that helps make subliminal judgments about the pleasantness and erotic potentials of our social world. Whether the AOS also mediates some human fears remains unknown.

Suggested Readings

Burrows, G. D., Roth, M., & Noyes, R., Jr. (eds.) (1990). *Handbook of anxiety*. Vol. 3, *The neurobiology of anxiety*. Amsterdam: Elsevier.

Denney, M. R. (ed.) (1991). *Fear, avoidance, and phobias*. Hillsdale, N.J.: Lawrence Erlbaum.

Dunn, A. J., & Berridge, C. (1990). Physiological and behavioral responses to corticotropin-releasing factor administration: Is CRF a mediator of anxiety or stress responses? *Brain Res. Revs.* 15:71–100.

Fann, W. G., Karacan, I., Pokorny, A. D., & Williams, R. L. (eds.) (1979). *Phenomenology and treatment of anxiety*. New York: Spectrum.

Gray, J. A. (1987). *The psychology of fear and stress* (2d ed.). Cambridge: Cambridge Univ. Press.

Klein, D. F., & Rabkin, J. (eds.) (1981). *Anxiety: New research and changing concepts*. New York: Raven Press.

Panksepp, J. (1990). The psychoneurology of fear: Evolutionary perspectives and the role of animal models in understanding human anxiety. In *Handbook of anxiety*. Vol. 3, *The neurobiology of anxiety* (G. D. Burrows, M. Roth, & R. Noyes, Jr., eds.), pp. 3–58. Amsterdam: Elsevier.

Panksepp, J., Sacks, D. S., Crepeau, L. J., & Abbott, B. B. (1991). The psycho- and neurobiology of fear systems in the brain. In *Fear, avoidance, and phobias* (M. R. Denney, ed.), pp 7–59. Hillsdale, N.J.: Lawrence Erlbaum.

Puglisi-Allegra, S., & Oliverio, A. (eds.) (1990). *Psychobiology of stress*. Dordrecht: Kluwer Adademic.

Soubrie, P. (1986). Reconciling the role of cental serotonin neurons in human and animal behavior. *Behav. Brain Sci.* 9:319–364.

PART III

The Social Emotions

Substantive understanding of social emotions has begun to emerge only recently. The first chapter of this part is devoted to the most primitive and exciting form of social engagement, sexual behavior, which is obviously already well represented in the reptilian brain. During the long course of mammalian evolution, driven partly by the sexual recombination of genes, a variety of behavioral strategies have emerged by which organisms select mates, and the existing diversity of sexual strategies is enormous. As summarized in Chapter 12, we now know that there are distinct LUST circuits for male and female sexuality, even though they also share many processes.

As we will see in Chapter 13, sexuality also established the possibility for nurturance. The emotional tendency to provide special care to the young, so impressive in mammals, is seen only in rudimentary forms in reptiles. Still, a primitive tendency to provide maternal care probably evolved before the divergence of mammalian and avian stock from their common ancestor. This is suggested by the strong parental urges of most avian species and by recent paleontological evidence suggesting that some dinosaurs may also have exhibited maternal tendencies. However, maternal devotion, through the evolution of CARE systems, has vastly expanded within the mammalian brain, while remaining rooted in the sociosexual processes that had evolved earlier.

Complex social feelings in mammals emerged hand in hand with the evolution of the limbic system. As summarized in Chapter 14, one of the most poignant advances in the evolution of emotionality was the capacity of the young to value social support. This social sense is closely linked to vocalization circuitry in the brain. Just as FEAR and RAGE systems allow organisms to cope with archetypal emergency situations that threaten survival, the separation-distress, or PANIC, system provides mammals with a sensitive emotional barometer to monitor the level of social support they are receiving. If social contact is lost, organisms experience a painful feeling of separation, and the young protest (cry) vigorously in an attempt to reestablish contact and care. The neuroscientific analysis of this system will have many implications for understanding everyday loneliness, as well as various psychiatric disorders, such as childhood depression and the emergence of panic attacks.

In the last chapter on a specific emotional system, I will delve into the subcortical circuits that generate playfulness. The rough-and-tumble PLAY system, described in Chapter 15, is important for learning various emotional and cognitive skills, including aspirations for social dominance and cooperation, which influence behavior with different intensities throughout the life span of each animal. The PLAY system promotes the establishment of social structures and helps ensure the learning of social skills, which can facilitate reproductive success. It is one of the major systems in the brain that can generate happiness and joy.

Finally, in Chapter 16, I will consider a variety of critical issues concerning higher brain mechanisms in emotionality, including such fundamental aspects of brain organization as the nature of "the self," which must be addressed by neuroscience if we are ever to understand how emotional feelings are actually generated by the brain. I will attempt to clarify some of the most difficult and important issues in neuroscience, but unfortunately they are ones that have barely been touched empirically. To scientifically consider such topics, we must work concurrently at high theoretical and basic empirical levels. Many have suggested that there is probably no coherent neural representation of "the self" within the brain, but here I will advocate the position that there is such a neural entity, and that it elaborates a basic motor representation of the organism as an active creature in the world. This neural representation may be essential for an animal to have affective feelings. To help us talk about such a complex function of the brain, I will refer to its primordial neural substrates, deep in the brain stem, as the SELF (Simple Ego-type Life Form). I will develop the idea that this mechanism is multiply rerepresented in the brain during development and that it provides the center of gravity for the emergence of affective consciousness in brain evolution. Although adult human emotional experience also relies on higher brain representations of emotional systems, the position advocated here is that those higher functions could not subsist without the integrity of the lower functions.

12

The Varieties of Love and Lust

Neural Control of Sexuality

"What kind of love . . . is it that sanctifies marriage?" he asked hesitatingly. . . .

"True love. . . . When such love exists between a man and a woman, then marriage is possible," she said.

"Yes, but how is one to understand what is meant by 'true love'?" said the gentleman with the glittering eyes timidly and with an awkward smile.

"Everybody knows what love is," replied the lady, evidently wishing to break off her conversation with him.

"But I don't," said the man. "You must define what you understand. . . ."

"Why? It's very simple," she said, but stopped to consider. "Love? Love is an exclusive preference for one above everybody else," said the lady.

"Preference for how long? A month, two days, or half an hour?" said the gray-haired man and began to laugh.

Leo Tolstoy, *The Kreutzer Sonata* (1889)

CENTRAL THEME

Male and female sexuality are subservient to distinct brain controls, although they also share many influences. The primordial plan for both female and male fetuses, in mammals but not in birds, is initially feminine. Some have called this the "default" plan, since masculinization results from the organizational effects of fetal testosterone, which, in humans, occur during the second trimester of pregnancy. Others would call it the "without fault" plan, since the female brain coordinates the use of both cerebral hemispheres more effectively than does the male brain. Contrary to some creation myths, in mammals maleness arises from femaleness, rather than the other way around. If all biochemical events go according to the masculinization plan during this phase of gender specialization, the initially feminine brain is masculinized in utero by the timed secretion of testosterone and its conversion to the active organizational hormone, estrogen. The developing female brain is protected by prophylactic molecules, such as alpha-fetoprotein, which neutralize the effects of maternal estrogens that would otherwise tend to masculinize the brain. To be masculinized means that certain areas of the brain, especially specific nuclear groups in the anterior hypothalamus, grow larger in males than in females, while other areas remain smaller, such as the corpus callosum, which connects the two cerebral hemispheres. These brain organizational effects of early hormone secretions go a long way toward explaining some homosexual tendencies, for the hormones that ultimately trigger the organization of the male brain (testosterone aromatized to estrogen) are distinct from those that trigger the organization of the male body (testosterone converted to dihydrotestosterone, or DHT, by 5α-reductase). Due to this branching of control factors for brain and body organization, it is quite possible for a male-type body to contain a female-type brain, and for a female-type body to contain a male-type brain. It has been repeatedly shown in animal models that maternal stress can hinder the normal process of brain masculinization by desynchronizing the underlying physiological processes: If neonatal testosterone is secreted too early, before receptors are available to receive the message, normal masculinization does not occur. Maternal stress also impairs aromatase activity, which retards conversion of testosterone to estrogen. These different gender potentials in the brain, laid down during fetal development, are activated by the maturation of gonadal steroid synthesis during puberty. It is also known that male and female sexual urges emerge from different neural systems. Perhaps this is clearest in songbirds, where male courting-song systems in the brain grow and shrink in phase with the breeding season. However, mammals also exhibit major brain functional differences between the sexes. For instance, preoptic area damage has more deleterious effects on male sexual behavior than on female behavior, while ventromedial hypothalamic damage has the opposite effect, compromising female urges more than those of males. These brain areas are organized differently in males and females. To have a male or female brain means many things, but among the best-established effects are the higher prevalence of arginine-vasopressin (AVP) circuits in males and more extensive oxytocin circuits in females. Several other neuropeptides control sexuality differentially between the sexes. The existence of such systems in the brain will eventually help explain many of the behavioral and emotional differences in male and female sociosexual tendencies. We are now on the verge of understanding the powerful feelings that control sexuality, but a great deal of affective neuroscience remains to be done before precise knowledge replaces credible hypotheses.

On the Nature of Sociosexual Feelings

Warm and friendly companionship is essential for mental health in humans, and probably most other mammals. Justifiably, some call the most fulfilling long-term relationships love, but sex is also essential to most vertebrate species.[1] Some humans are prone to call even the transient passions of sexual lust by the name of love. It is wonderful when the forms of "love" go together, but in humans all too often they do not, and in animals the concept of love is deemed to be highly suspect by the scientific community. Many confusions and disagreements have arisen from the failure to distinguish the two major forms of love. As Tina Turner sings: "What's love got to do with it?" And as that creative explorer of the human soul, Leo Tolstoy, expounded in *The Kreutzer Sonata*, a great deal of social chaos can emerge when we confuse the two. Members of our species regularly demonstrate that sex and social warmth or nurturance need not go together, and in primitive areas of the brain that elaborate such feelings, confusion also prevails. Sexuality and nurturance are to some extent independently and to some extent interdependently controlled. The Janus-faced nature of human passions and human warmth can only be understood by unveiling the underlying networks of the brain.

Clearly, humans can experience many social feelings. Some of them arise from our erotic nature, and some from the gentler feelings of friendly acceptance, nurturance, and social bonding. Filial love—the love between parent and child—seems outwardly quite distinct from sexual desire, but as Freud suspected, they may share important features. As we will see, findings from modern psychobiology can now be used to bolster this view; key molecules such as oxytocin are involved in both, albeit by actions on different parts of the brain. Although our cultural evolution has sought to bind our desire for sex and our need for social bonding together in an inextricable whole called the institution of marriage, there is no guarantee in the recesses of the brain that such cultural unions will succeed. And so, Tolstoy, through his protagonist in *The Kreutzer Sonata*, cries out in despair: "'Yes, I know,' the gray haired man shouted. . . . 'You are talking about what is supposed to be, but I am speaking of what is. Every man experiences what you call love for every pretty woman'" (p. 120). He proceeds to assert that many people marry only for the opportunity to copulate "and the result is either deception or coercion. . . . And . . . when the husband and wife have undertaken the external duty of living together all their lives, and begin to hate each other after a month, and wish to part but still continue to live together, it leads to that terrible hell" (p. 171) of mutually inflicted psychic pain and alienation.

Indeed, it seems likely that human bonding is not totally monogamous by nature, but our neurobiology is compatible with long-term serial and parallel relationships. The views fashioned by our cultural heritage may choose to disagree. In any event, evolutionary psychologists have now clearly demonstrated that men and women are typically looking for different attributes when they seek mates: Many surveys of human mate preferences indicate that females are seeking companions who are powerful and willing to invest resources in their behalf, whereas males are swayed more by youth and beauty, namely, external indicators of reproductive fitness.[2]

Sexual Feelings

Many psychobiological processes exist in the human brain to facilitate successful social and sexual connections. The tyranny of lust can lead one to feelings of moral degradation and physical dissipation, while acceptance of the power of lust can lead to incomparable ecstasies of psychophysical delight. Full acceptance of one's passionate nature, as elaborated in Tantric Buddhist philosophies, has even been touted as a path to enlightenment. In any event, it is an inescapable fact of life that evolution has built uncompromising feelings of sexual desire into the brain, as well as the potential for social devotion and deception, which can serve to maximize reproductive success. (This, of course, is an excessively casual way to express the matter, since evolution has no ends; it merely reels out endless patterns of reproductive possibilities—some successful, others not—depending on local social and environmental conditions.)

We experience the various feelings we call sexual love and lust because our biological nature has made us social creatures. Brain evolution has not given us, or any other animal, the innate cognitive appreciation that our sense of physical beauty and the pleasures of copulation are designed to service reproductive ends. That is something the human species had to learn through insight, and it is still a difficult lesson for many to accept. Cognitive insights commonly govern sexual behavior less than do the insistent feelings of lust, which diminish only with age, stress, and illness.

Although we cannot definitively explain how erotic feelings are created in the brain, during the past few decades, neuroscience has given us the essential pieces of the puzzle. Although we have yet to see PET or MRI images of sexual arousal or orgasm, the first evidence concerning the neural sources of human sexual feelings were provided by Robert Heath almost 30 years ago. He found that during sexual arousal humans exhibit massive changes in brain electrical activity, including spiking in the septal area. When he placed acetylcholine (ACh) into that brain area in one schizophrenic woman, she described feelings of imminent orgasm. Such feelings have also been evoked there by electrical stimulation of the brain (ESB).[3]

Paul MacLean mapped out the monkey brain for sites from which genital arousal (erections) could be evoked by localized ESB. He discovered a broad swath of tissue, in higher limbic areas, where sexual responses could be elicited.[4] They included, prominently, areas such as the septal area, bed nucleus of the stria terminalis, and preoptic areas, all of which converge through the anterior hypothalamus into the medial forebrain bundle of the lateral hypothalamus. These brain regions will figure heavily in our discussion of the neural substrates of sexual behavior in this chapter and of maternal behavior in the next. However, before I proceed to detail the mass of neurobehavioral evidence that is now available, let us briefly consider the broader social contexts in which sexuality must develop.

The Sociobiology of Sexual Attachments

The tortured protagonist of *The Kreutzer Sonata* contrasted the stark reality of male sexual urges with the softer fabric of feminine social expectations. Which view is correct—the image of the male who desires nothing but sex or the image of the female who seeks devotion? Obviously, both, but the desires of men and women are not as distinct as Tolstoy portrayed them. Women need sex as much as males need devotion, and it is hard to find devotion in marriage without sex. Only when one's sexual appetite is slaked with lots of reproductive activity, or perhaps when one has become wizened with age, is loving companionship enough. Thus, younger people need more sexual passion in their lives, while older ones tend to be more satisfied with friendly companionship. But everyone is capable of experiencing both commitment and deceit in the quest for reproductive success. Marriage, of course, is a human invention to assure that the former will generally outweigh the latter. Other species have gone to great lengths to minimize male philandering (Figure 12.1).

For marital relationships to last, the frailness of human commitments typically needs to be solidified by cultural mandates. Still, at present, some estimate that one marriage in every two ends in divorce. Why does this happen? Perhaps because nurturance, sexual motivation, and the quest for power are partially independent but also intertwined in the brain in ways that we do not yet fully comprehend. Evolution progresses via the continual magnification and reinforcement of strategies promoting reproductive fitness. In certain species and under certain circumstances, it may be a wise evolutionary strategy to reproduce and leave someone else to care for the offspring. Males make a smaller biological investment, not only because of their ability to produce exorbitant quantities of sperm but also because they do not get pregnant, and so are more likely to depart without establishing long-term commitments than are females, who carry and gestate the fetus. Hit-and-run tactics become counterproductive, however, when a single individual is bound to have great difficulty rearing offspring successfully to reproductive age. Thus, the amount of male investment varies enormously in mammalian and avian species. Some species make no lasting bonds, while others remain paired for life.[5]

Reproductive strategies have left indelible marks on the behavior of each creature. In certain fish, the male is more devoted to the offspring than the females; in many birds, males share responsibilities equally with females, while in most mammals the responsibilities are left more to the mother.[6] Some species are exceptional, such as humans, where the father has become an increasingly active participant in many cultures. There are even a few mammals, such as the titi monkeys of South America, where fathers naturally take greater care of the young than mothers, perhaps as a strategy to allow the mother adequate time to seek nourishment. Indeed, recent cultural thought in the West has sought to coax men increasingly toward an avian or titi monkey psychology, even though there is no assurance that the neural underpinnings of male nature are in total agreement with such a plan. Many human males remain satisfied with less commitment than society desires,[7] while others exhibit sustained devotion.

Since there is such marked variability in reproductive strategies among mammals, we should be cautious in generalizing from one species to another. Also, in some species there are great interindividual differences. There is, in fact, no single anthropoid plan that can be discerned among our brethren great apes: Whereas gibbons appear to mate for life with a single partner, gorillas prefer a harem-type family structure, orangutans tend to be social isolates, with the sexes coming together mostly for copulatory purposes, while chimpanzees are quite social and promiscuous, sharing partners rather indiscriminately. Thus, even our closest evolutionary cousins provide no clear insight about our intrinsic sexual nature.[8] Humans, with help from their rich imaginations, can partake of all these viewpoints.

Since human females exhibit "concealed estrus," with no seductive display of skin or smell to advertise ovulation, most assume that our sexuality has become strongly dissociated from immediate reproductive concerns. Human sexuality is probably as closely aligned with social bonding as it is with propagation. Thus, my discussion of "lower" species can only offer clarity in thinking about certain underlying issues. The biological constraints that all mammals share contain no prescription for what human sexual behavior should be. As always, in the subcortical reaches of the brain, the evidence can only tell us what *is*; it does not inform us about what *should* or *could* be, especially when it comes to creatures as complex as humans.

Although we cannot fathom the thoughts of other species, evolutionary psychologists have recently advised us that humans may have various intrinsic cognitive tendencies that guide our thinking about sexuality. Probably the most obvious fact is that the human male brain has many "simpleminded" feature detectors for various aspects of the female body, which easily generate sexual arousal. Female eroticism is not so visually captivated, but male bodies obviously also convey many sexual and other social messages. For instance, it has recently been argued that male-pattern baldness helps signal that one is relatively mild-mannered and not very threatening, while a large bush, especially on the face, tends to convey the opposite message.[9]

Sociobiologists have also suggested that the human brain is cognitively prepared to deliberate upon a large variety of reproductive issues—ranging from sexual competition to consummation, from parental care to social alliances that maximize inclusive fitness. Although it is unlikely that other mammals have similar thoughts, they appear to be spontaneously prepared to cope emotionally with very similar concerns. The tendency to help kin is widespread in nature.

It is now widely believed that reproductive urges have ruled the evolution of many subtle brain and bodily mechanisms. Indeed, the whole discipline of *sociobiology* is premised on the analysis of psychological, behavioral, and genetic complexities that have emerged in evolutionary history in the service of reproductive fitness.[10] Although sexual feelings cannot be observed directly, it is an inescapable fact that they exist, probably in all mammals, and they can be as intense as other bodily needs such as thirst and hunger. Indeed, sexuality lies at the very fulcrum of our attempts to distinguish processes that psychologists have traditionally called motivations, in which a bodily need is subserved by a behavior, from those called emotions, for which no bodily need is evident. Obviously, sex is not essential for the bodily survival of any individual member of a species, "merely" for the survival of the species itself. In other words, it is not just a peripheral bodily need but a brain need that has profound consequences for each species. Thus it is not surprising that it is a bodily and psychological function that is highly politicized in both animal and human societies.

We now know with considerable assurance that sexual feelings emerge from primitive hormonally regulated mechanisms of the emotional-limbic brain that we share to a substantial extent with other mammals. It was a remarkable feat of nature to weave powerful sexual feelings and desires in the fabric of the brain, without also revealing the reproductive purposes of those feelings to the eager participants. Unfortunately, routine sex education for young humans rarely attempts to clarify the types of neural fabric from which lust and erotic desires arise. Partly this is surely because most people are really not very interested in such neural details. Here, however, I will focus forthrightly on the brain substrates of those lusty passions that we have inherited from ancestral species. The little that we humans have learned about such matters—about the many erotic brain molecules and brain areas that fuel our sexual desires and behaviors—has emerged only during the past few decades. However, most of the peripheral hormonal mechanisms have been known for a much longer time.

The fact that gonadal hormones govern sexual behaviors has long been recognized and was experimentally characterized in the middle of the last century, starting with A. A. Berthold's studies of castrated roosters in 1849.[11] Berthold demonstrated that adult sexual characteristics did not emerge in roosters whose gonads had been removed, but that the roosters' full spectrum of male vigor was restored by reimplantation of the testes. During the early part of this century, the active factor controlling both the physical and the psychological expressions of male sexuality was demonstrated to be testosterone. However, almost a century passed before the role of specific brain systems in elaborating sexuality began to be recognized. Now we know there is really no other way to understand the basic nature of sexual lust and passion than through the intricacies of psychoneuroendocrinology and brain research. I will dwell no further on the peripheral genital and hormonal machinery, for that is well covered in many texts.[12] Instead, I will focus on the more recently discovered neuroanatomical, neurochemical, and neurobehavioral issues that are now ready to be linked to psychology.

Unfortunately, brain scientists are prone to restrict their discussions to sexual behavior and tend to ignore sexual feelings, for such neurodynamics cannot be directly observed. Thus, it will require some imagination and theoretical courage to discern the vague outlines of the primitive brain mechanisms that create the sociosexual feelings that are our foremost concern here. However, we can only scientifically probe such emotions in the context of objective behavioral and brain data. As previously argued, in affective neuroscience, these levels of analysis—the behavioral, psychological, and neurological—must always go together.

Varieties of Sexual Behaviors

It is wondrous to behold the varieties of courting and other sexual strategies that have evolved in the service of reproductive fitness.[13] For instance, the sexual skills and proclivities of various species of fish suggest that we should accept behavioral variety as the norm rather than the exception. For the deep-sea angler fish, the very limited male role is to bite into the body of the female, becoming a permanent sperm-donating "slave" that dangles from her more massive body, their reproductive functions under her hormonal command (Figure 12.1). On the other hand, sea bass have developed a strategy of "egg trading" in which pairs of animals reciprocally take male and female roles during successive reproductive episodes, so as to minimize the potential influence of male philandering (i.e., to minimize hit-and-run tactics in males that would provide no follow-up investment in rearing the young). Then there are hermaphrodites, such as killifish, which under adverse environmental circumstances indulge in self-fertilization. Such "peculiarities" are not restricted to lower animals.

Certain mammals also exhibit memorable sociosexual tendencies. For instance, as mentioned in Chapter 10, female hyenas have an enlarged clitoris (or pseudopenis) that, by any measure, is as impressive as the male organ and is quite capable of erectile activity. This appendage is used primarily for purposes of sociosexual communication, especially dominance displays. Baby hyenas are also delivered, perhaps quite painfully, via the narrow uterine canal that exits through this enlarged clitoral organ. The unusual reproductive apparatus of female hyenas highlights a key aspect of their social reality—the exceedingly powerful role of females in hyena societies. Females are consistently dominant over the males. How evolution promoted social power and dominion in female hyenas remains unclear, but it was probably achieved, at least in part, by hormonally induced masculinization of certain brain processes and body parts. In many mammals, the vigor of male sexuality and male assertiveness (i.e., social dominance) tend to go together, and we are finally beginning to understand the underlying neural conjunctions. The fact that male sexuality and aggression interact to a substantial extent in subcortical areas of the brain is now a certainty (see Chapter 10). The meaning of this interaction for human sexuality remains regrettably pregnant with ambiguities.

Most of our understanding concerning the brain substrates of sexuality has come from the analysis of how hormones modify brain activities in animals. There has been some puritanical resistance to accepting the implications of this work for the human condition, perhaps representing a culturally ingrained societal stance of separating the present cultural condition of humans from our animal past. The failure to recognize the common mammalian underpinnings of sexuality is also due in part to the dazzling diversity of sexual strategies in nature, as well as the obvious fact that many human strategies are cognitively mediated, yielding complex ideas and voluntary selection of gender stances that most smaller brains simply cannot assume. Accordingly, it is too widely believed that the underlying brain details may vary so markedly among species that useful translations are impossible. However, as more and more neurobiological evidence accumulates, such beliefs are becoming less and less tenable. It is unfortunate that in this important area of human experience, so many psychologists and other social scientists attempt to construct wishful belief systems that do not reflect physical realities.[14]

Still, surface variety is remarkable across species. For instance, the neural timing of sexual receptivity is dramatically different between animals that remain receptive throughout the year and seasonal breeders

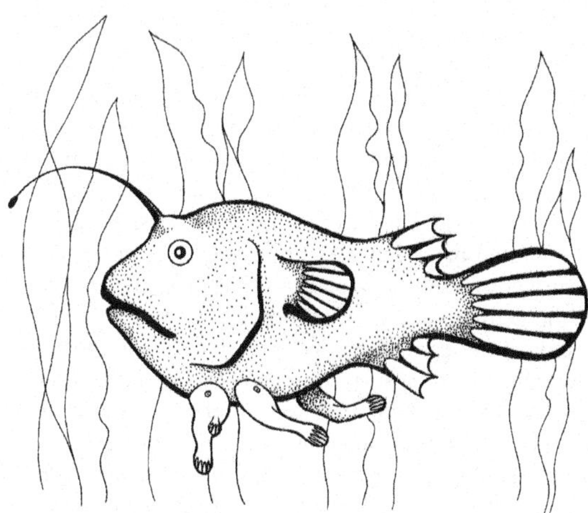

Figure 12.1. Drawing of a female deep-sea angler fish, with three males permanently attached to her body as ventral appendages. Through her hormones, she controls the testicular secretions of the fully "captivated" males. (Adapted from Crews, 1987; see n. 26.)

whose gonads grow and regress in early spring and autumn as the availability of daylight increases or decreases. Seasonal reproducers typically go to great lengths to advertise their receptive status, unlike humans and other species, including laboratory rats, that remain sexually active throughout the year. Despite such variety, we can be confident that many general principles of sexuality have been conserved in all mammalian species; here I will focus on those issues that seem most likely to apply to the human condition. This is not to say that humans cannot choose to override these mechanisms with their free will. They certainly can, especially if they are either skilled at deception or exceptionally saintly. Fortunately, other animals, which cannot lie and have no apparent urge to exercise willpower, speak their minds quite transparently through their behaviors.

To approximate the biological nature of things, the first tenet we need to accept is that male and female sexualities are as differently organized in male and female brains as they are in bodies. Although learning mechanisms are of obvious importance in generating the details of gender identity, the different sexes value substantially different things because of the distinct types of brain mechanisms and psychobiological values with which they are endowed. As already mentioned, human males are enticed by youthful beauty, while females are enticed by resource commitment. We also see this in other primate societies. Male chimpanzees usually fight over meat and sexual issues and also during social reunions, while females exhibit aggression largely in the context of seeking protection, competing for plant foods, and protection of the young.[15]

To some extent, especially in humans, the different gender expectations are culturally biased, but there are many psychobiological differences that are not simply a matter of choice or learning. For instance, males are more aggressive and power-oriented, while females are more nurturant and socially motivated. Indeed, recent brain metabolic evidence in humans indicates that temporal lobe areas (where aggression circuitry is concentrated) are more active in males, while cingulate areas (where nurturance and other social emotional circuitries are concentrated) are more active in females.[16] Such natural gender differences (at least at a population level) should no longer be a matter of debate, for the empirical facts seem overwhelming. However, we should doubt claims made for facts that have been poorly collected. For instance, in our estimation, rough-and-tumble play tendencies are quite comparable among males and females, at least in laboratory rats (see Chapter 15). Data on humans and other primates are not sufficiently well collected that we can exclude the effects of social learning on the gender differences that have been reported. In any event, we should come to terms with the fact that there are intrinsic neurochemical and psychobehavioral mechanisms in our brains that help create certain sex differences. Indeed, without the biological underpinnings, there would be no human sexuality or nurturance. It is truly remarkable how far back these differential controls go in brain evolution.

Evolutionary Sources of Mammalian Sexuality

If one places a small, naturally occurring, nine–amino acid peptide called *vasotocin* into the brains of male frogs and lizards, they begin to exhibit courting sounds and sexual behaviors. Given the opportunity, males treated with vasotocin mount and clasp females and copulate. In other words, a simple brain chemical system can trigger complex and coordinated sequences of sexual behavior.[17] It is not clear exactly what triggers the release of this transmitter in the reptilian brain under natural conditions, but it is clear that testosterone promotes vasotocin synthesis, and a host of social stimuli probably arouse the system into action. In fish the evolutionarily related hormone is *mesotocin*.

In mammals, two evolutionary offspring of these reptilian and piscine hormones (Figure 12.2), vasopressin and oxytocin, assume key roles in controlling certain aspects of sexual behaviors. Each differs from vasotocin by only one amino acid. Oxytocin has more effect on female sexual and social behavior, while vasopressin (which differs from oxytocin by only two amino acids) retains the ability to govern male sexuality.[18]

Intellectually, it is quite satisfying to discover that these descendants of more ancient molecules still control social and sexual behaviors in mammals. Vasopressin, which is more abundant in the male brain, is especially important in the mediation of many aspects of male sexual persistence (including courtship, territorial marking, and intermale aggression). Oxytocin, which is more abundant in female brains, helps mediate female social and sexual responsivity (especially the tendency of female rodents when mounted to exhibit lordosis postures, a characteristic, arch-backed, female receptivity reflex).[19] It is even more remarkable that after the birth of the young, these same synaptic modulators encourage parents, especially the mothers but at times also the fathers, to take care of their offspring (see Chapter 13).

To the best of our present knowledge, the segregation of male and female sex-related chemistries in the mammalian brain is incomplete. Vasopressin systems may help energize some of the more aggressive aspects of maternal behavior (i.e., protecting the young from harm); conversely, oxytocin systems may sustain some of the gentler aspects of male behavior (e.g., the tendency of fathers to be nonaggressive and supportive toward their offspring).[20] It cannot be emphasized too much that brain oxytocin is not completely reserved for female functions. It also has some role in governing male sexuality, just as vasopressin may have some role in females (i.e., reducing sexual readiness and increasing maternal aggressiveness).

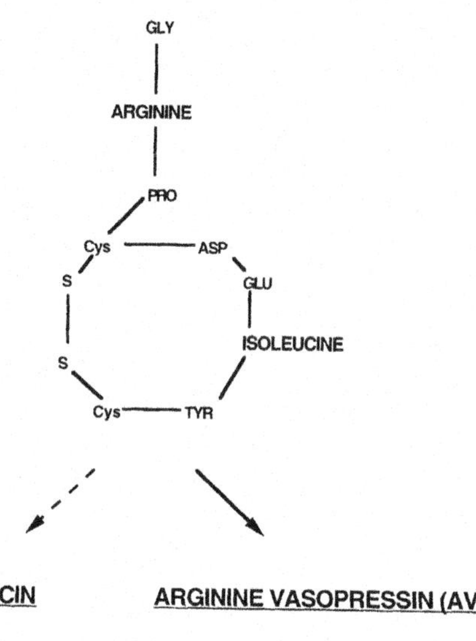

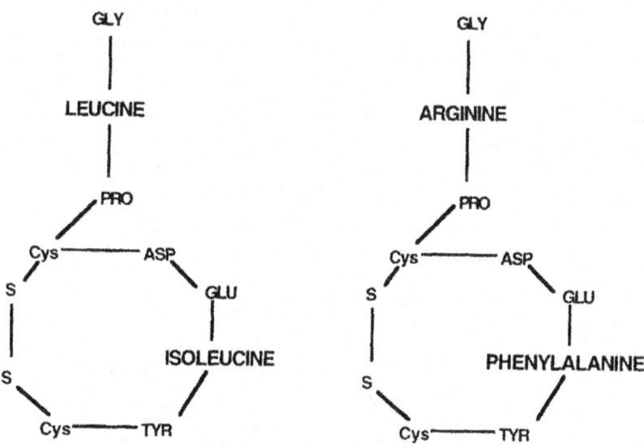

Figure 12.2. Summary of the structures of mammalian arginine-vasopressin (AVP) and oxytocin (OXY) as compared with the structure of the ancestral avian posterior pituitary neuropeptide arginine vasotocin (AVT). Each of the mammalian peptides differs from AVT by a single amino acid.

In males, oxytocin placed directly into many brain areas promotes sexual arousal (i.e., induces erections), ejaculation, and orgasm.[21] It is somewhat perplexing that the hippocampus would be a highly sensitive brain tissue to generate such effects, since it has generally been thought to function mainly in the conversion of short-term memories to long-term ones. This, of course, leads to the possibility that oxytocin produces erections there by activating sexual memories. In any event, brain oxytocin also appears to help mediate the behavioral inhibition, or "refractory period," that follows orgasm in males. Perhaps this peptide helps mediate postorgasmic feelings such as the "afterglow" that commonly follows copulation, at least in humans.[22]

It may seem paradoxical that the same brain chemical can mediate both sexual arousal and sexual satiety, but such subtleties no longer surprise neuroscientists. Reversals in behavioral effects are common in neuropeptide research and may correspond to the dynamics of the evoked psychological processes.[23] Just as a little alcohol can facilitate sociability, higher levels are bound to impair. As discussed more extensively in the following, similar effects can be obtained with endogenous opioids, where low doses of morphine can promote sexuality, while high doses impair it. Such effects may be mediated by slightly different circuits, receptor systems, or other yet unfathomed emotional dynamics of these systems in action as a function of how much of a given neuromodulator has been released over time.

There are many other situations in which social neuropeptides have one effect at low doses and a diametrically opposite effect at higher doses. One relevant example, which will be discussed more fully later, is the ability of low doses of oxytocin to solidify social memories, while high doses impair such memories.[24] Thus, at modest levels, brain oxytocin activity appears to help cement social bonds that may be the foundations for future reciprocities and "friendships," while excessive activity may lead to social aloofness.[25] One thing modern neuroscience has revealed is that the brain is full of apparent puzzles and paradoxes, and that logic is not as good a guide to knowledge in the natural sciences as careful observation!

Let us now consider how the basic impulses for male and female sexuality are organized in the mammalian brain. To understand sexuality, it is essential to recognize important differences in male and female brain organization, some of which occur during fetal development and some of which become apparent only when those differential plans are activated by the increasing hormonal tides of puberty. I will shift readily between animal data and human implications, since the evidence suggests that at the basic subcortical levels the neuronal machinery is remarkably similar.[26]

Genetic Sex and Fetal Sexual Differentiation

The ever-increasing appreciation of the differences between the *organizational* and *activational* components of sexuality has deepened our understanding of what it means to be male or female. A photographic analogy helps us envision these distinct processes. The hormonal patterns that are set in place during the organizational phase of fetal development help "expose" the imprint of maleness or femaleness on maturing brain circuits, as well as on bodily appearance. The hormones secreted at the onset of puberty eventually "develop" the exposed "negative," thereby activating the latent male or female sexual proclivities that have remained comparatively dormant within brain circuits since infancy. If brain and body organization do not match up, the individual will have to discover, through painful experience, which gender was predominantly imprinted within his or her brain, and to what extent. This can be a stressful and lonely psychological journey.[27]

Animal research has indicated that the male and female poles of brain sexuality reflect extremes of a gradient that allows for many intermediary types. Although male and female sexuality are distinct to a substantial extent, each sex does in fact possess circuits for both forms of behavior, but typically to different degrees. The fact that male and female brains have distinct but related psychosocial proclivities allows sexual urges to become quite complicated in the real world. The possible permutations allow for cross-sexual variants that society is still trying to reconcile with long-standing cultural expectations, which are sometimes based on ignorance and intolerance. This issue was poignantly highlighted when President Clinton attempted to open the doors of the military to homosexuals at the start of his presidency in 1993, but the forces of ignorance and discrimination prevailed.

Brain scientists have suspected for many decades that there are intrinsic brain organizational patterns that promote certain forms of homosexuality.[28] The remarkable confirmatory story that has now been worked out in animal models is only slowly percolating into our general cultural imagination. To highlight this story for my students, I typically ask them a seemingly inane question: "How many genders or sexes are there?" At first they look puzzled, but courageous students are willing to provide the reasonable and expected answer: "two." I tell them how curious it is that our modern society still holds on to such prescientific views, for "four or more" is certainly a more accurate answer. Indeed, this is the belief some Native American tribes held as the correct description of their social world. They believed that in addition to the prevailing variants of *man within man* and *woman within woman,* nature sometimes created a *man's mind within the body of a woman* and a *woman's mind within the body of a man.* The essential accuracy of this view has now been affirmed by years of scientific research on the development and expression of sex circuits inside the rodent brain. Indeed, one could argue that there can be an "infinite number" of permutations along the biochemically determined gradients of brain and body masculinization and feminization. However, for our purposes "four" is certainly a more accurate answer than "two" as an estimate of the major types of gender (brain/mind) and sex (body) identities that actually exist in the world. Although the details have been worked out in lower animals, existing evidence suggests that similar principles also operate in humans.

In simplest terms, the brain *organizational* story goes like this. One is typically born either genetically female (with the XX pattern of sex chromosomes) or genetically male (with the XY pattern). What the Y chromosome provides for the male is testis determining factor (TDF), which ultimately induces the male gonadal system to manufacture testosterone.[29] The XX pattern allows things to progress in the ongoing feminine manner, unless some external source of testosterone (or, more accurately, one of its metabolites) intervenes. The actual manner in which male brain and body development proceeds is determined by the timing and intensity of the resulting hormonal organizational signals, namely, testosterone and two closely related metabolic products, estrogen and dihydrotestosterone (DHT). These last two steroid hormones normally control the final trajectory of brain and body development, respectively, while the XY baby is still in the womb—still hidden from the cultural influences of its future social world (Figure 12.3).

These hormones can similarly affect female development if they happen to be present in sufficiently high levels during pregnancy. However, the XX sex chromosome pattern informs the female body to manufacture proteins such as the steroid-binding factor *alpha-fetoprotein*, which can thwart the cross-gender organizational influences of sex steroids during early development.[30] This protects the female fetus from being masculinized by the generally high levels of maternal estrogens. If there is not enough of this fail-safe factor, or if the maternal levels of estrogens are so high that they saturate the available alpha-fetoprotein, the female will proceed toward a male pattern of development—sometimes in both body and mind, sometimes in one but not the other, depending on the hormonal details that have transpired.

The four major types of organizational permutations can yield the obvious forms of cross-sexual gender identities: the presence of malelike brains in female bodies and of female brains in malelike bodies. The fact that individuals who look like men on the outside can come to feel like women on the inside, and individuals who look like women on the outside can come to feel like men on the inside, arises from a simple biological fact. The signals that trigger babies' brains and bodies to take the various possible gender and sex paths are separate (Figure 12.3). Initially, all fetuses are femalelike, and masculinity emerges from distinct prenatal signals that tell the brain and body to be masculinized. After the TDF gene has induced the male fetus to manufacture testosterone, several critical events must take place before the male brain and body phenotypes can be fully expressed (Figure 12.3). First, testosterone needs to be converted in two distinct one-step reactions to estrogen and DHT. The final organizational signal that tells the brain to masculinize is estrogen, and the signal that tells the body to develop along male-typical lines is DHT. Of course, these sexual potentials, laid down in the brain and body during gestation and infancy, do not become fully manifested until puberty.

With our current understanding of this organizational phase of psychosexual development, it is no longer a surprise that estrogen, a steroid hormone that is associated with female sexuality in the popular imagi-

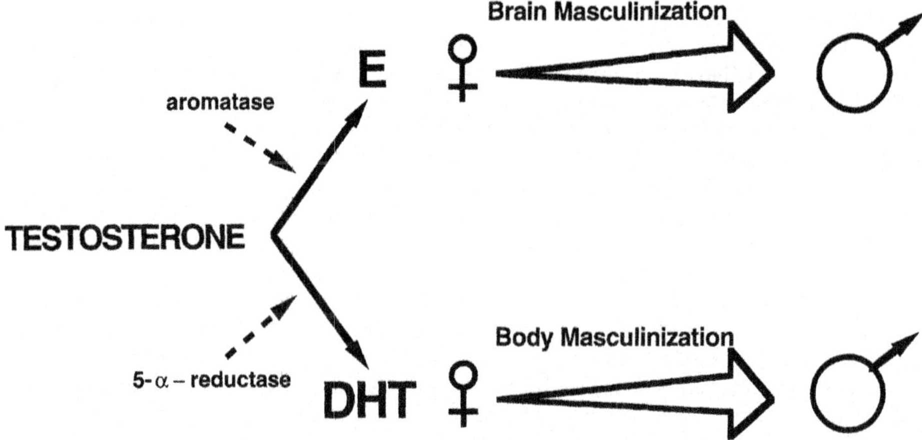

Figure 12.3. Both the brain and body of mammals are initially organized according to a female characteristic plan. Maleness emerges from two distinct influences of testosterone on body tissues—masculinization of the brain being mediated by estrogen (E) and of the body by dihydrotestosterone (DHT). Different tissues can convert testosterone to different products because of the enzymes they contain. DHT is manufactured in cells containing 5-α-reductase, and E is manufactured in those that contain aromatase.

nation, helps organize the intrinsic brain aspects of male gender identity in many species. To understand this, we need to consider the metabolism of testosterone (Figure 12.3). After testosterone has been synthesized from cholesterol, via many steps that include the intermediates progesterone and dihydroepiandrosterone, it can be biochemically modified in two distinct ways. Along one metabolic path, it can be converted into DHT with the assistance of the enzyme *5-α-reductase*. Along the other path, it can be converted into estrogen by the enzyme *aromatase*. These products of testosterone metabolism are critical ingredients that dictate whether a genetic male will continue along the male path in terms of body and brain development, both before and after puberty.[31] Various forms of homosexuality and bisexuality are promoted if "errors" occur in the various control points of these biochemical processes—if the developing male brain is not bathed in testosterone at the sensitive time or if it is missing the enzyme aromatase that converts testosterone to estrogen.

If the female brain is exposed to too much estrogen during the sensitive periods of development (the precise time varies from species to species), it will assume malelike characteristics while leaving the body feminine.[32] Females such as these will preferentially exhibit male-typical behaviors at maturity, but only if their brains are exposed to the activational effects of testosterone at that time. Indeed, in humans, tomboyishness in females has been promoted by maternal injections of diethylstilbestrol (DES), an estrogenic hormone that was given to pregnant mothers during the second trimester to prevent miscarriages in the 1940s and 1950s.[33]

Conversely, in the absence of fetal estrogen but with sufficient DHT, a male body can emerge with female-type circuits hidden within the brain. A naturally occurring instance of this type of organizational development has been found in a small group of individuals in the Dominican Republic. These boys, called *guevedoces,* which literally means "penis at 12," are genetically deficient in 5-α-reductase.[34] They have a female appearance at birth, with some enlargement of the clitoris and no apparent testicles (which are present but remain undescended within the body). However, their fetal gonads do apparently secrete testosterone at the usual time, and since they have normal aromatase activity, it is converted to estrogen but not DHT. Accordingly, their brains, but not their bodies, are fully organized along male lines. When such boys enter puberty and begin to secrete testosterone, they develop male-typical bodies—with an increase of body hair, deepening of the voice, enlargement of the penis, and, finally, the descent of the testes. Male-typical sexual urges also begin to emerge. Thus, the boys' pubescent erotic desires come to be directed toward females, even though they were reared as girls throughout childhood! This probably indicates that the male brain is instinctively prepared to respond to certain features of human femaleness, including facial and bodily characteristics, voice intonations, as well as ways of being.

There are yet other fascinating variants of psychosexual expression in humans that are probably biologically based but less well understood. For instance, some males have an extra female chromosome (i.e., XXY) and exhibit *Klinefelter's syndrome*, which is characterized by exceptionally small gonads. Such children are often temperamentally passive, socially dependent, and mentally slow. On the other hand, boys with an extra male chromosome (i.e., XYY) have been claimed to be more hostile and aggressive than normal males, even though these findings are debatable. In addition, many drugs can modify the normal progression of the underlying psychosexual organizational processes, which should caution women against taking any drugs or being exposed to environmental toxins during pregnancy.[35]

These fascinating details of early development inform us of a profound fact of nature: Although male and female are the most typical biologically ordained poles of sexual identity, a vast number of gradations can be produced by normally occurring variations in the underlying hormonal control mechanisms that guide gender differentiation. Because of this, the biological forms of homosexuality do not represent psychological perversity resulting from aberrant psychosocial experiences but simply represent natural variants that can occur in the course of development. Of course, this does not exclude the possibility that humans sometimes voluntarily select gender roles in accord with their whimsical or neurotic cognitive desires. It is possible for someone to be halfway on the biological gradient of masculinity-femininity, and we might expect such individuals to be highly bisexual, with a maximal choice as to which direction they wish to orient their erotic tendencies. Since the real causes are typically hidden in the brain, it will be difficult to distinguish who is who, and it should not matter. Obviously, one's erotic choices should remain an individual matter, as long as no coercion or child abuse is involved.[36]

In sum, the major role of sex chromosomes is to dictate which enzymes and hormones will be manufactured by the developing reproductive apparatus. The XY chromosome pattern tells the male's body to manufacture testosterone at critical periods of development, setting in motion a cascade of changes in the protoypical female-type brain. This type of brain masculinization can also occur in females, which can promote cross-sexual behavioral and erotic tendencies in adulthood. The traditional XX pattern of femaleness will emerge, even in genetic males, if such early hormone secretions do not occur. Thus, the brain substrates for sexuality that are organized by these early hormonal experiences help determine what type of gender identities, erotic desires, and sex behaviors individuals will exhibit at puberty, when the elevations in hypothalamic gonadotrophic hormones and gonadal sex steroids begin to "activate" sexual tendencies (Figure 12.4).

Although the exact details of the hormonal cascades controlling these early organizational events vary somewhat among species, they are sufficiently similar in rats and humans that work on the former has elucidated the patterns that were subsequently found in the latter. But there presumably are differences in the magnitude of the cross-gender effects that can be achieved in different species. For instance, existing evidence suggests that rats exhibit larger brain changes during fetal masculinization than do humans, which would be in line with the larger average differences in body size between males and females. Usually the average gender difference in body size is considered an index of the extremity of sex roles in a species. Thus, it is to be expected that "tournament species" such as elks and walruses, in which intermale competition and the seeking of dominion over females are extreme, will exhibit the largest dimorphism between the sexes. In comparison with such creatures, the relative biologically based gender differences are modest in humans. On the other hand, in such species as the spotted hyena, we would predict that the tables would be turned, but sufficient brain data have not yet been collected.

What Is Organized in the Male Brain by Fetal Testosterone?

Much confusion in earlier discussions of hormones and sexuality arose from the failure to draw a clear distinction between the ways hormones *organize* male and female brains during fetal development and how they later *activate* the physiological and neuropsychological changes that accompany puberty. Because of the bifurcation of hormonal control of body and brain development (Figure 12.3), we now understand why intrinsic gender identity and body morphology do not always match up. To summarize, both humans and rats can have female-type brains in male-type bodies (if DHT was present in sufficient quantities but estrogen was not) or male-type brains in female-type bodies (where estrogen was present but DHT was not).

Although such biological facts are unlikely to explain all homosexual tendencies, they probably account for many cases, especially those including explicit internal desires for transsexual transformations, which in our modern society can prompt individuals to have sex-change operations. Recent evidence indicates that transsexuals have demonstrable differences in the bed nucleus of the stria terminalis, one of many brain areas that control sexual motivation. Thus, many males who have sought to be surgically converted to females do have more female types of brain organization.[37] Understandably, most people would desire that their internally experienced sexuality and gender identity should match their external appearance. There are bound to be many variants in the organization of the underlying circuits, but at present we have woefully little detailed information on such matters.

Although socialization certainly influences the sexual roles individuals choose, it now appears less crucial than has been widely believed in the arena of basic sexual feelings. For instance, the Dominican XY males who lacked 5-α-reductase did not experience extreme difficulty in reorienting their lives as males following puberty, even though they had been reared as girls. In

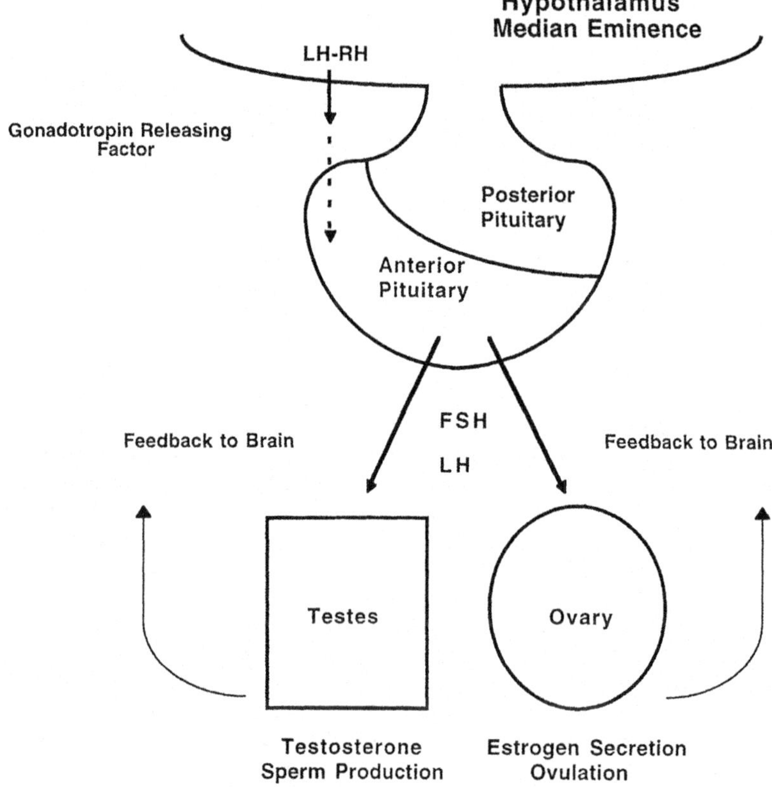

Figure 12.4. Overview of the hypothalamic and anterior pituitary control of sex steroid secretion. Hypothalamic gonadotrophin-releasing hormone, also known as LH-RH (leutenizing hormone-releasing hormone), activates the release of leutenizing hormone and follicle-stimulating hormone, which promote estrogen secretion from the ovary and testosterone production in the testes.

contrast, boys who have lost their genitalia early in life and have been reared as girls throughout their childhood have been found to experience considerable emotional distress and confusion at puberty when they are expected to behave like women. This is probably because they have the imprint of maleness stamped firmly in their brains.

What does it mean precisely when we assert that a brain has been masculinized? Although all the details have not been resolved, male and female brains differ in many important respects. For instance, females generally exhibit greater hemispheric coordination, since their right and left lobes are integrated more extensively via the larger fiber connections of the corpus callosum. This may have important implications for higher brain functions, such as the tendency of females to use both hemispheres in speech while males tend to use only the left side of their brains.[38] Accordingly, females often recover speech more readily after left hemisphere strokes than do men. Unfortunately, because of the lack of appropriate animal models, this is not well understood at the neuronal level. The most widely studied sex-related brain differences are found in subcortical areas. Remarkably clear neuroanatomical and neurochemical distinctions are found in neural systems that contain high levels of sex-steroid receptors, which are known to exist in all of the distinct varieties that one might expect—including different ones for testosterone, DHT, estrogen, and progesterone.

The largest subcortical differences have been found in the anatomy and chemistry of the medial *preoptic area* (POA), where males in practically all species studied have significantly larger neuronal densities than females.[39] In rats, the most highly masculinized zone is called the sexually dimorphic nuclei of the preoptic area (SDN-POA). In females, many neurons in this part of the brain die during fetal development for lack of testosterone, or more precisely its product estrogen, which is a powerful growth factor for these neurons. In humans the homologous brain areas are called the interstitial nuclei of anterior hypothalamus (INAH). Several studies have now documented that sex differences in specific INAH nuclei of human brains closely resemble those found in rats, albeit the sexual dimorphic growth of these areas is not as great.[40] This probably helps explain why behavioral sex differences are not as great in humans as in some other species, in which these hypertrophied hypothalamic circuits do participate in the elaboration of male-typical sex behaviors. Even though a great deal is known about such matters in rats, there is, at present, little direct evidence in humans. Hence, generalizations are hazardous, but they may help guide our thinking.

Brain Control of Male Sexual Behavior

Following puberty, these organizational effects in the POA influence male sexual tendencies in all mammals that have been carefully studied. If the POA area is damaged, male sexual behavior is severely impaired (Figure 12.5).[41] In certain creatures, such as rats, lots of early play experience can partially overcome such deficits.[42] In others, such as cats, play does not promote restoration of sexual functions.[43] Overall, the influences of this area on sexuality presently appear to be more evident in the behavioral than the psychological realms, as highlighted by studies that have contrasted POA lesion–induced changes in sexual behavior and sexual motivation.

In sexually experienced rats, this area is more important for the generation of sexual *behavior* than sociosexual *motivation*. Following lesions of the POA, male rats that have had abundant sexual experience still seek access to receptive females, even though they do not attempt to copulate with them.[44] In other words, their social memories, situated perhaps in the cingulate cortex, amygdala, and nearby areas of the temporal lobes, are still capable of motivating social approach, although sexual engagement is no longer initiated. Perhaps this is because they can no longer experience sexual pleasure. Neurophysiological studies in primates indicate strong neural arousal in the POA not only when animals are copulating but also when males are approaching the subject of their desire.[45] Comparable effects are not seen when they approach other objects of desire, such as a bunch of bananas!

The SDN-POA of male rats contains abundant testosterone receptors, which activate male sexual tendencies at maturity.[46] In some species the less abundant DHT receptors also contribute to arousal. Castrated male rats that have lost their sexual ardor can be reinvigorated simply by placing testosterone directly into the POA. Indeed, male rats that are not very active sexually (so-called duds) have fewer testosterone receptors in this part of the brain than sexually vigorous animals (the so-called studs).[47] Estrogen, although it helped organize this tissue in male-typical ways during infancy, has no apparent role to play in activating adult male sexuality.

Major sex differences in brain anatomies and neurochemistries have also been found in various other brain areas such as the amygdala, especially in medial areas, where high concentrations of sex steroid receptors are found (areas that also play an important role in elaborating rage and intermale aggression). Neurons in the anterior areas of the medial amygdala of male rats respond equally to copulatory experiences as well as aggressive ones, while some of the cells in more posterior areas appear to respond selectively to the ejaculatory, and hence perhaps their orgasmic, experiences.[48] Androgen as well as estrogen receptors are concentrated in many of the same brain areas, including the POA,

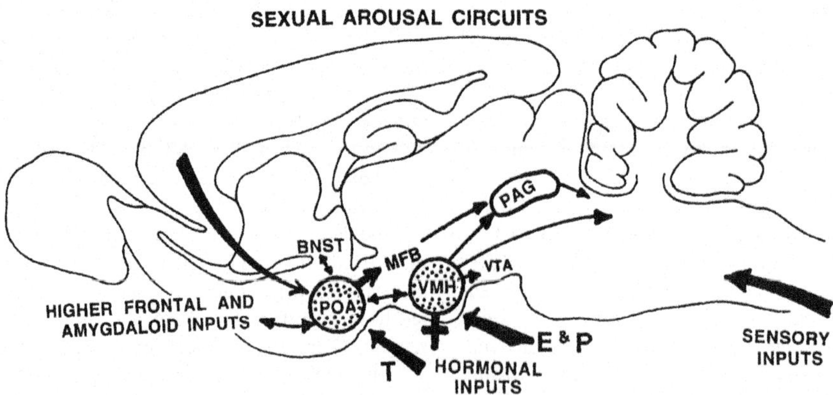

Figure 12.5. Lateral view of the rat brain summarizing two major areas that provide differential control over male and female sexual behaviors. Males contain a larger POA, and this area is essential for male sexual competence. The VMH is clearly more influential in female sexual responsivity. These systems operate, in part, by sensitizing various sensory input channels that promote copulatory reflexes. The extent to which these circuits control the affective components of sexual behavior remains uncertain.

the ventromedial hypothalamus, the periaqueductal gray, and down to the lower reaches of the spinal cord, where both male and femal sexual reflexes are controlled.[49] There are fine anatomical and neurochemical differences between males and females in all these areas, with the most striking one in the lower spinal cord being the *nucleus of the bulbocavernosus*, which is distinctly larger in males than in females. As already indicated, there are also some differences in the cortex, as well as in the commissures that connect the two hemispheres, which no doubt contribute to distinct cognitive styles in men and women.

Many brain areas exhibit neurochemical differences, but we are just beginning to fathom which of them control the various aspects of sexual behavior, sexual desire, sexual pleasure, and the many other sex differences documented in the behavioral tendencies of animals and humans—especially in urges such as aggressiveness, exploration, fear, and nurturance.[50] It is also reasonable to assume that comparable brain differences in humans control the strength of psychological and behavioral strategies that human males and females employ in seeking reproductive success, but there is precious little objective evidence to bolster such beliefs. Indeed, it is hard to imagine how documentation could be obtained, not only because of the pervasive methodological difficulties (e.g., it is impossible to control for differential learning factors in humans) but also because of the pervasive influence of issues of political correctness in this arena of knowledge.

In our society, many find it difficult to accept any intrinsic differences among the sexes. It also seems that others would be delighted to embellish any intrinsic differences with "naturalistic phallacies" that attempt to transform factual "is" statements into ethical "should" statements, thereby promoting various reactionary gender-biased political agendas. Abundant neuroscience data now suggest how brain and neurobiological differences between the sexes can promote or hinder certain psychological and behavioral tendencies—from aggression to nurturance. These are bound to have consequences for the emergence of long-term changes that we might seek in the sociopolitical arena of human affairs. How we will deal with these emerging facts, and incorporate them into our worldviews gracefully, remains a major challenge to our culture. Obviously, our search for equity must increasingly empower pro-social human qualities that ennoble us as caring creatures (see Chapter 13 and "Afterthought," Chapter 16).

Stress-Induced Suppression of Brain Masculinization

Although nature is strongly disposed toward creating relatively clear-cut male brains within male bodies and female brains within female bodies, we have now seen that it can easily produce other permutations. These may have adaptive consequences under certain circumstances. For instance, they can lead to different courting strategies that might actually increase reproductive fitness: Less strongly masculinized males might succeed with females by exhibiting behaviors that some would find more attractive than the tendency toward male brutishness that is so evident in many tournament species. Alternatively, the presence of such individuals in the social group may provide psychological dispositions that increase the reproductive advantage of their relatives (e.g., increased helping behaviors in male homosexuals). One additional idea is that under certain conditions, such as periods of high social and environmental stress, increased levels of homosexuality may be adaptive by limiting reproduction that could prove wasteful.[51] In any event, it is now well established that mother rats who have been heavily stressed during pregnancy tend to have a high incidence of homosexual male offspring. Maternal stress sets in motion internal neurochemical changes that tend to leave the brains of male offspring in their primordial femalelike condition.

When a pregnant rat is exposed to any of a variety of stressors during the last trimester (third week) of the three-week gestation period, many of the male offspring exhibit gender ambiguity when they reach puberty. Commonly, the experimental stress imposed on such mothers has consisted of prolonged immobilization, with continuous exposure to bright light, which rats dislike and which also generates thermoregulatory discomfort. However, many other stressors, such as foot shock or overcrowding, have also been used with comparable results. In a normal litter from unstressed mothers, approximately 80% of the males become "studs" at puberty, while the rest remain asexual "duds," which exhibit little male- or female-typical sexual behavior. Among the male pups of stressed mothers, however, only about 20% become "studs," while about 60% either are bisexual (exhibiting male behavior with a highly receptive female, and female behavior in response to a "stud" male) or else exhibit exclusively female sex behaviors (i.e., they exhibit lordosis, the characteristic female-specific receptivity pattern, when mounted by a sexually aroused male). The remaining 20% are asexual, as in unstressed litters. From the perspective that homosexuality may promote nurturance, it is noteworthy that the homosexual and bisexual males from stressed mothers are also more likely to exhibit maternal behaviors than their normal counterparts.[52]

These ratios can be altered substantially by the pups' social rearing conditions: The male offspring of stressed mothers exhibit more "normal" sexual behavior if they are housed continuously during adulthood with sexually experienced females. Although the expression of homosexual tendencies varies as a function of environmental conditions, the dramatic increase in the potential for this kind of gender ambiguity is now known to arise from the fact that maternal stress causes physiological changes that work against the normal masculinization of the male brain.

The fetal spurt of testosterone that normally masculinizes male rats occurs several days prior to birth (around 19 days of fetal age).[53] Under conditions of maternal stress, the critical cascade of events is disrupted so that the peak of testosterone secretion occurs several days earlier than it should, when brain tissues are not yet ready to receive the organizing message. It is as if the organizational camera shutter had been clicked without the lens cap being removed: Although enough testosterone is secreted, it simply comes too early, and the neural image of maleness is not adequately imprinted upon the brain. In addition, maternal stress impairs enzymes that help synthesize testosterone in the gonads. Delta^5-3ß-hydroxysteroid dehydrogenase is inhibited, especially around days 18 and 19 of gestation, when the enzyme is normally available in highest levels. Likewise, brain aromatase, which allows testosterone to be converted to estrogen, is inhibited at the same time. These factors combine in such a manner that the brains of the affected males remain more femalelike. For instance, the SDN-POA becomes feminized because of the normal female-typical progression of cell loss in that area, since the effect of estrogen in promoting nerve growth is absent.[54]

Recent work has clarified whether it is the psychological consequences of maternal stress that cause demasculinization or whether stress-related physiological changes suffice: The effect seems to be a direct result of the mother's bodily stress response. Of the several prominent stress hormones, excess opioid (perhaps ß-endorphin) secretion appears to mediate the demasculinizing effect of stress. Pituitary ß-endorphin release is partly a counterregulatory hormonal mechanism that helps prevent other excessive stress responses, such as those arising from adrenocorticotrophic hormone (ACTH) secretion. The possible role of an opioid component in stress-induced neurodevelopmental changes has been evaluated simply by blocking opioid receptors during maternal stress with long-acting drugs such as naltrexone; the result was a complete restoration of masculinization. Stress-induced abnormalities in various biochemical parameters, such as reduced aromatase production, were also rectified.[55]

Since opiate receptor blockade can mildly increase the psychological perception of stress in humans, these results suggest that the opioid component of the stress response, as opposed to any psychological response to the stressor, is the critical element in the cascade of events that lead to the failure in fetal masculinization. This line of research also suggests that external administration of opioids to pregnant mothers may demasculinize males, and there is some evidence for this in animals.[56] One must wonder whether similar changes would occur in the male offspring of women addicted to opiates during pregnancy. At present we do not know, but the prediction is clear: Boys born to mothers using opiates during the second trimester would be expected to have a higher incidence of homosexuality than the offspring of nonaddicted women.

Does maternal stress also affect the development of the female offspring? The answer was thought to be no, but some behavioral differences in females have now been detected. The most noteworthy, in the present context, is that female offspring of stressed mothers exhibit weaker maternal tendencies than those from nonstressed mothers—just the converse of the pattern seen in males, who tend to become more nurturant.[57] Such changes in nurturance have been evaluated using a "sensitization" or "concaveation" procedure, whereby virgin animals (either male or female) are given free access to rat pups. Across several days of exposure, these initially nonmaternal animals begin to exhibit such behaviors as retrieving pups and huddling over them (see also Chapter 13). The females from stressed mothers take longer to exhibit this type of sensitization, while the males begin to exhibit nurturant behaviors more rapidly than controls.[58]

Another urgent question is whether human babies exhibit similar brain changes when their mothers are confronted by stress. Although several positive findings are available, they are generally deemed controversial. For instance, it has been documented that one highly stressful historical period, namely, the years of declining fortunes for Germany during World War II, led to a higher incidence of homosexual individuals, as measured by their sexual preferences in later years. In other words, boys born during the peak years of wartime stress were reported to have a higher incidence of homosexuality than those born during the years of peace before and after the war.[59] Also, there has been some work relating the levels of perceived stress during the various trimesters of pregnancy to homosexuality in male offspring. Elevated stress during the second trimester has been reported by some investigators to be related to a higher incidence of homosexuality in the offspring.[60]

Of course, scientific caution is always advised in trying to extrapolate from animal data to the human condition. As one scientist who has done much of this work points out, "The optimistic conclusion . . . that this (i.e., stress) syndrome provides a direct explanation of homosexuality in human males should be greeted with some caution."[61] At the same time, however, to insist that such findings have no implications for human issues is to sustain an excessively cautious stance about the underlying dynamics of the human body and brain.

In sum, even though environmental effects clearly modify one's self-perceptions, the sources of gender identity, as genetic sex itself, are heavily rooted in biology. Although it would be foolish to conclude that sexual preferences are completely controlled by nature, we can no longer discount innate biological influences. The reason such factors were not considered more fully during earlier eras of cross-sex research was because the efforts of most investigators were focused on the role of hormone patterns that occur during the activational phase of sexuality at the onset of puberty rather than those that guide the organizational phases of fetal development.[62] Obviously, those early hormone secretions are still difficult to study in humans, so we must be satisfied with the snippets of indirect evidence that may be gleaned from clinical evidence.

Female and Male Sexual Behaviors: The Activational Phase

The imprint that is made on male and female fetal brains by early hormonal tides is finally developed at puberty (Figure 12.4). The passionate potentials of the nervous system are brought to life by renewed tides of hormone secretion. When animals copulate, neurons in widespread areas of the brain "light up," as seen through Fos immunocytochemistry. The areas are widespread in medial subcortical zones, but especially in areas that have high concentrations of hormone receptors.[63] These brain areas manufacture transmitters, partly under the control of sex hormones, that are especially important for normal sexuality. Obviously, a multiplicity of controls—emotional, cognitive, behavioral, and physiological—must be synchronized for competent sexual behavior in both males and females. Thus, scientific progress in this area will arise from our ability to follow and quantify these various components objectively, rooting out pervasive methodological problems, not to mention cultural biases. This makes the relevant human research remarkably difficult.

The most evident features of sexuality are behavioral, and excellent techniques exist to study the appetitive (proceptive) and consummatory (receptive) aspects of sexual behavior in lower animals. Accordingly, my focus here will be largely on the behavior of laboratory rats. However, we must remember that even in the brain research laboratory, much more work has been devoted to the consummatory (i.e., copulatory) components than to the proceptive, courting, or appetitive components of sexual behavior. Even more regrettably, more empirical work has been done on male than female sexual proclivities, and hence our factual coverage will remain a bit lopsided. This sex bias in the questions being asked has gradually been changing as increasing numbers of female investigators have entered this field of inquiry.

In general, experienced male rats housed alone in their cages are always ready for a little sex. Females, on the other hand, are not. Female rats typically have four-day sexual (estrus) cycles, and only for several hours on the day of estrus are they willing to participate in copulation. Nature has assured, for most species, that sexual arousal in females is tightly coordinated with peak fertility.

A few species, including humans, exhibit no such correspondence, and human females can remain receptive throughout the monthly cycle. In other words, human females exhibit a "concealed ovulation" with no clear "estrus cycle," which makes sexual behavior around the peak of the monthly cycle a less probable event than it is in most other species. This means that sexual urges and the likelihood of fertilization have been dissociated to a substantial extent in our species, which may help promote male investment and pair-bonding with individual women. In other words, a human male cannot identify which female is ovulating by any external sign. Hence, for reproductive success, he needs to be more attentive to one female's needs for longer periods of time than is characteristic of most mammals.[64]

If a human female is willing to offer sufficient sexual gratification to one male, the probability that he will squander or invest his resources elsewhere is reduced. This would obviously set female sexuality in humans apart from that found in most other species. However, this could have been effected by fairly modest shifts in the motivational substrates, such as a shift toward a male pattern of testosterone-mediated eroticism, while sustaining the other subcortical principles of female sexuality summarized earlier. We also must remember that the neural programs for sexuality are much more "open" to higher mental influence in humans than in other species. This is especially important when we come to the stereotyped sexual behavior exhibited by males of most species.

In rats and most other mammals, the general male strategy (facilitated by testosterone) is to exhibit fairly persistent searching for numerous sexual interactions (the word *cruising* has been used for this behavior pattern), followed by the emission of vigorous overtures (*courting* patterns, with characteristic 50 KHz vocalizations), which, if the female does not object, culminate in stereotyped consummatory (or *copulatory*) behavior.[65] During this final phase, the male mounts the female from the rear, palpating her flanks with his forepaws to arouse an arched-back, rump-raised receptive posture called *lordosis*. Whereupon, the male rat exhibits sets of rapid thrusting movements called *intromissions*, which, if well guided, lead to entry of the penis into the vagina. After a series of intromissions, the male ejaculates, which is accompanied by a "deep thrust," and then he pushes off, often falling over in the process. He then attends to personal matters, with intense grooming of his genital area, with a shift to 22 KHz defeat-type (or "I'm not in the mood") vocalizations. Presumably, all this is accompanied by various emotional shifts, but we can only infer such states from external signs such as changes in vocal patterns and specific affective measures, such as place-preference tests.

The sexually aroused female rat also has a variety of active behaviors to attract males. These "flirtatious" appetitive or *proceptive* behaviors appear designed to capture the attention of a male and entice him to pursuit. The most evident behaviors in the rat are repeatedly running toward and away from the male, or past him in a hopping, darting fashion with the head wiggling and many 50 KHz vocalizations.[66] Many of these behaviors also characterize play solicitation behaviors, which precede rough-and-tumble juvenile wrestling (see Chapter 15). If the male is aroused to pursue and mount the female, she makes entry easy for him: As he palpates her flanks, she assumes the lordosis posture—which, to amplify on the previous description, consists of a momentary rigid immobility, with a helpful arching of the back in such a way that the rump is elevated and the tail is flexed laterally to permit intromission and ejaculation by the male.

One common measure of female sexual receptivity is the *lordosis quotient*, which is the ratio of the number of mounts required to evoke the lordosis reflex. A great deal is known about how the rodent brain elaborates this reflex, but there is an unfortunate paucity of information about brain mechanisms that mediate the active appetitive components of female sexual behavior. Because the female shows no behavioral component similar to ejaculation (whether they experience anything like orgasm is unknown), it is more difficult to speculate about the nature of sexual experiences in female rats than in males. In short, the nature of sexual reward in the female remains less well understood than similar processes in males.

Physiological Substrates of Sexual Activation in Females

In most species (perhaps even humans), the hormonal changes that periodically prepare an egg for fertilization (i.e., gradually increasing estrogen followed by a rapid rise of progesterone) also prepare the female brain for heightened sexual receptivity. This consists of several discrete neuropsychological changes, including (1) a decrease in aggressiveness toward sexually aroused males, (2) an active tendency to solicit male attention, and (3) a sensitization of the female copulatory reflex of lordosis.[67] In many species, ovulation is accompanied by evident external signs of sexual readiness, such as a swelling and reddening of the anogenital region or the production of attractive odors. In the laboratory, one can use an experienced male rat as a detective to identify females that are in heat: He will spend a great deal more effort investigating the anogenital region of receptive females than nonreceptive ones, and, if permitted, copulation will follow rapidly.[68]

It is clear that the female lordosis reflex involves a spinal mechanism that is presensitized by higher brain mechanisms to respond to hormone patterns that help constitute sexual receptivity. This is because the latency of the lordosis reflex from the moment of flank stimulation is shorter than the conduction speed necessary for spinal neurons to send information up to the brain and back to the spinal cord.[69] Thus, female physical receptivity is imposed by readiness potentials emerging from higher brain areas. Critical circuits that sensitize the lordotic spinal reflex via tonic descending influences arise from the central gray of the midbrain and the ventromedial hypothalamus (VMH)—brain areas that, as we have seen, figure heavily in energy-balance regulation, as well as the elaboration of many other emotions (suggesting a way in which sexual readiness might be influenced by other emotional and motivational processes). It appears likely that females' diminished food intake and heightened sexual receptivity during estrus may reflect the common effect of hormonally induced sensitivity changes in these parts of the brain.[70] It may also be worth noting that starved animals are much less likely to mate than are well-fed ones, and the linkage between energy balance and mating readiness may be neurally negotiated directly within the VMH. Obviously, it is unwise to seek reproduction when energy resources are low, and nature has assured that this is unlikely to happen.

As already indicated, the hormonal patterns that induce receptivity in females are high circulating levels of estrogen followed by a rapid rise in progesterone (which typically occurs when the egg arrives in the fallopian tubes). Sexual receptivity can be reliably evoked in rats if one simulates this hormonal pattern by the appropriate regimen of injections.[71] In contrast, human females are more willing than most other mammals to indulge in sex independently of their hormonal status, but it is also clear that better studies concerning the sexual-emotional motivation of women need to be done before we exclude the importance of hormonal fluctuations. At best, human females exhibit only a modest trend for increased receptivity during ovulation.[72] Indeed, as we will see, the hormonal control of female sexuality in humans may be considerably different than in other species. Also, at present there are not enough studies analyzing feelings of eroticism in humans as a function of the menstrual cycle to draw any definitive conclusions concerning the role of ovarian hormones in modulating psychological responses related to sexuality.

Neurochemical Activation of Adult Sexuality: Male and Female Erotic Hormones in Action

Although we are beginning to understand what it means for the brain to be masculinized or feminized, what types of dynamic neurochemical changes actually mediate male and female sexual desires at maturity? Since this story is complex, and still in the preliminary phases of development, I will restrict my discussion to several key examples from brain chemistries that have been considered on previous pages. These same chemistries will also be important in subsequent chapters on the other social emotions.

As noted in Chapter 11, the male brain has more AVP, especially in neurons situated in several parts of the brain, including the amygdala, septal area, and anterior hypothalamus. The levels of AVP in some of these circuits increase as juveniles go through puberty and sexual urges begin to emerge.[73] These chemical systems help invigorate persistent male-characteristic behaviors, both aggressive and sexual. Indeed, when extra AVP is placed into the POA of male rodents, they obsessively patrol and mark their territory, and become substantially more combative. These are the same behaviors that are elevated by the onset of puberty and testosterone. They are also diminished after castration. Indeed, as mentioned earlier, when this part of the brain is damaged, male sexuality rapidly diminishes, while female sexuality remains largely unaffected.[74] In males who have been made sexually sluggish through castration, sexual eagerness can be restored by placing testosterone directly into this brain area.[75] This may occur in part because testosterone stimulates the manufacture of AVP in sex-control circuits through a direct effect on the genetic machinery that codes for the expression of AVP. The proximity of sexual and aggression control circuits in the male brain should also lead us to pause and wonder about possible functional relationships.

In a certain sense, this is the male dilemma: The hormonal stimuli that promote sexuality also increase certain types of aggressiveness.[76] If male animals are castrated, both their sexual ardor and their pugnacity diminish gradually, as do levels of AVP in approximately half the neural systems of the brain. Although sexuality can continue without brain AVP, it is sluggish, lacking the high level of persistence characteristic of sexually aroused males. While castration leads to a gradual decrease of sexuality in normal males, it leads to a rapid cessation of sexuality in genetically impaired animals that have little vasopressin in their brains to begin with (e.g., rats of the Brattleboro strain).[77]

During sexual activity, AVP is released from the pituitary into the circulation during the anticipatory phase of male sexual arousal that precedes ejaculation (Figure 12.6), and AVP appears to be more important in male than in female sexual craving. Indeed, when AVP is artificially increased in the female brain, sexual receptivity plummets.[78] Perhaps the presence of this male sex factor impairs female sexuality by making the females more aggressive (see Chapter 10). Indeed, soon after giving birth, brain AVP is elevated in females, and perhaps this neurochemical change helps pave the way for maternal aggression.[79] Of course, AVP has other functions in the brain, including overall arousal, attention, and perhaps some forms of memory, especially social memories. It should come as no surprise that quite a few circuits in the female brain contain this peptide. Thus, when investigators deem AVP to be predominantly a male sexual factor, it must be kept in mind that they are speaking only in relative terms.

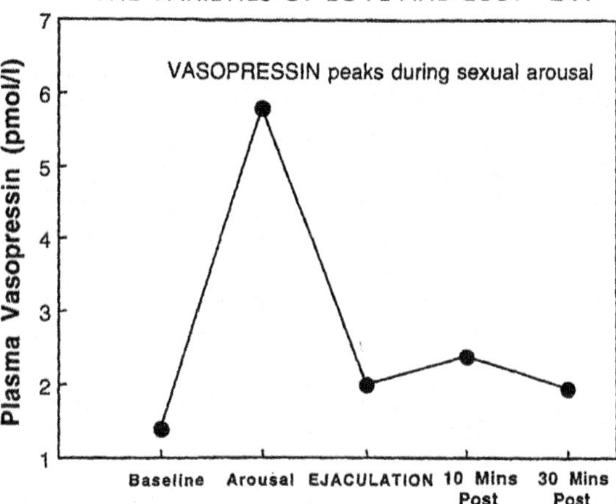

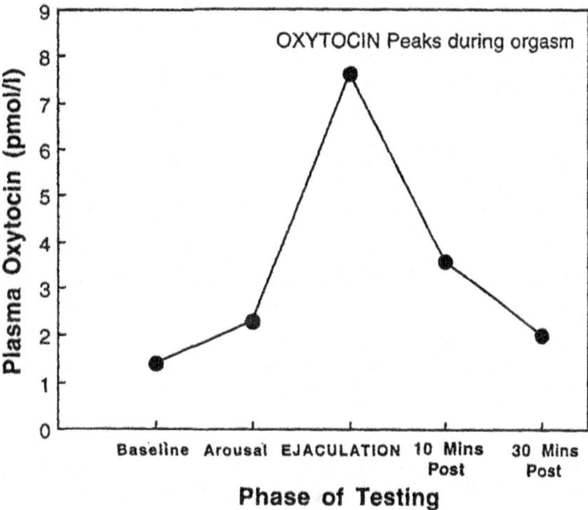

Figure 12.6. Effects of sexual arousal, ejaculation, and postejaculatory interval on average plasma oxytocin (OXY) and arginine-vasopressin (AVP) levels in human males. (Adapted from Murphy et al., 1987; see n. 87.)

By contrast, the female brain contains more oxytocin neurons than the male brain, and the genetic manufacture of oxytocin is under the control of the ovarian hormone estrogen.[80] The role of this neuropeptide in sexuality is not as lopsided as that of vasopressin in the male brain. Administration of oxytocin directly into the brain can increase both male and female sexuality, but seemingly in different ways. In males, oxytocin promotes erectile capacity, and it is released into the circulation in large amounts at orgasm (Figure 12.6). Unfortunately, no comparable data appear to be available for females. In any event, at present, brain oxytocin release is a key candidate for being a promoter of orgasmic pleasure and hence one of the mediators of behavioral inhibition commonly seen in males following copulation.[81]

There is a certain beauty in the fact that oxytocin, a predominantly female neuromodulator, is an especially important player in the terminal orgasmic components of male sexual behavior. In that role it may allow the sexes to better understand each other. Indeed, we shall see that sexual activity can invigorate this chemical system in the male brain, thereby helping to promote nurturant behaviors (see Chapter 13). While oxytocin does modulate the orgasmic phase of male sexual activity, in females it appears to be important for both the courting and copulatory phases. In less clinical terms, it activates female flirtatiousness as well as sexual ardor. These urges are probably promoted by specific changes in specific parts of the brain.[82]

As already mentioned, a major area of the brain where sensitization of female sexual eagerness transpires is the ventromedial nucleus of the hypothalamus (see Figure 12.5). It has long been known that this area is uniquely important for normal female receptivity. Damage can seriously impair female sexual responsivity while having little effect on male sexuality. We now understand how this happens. The sex hormones that prepare the body for fertilization also dramatically change neurochemical sensitivities in this part of the brain. Indeed, hormonally induced receptivity (i.e., estrogen injections for several days, followed by progesterone a few hours before behavioral testing) leads to clear-cut anatomical and neurochemical changes in the medial hypothalamus.[83] A major neurochemical principle mediating this change is oxytocin. Hormone priming (just like normal estrus) leads to a proliferation of oxytocin receptors in the medial hypothalamus, as well as an expansion of the dendritic fields, which physically expand, reaching out toward the incoming oxytocinergic nerve terminals arising from more rostral neurons. This completes a circuit that sensitizes the lordosis reflex of the spinal cord (and presumably prepares the female psychologically to interact seductively with males). It is to be expected that the opening and closing of this gate will have substantial effects on the affective erotic feelings of a female.

Female receptivity can be markedly increased by administering oxytocin into various brain areas that normally contain oxytocin circuits, but only if the females have been adequately primed with estrogen. Conversely, sexual receptivity is compromised by administration of oxytocin antagonists into these brain areas.[84] Following brain oxytocin receptor blockade, females exhibit no sexual receptivity and actively reject the eager advances of males. Indeed, they squeal and complain if a male attempts to mount them, and they may even attack.[85] Of course, the befuddled males remain in hot pursuit, for their olfactory senses convince them that the female must be in a receptive state. Male sexual behavior is also strongly diminished with oxytocin antagonists,[86] again indicating that males and females do share some factors in the control of their sexual urges. We should note that, unlike the case of visual titillation in human males (which presumably reflects well-processed visual input into amygdalar tissue in the medial temporal lobes), in rats the smell of a female is more essential than physical appearance in the control of sexual urges.

At present, we know very little directly about the role of these chemical systems in the control of human sexuality (because of the difficulty of obtaining such evidence), but, as already noted, some interesting parallels have been obtained from an analysis of plasma peptides in males. AVP is elevated during the arousal phase of masturbation but declines rapidly at orgasm. Oxytocin, on the other hand, remains low during the preliminaries of sexual arousal but is released vigorously during orgasm and remains high for some time thereafter (Figure 12.6).[87] These changes probably correspond to erotic mood changes that are transpiring within the brain—with AVP promoting sexual eagerness and oxytocin promoting sexual pleasure.

Primitive areas of all mammalian brains contain affective systems designed to assure that males and females seek each other's sexual companionship. As we will see in the next chapter, these same chemistries have been utilized to construct circuits through which parents are eventually coaxed to take care of their offspring. These same chemical systems also appear to establish attachment bonds between mother and child, and they may also cement love, friendships, and social preferences among adults (see Chapters 13 and 14). However, there is a darker side to this story.

Sexual arousal may set the stage for sexual jealousies. For instance, one especially intriguing finding is that a male's "jealous" attachment to a female may be dependent on the fact that AVP was active in his brain during sexual activity. At least in prairie voles, the only species studied so far, sexual activity can increase the likelihood that a male will attack potential interlopers. Males that are allowed to copulate will become aggressive toward other males that enter their territory. However, if an AVP antagonist is placed into the brain just prior to the sexual activity, these field mice do not develop such a jealous attitude. On the other hand, if one simply puts AVP into the brain of a male in the presence of a female, with no sexual activity allowed, the males still begin to treat other males in threatening ways.[88] If one is willing to generalize from these behavioral results to human feelings, one might hypothesize that tendencies for sexual jealousy are promoted in the male brain by the release of AVP during sexual activity. Of course, animal behaviorists are unlikely to use such subjective terms as *jealousy* in the interpretation of their work, for such subtle emotional issues can only be evaluated through human research. However, the likelihood that such work will ever be done in humans seems remote, but if an orally effective AVP antagonist is discovered, we might anticipate that it will take the edge off sexual jealousy in men.

The Neurochemistry of Sexual Pleasure

A key emotional question related to sexuality is: What does it mean, in neurochemical and neurophysiological terms, to have experienced sexual pleasure? This is a difficult question to answer on the basis of available evidence, and to a substantial extent we must rely upon mere speculation. Indeed, sexual pleasures should probably be subcategorized into neurologically distinct pre- and postorgasmic phases. At present, we have no absolute assurance that other animals even experience orgasm. It might be easier to argue that males do, since they exhibit the explicit response of ejaculation, which in humans is highly related to the emotional experience of orgasm, but the issue is much harder to judge for females. There is no outward sign as clear as ejaculation in females. Indeed, it could be argued that there is no clear adaptive value for female orgasm in creatures that are as hormone-bound in their sexual appetites as are the females of most other mammalian species. Only when there emerged a major social payoff for extended sexuality (as is the case in humans) was there significant evolutionary pressure for the emergence of reasonably stable pattern of female orgasms. As will be discussed more extensively in a subsequent section, perhaps orgasms evolved as an internal signal that one had found "Mr. Right." Even though females of other species may not experience orgasm, this is not to say that they do not enjoy sex. Obviously, positive erotic feelings in both sexes are likely to be critical in sustaining sexual activities.

Although brain oxytocin and vasopressin circuits are excellent candidates for organizing both the behaviors and the emotional feelings associated with sexuality, they are only two especially prominent candidates in a growing list of chemistries that elaborate libido. For instance, one neuromodulator we have yet to mention is luteinizing hormone releasing hormone (LH-RH), which controls secretion of gonadotrophins from the pituitary (see Figure 12.4) and is represented by extensive systems within the brain that generally parallel the oxytocin neural system. Administration of LH-RH into the brain can selectively increase female sexual receptivity in rats, and it has been of some clinical interest to determine whether this agent can increase libido in humans.[89] Some success in treatment of sexual disorders has been achieved by administration of this agent peripherally in both females and males (with more positive effects observed in females), but no one has yet injected it directly into the human brain to ascertain if subjective effects are produced.

At present, one of the few ways we can determine which chemistries participate in sexual reward is through the conduct of place-preference studies in animals. One approach that has been taken is to evaluate preferences for those locations where animals have had the opportunity to copulate. (In such studies, animals were allowed to have sex in one of two environments, and male animals chose to spend more time in the environment in which they have had sex.)[90] Since both dopamine and opioids have been implicated in the mediation of brain reward, investigators have determined whether the sex-induced place preference could be modified by either dopamine- or opiate-blocking agents. Such experiments have clearly indicated that opiate blockade is more effective than dopamine blockade in attenuating sexual reward in males. Indeed, this effect has been obtained by the restricted blockade of opiate receptors within the preoptic area, where the sexually dimorphic nucleus is situated.[91]

In this context, it is also noteworthy that opiate addicts who "mainline" strong drugs such as heroin report feeling an orgasmic rush, with a warm erotic feeling centered in the abdomen, when the drug hits their system. Thus, it seems that both sexual pleasure and taste pleasure (see Chapter 9) are mediated by similar chemistries, but perhaps in different brain areas. But surely other chemistries are also involved. For instance, as mentioned at the outset of this chapter, administration of ACh into the septal area has induced orgasmic feelings in humans. However, since ACh is important in so many brain functions, it will not be of much use in the treatment of sexual or erotic disorders. Also, as previously indicated, the probability that oxytocin secretion contributes to orgasmic feelings is high, but it may well be that the larger part of the orgasm-correlated secretion (e.g., Figure 12.6) is due to concurrent opioid release within the brain.

What is needed now are more animal studies that concurrently evaluate the role of several neuropeptide systems, such as vasopressin, oxytocin, and LH-RH, in this type of reward. All such studies need to control for social-reward effects that are independent of sexual reward. In addition, we desperately need more studies along these lines that focus on the female side of the sexual interaction. Until such work is more vigorously pursued, the subjective erotic effects of sex behavior–mediating systems of the brain will remain veiled in mystery.

Some Evolutionary Issues concerning Orgasmic Responses in Humans

Presumably, reproductive issues have helped guide the evolution of various sexual interactions, as well as sexual pleasure mechanisms in each species. For instance, why is it that human females are capable of multiple orgasms, while human males need periods of repose (i.e., postejaculatory pauses) before they can resume sexual activity? We do not know, but perhaps it is because the male body must have time to restore sperm resources before it makes biological sense to continue sexual activity, while females have no such constraint. Why is it that males can generally achieve orgasm more rapidly and reliably than females? We do not know, but perhaps it is because essential reproductive reflexes (i.e., ejaculation) are more tightly linked to orgasmic experiences in males than in females. Reproduction would not be possible without male ejaculation, and it is easy to understand why the approach of orgasm in males would further invigorate sexual activity. Egg fertilization, on the other hand, apparently can proceed effectively without female orgasm, although it remains possible that such responses promote sperm extraction and propulsion up the uterine canal and even into the fallopian tubes.

Since the human female's orgasm appears to be largely independent of simple reproductive issues, it may be related to more complex social ones such as bonding. From this vantage, it might be understandable why females would be capable of multiple but less predictable orgasms (at least during interpersonal sex) than males. Orgasm may provide a novel emotional route for identifying and reinforcing certain male qualities. Mechanistically, the female orgasm may simply arise from the brain mechanisms that evolved to mediate male orgasm; alternatively, it may be an evolutionarily emerging state, perhaps as an exaptation derived from aspects of male orgasmic mechanisms. Obviously, it is attractive to believe that male and female orgasms are fundamentally similar in terms of brain neurophysiology (just as the penis and clitoris develop from the same primordial tissue), but such a commonality remains to be demonstrated.

One important line of evidence that supports the idea that male and female eroticism have converged in humans is the finding that sexual desire in females is more dependent on adrenal testosterone than in other mammals,[92] whose receptivity relies more critically on ovarian estrogen and progesterone. If, in fact, female orgasm is a process that is presently emerging in an evolutionary sense, one provocative idea is that it may help females identify males who have the right characteristics for social bonding and hence are likely to support the woman's future needs. However, the bottom line is that, at present, we simply do not know.

It still remains possible that male and female sexual reward differ in some fundamental ways in the brain, and a large number of neurochemistries, from galanin to cholecystokinin in the preoptic area, may eventually shed light on this important facet of human life. However, without a good animal model of female sexual gratification, it will be most difficult to evaluate such issues. Also, since the hormonal control of sexual urges is so different in human females than in other animals, it may be impossible to devise a simple laboratory model for such processes.

Learning within the Sexual Systems of the Brain: The Case of Birdsong

As has been observed with all of the other basic emotional systems, sexual circuits of the brain can promote learned behaviors. Indeed, for a long time it was commonly assumed that gender identity was learned, but we now recognize that to be, at best, only half true. Although human choice cannot be denied, the greatest part of sexuality is guided, as in other animals, by the types of neural systems nature has provided within male and female brains. Of course, how each organism uses sexuality in the world is subject to a great deal of learning, especially with respect to courting rituals and specific sexual preferences. Such issues are most provocatively highlighted by recent discoveries about how song is elaborated in the avian brain (also see Appendix B).

It is typically the case that males sing, both to attract females and to ward off competing males that would enter their living space. Song usually occurs at the time of year, namely, springtime, when birds' gonads are rapidly growing to their maximal size, following the shrinkage that occurred during the previous fall and winter. It has been a remarkable observation that along with the changing size of the gonads, the circuits of the brain that mediate singing also sprout forth and recede with the seasons.[93] Unlike brain tissues in mammals, avian brains sustain the ability to manufacture new neurons even in adulthood. During springtime, males are endowed with increasing amounts of neural tissue especially in the areas of the brain that generate singing. These events are mediated by fluctuating testosterone levels. When testosterone falls, the areas of the male brain that mediate singing regress and remain, in relative terms, as small as their gonads.

A series of higher brain structures in birds have now been found to be under the neurotrophic control of testosterone, and it has been demonstrated that these structures acquire much of their eventual behavioral competence as a result of early learning.[94] Although there is considerable variability from one species of bird to the next, the most common theme is that birdsong is not completely formed within the genetically connected components of their song circuits; rather, in most species, there is only a rudimentary form of the species-characteristic "score" embedded within the genetically dictated connections of those circuits. To become complete, circuit functions need to be optimized through learning, and the birds need to be able to hear their own fledgling attempts at song production. Without early exposure to their own song, the males of most passerine species (i.e., songbirds) will exhibit only a few fragments of their ancestral tunes.[95] In the absence of any better role model, some species are able to approximate the songs of other species heard during their youth, but most will fully perfect only the song of their own species. And this perfection requires experience. The refinement process occurs in those specific areas of the brain where neural circuits can be invigorated by increasing tides of testosterone.

In the sexual arena, as elsewhere, it is clear that nature and nurture go hand in hand, with experience bringing the organic potentials of genetically ingrained systems to their full potential. Human courtship and sexual styles are obviously learned. The passions that accompany them are not. It seems likely that biological factors are as influential in the hidden desires of the human heart as they are in the birdsong of springtime.

AFTERTHOUGHT: More On the Nature of Sexual Pleasure

So, let us ask once more: To what extent do the animal studies summarized here have implications for the human condition? While the higher levels of cortical influence in the human brain provide overriding principles of cultural control, the power of subcortical emotional circuits may be decisive in the sexual quality of individual lives—the ability to sustain receptivity and potency and to have experiences of intimacy and pleasure. Neuroscience will eventually provide new forms of assistance to such aspirations of the human heart, and future remedies will be much more effective than the aphrodisiacs of the past.

Already there have been anectodal reports that intranasal oxytocin is able to facilitate sexual performance in humans.[96] As mentioned earlier, this peptide is quite effective in increasing both male and female sexual activity in rodents. Could this type of knowledge be used routinely to promote sexual functioning in humans? We can be sure that many pharmaceutical firms are presently searching for new aphrodisiacs based on a solid knowledge of the mammalian brain as opposed to wild hunches from folklore and the approximations of ancient traditions. Powdered rhinoceros horn may continue to be sold in some part of the world as long as there is a market for superstitions and the body parts of endangered animals, but such practices are based more on faith and the power of placebo effects than on solid knowledge. As we saw in Chapter 8, the mammalian brain is designed to construct belief systems, and once they are solidified, they are as hard to move as mountains.

One molecule with scientifically established aphrodisiac qualities is yohimbine,[97] which blocks brain norepinephrine receptors of the alpha-1_A variety. In addition, the MAO-B inhibitor l-deprenyl has been found to sustain sexual vigor and longevity in aging male rats.[98] Although more needs to be learned about these fascinating systems before useful connections to psychiatric issues can be formulated, it does seem that basic sexual urges are controlled by similar neurochemistries in both rats and humans. But this is not to say that the road from biology to behavior is a one-way street. There is also feedback from behaviors to biological processes. As with most complex brain systems, there are complex two-way interactions between the brain and the environment in which it operates. Several fascinating phenomena have been discovered when people have monitored changes in the sex hormones as a function of various social challenges.

Animals have been found to exhibit remarkably consistent hormonal fluctuations as a function of their social successes, and similar changes are also evident in humans. As mentioned in Chapter 10, the winners of social encounters typically exhibit elevations in circulating testosterone, while losers exhibit declines.[99] It is reasonable to expect that such changes would promote neurochemical activities that facilitate male libido (and thereby increase their reproductive success), even though such effects remain to be documented.

Conversely, it is also interesting in this context to consider how environmental psychosocial variables might modify the physiological substrates of sexual and reproductive tendencies in females. Many fascinating observations have been made: (1) Young females, including humans, typically become sexually mature more rapidly when strange males enter their environments. (2) Social stimulation can modify levels of bodily enzymes controlling the manufacture and processing of sex steroids. (3) Groups of female primates, as well as wolves and other species, exert physiological influences over each other to control which animals will reproduce in the group (perhaps via olfactory cues). (4) Finally, we are beginning to find that the olfactory senses of human beings may also be acutely sensitized to certain smells that can synchronize sexual cycles and hence may coordinate sociosexual activities.[100]

Humans are generally less dependent on olfactory cues for sexual arousal than are most other mammals, but recent work indicates that human sexuality is still linked to certain bodily odors.[101] Visionary entrepreneurs in the perfume industry are paying close attention to these findings, hoping to profit through the manufacture and distribution of smells that can amplify moods that control our behaviors at the affective fringes of our consciousness. The emerging knowledge concerning the existence of a vomeronasal organ and an accessory olfactory system in humans will undoubtedly figure heavily in the success of such efforts.[102]

Suggested Readings

Allgeier, R. A., & Allgeier, E. R. (1995). *Human sexuality* (4th ed.). Lexington, Mass.: Heath.

Becker, J. B., Breedlove, S. M., & Crews, D. (eds.) (1992). *Behavioral endocrinology.* Cambridge, Mass.: MIT Press.

Campbell, B. (ed.) (1972). *Sexual selection and the descent of man.* Chicago: Aldine.

Crews, D. (ed.) (1987). *Psychobiology of reproductive behavior.* Englewood Cliffs, N.J.: Prentice-Hall.

Dorner, G. (1976). *Hormones and brain differentiation.* Amsterdam: Elsevier.

Kincl, F. A. (1990). *Hormone toxicity in the newborn.* Berlin: Springer-Verlag.

Le Vay, S. (1993). *The sexual brain.* Cambridge, Mass.: MIT Press.

Money, J. (1980). *Love and love sickness: The science of sex, gender difference, and pair-bonding.* Baltimore: Johns Hopkins Univ. Press.

Symonds, D. (1979). *The evolution of human sexuality.* New York: Oxford Uni. Press.

Ziegler, T. E., & Bercovitch, F. B. (eds.) (1990). *Socioendocrinology of primate reproduction.* New York: Wiley-Liss.

13

Love and the Social Bond

The Sources of Nurturance and Maternal Behavior

> Love comes quietly . . .
> but you know when it is there,
> because, suddenly . . .
> you are not alone any more . . .
> and there is no sadness
> inside you.
>
> J. W. Anglund, "Love Is a Special Way of Feeling" (1960)

CENTRAL THEME

Although there are many bad forms of parenting, there are also good and nurturant forms. An age-old concern of pregnant women is the doubt they feel about their ability to nurture and love their first baby. However, nature tends to spontaneously take care of such concerns, at least in lower animals, as the sequence of biological events leading up to the delivery of the baby unfolds. The ongoing physiological changes that prepare the body for birth also prepare the mother's brain for nurturance. In most animals this includes her role as the primary caregiver. Males can be trained to exhibit a high level of nurturance, but their care is rarely as natural or as intense a motive as it is for the mother. Only in species where male participation is absolutely essential for offspring survival, as in some birds and perhaps in humans, where the child is helpless for longer than any other animal, can nurturant behavior be as vigorous in males as it is in females. On the other hand, in many species of fish where external fertilization is the norm, the fathers typically remain to tend and protect the eggs while females depart to entice another receptive male. Nurturance may have emerged independently several times in the evolution of different species, but in mammals the basic urge probably comes from homologous brain circuits, even though the specific behaviors that constitute parenting can vary markedly from species to species. Humans obviously exhibit more behavioral complexity in child care endeavors than other species, but our behavior is still motivated, in part, by primitive emotional systems we share with the other mammals.

When did nurturant motivation emerge in mammalian brain evolution? Momentous evolutionary changes must have occurred when animals with an urge to take care of their offspring emerged on the face of the earth. Presumably this was achieved because parental care provided a decisive competitive edge for the survival of certain species. But how could nurturance have evolved from a state of nonnurturance? We cannot go back in evolutionary history, but we know that part of the script was written with the same ancient chemistries that generate sexual urges. In mammals, brain oxytocin circuits lie at the neural core of the incipient maternal intent that follows the first birth. As we saw in the previous chapter, this chemistry is important for regulating both male and female sexuality. The nurturant circuits in the mother's brain and care-soliciting circuits in infants are closely intermeshed with those that control sexuality in limbic areas of the brain. This confluence lends modest support to controversial and widely debated Freudian notions of infantile sexuality and the possible relations between maternal love and female sexuality. Nurturance circuits can lead to the rapid learning of maternal behaviors, which then become permanent parts of a mother's behavioral repertoire. Males can also learn nurturant behaviors, and it is intriguing that sexual activity can strengthen antiaggressive, caregiving substrates in male brains. We are finally deciphering the ancient neurosymbolic processes that first led to nurturance and social attachments in the mammalian brain. This work has important implications for the biological sources of friendship and love, as well as for sociopathy and psychiatric disturbances of affective contact such as autism. Although as yet there is little information about the operation of these systems in the human brain, our understanding of these issues in the animal brain is impressive. In this chapter, I will again entertain the working assumption that the information obtained from animals will apply reasonably well to understanding basic emotional tendencies in humans. Of course, the emotional feelings that accompany nurturance are subtle, warm, and soft, and in the complex, cortically mediated politics of human societies, such social feelings can easily be overridden by other concerns. Also, in humans, where child care is accompanied by various unpleasant chores like changing diapers, it is sometimes difficult to view the emotional pleasures of nurturance with a completely unjaundiced eye.

An Overview of Human Nurturance

Human societies have seen many forms of parenting down through the ages. At present, we live in a child-oriented era, whereas in many previous ages, child care was more harsh, producing emotional harm that may have had untold effects on the course of human history. As Robert Burton wrote in his classic, *The Anatomy of Melancholy*: "If a man escape a bad nurse, he may be undone by evil bringing up. . . . Parents . . . offend many times in that they are too stern, always threatening, chiding, brawling, whipping, or striking; by means of which their poor children are so disheartened and cowed, that they never after have . . . a merry hour in their lives."[1] It is generally believed that harsh early experiences can modify emotional traits for a lifetime. Could the many wars and other human tragedies caused by the megalomaniac tendencies of certain individuals and groups throughout history have been avoided if the leaders had been more warmly parented as children?

Parenting styles still vary enormously from culture to culture, depending on existing traditions and ecological necessities confronted by various societies. For instance, not too long ago in certain arctic aboriginal groups, such as the Netsilik Eskimo of northern Canada, long-term social concerns often overrode short-term emotional ones. Female babies who had little hope of finding an appropriate mate, because no male babies of comparable age had been born in the tribe, would be left to die in the snow, with little outward distress or remorse exhibited by the parents.[2] In our culture, such behavior is deemed criminal. This indicates once again that among humans, biology is not necessarily destiny, because we have the ability to make cognitive choices.

For humans, the rearing of a child is as much an economic question as an emotional one, and economic concerns often prevail. Antecedents of this are evident even in some lower species, where mothers kill some of their weaker pups. When environmental resources are scarce, this practice can increase the probability of success for the surviving offspring. Thus, the amount of investment made in offspring is only partly an emotional issue. This is one of the reasons there is so much confusion and variety in child care practices, in human cultures as well as across species.

While we presently accept a long period of childhood dependence, certain African tribes have encouraged levels of early independence unheard of in our culture. In the Digo tribe of East Africa, most babies are toilet trained by 1 year of age, and soon thereafter they are encouraged to behave as relatively independent members of their tightly knit, extended-family group. In our nuclear-family culture, parents of 1-year-olds are just beginning to think about toilet training. Much older children are still closely supervised and are afforded little opportunity for independent action within the larger community. Obviously, Digo types of nurturance can occur only in social situations where the whole village cares for children. As the African proverb says: It only takes one woman to bear a child, but it takes a whole village to raise it.[3]

The variety of parenting in other species is also vast, ranging from frequent, highly attentive parenting, as in rats, which feed their offspring every few hours and exhibit intense search and retrieval behaviors if infants are lost or dispersed, to very brief and infrequent parenting, as in rabbits, which feed their sequestered litters only once a day and seem not to possess the motivational or neurobehavioral equipment to retrieve little bunnies that are dispersed from the nest.

It is widely believed in our culture that children who come from loving and supportive families, and who are given progressive age-appropriate educational challenges, have the best chance of growing to a vigorous and independent adulthood. Put another way, many experts agree that a "secure base" is essential for optimal personality development in children.[4] Chronic insecurity is likely to yield adults who have difficulties with intimacy and trust and are more likely to act out their lack of confidence by burdening others with their insecurities. But what is the nature of this loving and supportive "secure base" that psychologists speak of? Obviously, it is partly a matter of how parents behave toward their children, but it also runs deeper into our affective nature as biological creatures.

The Physiology of Nurturant Behavior

Although child-rearing practices vary greatly, the emotional dimensions of social bonds are probably controlled by highly conserved biological processes that guide expressions of both parental and infantile behavior and the consequent feelings that parents and children develop for each other. Before the birth of their first child, women commonly worry about their future adequacy as mothers, but such doubts typically vanish, as if by magic, soon after the birth of the baby.

Recent brain investigations suggest that social bonding is rooted in various brain chemistries that are normally activated by friendly and supportive forms of social interaction. As will be elaborated in this and the ensuing two chapters, such urges are controlled by neuropeptides such as oxytocin and prolactin, as well as endogenous opioids such as endorphins (*endo-* meaning produced inside the body rather than coming from outside, and *-orphins* meaning like morphine).[5] For instance, opioids mimic the action of heroin in the brain and have powerful influences over our feelings, especially our negative responses to social isolation. Animal research indicates that both brain opioid and oxytocin circuits are activated by various pleasurable pro-social activities, such as grooming, play, and sexual interchange. Accordingly, such neurochemical changes in the brain may promote feelings of security in children, as well as nurturant and sexual behaviors and related social emotions, perhaps even love, in adults.

Of course, because of our cognitive abilities, humans begin to prepare for the baby months before its arrival, but there still seems to be a special time just preceding delivery where strong biologically based motivations take hold. This is probably because of the many hormonal changes, such as those summarized in Figure 13.1, that herald birth. Although such data are from the rat, the general patterns are quite similar across all mammals, and these changes, artificially produced, are known to promote nurturance.[6] In other words, evolution has not left the important events of birthing and the ensuing nurturance and bonding either to chance or to the vagaries of individual learning.

All mammals have neuronal operating systems that evolved to help prepare them to take care of infants, even though some, such as the Netsilik mentioned previously, do not exercise the option of warm social acceptance in circumstances they believe compromise the long-term stability of their culture. Presumably the Netsilik, as well as other parents who abandon their infants, do so before the bonding process has progressed too far. Some species, such as rats and humans, have a bonding window that remains open for a long time, while for others, including herbivores such as sheep and many avian species, the entry window is closed within a few hours of birth. This variability appears to reflect the motoric maturity of the young when they are born. Prey species are typically born rather mobile, so they can run away from predatory dangers soon after birth. They also tend to live in herds where the young can easily get separated from parents. Thus, out of sheer necessity, mothers and infants must bond rapidly. Predators, on the other hand, are typically born relatively immature, and the bonding process, at least from viewpoint of the offspring, can be extended across longer periods without compromising their chances of survival.

Some animals, such as infant rats, bond as much to their nest sites as to their mothers.[7] Likewise, rat mothers readily accept strange pups into their nests and begin to provide care without much fussing or aggression. Sheep and other ungulates, on the other hand, will re-

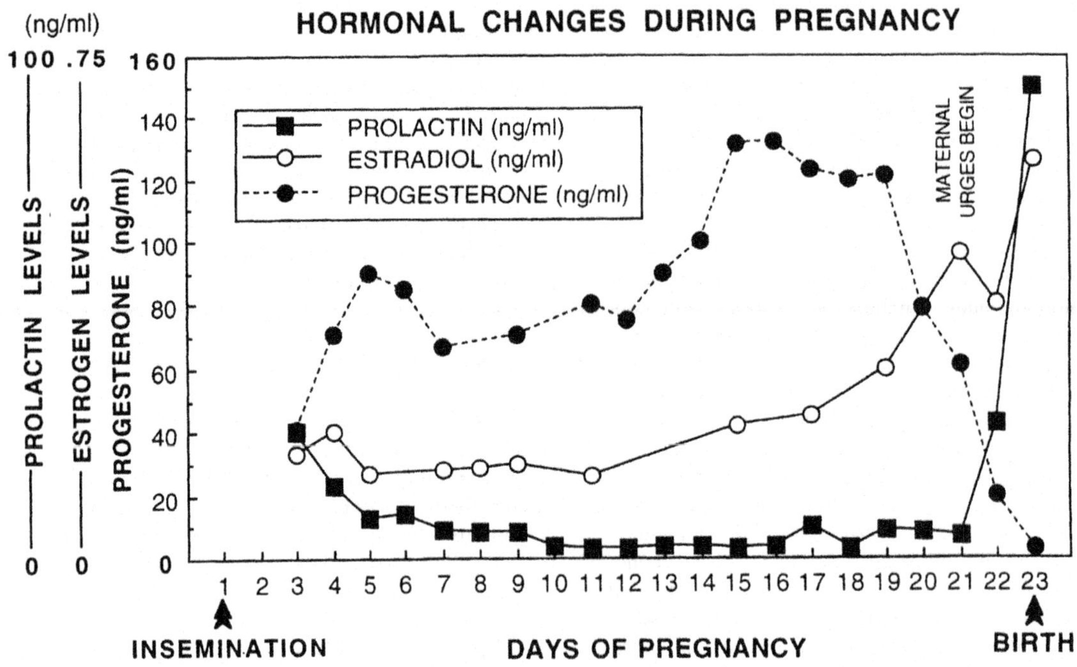

Figure 13.1. Circulating levels of progesterone, estradiol, and prolactin during pregnancy in the rat. (Adapted from Rosenblatt, 1990; see n. 6).

ject others' young. Despite these outward differences among species, it presently seems likely that their bonding chemistries are quite similar. They simply operate in different time frames and within different ecological constraints. These fascinating species differences shall receive little additional attention here, for my aim will be to summarize underlying physiological principles that may have substantial cross-species generality, extending hopefully even to the human level.

We now know a great deal about the nurturance systems of the mammalian brain, and this chapter covers some recent information that now needs to be integrated into modern psychological thought. Some remarkable neurochemical systems, which promote both sexual and maternal behaviors and even more subtle social processes, have been revealed within the subcortical reaches of the visceral nervous system, including areas like the cingulate cortex, septal area, bed nucleus of the stria terminalis, and preoptic and medial areas of the hypothalamus, along with their respective mesencephalic projection areas. At present, brain oxytocin, opioids, and prolactin systems appear to be the key participants in these subtle feelings that we humans call acceptance, nurturance, and love—the feelings of social solidarity and warmth.[8] Although many human interactions and cognitive experiences also contribute to maternal states, without the underlying mood- and behavior-altering neuropeptides, those experiences would probably remain shallow and without emotional intensity.

When humans have imbalances in these chemical systems, they experience emotional problems, which, if sufficiently severe, can be deemed psychiatrically significant bonding disorders. For instance, postpartum depression and psychosis, which have been correlated with high levels of a circulating ß-casomorphin (an opioid peptide derived from milk), are not uncommon in humans.[9] Perhaps tendencies toward sociopathy, characterized by the inability to share the emotions of others, are also accompanied by abnormalities in these social chemistries. The same may apply to psychiatric conditions characterized by social and emotional deficiencies, such as early childhood autism.[10] Both of these problems are much more common in males than in females, suggesting striking gender-related differences in the underlying brain circuits. Unfortunately, our understanding of these systems in the human brain is meager, but knowledge concerning such systems in animal models is growing rapidly.

Sex Differences in Nurturance Circuits

I use the term CARE circuits to acknowledge the existence of intrinsic brain systems that promote nurturant behaviors of mothers, and occasionally fathers, toward their offspring. In rats, full maternal behavior consists of building nests, gathering all dispersed pups together, hovering over them to provide warmth, and, in the presence of lactation, sustaining pups through nursing. In most species, mothers are more adept at these behaviors than fathers, presumably because of the more vigorous CARE systems in their brains, but this is not to suggest that males cannot exhibit nurturance. As we will see, even male rats, especially if they are young, will exhibit maternal-type care under the right conditions.

Obviously, humans, contrary to most other animals, can consciously appreciate the importance of child care, but despite such cognitive assistance, fathers probably provide child care more instrumentally than mothers. Mothers are more prone to get intensely involved with babies than fathers, and they exhibit a more natural persistence, warmth, and desire to communicate affectively with the baby. They typically get more concerned when babies are in distress; this is also evident in animals.[11]

Thus, the biggest differences in human nurturance probably exist at the emotional level—with most mothers generally having stronger and more positive emotional responses in nurturant situations than fathers. Of course, there are bound to be exceptions to this rule, depending upon one's early brain organization (see previous chapter), early rearing experiences, prevailing cultural rules, and individual philosophical perspectives. However, because of evident sex differences at the biological level, I will occasionally call nurturant CARE circuits maternal behavior circuits, in the context of the present discussion.

Because of our ability to conceptualize social rules, human mothers and fathers can care for a child equally well, but only a mother can provide sustenance from her breasts. She is also more likely to offer affective engagement from emotional depths unfamiliar to most men. We now know that among all mammals that have been closely studied, the female brain is more prepared than the typical male brain to care for infants. Indeed, it may have been the evolution of the maternal circuits that initially led creatures down the mammalian path that now makes us humans the sophisticated social creatures that we are. Not surprisingly, if we dwell on the matter, maternal urges probably emerged (i.e., were *exaptations*) from a subset of subcortical systems that initially governed female sexual urges. It would also have been reasonable to couple parental emotions to the preexisting psychobehavioral systems that encourage individuals to come together for mating. Thus, maternal nurturance and social bonding may have emerged from evolutionary tinkering with preexisting processes, rather than through totally new forms of brain "engineering." As François Jacob, the Nobel Prize–winning molecular biologist, put it: "Natural selection . . . works like a tinkerer . . . who does not know exactly what he is going to produce but uses whatever he finds around him . . . to produce some kind of workable object. . . . Evolution makes a wing from a leg or a part of an ear from a piece of jaw. . . . Natural selection . . . does not produce novelties from scratch. It works on what already exists."[12]

This is the essential meaning of an *exaptation*—the utilization of an existing function for some other purpose. Indeed, modern neuroscience highlights the possibility that the neural dictates of the sexually passionate parts of the limbic system set the stage for parental nurturance. The evolution of such systems also led females to be especially sensitive and responsive to calls of distress from infants (see Chapter 14) and to interact with them more intimately, and probably more playfully, throughout childhood (see Chapter 15).

Although we have no firm data for humans, on the assumption that similar neural dictates still govern our deepest social feelings, I will devote the next two chapters to a detailed discussion of the relevant animal brain issues. Because of the reciprocity between maternal behavior and infant need systems, and the importance of these systems for understanding normal human behavior and its pathologies, there will be some overlap of materials. The premise will be that when we nurture our children well, they have a secure base because their brain chemicals evoke the comfortable feeling that "everything is all right." When children are neglected, other chemical patterns prevail in their brains. The latter patterns do not promote confidence and social efficacy but rather motivate behaviors based on persistent feelings of resentment and emotional distress. If these feelings prevail for too long, depression emerges, personality changes may occur, and the most sensitive individuals may be psychologically scarred for life.[13]

Let us first pause to consider how the new forms of mammalian social behavior could have emerged from preexisting solutions in the brains of ancestral vertebrates that did not care for their offspring. After all, parental care evolved from a mode of life that was nonparental, a mode that still predominates in the reptilian world. Most reptiles produce their young and leave them to fend for themselves. Although a number of species—for instance, crocodiles—do exhibit some parental care, it is meager by mammalian standards. If we simply consider that all infants enter the world through a well-regulated birth process, it would be reasonable to suppose that the initial impulse for nurturance might have been closely linked to the biological mechanisms that already existed to deliver the young into the world. Indeed, as we shall see, nurturance probably initially arose from neurochemical processes that controlled mating and egg laying in reptiles.

The Evolutionary and Sexual Sources of Maternal Intent: Pituitary Peptides and Parental Behavior

As mentioned in the previous chapter, vasotocin is an ancient brain molecule that controls sexual urges in reptiles. This same molecule, the precursor of mammalian oxytocin, also helps deliver reptilian young into the world. When a sea turtle, after thousands of miles of migration, lands on its ancestral beach and begins to dig its nest, an ancient birthing system comes into action.[14] The hormone vasotocin is secreted from the posterior pituitary to facilitate the delivery of the young. Vasotocin levels in the mother turtle's blood begin to increase as she lands on the beach, rise further as she digs a pit large enough to receive scores of eggs, and reach even higher levels as she deposits one egg after the other. With her labors finished, she covers the eggs, while circulating vasotocin diminishes to insignificant levels (Figure 13.2). Her maternal responsibilities fulfilled, she departs on another long sea journey. Weeks later, the newly hatched turtles enter the world and scurry independently to the sea without the watchful, caring eyes of mother to guide or protect them.

In mammals, the ancient molecules that control reptilian sexuality and egg laying evolved into the oxytocin and arginine-vasopressin (AVP) social circuits of the brain (see Figures 6.7 and 12.2). As discussed in the previous chapter, oxytocin came to prevail in female sexual behavior, and AVP prevails in that of males. Now we also know that oxytocin—the hormone that helps deliver mammalian babies by promoting uterine contractions and helps feed them by triggering milk letdown from mammary tissues—also serves to facilitate maternal moods and related action tendencies in the brains of new mothers. However, these psychobehavioral effects can emerge only if a variety of physiological and hormonal changes related to parturition have first occurred in the brain and body of the mother.

The initial clue that there is an intrinsic bodily signal to promote maternal behavior was the fact that transfusion of blood from a female rat that had just given birth could instigate maternal behaviors in a virgin female.[15] It is not yet known exactly what the blood-borne signals are, since oxytocin alone cannot perform this function. It may be the full symphony of hormonal changes that precede birth. As summarized in Figure 13.1, estrogen, which has remained at modest levels throughout pregnancy, rapidly increases as parturition nears. Progesterone, which has been high throughout pregnancy, begins to plummet. And, of course, there is a precipitous rise in prolactin, which induces the mother's acinar glandular tissues to manufacture milk.

These hormonal changes heralding imminent birth also prepare the mother to exhibit maternal urges before the actual arrival of the infant(s). Human mothers commonly exhibit a compulsive flurry of house preparation several days before the baby is due, and rat mothers begin to build nests and become substantially more eager to interact with baby rats. Such tendencies are common in many species and are especially clear if the mother has given birth before. This heightened maternal desire corresponds to the peak of the three previously mentioned hormonal changes, reaching an apex several hours before birth in rats. As mentioned earlier, if one produces this pattern of hormone change via injection, one can also instigate expressions of maternal

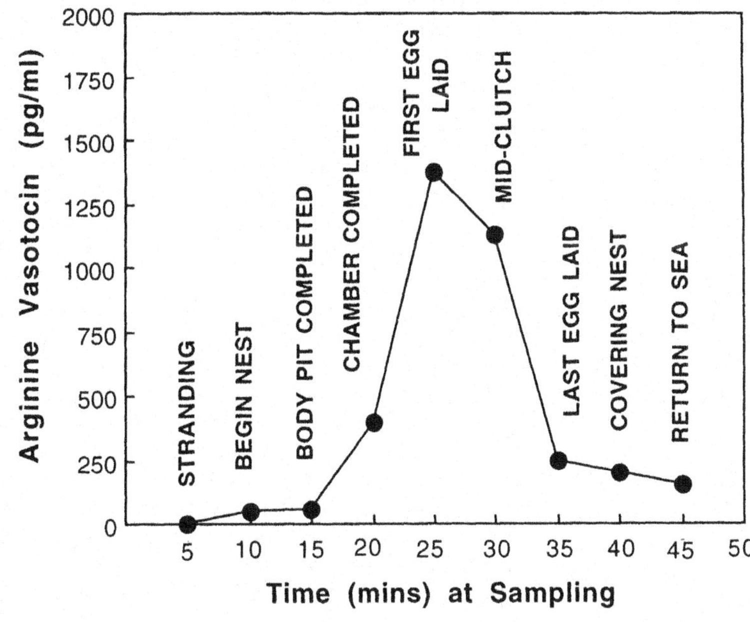

Figure 13.2. Mean serum vasotocin levels in loggerheads and ridley olive sea turtles. (Adapted from Figler et al., 1989; see n. 14.)

care in virgin rats.[16] Prolactin may be the critical ingredient in sustaining the natural behavior sequence, not only because brain injections of prolactin promote nurturance,[17] but females who are nonmaternal because they have been surgically deprived of their pituitary glands do gradually become maternal when replacement injections of prolactin are provided.[18] But what are the relevant changes in the brain that result from these hormonal manipulations?

Although many neural changes result from such peripheral hormonal fluctuations, the increased responsivity and sensitivity of brain oxytocin circuits is a major event. During the last few days of pregnancy and the first few days of lactation, there are remarkable increases in oxytocin receptors in several brain areas, as well as increases in the number of hypothalamic neurons that begin to manufacture this neuropeptide. Both of these effects are controlled by the elevations of estrogen at the end of pregnancy, and the induction occurs in circuits that promote nurturance.[19] These estrogenic effects on the genetic expression of oxytocin synthesis and receptor expression may be further reinforced by the stimulating effects of the newborn pups, as well as other hormonal shifts in the body.

These changes are accompanied by additional adjustments in oxytocin circuitry. During lactation, oxytocin cells begin to communicate with each other directly via the development of *gap junctions* between adjacent oxytocinergic neurons, allowing them to synchronize their neural messages precisely.[20] This helps suckling stimuli from nursing babies to more effectively trigger oxytocin secretion in the brain of the mother, presumably to sustain a maternal mood, as well as release from the pituitary gland, which is essential for milk to be released from the breasts (Figure 13.3).[21]

Brain Oxytocin and Maternal Competence

A critical question is whether and to what extent these brain changes do, in fact, mediate the affective and behavioral components of maternal urges. For a long time it was believed that oxytocin was not essential for mothering, since elimination of peripheral oxytocin (by removing the posterior pituitary in nursing mothers) did not eliminate subsequent maternal behavior.[22] It was only when distinct oxytocinergic neural systems were discovered in the brain (see Chapter 6) that a role for oxytocin was entertained once more. Most of the pertinent work to date has been done in rats and sheep, and hence substantive conclusions must be restricted to those species; but considering the ways of evolution, the probability that the results do not apply to others, including humans, is remote.

The initial studies that evaluated the ability of oxytocin to mediate maternal behavior found strikingly rapid onset of maternal tendencies in female rats when this peptide was administered directly into the brain's ventricular system.[23] Similar effects were obtained in sheep.[24] However, the evidence rapidly became confusing and contradictory. While a few investigators were

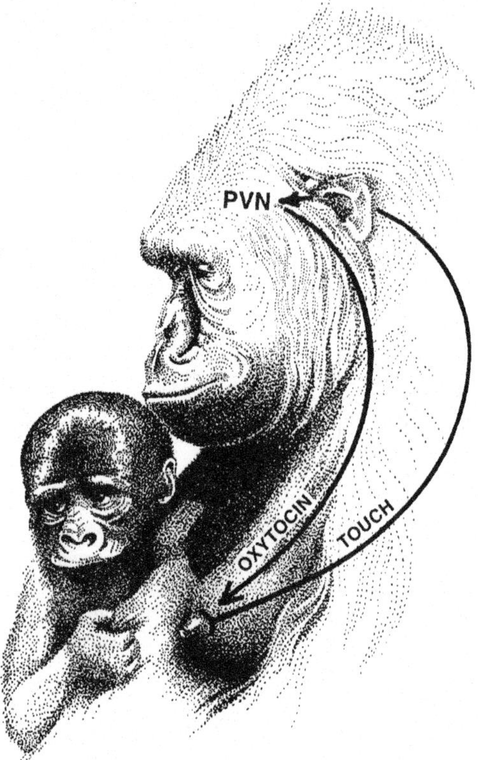

Figure 13.3. Depiction of suckling reflex. The infant's suckling stimulation of the nipple sends messages to the paraventricular nucleus of the hypothalamus (PVN), which instigates the release of oxytocin from the posterior pituitary into the circulation, leading to the contraction of smooth muscles of mammary tissues, which pumps milk from the breast. This reflex becomes easily conditioned to various behavioral cues from the infant.

able to trigger full maternal behavior (nest building, retrieving, and attempts to nurse) in virgin female rats, others had no success.[25] Such failures to replicate were very troublesome, but more recent work has revealed that many of the problems were methodological.

Normally, virgin female rats tend to find the odors of newborn pups aversive, perhaps to dissuade them from wasting time interacting with strange babies.[26] Thus, even if such animals were in a maternal mood, they might not exhibit nurturant behaviors if the aversion outweighs the maternal urges. Oxytocin alone is apparently not able to overcome this olfactory "disgust," even though the complex of physiological changes that accompany birth accomplishes that quite well—changing the olfactory aversion to an attraction.[27] In other words, oxytocin triggers rapid maternal behavior in virgin female rats only if they are first prevented from smelling the pups.[28]

In addition, to get a robust maternal effect from oxytocin infusions into the brain, virgin females need to be primed with injections of estrogen so that the appropriate oxytocinergic receptor fields have a chance to proliferate (natural mothers, of course, provide their own estrogen, as described earlier). Finally, and quite perplexingly, oxytocin is effective only if animals have been habituated to test chambers for a few hours but not if they have been fully habituated for a day or more.[29] This may mean that if animals already have a reasonably well-established place attachment, they have difficulty forming new social attachments. Perhaps test animals that are just becoming familiar with a situation are in a transient neuropsychological state that enhances their motivation to start a new family and to modify their environment appropriately. In any event, the likelihood that endogenous oxytocin does in fact normally promote such behavioral tendencies is affirmed by the ability of oxytocin receptor antagonists to reduce the onset of maternal behavior following the first delivery.[30] Surprisingly, this manipulation does not disrupt maternal behavior that has already been fully developed.[31]

Thus, if all the conditions are right, oxytocin administered directly into the brain can provoke maternal behavior, but it is certainly not the only ingredient that can do this. As mentioned, administration of prolactin into the brain also facilitates maternal tendencies. In fact, we now know that there are prolactin-based neural systems in the brain, and, as indicated, there is active uptake of this rather large peptide hormone into the brain from the circulation.[32]

As will be discussed more fully in the next chapter, maternal competence can also be increased by mild facilitation of opioid activity, even though high levels of opioids diminish maternal interest, as well as gregariousness in general.[33] It presently seems likely that part of the gratification derived from the primal act of nursing emerges from the concurrent release of oxytocin and opioids within the limbic system, as well as other chemistries that remain to be identified. While oxytocin may be especially important in the initial triggering of maternal behavior, prolactin, opioids, and social learning are important in sustaining it once the behavior pattern has developed.

Experience-Induced Solidification of Maternal Behavior

It should be emphasized that well-established maternal behavior no longer requires brain oxytocin arousal; oxytocin blockade impairs maternal behavior only if administered to mothers during the birth of their first litter of pups. In animals that have been allowed to exhibit maternal behavior for several days, oxytocin antagonists have no outward effect on maternal competence. In other words, they cannot block previous social learning.

The ability of several days of normal maternal experience to solidify maternal competence is also evident in studies that have focused on nurturance after lesions of one of the primary sources of brain oxytocin, the paraventricular nucleus (PVN). PVN lesions administered prior to parturition weaken subsequent maternal behavior, but those administered after several days of normal maternal functioning do not.[34] It seems that learning that transpires from the spontaneous use of this intrinsic brain operating system rapidly becomes functionally autonomous, at least in the short run. In other words, once the habit has solidified, maternal behavior can proceed independently of the original initiating processes.

Analysis of this learning mechanism deserves more experimental attention than it has yet received. Similar to the pattern seen with other emotions, a great deal of learning is probably controlled in the higher reaches of CARE circuits such as the anterior cingulate cortex and bed nucleus of the stria terminalis. It is still an open question whether ongoing brain oxytocin activity is essential for continuation of efficient maternal behavior in the long term. Although there are no relevant human data on such issues, perhaps the oxytocin secretion during each successful nursing episode continues to reinforce the affective experience of a satisfying social interaction. Temporary absence of such satisfaction (as might occur with centrally administered oxytocin antagonists) is apparently not sufficient to dissuade the mother from carrying out her maternal responsibilities, once she has established the social bond and can cognitively mediate social commitments.

However, it would come as no surprise if maternal vigor diminished gradually without the reinforcement provided by periodic oxytocin release within the brain. If that is the case, *long-term* sustained oxytocin blockade may lead to the gradual deterioration of maternal care. It might also be expected that chronic oxytocin blockade would reduce the experience-induced maternal behavior that can be normally evoked in nonmaternal animals by long-term exposure to young pups. As will be discussed later in this chapter, social experience itself, without the physiological act of parturition, is sufficient to arouse nurturant motives in virgin rats, both male and female.[35] However, the role of oxytocin in such processes remains to be evaluated empirically.

It also remains to be determined whether the absence of oxytocinergic transmission in the brain makes the maternal experience less satisfying. This could be tested by allowing mothers to nurse in one environment while their brain oxytocin systems are blocked with an appropriate receptor antagonist and in an adjacent distinct environment without blockade. At present, most investigators would predict that such animals would exhibit a place preference only for the environment in which they fully experienced their brain oxytocin systems in action, but we do not yet know that to be the case. Indeed, in our lab, we have tried repeatedly to obtain a robust conditioned place preference with centrally administered oxytocin, but we have not been successful. Oxytocin only works when supplemented with other social stimuli. By comparison, it is easy to obtain simple reward effects with opiates and psychostimulants.

In sum, it seems that maternal behavior is initially aroused by changing responsivity and synaptic sensitivity in brain oxytocin systems. This sensitivity is due, to a substantial extent, to the proliferation of oxytocin receptors, a change resembling that which occurs in the uterus just before the onset of labor.[36] In the brain, the greatest oxytocin receptor proliferation is observed in the bed nucleus of the stria terminalis (BNST); when that area is damaged, maternal behavior is severely impaired.[37] These kinds of studies are beginning to clarify the details of maternal CARE circuits in the mammalian brain.

The Neural Circuitry for Maternal Behavior

The actual brain circuits that control the various components of full maternal behavior extend far and wide in subcortical regions of the brain (Figure 13.4). Part of the circuitry descends from the preoptic area along a dorsal route through the habenula to the brain stem, and part through a hypothalamic route to ventral tegmental area (VTA) dopamine systems and beyond.[38] The VTA component may facilitate general foraging tendencies that are essential in retrieval and nest building, while the other routes may be more important in up-close nurturance and nursing. For instance, a distinct neural circuit that controls milk letdown descends from the lateral midbrain area down to segments of the spinal cord that innervate the nipples.[39]

It is especially noteworthy that neural circuitry for maternal behavior (and estrogen-responsive populations of oxytocin cells) are situated within the dorsal preoptic area (POA) just above the brain areas that elaborate male sexuality. These cells probably control nurturance in both males and females, but there are more of them in females, partly because of the inductive effect of estrogen.[40] The specific ventromedial hypothalamic zones that control female lordosis behavior (where oxytocin systems also proliferate under the influence of estrogen and progesterone) do not appear to be essential for maternal behavior. However, lesions of the BNST and the nearby POA can eliminate essentially all aspects of maternal behavior.[41] As mentioned, the relevant neural pathways exit from the POA laterally and descend in the medial forebrain bundle, with key terminals being in the VTA.[42]

It has been established that the oxytocinergic synapses that terminate on dopamine cells of the VTA do, in fact, promote maternal behavior. Oxytocin injections into the VTA can induce maternal behavior, whereas comparable injections are not effective in amygdala, septum, or POA.[43] Damage to these ascending dopam-

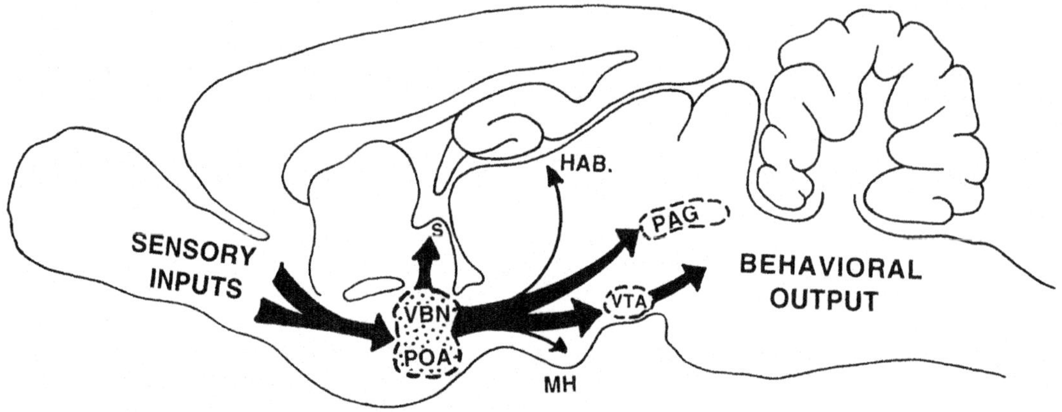

MATERNAL BEHAVIOR CIRCUITS

Figure 13.4. General overview of maternal behavior circuits in rodents. The central integrator is in the dorsal preoptic area (POA) and the ventral bed nucleus of the stria terminalis (VBN), which receives various sensory cues for maternal behavior and distributes controls into widespread brain areas, including the medial hypothalamus (MH), the ventral tegmental area (VTA), the periaqueductal gray (PAG), the habenula (HAB), and the septal area (S). The precise functions of these various areas remain to be identified.

ine systems can also severely impair maternal behavior, including dopamine-selective neurotoxic lesions of the VTA, as well as the lateral hypothalamic and dopamine target zones in the nucleus accumbens.[44] Of course, these forms of damage compromise many other sorts of appetitive behavior. As discussed in Chapter 8, the VTA-centered SEEKING system is a nonspecific appetitive system that can mediate many goal-directed behaviors. If this oxytocin-VTA interface is relatively nonspecific, the additional oxytocin influences, perhaps lower in the brain stem, may be essential for engaging specific motivational circuits for maternal behavior, such as sensitization of affective responses to specific forms of somatosensory stimulation such as suckling. We do not yet know where those circuits are situated, although there are some clues.[45] Alternatively, it is possible that oxytocin input to the VTA can intrinsically code a subtype of appetitive eagerness that is specifically directed toward expressions of nurturant behaviors.

To what extent are the brain circuits for social bonds coextensive with those that mediate maternal behavior? It is reasonable to suppose that the neurochemical satisfactions of giving birth and the natural urges of motherhood would prepare the brain for the formation of social attachment to the infant. However, we also need to look at the social bond from the infant's side, and the mechanisms there may be slightly different (see the next chapter for a fuller discussion of this distinction). Work on such questions is just beginning, but there appears to be a substantial overlap between the two processes, at least at the neurochemical level, even though we do not know yet exactly where in the brain the bonding process transpires. The prime neurochemical candidates at present are the endogenous opioids, oxytocin, and AVP. Neuroanatomically, the best candidate areas are the higher brain zones, where damage can disturb maternal competence: the amygdala,[46] the septal area,[47] and the cingulate cortex.[48] What these specific brain areas contribute to maternal competence will have to be solved by more sophisticated psychobiological research than has yet been conducted. We will certainly have to pay more attention to issues such as which brain mechanisms mediate social attachments, friendly interactions, gregariousness, and various social memories, in addition to specific perceptual and behavioral abilities.

Brain Systems for Social Bonds

Social bonding is of enormous psychiatric importance, for if it is inadequately established, the organism can suffer severe consequences for the rest of its life. A solid social bond appears to give the child sufficient confidence to explore the world and face a variety of life challenges as they emerge. As John Bowlby poignantly documented in a series of books,[49] a child that never had a secure base during childhood may spend the rest of its life with insecurities and emotional difficulties.

Until recently, we knew nothing about the neurochemical nature of social bonds. Even though all humans feel the personal intensity of their friendships, family attachments, and romantic relationships, there was practically no way of studying how these feelings might be constructed from specific brain activities. In the past score of years there have been several breakthroughs: the discovery that neural circuits mediating separation distress are under the control of brain opioids,[50] and, as already discussed, the developing understanding of the neurochemical basis of maternal and sexual behaviors.[51] In addition, several groups of investigators have started to decode how filial imprinting and sexual bonding are neurochemically mediated within the brain.[52] These lines of inquiry proceeded separately for some time, but they are coming together now in quite interesting ways.

The first neurochemical system that was found to exert a powerful inhibitory effect on separation distress was the brain opioid system. This provided a powerful new way to understand social attachments.[53] There are strong similarities between the dynamics of opiate addiction and social dependence (see Figure 13.5), and it is now clear that positive social interactions derive part of their pleasure from the release of opioids in the brain. For instance, the opioid systems of young animals are quite active in the midst of rough-and-tumble play, and when older animals share friendly time grooming each other, their brain opioid systems are activated (see Chapters 14 and 15). Finally, sexual gratification is due, at least in part, to opioid release within the brain.[54] From all this, it is tempting to hypothesize that one reason certain people become addicted to external opiates (i.e., alkaloids, such as morphine and heroin, that can bind to opiate receptors) is because they are able to artificially induce feelings of gratification similar to that normally achieved by the socially induced release of endogenous opioids such as endorphins and enkephalins. In doing this, individuals are able to pharmacologically induce the positive feeling of connectedness that others derive from social interactions.[55] Is it any wonder that these people even become intensely attached (classically conditioned) to the paraphernalia associated with their drug experiences, or that addicts tend to become socially isolated, except when they are approaching withdrawal and seeking more drugs? Indeed, opiate addiction in humans is most common in environments where social isolation and alienation are endemic. Investigators have been able to increase opiate consumption in experimental animals simply by separating them from companionship.[56] These social problems are more understandable in light of the fact that positive social emotions and social bonds are, to some extent, mediated by opioid-based, naturally occurring addictive processes within the brain (see Figure 13.5 and Chapter 14).

One of the methodological difficulties in studying social-bonding in mammals has been the lack of efficient laboratory models. By comparison, excellent models exist in birds. Konrad Lorenz originally described the powerful form of social learning that can occur in infancy, whereby young animals strongly "imprint" upon available social stimuli.[57] Newborn birds of species that are born relatively mature (i.e., precocious species such as chicks, ducks, and geese) will typically learn to follow the first moving object they encounter. In this way, young animals normally come to follow eagerly after their mothers, and Lorenz easily trained young greylag geese to treat him as their surrogate parent. In other words, newborn geese that

SIMILARITIES BETWEEN

OPIATE ADDICTION & SOCIAL DEPENDENCE

OPIATE ADDICTION	SOCIAL DEPENDENCE
1) Drug Dependence	1) Social Bonding
2) Drug Tolerance	2) Estrangement
3) Drug Withdrawal	3) Separation Distress
a) PSYCHIC PAIN →	a) LONELINESS
b) LACRIMATION →	b) CRYING
c) ANOREXIA →	c) LOSS OF APPETITE
d) DESPONDENCY →	d) DEPRESSION
e) INSOMNIA →	e) SLEEPLESSNESS
f) AGGRESSIVENESS →	f) IRRITABILITY

Figure 13.5. Summary of the major similarities between the dynamics of opioid dependence and key features of social attachments.

were separated from other geese and allowed to spend a lot of quality time with Lorenz developed a special fondness for him and would persistently follow him about as if he were the matriarch of the group. In adulthood, sexual desires could also be guided by these early imprints to take a cross-species course that seemed comical from a human, albeit not an evolutionary, perspective. For instance, Lorenz vividly described how he was courted by a blackbird he had hand-reared from infancy. A great deal of neuroscientific information is available on imprinting, including the demonstration of specific brain changes (see next chapter), but we still do not satisfactorily understand the neuroanatomical pathways and the neurochemical factors that mediate these effects. Many researchers believe vasotocin in birds and oxytocin in mammals are key factors, but pertinent evidence is scarce.

However, due to the recent development of an efficient mammalian model for studying bonding, compelling evidence from laboratory rats indicates that central oxytocin may mediate the attachment of an infant to the mother. Basically, the experimental design was to separate pups from their mother for several hours and then reunite them for half an hour. Just before each reunion, the mother's ventral surface was sprayed with a distinct odor (either lemon or orange), which imparted a distinct sensory quality to the reunion episodes. In contrast, control animals were simply reunited with a cotton wad permeated with those same odors. This was done for three successive reunion trials, all occurring during a single day. The following day, the attraction of the pups to the conditioned odor and other odors was evaluated using various measures, including approach in runways and place preference tasks. Clearly, only the pups that had been reunited with mom exhibited a selective approach and an attraction to the odor associated with maternal reunion. This attraction was blocked completely in animals that had been given oxytocin antagonists. However, giving animals oxytocin when they were "reunited" with the cotton wad was not sufficient to induce such an attraction.[58]

Considering the importance of oxytocin for maternal behavior, it has also been of great interest to determine whether the molecule modulates negative emotions that arise from separation. Indeed, as discussed in detail in Chapter 14 oxytocin and vasotocin have turned out to be extremely powerful inhibitors of the separation call in various species, affirming that social comfort is produced by the same brain chemistries that help mediate maternal and sexual behaviors.[59]

Moreover, it is noteworthy that the oxytocin molecule has special properties to increase the sensitivity of brain opioid systems. Organisms typically exhibit tolerance to opiates, as in the case of addicts who must administer ever-increasing amounts to obtain the same psychological response. Oxytocin can inhibit the development of this tolerance.[60] Perhaps the secretion of oxytocin in nursing mothers blocks tolerance to opioid reward, and thus provides a dual way for the maternal experience to sustain social pleasures: not only by directly activating oxytocin-based social reward processes but also by sustaining high affective arousal in the brain's opioid experiences. It would be disastrous if mothers lost their ability to feel intense social gratification from nurturance when children were still quite young. Parenthetically, it should be emphasized that the male sex factor, AVP, has little ability to reduce separation distress, but as we will see later, it can facilitate social memories. Recent work in males also suggests that AVP is an important ingredient in sexual bonding, as demonstrated in the tendency of field mice to defend and prefer the company of certain female partners. Male *prairie voles*, an especially gregarious mouse strain, will choose to spend time with those females in whose company they have experienced elevated levels of AVP.[61]

At the present time, AVP, oxytocin, and opioid systems appear to be prime movers in the construction and maintenance of social bonds in mammals. Vasotocin, which is the homologous peptide in birds, may also be important in guiding social preferences, but this has not been demonstrated yet. Animals also prefer to spend more time with other animals in whose presence they have experienced high brain oxytocin and opioid activities.[62] Thus, it seems as if friendships are cemented by the same chemical systems that mediate maternal and sexual urges. Perhaps this is one of the primitive emotional reasons we are more likely to help family and friends than strangers (a phenomenon called *kin selection* by sociobiologists). Not only do we simply feel better about those we already know than we do about strangers, but even their faces, voices, and ways of being are engraving more powerful affective imprints in our memories. How does this engraving process occur?

Oxytocin, AVP, and Social Memories

How do we come to recognize and value friends above strangers? Although the answer to this question remains complex and poorly understood, we can assume a central role for brain chemistries that help strengthen and consolidate memories made up of positive social experiences. Emotionally, there are bound to be connections to the mother-infant type bonding processes discussed here, as well as the emotional systems that mediate separation distress (see Chapter 14) and social play (see Chapter 15). However, these affective issues interact with various special-purpose cognitive mechanisms.

While humans recognize each other very well by sight and sound, with the aid of special-purpose face and voice recognition networks situated in specialized areas of the temporal lobes, rats generally accomplish this by smell. This mode of social recognition has been used to develop an effective animal model for the analysis of social memories, relying on the fact that rats get acquainted through mutual investigation, especially of the ano-genital region (as do dogs). If animals already know each other well, they spend considerably less time investigating each other than if they are strangers.[63]

The decrease in social investigation as familiarity increases reflects social memories, and provides a simple way to analyze neurochemistries of the underlying brain processes. It has been found that administration of AVP soon after a social encounter strengthens social memories (at least in males; again, females remain to be tested!). Conversely, administration of AVP antagonists (various molecules that prevent communication at AVP synapses) can obliterate the memories.[64] While data indicated that oxytocin also impairs the consolidation of such memories, more recent work has demonstrated that only very high doses produce such effects. In fact, low doses of oxytocin, which are more likely to be in the natural physiological range, also strengthen social memories.[65] Thus, the same brain chemistries that facilitate various friendly social and sexual behaviors also help solidify the memories that emerge from those experiences.

It remains a mystery exactly where and how memories promoted by oxytocin are solidified in the brain. Interestingly, however, the hippocampus, which is a key brain area for the consolidation of memories, has high oxytocin and AVP sensitivity. It is also noteworthy that the ability of oxytocin to promote erections in male rats is especially easily obtained by infusion of the neuropeptide into the hippocampus.[66] This is perplexing, since the hippocampus is not generally thought to control sexuality. However, the dilemma may be easily resolved if one is willing to entertain the possibility that the manipulation can evoke sexually arousing memories in the rat's "mind."

Oxytocin and Peaceful Coexistence ("Make Love Not War!")

Additional research on oxytocin provides yet another intriguing piece to the neurosocial puzzle. The chemistries that promote pleasure and family values are also able to dramatically reduce irritability and aggressiveness. It has long been known that human societies that encourage physical closeness, touching, and the free flow of intimacy tend to be the least aggressive in the world. For instance, it has been documented that societies that exhibit high levels of physical affection toward infants and children and permit premarital sex are generally low in adult physical violence, while those that are low in physical affection and punish premarital sex tend to be more violent.[67] This, of course, makes a great deal of evolutionary sense: If one is socially well satisfied, there is little reason to fight. However trite this may sound, the principle is profound and supported by brain research. Both opioids and oxytocin (but not AVP!) are powerful antiaggressive molecules,[68] and they also have a powerful inhibitory effect on separation distress. For the present purposes, let us focus on the oxytocin part of the story.

Oxytocin administration reduces all forms of aggression that have been studied. Perhaps the most intriguing one is infanticide—the tendency of animals, especially strange males, to kill the young in a territory they have successfully invaded;[69] this is an especially common (mis)behavior in male rats. Oxytocin, whether given peripherally or centrally, dramatically diminishes this tendency.[70] Since it has been found that sexual experiences promote oxytocin synthesis in the male brain, we might expect that access to sexual contact would also make males less aggressive. Indeed, as mentioned in Chapter 10, it has recently been discovered that sexual activity diminishes the tendency of male rats to exhibit infanticide. This peaceful tendency grows as a function of the number of weeks that have followed copulation, peaking at three weeks after the sexual encounter.[71]

This curious fact makes good evolutionary sense: The male rat has a mechanism in its brain that decreases the likelihood that it will kill its own young. In rats, it typically takes three weeks from the time of successful fertilization to the time of birth. Thus, it would behoove a male rat to restrict its pup-killing ways maximally at about 21 days following sexual activity. As mentioned in Chapter 10 (see Figure 10.7), this is exactly what happens.[72] Although it has not yet been demonstrated that this effect is directly attributable to the lingering effect of brain oxytocin dynamics, it is certainly a reasonable place for investigators to search for a physiological explanation. In rodents, however, it has been shown that free access to sexual gratification can lead to an enormous threefold elevation in oxytocin levels in some parts of the male brain. Apparently, sex promotes the synthesis of nurturant and antiaggressive neurochemistries in the male. Of course, the female is already endowed with abundant activity in this system. Perhaps this brain change, which brings male chemistries closer to those of the female, is one that coaxes males to become supportive and nurturant fathers. This is a socially attractive idea, but only future research will tell us to what extent it can subvert the strong positive linkage that also exists between sexual desire and the arousal of male jealousies and ensuing tendencies toward aggression (see Chapter 10).

Experience-Induced Maternal Behavior

It makes good evolutionary sense for an animal not to "waste" much effort taking care of another animal's offspring—time that would be better spent looking after the welfare of one's own genes. Thus it is perplexing that the mere exposure to young infants can induce nurturant behaviors in some animals, a phenomenon that has been studied extensively in rats.

Since work on this question can only be conducted in animals that normally do not exhibit infanticide, only certain individuals can be tested for the induction of nurturance. Those laboratory rats that do not exhibit infanticide can be induced to gradually exhibit maternal behavior by the simple maneuver of repeatedly exposing them to infant rats. Although they are not attracted by this opportunity at the outset (due, in part, to the smell aversion discussed earlier), the animals gradually begin to show interest in the pups, and eventually most will exhibit well-organized maternal behaviors.

This artificial induction of maternal behavior has been termed *concaveation* or *sensitization* by different authors.[73] It should come as little surprise that mature virgin female rats typically exhibit the behavior more rapidly (about four to seven days) than males (about six to eight days).[74] This finding indicates that adult female brains can be sensitized more readily, but we do not yet know how or where in the brain this phenomenon is elaborated. It does seem to correspond to an increase in prolactin and oxytocin output of the pituitary. One reasonable hypothesis is that the experience with the pups gradually leads to increased genetic expression of these neuropeptides within the relevant brain circuits, but that remains to be empirically demonstrated. It is noteworthy, however, that among juvenile rats, which normally exhibit a brief natural period of great interest in small pups (maybe the rat analog, or even homolog, of playing with dolls), sensitization progresses very rapidly, and slightly more rapidly in young males than in females.[75] However, this period of heightened "intrigue" with infants is short-lived, and throughout most of adolescence, juvenile rats are not as strongly attracted to baby rats.

The tendency of young male rats to sensitize more rapidly than females suggests that the organizational effects of early hormones that lay down a male brain do not inhibit the sensitization process. Indeed, the faster sensitization may be an adaptive way for males to obtain early experience with nurturant behaviors that they may need later in life. In this context, it is worth reemphasizing that males from prenatally stressed mothers (i.e., those with homosexual tendencies described in the previous chapter) exhibit sensitization faster than their "normal" nonstressed counterparts. On the contrary, females from these same stressed mothers show the opposite trend; their acquisition of maternal tendencies is impaired.[76]

Whether these effects are present in other species, such as humans, and whether they are caused by changes in the responsivity of brain oxytocin systems remain unknown. However, the potential implications of such findings for understanding the learning processes that contribute to human social bonding, as well as problems in nurturant motivation, deserve wider attention. Might such processes explain the emotional difficulties and temperamental differences that exist among human mothers? Can difficulties in human bonding be explained by the disruption of such neural dynamics? Do human mothers have a special window of opportunity when they would bond most effectively with their infants? Do mothers who exhibit bonding problems have difficulties in recruiting the relevant brain chemistries? Can medical assistance be provided in such cases? And, perhaps most important, can fathers, who seem to be instinctively less nurturant than mothers, be induced to be more nurturant by facilitating certain neurochemical processes? We simply do not know at the present time, but we can begin to entertain such questions. The probability that simple administration of oxytocin (in a brain-accessible form) would promote social tendencies seems remote. Many of the dynamic changes in sensitivity within this system reside in the proliferation and location of oxytocin-receptive fields, which vary widely as a function of species and a host of physiological variables.[77]

Species also differ widely in the temporal dynamics of the social bonding processes. To some extent this is related to how mature the offspring are at birth. As already indicated, animals that have very altricial (i.e., immature) offspring, like rats and humans, generally exhibit a wider "window of opportunity" for social acceptance than precocious species, like sheep, whose young are born very mature.[78] Generally, rat mothers sequester their offspring in nests and exhibit a great deal of tolerance if their babies are replaced with strangers. They appear to be satisfied as long as some young remain in the nest, for they seem to be attached more to the general concept of having babies in their nests than to their own specific babies, presumably because the appearance of strangers has been a rare event in their evolutionary history. On the other hand, in most herbivores, babies are born motorically precocious, and the mothers must rapidly establish discriminating bonds. Sheep are an interesting species in this regard. Mothers typically tolerate and feed only their own lambs, or only those lambs with which they have developed social bonds within the first hour or two after birth. This is based primarily on olfactory recognition processes. If ewe and lamb are separated for several hours after birth, the window of bonding opportunity passes, and mothers will then reject the care-soliciting overtures of their own lambs, butting them and refusing them opportunities to nurse.[79]

However, as previously indicated, once the window of opportunity has closed, it can be opened once more by two manipulations. First, "reminding" mother sheep of the birthing experience, via artificial vaginocervical stimulation, puts the mother in a mood to accept lambs once more for another hour or two.[80] They become bonded and exhibit full maternal care. As we know from sex research summarized in the previous chapter, this type of stimulation activates oxytocin systems in the female brain, and perhaps that is the key. Indeed, the other method of reinducing bonding is to simply administer oxytocin into the mother's brain; this will reopen the window of maternal acceptance.[81] Parenthetically, it should be noted that in sheep, opioids do not promote active acceptance of lambs, but they do reduce the tendency of female sheep to actively reject strange lambs.[82] Thus, it is likely that oxytocin is more important than endogenous opioids in the mediation of maternal responsivity at least in sheep.

Considering the importance of oxytocin in sexual behavior and the mediation of mother-infant bonds, we must suspect that sexual interactions among consenting adults may neurophysiologically facilitate the consolidation of social attachments, thereby promoting the more nurturant forms of human love. However, before the final story is told, we will have to work through many complex empirical details, including issues related to the nature of altruism and emotions such as possessiveness and jealousy.[83]

Thoughts on Altruism

Since there are circuits and neurochemistries for nurturance in the mammalian brain, and since social bonding in mammals is largely a learned phenomenon, the possibility arises that humans may be able to sincerely extend love and altruism toward strangers. Indeed, we were all impressed recently when Binti the gorilla, of the Brookfield Zoo on the outskirts of Chicago, saved a young boy who fell into her "home." This act of concern impressed many, and it surely emerged from the types of CARE circuits that we share as mammals. To help commemorate such events, and to highlight the very nature of maternal instincts and the social bond, the portrait of motherhood depicted in Figure 13.3 was commissioned. The existence of maternal care should broaden our thinking about altruism.

However, sociobiologists have advised us that "true altruism" cannot exist in any animal, for to sacrifice one's good for the sake of others would be a self-defeating genetic strategy. Self-sacrifice typically occurs only in relation to kin, when it helps one's own gene pool. Although all this is true, we should remember that in mammals the social bonding mechanisms are based on learning and are certainly more pervasive than the *innate* mechanisms for "kin recognition."[84] We can learn to love other animals. It is especially important to emphasize that the experience of motherhood is a powerful force in promoting future nurturance. Thus, while a virgin female rat's nurturant urges require many days to become sensitized, those of a female who has once been a mother are engaged rapidly, usually in less than a day. Similar processes exist in humans.[85]

The acquisition of nurturant behavior leaves a seemingly indelible imprint on a creature's way of being in the world. Although learning is most likely to operate in the presence of genetic kin (for simple geographic reasons), in a cosmopolitan human world, bonding can become broader. Mass communication can potentially promote wider networks of bonding than is common in nature, assuming, of course, that a long-term "bonding window" remains partially open for humans as they mature. This broad albeit frail window of opportunity may be the best hope for the future of humankind.

In any event pro-social affiliative and bonding tendencies should be cultivated and accorded a value on a par with testosterone-driven power-urges. Indeed, the two can sometimes be productively joined, as they are in international efforts such as the Olympic Games. How this might be achieved in other arenas of human life deserves more attention from sociologists and political scientists (see "Afterthought," Chapter 16). Whether and how we shall choose to promote or hinder nurturance across cultural and geographic borders remain societal and political questions of momentous proportions.

AFTERTHOUGHT: The "Mere-Exposure" Effect

One of the most intriguing general psychological phenomena related to those discussed here is called the "mere-exposure" effect. If one simply exposes animals to various stimuli, they begin to develop a preference for those stimuli, especially if they have been paired with positive affective experiences.[86] This effect is pervasive and applies to all species and most objects that have been studied.[87] If one has been exposed to certain foods, one begins to prefer those foods.[88] If one has been exposed to certain objects and places, one begins to prefer those objects and places.[89] Indeed, place attachment arises from mere exposure, which may have been one of the antecedent processes for social bonding. Much of the mere-exposure effect operates at a subconscious level and may be related to other preconscious evaluative effects of emotional stimuli. For instance, it has been demonstrated that if one simply exposes American students to written Chinese characters they do not understand, some of which are preceded by a brief subliminal presentation of a smiling face, subjects will later prefer those characters as opposed to ones that were shown without affective priming.[90]

The attraction of familiar experiences may have far-reaching consequences: Humans who have been exposed to certain ideas often begin to prefer those ideas. Perhaps the most poignant example of this is the ease with which people can defend ideas they have held dear since childhood or even a short while, and how easy and natural it is to contradict the new ideas of others. Although one can readily conjure up exceptions to this pattern (e.g., as encapsulated in the phrase "familiarity breeds contempt"), the mere-exposure effect is a remarkably robust experimental finding. Indeed, some have suggested that social bonding or imprinting may simply reflect this type of process.[91]

The effect has also been used to focus investigators' attention on the possibility that unconscious evaluative processes may be important in the generation of emotional states and judgments.[92] Indeed, it is possible that this phenomenon may be reflected in the many psychobehavioral processes described in this chapter. If so, it would be important to clarify the neurobiological underpinnings of the mere-exposure effect, but relevant research is scarce.

It might be worthwhile to consider whether some of the chemistries that participate in the elaboration of social processes may also play a role in the generation of this interesting phenomenon.[93] Might opioids and oxytocin, as well as other bonding chemistries, be important in molding and modulating the mere-exposure effect? Conversely, what might be the role of other affectively positive neurochemistries such as dopamine, which do not appear to be important for bonding? If we begin to understand the mere-exposure effect, we may also shed light on what it means to feel relaxed and comfortable in a given situation. The mere-exposure effect may be a major affective process that allows animals to become accustomed to new situations efficiently. Is the feeling of déjà vu generated by the release of such chemistries? The mere-exposure effect may be an especially beneficial adaptation for animals that migrate, as well as for ones that are exposed to a variety of social stimuli.

Indeed, social tolerance may be promoted by mere exposure. Recall the young cats that were brought up with rats (see Chapter 2); they did not attack rats when they became adults. This speaks strongly for the benefits of exposing children to a diversity of other individuals and cultures when they are young. The more they have experienced of the world, the more accepting they will be of diversity. Wise governments will promote the use of mass media for such purposes, rather than undermining support for public broadcasting, educational endeavors, and endowments for the humanities, as is popular in some reactionary quarters.

In sum, specific brain systems lie at the heart of complex neuroevolutionary programs that generate the deeply social nature of mammals. Psychobiologists have started to recognize and untangle the neural underpinnings that control social motivation within the old mammalian brain. Nurturant behaviors can become a habit, at least partly independent of the basic brain substrates from which they were initially constructed. The potential implications of such lines of investigation are profound.

Suggested Readings

Alexander, R. D. (1987). *The biology of moral systems.* Hawthorne, N.Y.: Aldine de Gruyter.

Bowlby, J. (1972). *Attachment and loss.* Vol. 1, *Attachment.* New York: Basic Books.

Emde, R., & Harmon, R. (eds.) (1982). *The development of attachment and affiliative systems.* New York: Plenum Press.

Fletcher, D. J. C., & Michener, C. D. (eds.) (1987). *Kin recognition in animals.* London: Wiley.

Harlow, H. F. (1971). *Learning to love.* San Francisco: Albion.

Klaus, M. H., & Kennell, J. H. (1976). *Maternal-infant bonding.* St. Louis, Mo.: Mosby.

Knobil, E., & Neill, J. D. (eds.) (1988). *The physiology of reproduction.* New York: Raven Press.

Krasnegor, N. A., & Bridges, R. S. (eds.) (1990). *Mammalian parenting: Biochemical, neurobiological, and behavioral determinants.* New York: Oxford Univ. Press.

Pedersen, C. A., Caldwell, J. D., Jirikowski, G. F., & Insel, T. R. (eds.) (1992). *Oxytocin in maternal, sexual and behaviors.* Special issue of *Annals of New York Academy of Sciences*, Vol. 652. New York: New York Academy of Sciences.

Winberg, J., & Kjellmer, I. (eds.) (1994). *The neurobiology of infant-parent interaction in the newborn period. Acta Paediatrica*, Vol. 83, Suppl. 397. Oslo: Scandinavian Univ. Press.

14

Loneliness and the Social Bond

The Brain Sources of Sorrow and Grief

I have perceiv'd that to be with those I like is enough,
To stop in company with the rest at evening is enough,
To be surrounded by beautiful, curious, breathing, laughing flesh is enough, . . .

I do not ask any more delight, I swim in it as in a sea.
There is *something* in staying close to men and women and looking on them,
and in the contact and odor of them, that pleases the soul well,

All things please the soul, but these please the soul well.

Walt Whitman, "I Sing the Body Electric" (1855)

CENTRAL THEME

One of the great mysteries of psychology is the nature of the "something" that Walt Whitman extols in his masterpiece "I Sing the Body Electric." That subtle feeling of social presence is almost undetectable, until it is gone. We simply feel normal and comfortable when we are in the midst of friendly company, and that same feeling becomes warmer when we are among those we love deeply, especially when we have not seen them for some time. We often take these feelings, like air itself, for granted. But we should not, for when this feeling of normalcy is suddenly disrupted by the undesired loss of a lover or the unexpected death of a loved one, we find ourselves plunged into one of the deepest and most troubling emotional pains of which we, as social creatures, are capable. In everyday language, this feeling is called sorrow or grief, and it can verge on panic in its most intense and precipitous forms. At a less acute but more persistent level, the same essential feeling is called loneliness or sadness. This psychic pain informs us of the importance of those we have lost. In psychological terms, "importance" is not easy to define, but in evolutionary terms it is. We grieve most when we lose those in whom we have invested a great deal of genetic effort (our children) or those who have helped us to thrive (our parents, friends, and relatives)—in short, when we lose those with whom we have social bonds. Obviously, the loss of a parent is most acute when one is young and still dependent; the pain is less intense and protracted when a grown child loses an elderly parent. On the other hand, when adults lose a child, their genetic and emotional future is compromised forever, and their pain is as intense and lasting as that of a child who loses a nurturant caregiver. This type of psychic pain probably emerges from a brain emotional system that evolved early in the mammalian line to inform individuals about the status of their social environment and to help create our social bonds. Neuroscience is struggling to come to terms with the nature of such intrinsic brain processes, and it is becoming clear that several ancient emotional systems control our social inclinations. In the course of brain evolution, the systems that mediate separation distress emerged, in part, from preexisting pain circuits. Here we will call this neural system the PANIC circuit. It becomes aroused when young animals are separated from their social support systems. We can measure this arousal in several ways, perhaps most effectively by monitoring the separation calls young animals emit when left alone in strange new places. Since opioid systems had already evolved to modulate the intensity of physical pain, it is not surprising that these same neurochemistries can soothe the pain evoked by social isolation. As mentioned in the previous chapter (see Figure 13.5), this work was initiated by the realization that there are remarkable similarities between the dynamics of opiate addiction and social dependence. Other systems that are important in quelling this emotion are oxytocin- and prolactin-based neural activities. We now know where PANIC circuits are situated in the brain, and which neurochemistries transmit the message of distress. This knowledge addresses the essence of our nature as social creatures, allowing us to construct credible hypotheses about which neurochemistries contribute to creating the emotional bonds that link us with our fellows. The existence of such brain systems may eventually help explain the sources of human empathy, altruism, and love, as well as depression and autism.

On the Nature of the Social Bond

Imagine an archetypal situation: The life of a young sea otter is completely dependent on the care provided by its mother. After his sexual contribution, the father pays little heed to his young. It is the mother's job to be both caretaker and food provider, as often as not, on the open sea. The pup's life revolves around maternal devotion. When she dives beneath the dark surface of the water for food, being absent from her infant's side for many minutes at a stretch, the young otter begins to cry and swim about in an agitated state. If it were not for those calls of distress among the rising and falling waves, young otters might be lost forever. Their security and future are unequivocally linked to the audiovocal thread of attachment that joins them to their mothers. It is the same for all mammals. At the outset, we are utterly dependent creatures whose survival is founded on the quality of our social bonds—one of the remaining great mysteries, and gifts, of nature.

Only a few decades ago, behavioral scientists believed that social bonds emerged from an animal's experience of reinforcement contingencies arising from the receipt of conventional rewards. The idea was that young children loved their parents simply because they provided food, water, shelter, and warmth. There was no evidence that the brain contained emotional systems to directly mediate social bonds and social feelings. This behaviorist view began to change when it was shown that human babies fail to thrive if they do not receive physical affection. The classic studies of René Spitz in the 1940s demonstrated that babies in orphanages needed types of sustenance other than simply food and water to thrive.[1] Without caring human contact, many died prematurely, and the lesson is being learned once again in the orphanages of Rumania and other former eastern block countries. It is now widely accepted that all mammals inherit psychobehavioral systems to mediate social bonding as well as various other social emotions, ranging from intense attraction to separation-induced despair.

This same phenomenon has now been seen in many other creatures, ranging from primates to birds, but the details vary considerably from one species to another. The diversity of behavioral and physiological changes that accompany social isolation have been most completely studied in rats and primates, and the responses are quite similar. For instance, although young rats exhibit a very short period after separation when they emit separation calls (see Figure 2.1), they show many other long-lasting changes, including decreases in body temperature, sleep, and growth-hormone secretion, along with increases in brain arousal, behavioral reactivity, sucking tendencies, and corticosterone secretion.[2] The patterning of these responses is influenced by complex physiological controls, but an understanding of brain emotional changes also will be essential to explain this symptom complex.

We are beginning to understand the neural nature of separation distress and closely intermeshed social attachment systems. Not surprisingly, they are closely related evolutionarily and neurochemically to the emotional systems discussed in the last two chapters. My premise here is that a detailed analysis of the brain mechanisms that generate separation distress—as indexed by separation calls and the physiological consequences of social isolation—provides a significant way for us to understand the neurobiological nature of social bonds. Here I will focus on the primal brain system that mediates the emotional anguish of losing someone you love.

There are good reasons to believe that neurochemistries that specifically inhibit the separation-distress or PANIC system also contribute substantially to the processes that create social attachments and dependencies—processes that tonically sustain emotional equilibrium and promote mental and physical health throughout the lifetime of all mammals.

The mammalian brain contains at least one integrated emotional system that mediates the formation of social attachments. The affective components of this system are dichotomous—behaviors and feelings of separation distress on one hand, and those of social reward or contact comfort on the other (Figure 14.1). The existing data suggest that arousability in this system is controlled by multiple sensory and perceptual inputs, and that the evolutionary roots of the system may go back to more primitive control mechanisms such as those elaborating place attachments in reptiles, the basic affective mechanisms of pain, and fundamental creature comforts such as thermoregulation.[3]

One of the key issues for future research will be whether social reward processes exist independently of the neurochemistries that can inhibit separation distress. It is remotely possible that there is no distinct social reward process, since the candidate systems—the opioids, oxytocin, and prolactin—all inhibit separation distress quite well. Perhaps the rewards obtained from interactions such as rough-and-tumble play (see Chapter 15) may eventually yield such a unique reward system, but there is insufficient neural evidence to allow us to reach any definitive conclusions. At present, the most workable approach to understanding the nature of social attachments is through the brain mechanisms that control feelings of separation distress.

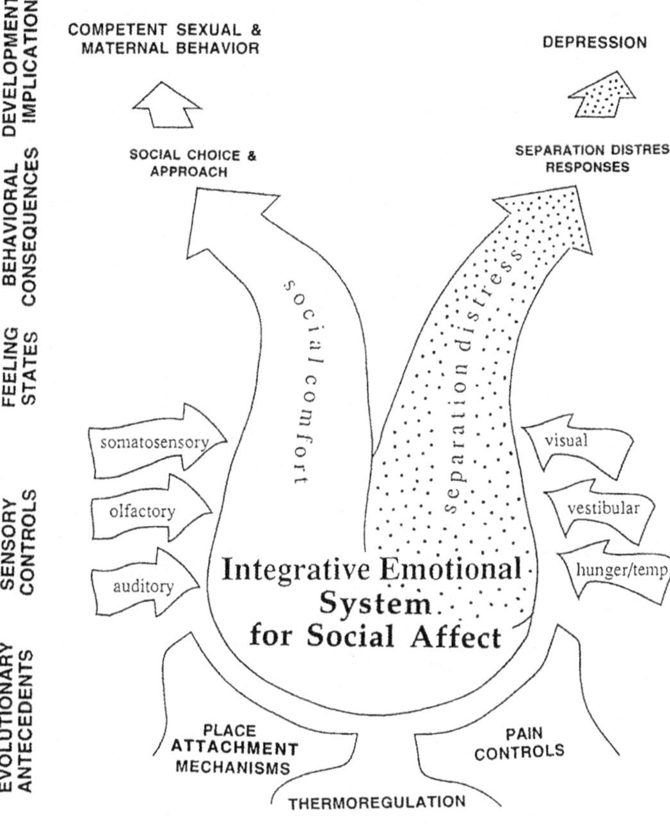

Figure 14.1. Schematic summary of the various influences and levels of analysis that are important in analyzing the potential nature of an integrative emotional system for social affect. (Adapted from Panksepp et al., 1997; see n. 3.)

The Experience of Loneliness and Nonsexual Love

Social bonding in the mammalian brain probably goes hand in hand with the experience of loneliness, grief, and other feelings of social loss. To be alone and lonely, to be without nurturance or a consistent source of erotic gratification, are among the worst and most commonplace emotional pains humans must endure. Indeed, as noted in Figures 13.5 and 14.1, the brain mechanisms of separation distress probably evolved from more ancient pain mechanisms of the brain. Love is, in part, the neurochemically based positive feeling that negates those negative feelings.

Social attachments are probably promoted by the ability of certain interactions (and their attending neurochemistries) to alleviate that mild form of separation distress that we call loneliness. Brain opioids were the first neurochemistries discovered to powerfully reduce separation distress. As predicted by the opiate theory of social attachment (see Figure 13.5), drugs such as morphine that powerfully reduce crying in animals (Figure 14.2) are also powerful alleviators of grief and loneliness in humans.[4] Indeed, as mentioned in Chapter 13, opiate addiction may emerge largely because we have brain systems that were designed by evolution to mediate various pleasures, including those that arise from friendly social relationships; individuals who cannot find those satisfactions in their personal lives will be tempted to succeed by pharmacological means, and this can lead to social isolation. For instance, the French artist Jean Cocteau recollected in his diary how opium liberated him "from visits and people sitting round in circles."[5]

Indeed, the fact that such molecules can alleviate sadness was documented many millennia ago: In Homer's *Odyssey,* we share in a reunion of warriors who had participated in the Trojan War, to rescue Helen of Troy. Although Helen was returned to Greece, many warriors, including Odysseus, did not return home across the wine-dark sea. At a memorial gathering, to Helen's dismay, the thoughts and feelings of the celebrants turn darkly to their lost compatriots, and

> A twinging ache of grief rose up in everyone . . .
> But now it entered Helen's mind
> to drop into the wine that they were drinking
> an anodyne, mild magic of forgetfulness.

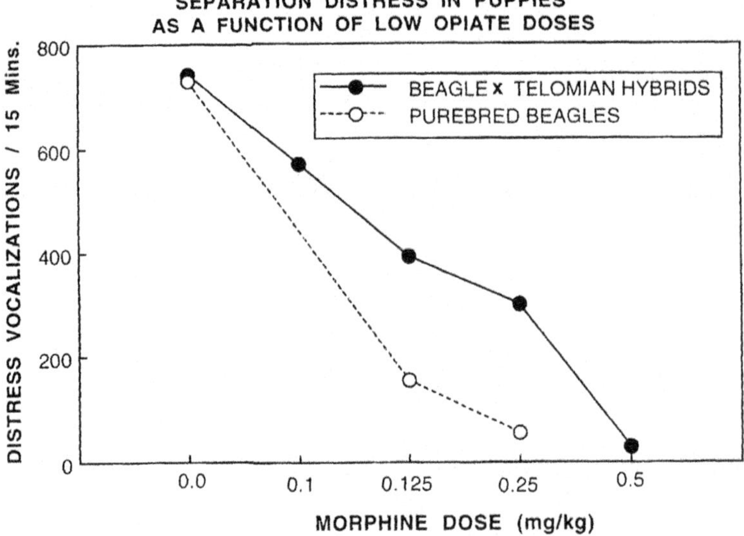

Figure 14.2. Dose-response analysis of the ability of very low doses of morphine to reduce separation distress in 6–8-week-old puppies of a hybrid beagle × Telomian hybrid cross and purebred beagles. (Adapted from Panksepp et al., 1978; see n. 4.)

> Whoever drank this mixture in the wine bowl
> would be incapable of tears that day—
> though he should lose mother and father both,
> or see, with his own eyes, a son or brother
> mauled by weapons of bronze at his own gate.[6]

It is likely that the anodyne Helen used was either tincture of opium or cannabis. Most believe it was the former, and modern pharmacological evidence clearly supports that conclusion.[7] With the limited pharmacopoeia of the times, Helen could only have sustained the convivial spirits of the celebrants with a substance that activates the large synaptic membrane protein that we now know to be the *mu* and *delta* opiate receptors (for distribution, see Figure 6.8). These receptors are among the brain's most powerful modulators of pain, as well as the very source of opiate addiction in humans. In fact, three major varieties of opiate receptors and opiate transmitters have been identified in the brain: The endorphins interact primarily with *mu* receptors, the enkephalins with *delta* receptors, and the dynorphins with *kappa* receptors. Separation distress is most powerfully inhibited by brain opioids that interact with *mu* receptors, which also mediate opiate addiction. The most powerful endogenous opiate-like molecule that interacts with the *mu* receptor is ß-endorphin, which also has the most powerful ability to alleviate separation distress.[8]

There is good reason to believe that several endogenous opioids are important in the control of social emotions, the elaboration of social attachments, and various forms of human love, both nurturant and erotic.[9] Nurturant love emerges between parents and children and seems different in obvious respects from sexual love. But are they really so vastly different in the deeper recesses of the brain? We simply do not know, for love is a difficult concept to biologize, unless we are willing to take some conceptual risks. There has been some theoretical speculation, although no hard data, suggesting that emotional infatuation and erotic love may be promoted by brain dopamine systems and mild dopamine-type psychostimulants such as phenethylamine, which occurs in fairly high levels in chocolate (which many of us "love"). The same type of argument could be made for *anandamide*, the endogenous cannabinoid-type molecule, also present in chocolate.[10] The database for such assertions remains nonexistent, and the argument that such molecules may reduce feelings of social isolation is further weakened by the fact that these molecules are not very effective in quelling separation distress in animals. Perhaps chocolate and other tasty foods help lonely people to cope better psychologically because pleasurable tastes activate endogenous opioid systems (see Chapter 9).

As we saw in the previous two chapters, one plausible way of thinking is that nurturant love emerges from brain systems that promote parental attachments, while erotic love may emerge from brain systems that generate sexual seeking. If so, the first might be more opiate- and oxytocin-based, while the latter is more dopamine- and vasopressin-based. But even if such hypotheses are on the right track, the two could not be completely distinct in the tangled neurochemical skein of the brain. Dopamine and opioid systems interact in several interesting ways, including through the arousal of brain dopamine by opiate receptors within the ventral tegmental area (VTA) and opiate inhibition of dopamine activity in the terminal fields of the striatum. Likewise, oxytocin has a diversity of neural interactions, including complex interactions with opiate and psychostimulant effects in the brain.[11]

If credible experimental approaches to disentangling such questions are ever developed, it will be remarkable to behold how erotic love and nurturant love are dynamically intertwined within subcortical neural circuits, and we may begin to understand why they are often tangled in the higher cognitive reaches of our minds. Fortunately, there are some more basic questions that can be answered definitively at the present time.

Attachment Styles and an Overview of the PANIC System

During the past several decades, developmental psychologists have constructed a coherent theoretical view of the nature of social attachment. They have observed that children exhibit a variety of attachment "styles," or temperaments, that have strong genetic and environmental antecedents.[12] Some are securely attached, while others are not. Securely attached children are confident of receiving social support from their parents or other caretakers. They are generally outgoing and tend to confront life with optimism and enthusiasm. By comparison, insecurely attached children are timid and do not readily become engaged with new situations. In fact, children who are insecure about their social support exhibit two major emotional and behavioral patterns of "neediness." Some are excessively clingy and seem to need more than the usual amount of attention from their caretakers. Others choose to distance themselves from social contacts, avoiding social situations presumably because they are not confident of receiving the positive support and feedback they crave. Perhaps they have felt rebuffed so often that they no longer reach out to others. In order to subsist comfortably, they have become cognitively detached from their emotional desires.[13]

How these attachment tendencies emerge from the fabric of the brain has remained a mystery until recently. Now, work on animal emotionality is beginning to reveal the neuromotivational forces that may mediate such social feelings. An especially promising line of work is emerging from the detailed analysis of one behavioral measure—the vocal "crying" aroused by social isolation in young animals. Some label these "isolation calls," others refer to them as "distress vocalizations," and others simply call it "crying" (a label that many behavioristically oriented investigators deem too anthropomorphic). The label is less important than the fact that there is an intrinsic neural system in the brain, here labeled the PANIC system, that mediates this strong emotional response.

As we will see, the PANIC circuits have been mapped out with localized electrical stimulation. To the best of our modest knowledge, such circuits help create the emotions organisms experience as a result of social isolation and loss of social comfort. Presumably, social attachments emerge, in part, from environmental events activating brain chemistries that can reduce arousal in these distress circuits.

The Separation-Distress System and Social Attachments

Since the infants of all mammalian species remain quite helpless for a variable period of time following birth, they must have strong distress signaling mechanisms to solicit and sustain parental care. Isolation calls, or distress vocalizations (DVs), as they will be called here, are one of the most primitive forms of audiovocal communication (Figure 14.2); the underlying brain mechanisms are probably shared homologously in all mammals, even though there is bound to be substantial variation among different species depending on their socioecological circumstances. For instance, socially deprived young rats do not vocalize in response to separation as much as many other species (see Figure 2.1), presumably because their underlying affective response system is comparatively rudimentary. This is true for most animals that are born very altricial (i.e., developmentally immature), since the probability that they will stray from the nest is remote. Young rats also are not strongly attached to their mother (i.e., any mother will do as heater and "feed bag"). Only when they become mobile do they exhibit a period of clear social bonding, but their responses still do not compare with the vigor seen in other species, ranging from birds to primates, that exhibit powerful, unambiguous, and long-lasting social bonds.

Human infants are also born very immature, and they do not begin to exhibit true separation distress and specific social attachments until their motor system has matured sufficiently for them to wander off and get lost. At about half a year of age, human babies begin to make sad and sometimes angry sounds of protest in order to attract the attention of caregivers when they are left alone for too long. This emotional response is a robust feature of childhood for many years, but it persists for only a few months in most other mammals because, in relative terms, their "childhood" is much shorter than ours.

In any event, DVs emerge quite promptly whenever young animals are left alone in strange new places. The proximity of a caretaker is typically sufficient to totally inhibit the calls in both humans and other species (Figure 14.3).[14] The home location can also inhibit separation distress to a modest extent, suggesting that separation-distress systems may be evolutionarily related to ancient mechanisms of place attachment. In most species, the mother is more effective in quelling distress than the father, but there are exceptions: As mentioned in the last chapter, among the titi monkeys of South

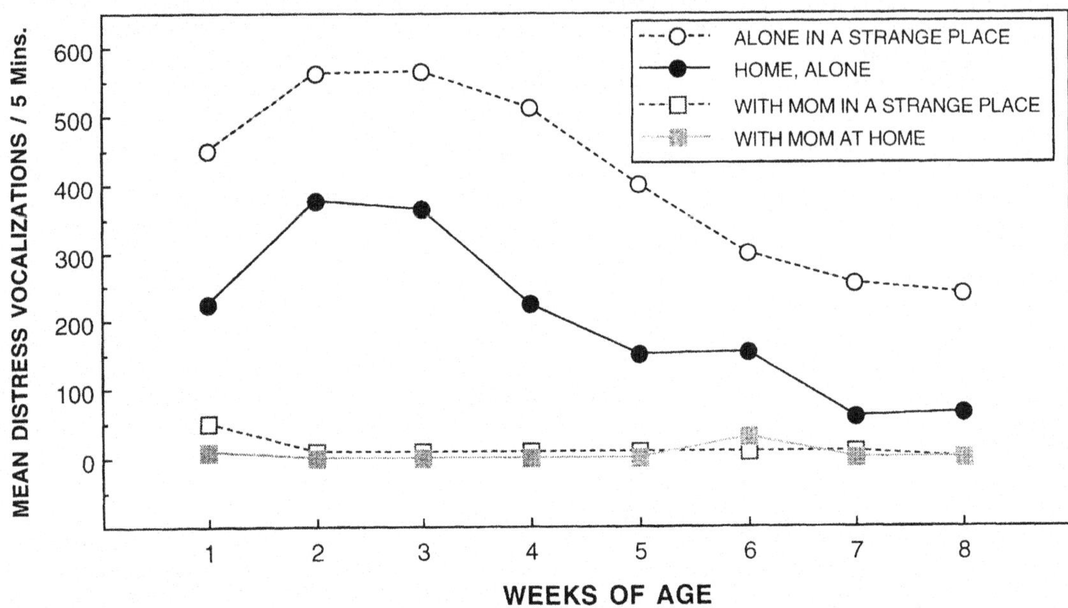

Figure 14.3. Distress vocalizations of young guinea pigs as a function of age, tested either alone or with mother in familiar and unfamiliar environments. (Adapted from Pettijohn, 1979; see n. 14.)

America, the young are more attached to fathers, even though mothers provide most of the food. Indeed, in this rare species, mothers tend to become agitated if left alone with infants, apparently because they are more strongly bonded to their mates than to their own infants.[15] These mothers just don't seem to like being alone with their young.

The fact that the neural systems for separation-induced crying emerged from more primitive distress mechanisms, such as those that mediate pain and feelings of coldness (Figure 14.1), raises a major methodological issue: How shall we discriminate the various types of cries? Even before they fully recognize their social circumstances, infants of most species respond to pain, hunger, and irritation by crying. In animals, there is evidence to suggest that separation-induced DVs can be distinguished from cries of pain on neuroanatomical and neurochemical bases, as well as via an analysis of sound spectrum characteristics.[16] However, because of the evolutionary relations between separation and pain mechanisms, they also share many controls—such as opioid-induced inhibition, as already mentioned.

In the presence of adults who have bonded with the young, DVs have the common effect of arousing the attention and typically the caregiving motivations of caretakers. Many experiments have now shown that the infant's call of distress is highly arousing and a powerful attractant to the parents. They investigate locations from which such sounds emanate, even if they are only tape-recorded, with mothers typically exhibiting stronger responses than fathers.[17] Is it because the cries of infants arouse resonant feelings of distress more readily in mothers than in fathers? Since no one has made the appropriate brain measurements, we do not yet know. However, we do know that specific locations in the auditory system, in both the inferior colliculi and the medial geniculate nuclei, are highly tuned to receive and process these primal communications.[18]

Even though there are many species differences in the detailed expression of bonding and distress mechanisms in the brain, it is assumed that the arousal of PANIC circuits is one of the major forces that guides the construction of social bonds. When these circuits are aroused, animals seek reunion with individuals who help create the feeling of a "secure neurochemical base" within the brain. Presumably, the young animals that exhibit the most intense separation responses will be the ones that exhibit the strongest social dependencies and are the most susceptible to psychiatric disorders that emerge from feelings of social loss.

It is reasonable to assume that the underlying neural dynamics within the PANIC system are especially important in allowing organisms to care for each other. Exactly how a concerned attitude is promoted within caretakers' brains by hearing distress calls from their infants remains unknown, but I would suggest that the sounds of crying arouse distress circuits in parents that parallel the distress of the children. If so, associated learning systems may rapidly establish the knowledge that an optimal way to reduce distress in both is for the parents to provide care and attention to their offspring. One of the most powerful sensory signals of care is direct contact, and touch appears to activate endogenous opioid systems, thereby reinforcing the social bond.[19]

If no bonds exist, the sound of distress calls may simply be perceived as an irritation, which in humans could easily lead to child abuse. Through a poorly understood reciprocity of social emotional systems, pro-social activities are initiated and sustained between parents and their infants. Pro-social acts are the instantiation of social bonds, and at present they are the only way we can monitor the underlying feelings. Obviously, in humans the role of cognitive factors, for better and worse, can often override emotional concerns. As we saw in the example of Netsilik behavior in the previous chapter, humans sometimes must make very difficult choices in caring for their offspring. In any event, when care is provided, emotionally distressed children rapidly exhibit responses of comfort and satisfaction, even though, if the care has taken too long to arrive, they may also harbor some resentments, as indicated by a transient phase of social detachment upon reunion. Adults often do the same. Apparently, through such social reciprocities, the social bond between related animals is first established and periodically strengthened.

Thanks to the clarity of separation-distress patterns, a study of this emotional processes in animals provides one of the most powerful lines of evidence for guiding our thinking about the deep neural sources of loneliness and social attachments in humans. These lines of thought also have the potential to highlight the primal biological nature of certain forms of love and friendship.[20]

Brain Circuits for DVs and PANIC

One of the best ways to identify the general locations of PANIC circuitry is by administration of localized electrical stimulation of the brain (ESB) into specific areas. This type of work has now been conducted in a large number of species, including primates, cats, and chickens,[21] and has yielded a remarkably similar picture. As depicted in Figure 14.4 from work with guinea pigs, the PANIC system appears to arise from the midbrain PAG, very close to where one can generate physical pain responses. Anatomically, it almost seems that separation has emerged from more basic pain systems during brain evolution (as is also highlighted in Figure 14.1). This affirms that separation distress is related to perceptions of pain, and this relationship remains codified in our language (i.e., to lose someone is a "painful experience").

The PANIC system is also well represented in the medial diencephalon, especially the dorsomedial thalamus. Even farther forward, one finds a high density of active DV sites in the ventral septal area, the preoptic area, and many sites in the bed nucleus of the stria terminalis (areas that figure heavily in sexual and maternal behaviors). In some higher species, one can also obtain separation calls from the very anterior part of the cingulate

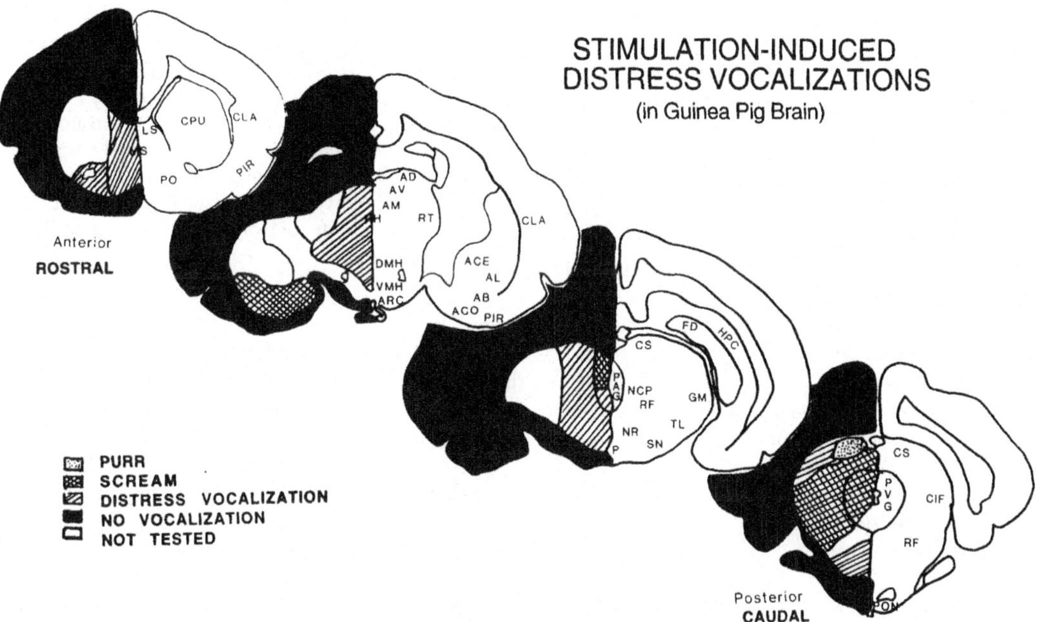

Figure 14.4. Schematic representation of electrically induced separation-distress vocalization sites in the guinea pig brain. (Adapted from Panksepp et al., 1988; see n. 27.)

gyrus, as well as some sites in the amygdala and scattered ones in other areas, including the hypothalamus.[22]

There is a remarkable resemblance between the neuroanatomy of this behavioral control system and those for the corticotrophin releasing factor (CRF) and ß-endorphin systems (see Figure 6.7). Endogenous opioids clearly suppress arousal of this system, not only as measured by natural DVs but also as measured by ESB techniques, and at least in some species CRF increases DVs.[23] Such neural systems extend branches to many other brain areas, suggesting how a variety of psychological processes are affected by the experience of separation and reunion.

It is a common assertion that human females are prone to cry more than males. There may be some neurobiological truth to this stereotype. Work on the isolation cries of guinea pigs and chickens indicates that administration of testosterone diminishes crying in young animals. This appears to be due to a change in the underlying sensitivity of the PANIC system. We have evaluated this possibility using ESB techniques in guinea pigs and have found that as animals get older, the sensitivity of the DV system diminishes; this effect is larger in males than in females.[24]

The age-related decline in males appears to be partly due to the maturation of the pituitary-gonadal axis. Male and female guinea pigs that have had their sexual glands removed exhibit smaller declines than animals with intact testes and ovaries, with the effects varying as a function of the brain region being studied. There are bound to be many other factors that contribute to the decline of separation-induced crying with age, but this natural decline clearly is not simply caused by the gradual degeneration of DV circuits: Strong crying can still be induced in mature animals, which no longer exhibit spontaneous DVs, by applying ESB directly into the trajectory of the crying circuits. The decline is largely the result of reduced sensitivity of the system. This appears to be more precipitous in males than in females, at least partly because of the powerful neural influences of testosterone on DV circuitry.[25] Likewise, young chicks that receive daily testosterone injections begin to vocalize less than controls, an effect that is especially prominent in the presence of social stimuli such as mirrors (Figure 14.5). From this perspective, it is not surprising that crying and panic attacks are more common among women than among men.[26] Such gender differences in emotionality may not simply be learned or culturally created phenomena.

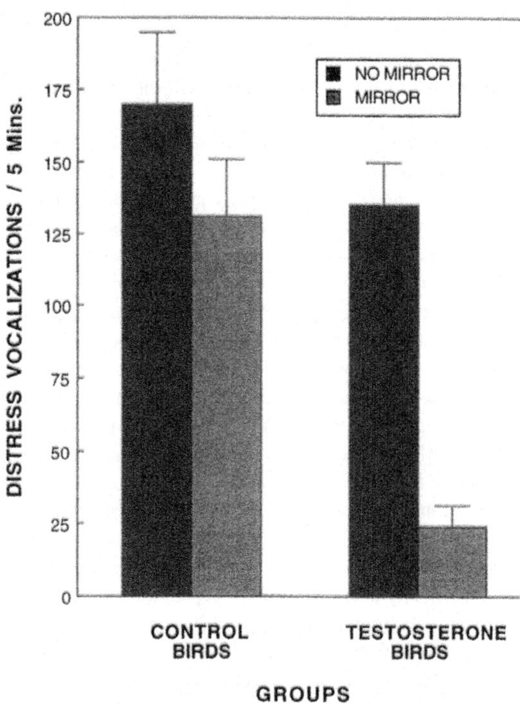

Figure 14.5. Summary of mean (±SEM) distress vocalizations in 14-day-old male chickens treated with testosterone (2 mg) or peanut oil vehicle for the previous eight days when they had been individually housed to reduce aggression. Animals were tested as in Figure 14.8 except for five-minute periods of no mirrors, mirrors, no mirrors, and mirrors. It is noteworthy how high the vocalization rates are considering that the animals are being moved from their isolated housing conditions to new isolation chambers. This may reflect the fact that animals had established place attachments and that separation from those conditions was sufficient to evoke emotional distress. In any event, the testosterone reliably reduced vocalization rates ($p < .001$), and the mirror effect was somewhat larger in them also ($p < .05$). It is noteworthy that usually one sees a larger mirror effect in control birds that are socially housed. (Unpublished data, Panksepp, 1995.)

The Neurochemistry of the PANIC System

We know approximately where in the brain DV circuits are situated, which neurochemistries provoke arousal of these distress systems, and also which chemistries soothe and calm the overarousal.[27] In addition to opioids, other neuropeptides that can greatly relieve the process are oxytocin and prolactin (Figure 14.6). Presumably, there are distinct chemistries for the many sensory and perceptual modulators of this emotional response, such as hearing, smell, and especially touch (see Figure 14.1). Nonpeptide neurochemistries that are effective include such drugs as *clonidine*, a norepinephrine (NE) receptor agonist, which both facilitates (postsynaptically) and suppresses (presynaptically) NE activity in the brain. Nicotine and various glutamate receptor antagonists also relieve DVs effectively. Many other chemistries have weaker, but statistically significant effects, such as some antidepressants, minor

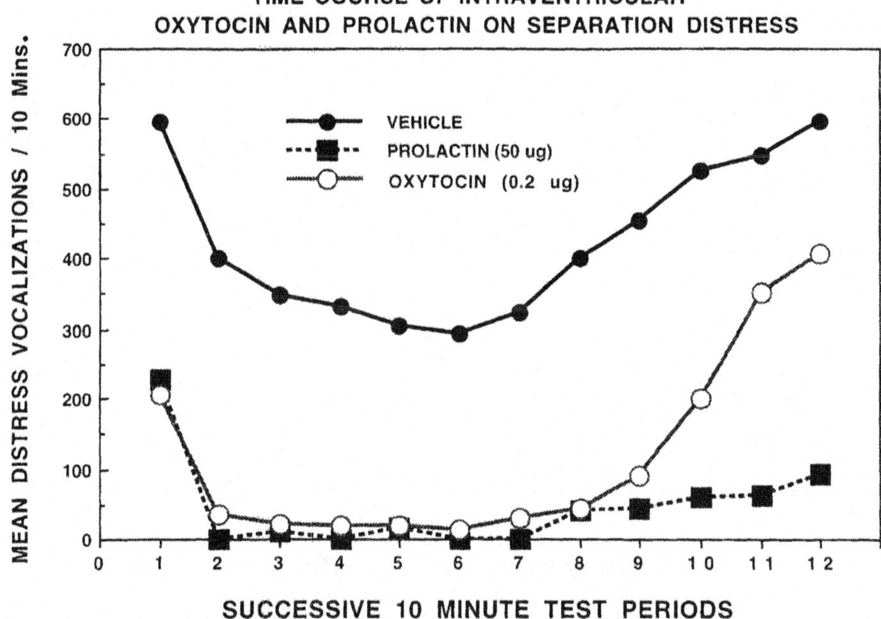

Figure 14.6. Effects of intraventricular oxytocin and prolactin on the separation distress calls of 5–6-day-old chicks socially isolated from their flock for a two-hour period. (Adapted from Panksepp, 1996; see n. 30.)

tranquilizers, and other sedatives. However, the vast majority of neuroactive drugs have minimal effects on this emotional response, including such powerful sedating drugs as the antipsychotics (i.e., the major tranquilizers).[28]

The major chemistries that have been found to activate crying in young animals are CRF, certain types of glutamate receptor stimulants (especially those that act on NMDA and kainate receptors), and also central administration of curare, a drug that normally blocks the nicotinic cholinergic system in the periphery, leading to paralysis, although in the brain it appears to do something else, perhaps activating glutamate receptors. All three of these agents can turn on the crying response, even if animals are housed with social companions.[29] At present, the best estimate is that the neuronal "command transmitter" for the PANIC system, as for so many other basic emotional systems, is glutamate. This is the only system (except for CRF) in which receptor activation can dramatically increase DVs, even in the presence of other animals, and receptor blockade can dramatically decrease DVs (Figure 14.7), even those induced by electrical brain stimulation.[30]

Many other drugs can promote crying that has already been initiated, including reductions in acetylcholine, serotonin, and opioid activity, but these are clearly modulatory, since they cannot evoke crying all by themselves. Hence, they do not directly arouse the primary pathways mediating the neural impulse to cry. Unfortunately, we presently know next to nothing about the specific types of environmental and internal information related to social loss that these various neurochemistries help mediate.

Before proceeding, let me share a methodological point. The aforementioned elevations of crying have been most extensively studied in newborn domestic chicks,[31] and it is easiest to see increases when baseline levels of crying have been reduced by providing social stimuli. One of the easiest ways to reduce the crying is to put mirrors on the wall of the test chamber. The chicks appear to behave as if they are in the company of others and cry less (see Figure 14.5).[32] Similar reductions can be induced with music (see Figure 14.8), which may simulate the comfort derived from audiovocal contact with other animals. This may be one of the reasons people love music—it keeps them company. Both of these comforting effects can be almost completely eliminated by stimulating the glutamate receptor system with intraventricular injections of kainic acid and NMDA, which, as mentioned earlier, can also increase vocalizations in the absence of mirrors. Comparable effects are produced with curare and CRF.

Although most of the early pharmacological work was done in young chicks, there is now considerable corroboratory work with mammals, including primates. This work provides confidence that many of the pharmacological effects reported here may be generalizable to most mammals; it also highlights nature's conserva-

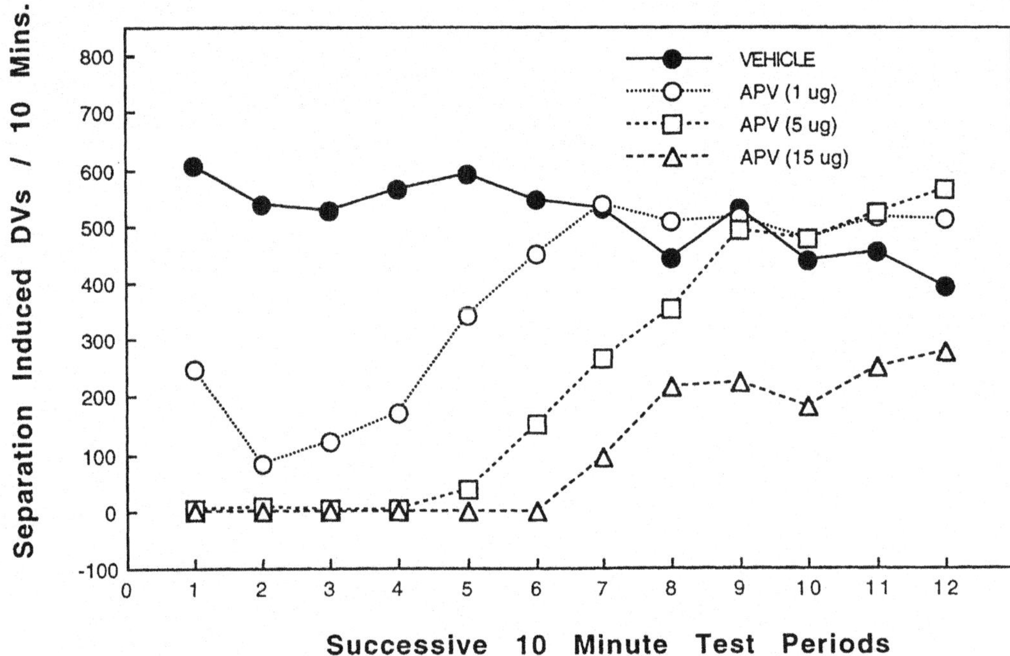

Figure 14.7. The glutamate receptor antagonist 5-amino-2-phosphonovalerate (APV) specifically blocks the NMDA receptor, which appears to be a key transmitter in the production of separation DVs. The animals tested here were 12-day-old domestic chicks that received APV injections into the 4th ventricle region just prior to being separated from their companions (a flock of 20 birds). The magnitude and duration of DV inhibition were directly related to the amount of APV injected. (Adapted from Panksepp, 1996; see n. 30.)

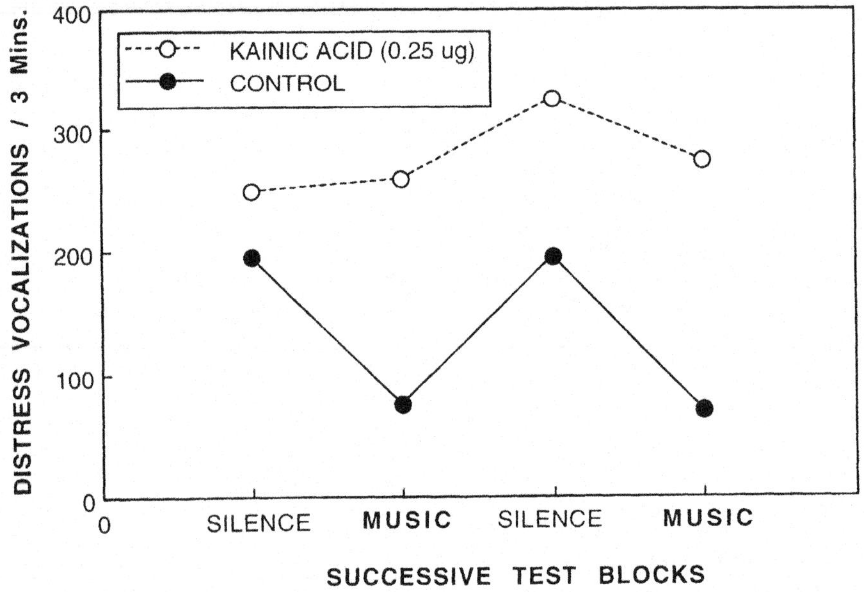

Figure 14.8. Mean number of vocalizations in 4–5-day-old chicks during successive three-minute testing blocks either in ambient silence or during exposure to music. Half of the animals were administered 0.25 μg of kainic acid (KA) into their ventricular systems just before testing. Not only did the KA markedly increase vocalizations, but the "comforting" effects of music were totally eliminated. The same pattern of results is obtained if one uses mirrored environments to reduce the vocalization. (Adapted from Normansell, 1988; see n. 30.)

tism when it comes to the organization of ancient emotional systems. However, there are certain exceptions to these patterns. Perhaps the most problematic ones come from the infant rat, which, as discussed earlier and highlighted in Figure 2.1, is not an ideal subject for separation-distress studies.[33]

On the Nature of Gregariousness

Programmatic research into the neural nature of gregariousness and social investigation has been sporadic, except for the study of social choices motivated by sexual urges. A great deal of work has focused on how gonadal hormones modulate social interest. The results have been fairly straightforward: Males and females seek out each other's company primarily as a function of hormonally primed states. Young intact males generally prefer the company of estrus females, but gonadectomized ones or elderly ones do not.[34] As mentioned in Chapter 12, the social preferences of estrus females are not as well studied, but we do know they seek out the companionship of sexually active males.

Little is known about the brain systems that motivate gregariousness independently of sexual motivation, even though it is recognized that certain interesting social patterns emerge from animals' tendency to congregate. For instance, mountain sheep (and many other herding animals) exhibit defensive group patterns in which the young animals keep to the center of a circle while adults line the periphery. Although it is attractive to see this as an ecologically important cognitive strategy, it may simply be a by-product of gregarious tendencies at different stages of development. For instance, the pattern could emerge simply from the fact that young animals are more gregarious than older ones, which would lead them to form a tighter nucleus, leaving adults to patrol the periphery because they do not prefer to be as close to each other.[35] This is a neat explanation for a factor that promotes defensive tactics in herding species, but it is only a distal explanation because the proximal neural and psychological dynamics are controlled by emotional circuits within the brains of these animals.

To experimentally analyze gregariousness requires systematic laboratory measurements that are relatively straightforward. The most common approach has been to measure the amount of time animals voluntarily spend in proximity to each other. In the 1960s and 1970s, social psychologist Bib Latane and colleagues extensively characterized gregarious tendencies in rats,[36] but they failed to extend their analysis to the brain. This was partly remedied by later investigators who demonstrated that gregariousness increases following septal damage and declines following amygdala damage,[37] and that these effects cancel each other out when both types of brain damage are inflicted.[38] Although these findings indicate that the limbic system is important in motivating animals to spend friendly time together, the underlying neurochemical mechanisms remain to be clarified.

One attractive hypothesis is that neurochemistries modulating separation distress will be important in motivating gregariousness and social reward (Figure 14.1). Thus, manipulations that increase distress should increase social motivation, and vice versa. For instance, reductions in opioid activity should increase desire for social companionship, and increases in this system should reduce the need for gregariousness.[39] Observations consistent with this interpretation have been collected from a large variety of species using several distinct behavioral measures. Animals treated with moderate doses of opiates tend to socially isolate themselves. Rodents reduce the amount of time they spend in proximity to each other,[40] dogs exhibit reduced tail wagging,[41] primates exhibit decreased social grooming, and humans have also reported a decreased need to socialize.[42] In other words, high opiate activity diminishes the underlying emotional need for companionship. Less work has been done with oxytocin, and at present the pattern of results is a bit more confusing, with oxytocin reducing gregariousness in short-term tests but increasing it in long-term conditioning tests.[43]

Conversely, opiate antagonists increase social motivation. Rodents have been observed to exhibit increased social proximity, dogs exhibit increased solicitous tail wagging, and primates groom each other more.[44] It is especially noteworthy that young primates exhibit more social clinging to their mothers and also make more social solicitations to other members of their troops when their opioid systems are blocked with drugs such as naloxone.[45] On the other hand, when mothers are given the same drug treatment, they often exhibit a strong decrease in social affiliation, possibly because they are not able to obtain the proper emotional feedback from their caregiving efforts.[46] In general, though, when animals cannot experience opioid activity in the brain, they are more likely to socialize, if prevailing conditions are nonthreatening. As I will elaborate later, this effect may also be present in humans, since opiate antagonists can induce moderate increases of social responsivity in autistic children.

On the Nature of Contact Comfort

As mentioned earlier, there is little clear-cut evidence for a unique social reward system independent of separation-distress and sexual urges (Figure 14.1). However, it is reasonable to believe that a substantial amount of social motivation emerges from the pleasures of touch, and the pleasure of play is strongly dependent on the sensation of touch. Indeed, it is possible that the mammalian skin contains specialized receptors, such as in "tickle-skin," for detecting social contact (see Chapter 15).

However, the ability of petting to comfort domestic animals and to produce powerful physiological effects is both obvious and poorly studied.[47] One easy way to study such effects objectively is to monitor crying in young animals that are held or not held. The effects are, of course, dramatic. Animals stop crying rapidly when gently touched. There is some evidence that this contact comfort is mediated, in part, by activation of brain opioid systems. For instance, one can also measure the latency of eye closure in response to holding, and opiate receptor antagonists reduce the ability of animals to settle down (Figure 14.9).[48] However, even with complete blockade of the opioid systems by naloxone or naltrexone, birds held gently in this way do eventually settle down and cry much less than unheld control birds. Clearly, neurochemistries other than opioids contribute to the feelings of contact-comfort.

The fact that touch can release opioids in the brain has also been confirmed in primates.[49] Indeed, administration of naloxone tends to increase grooming in primates, while administration of opiates reduces the desire to be touched.

The likelihood is high that prolactin and oxytocin participate in aspects of contact comfort, simply from the perspective that these hormones mediate milk production and the efficacy of the suckling reflex, but empirical data are scarce. However, in this context it is worth noting that the brains of mice with different social temperaments exhibit dramatically different oxytocin receptor distributions, which also change as a function of age.[50] The developmental changes in brain oxytocin receptor distributions are so striking that they suggest this chemical system may mediate different social affective processes at different times in the animal's life cycle (Figure 14.10). With respect to strain differences, the highly social prairie vole exhibits more "infantile" distribution of oxytocin receptors than does the montane vole, which prefers a solitary lifestyle.

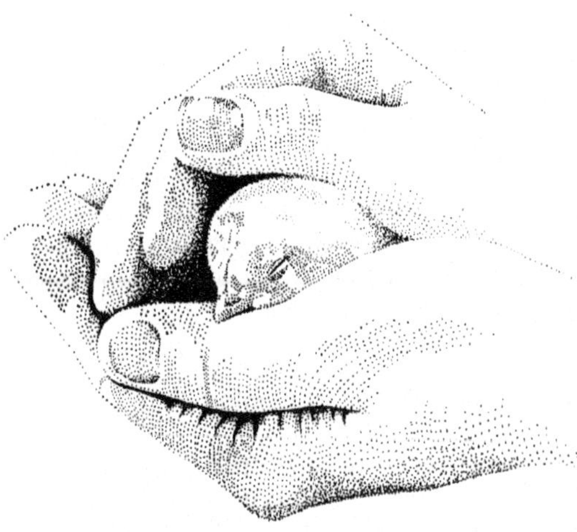

Figure 14.9. When held gently in human hands, newborn chicks exhibit a comfort response consisting of the cessation of vocalizations and eye closure. These effects are attenuated by opiate receptor blockade with naltrexone and amplified by low doses of opioids. (Adapted from Panksepp et al., 1980; see n. 32.)

Thus, different species, and even substrains of a single species, exhibit differential constitutional levels of arousability of different emotional systems, and it appears that one of these may function as a social reward system. Such differences also exist in humans and reflect intrinsic genetic variability in temperaments, as well as the differential impact of early experiences on the emergence of various personality dimensions.[51] Unfortunately, substantive knowledge at this level remains meager. Nonetheless, the search for a unique social reward system should yield future dividends in understanding social attachment processes.

Social Attachments and Imprinting: A Role for Opioids and Oxytocin

As we saw in the previous chapter, the most important work on the underlying nature of the social bond is emerging from empirical investigations based on two premises: the likelihood that the peripheral physiological processes that accompany birth may also control attachment processes in the brain, and that there are neurochemical similarities between opiate dependence and social dependence. Here I will amplify on these premises and also introduce a third, namely, that all neurochemistries that normally inhibit separation distress may also promote bonding. Obviously, all these factors are intermeshed, perhaps inextricably, within the brain.

The amount of evidence for neurochemical control of attachment processes in mammals is remarkably limited. As noted in the previous chapter, oxytocin clearly promotes bonding, and in unpublished data, we have also found evidence that vasopressin may be equally important.[52] How opiates participate in this process remains ambiguous,[53] but they probably provide a mechanism for making fine discriminations among the available bonding objects—for instance, whether a youngster develops strongest ties with mom, dad, or one of the aunts or uncles at the perimeter of the clan. However, it is clear that when animals have exogenous opiates in their bodies, they exhibit less social activity in general, except at very low doses.[54]

At present we know very little about the brain areas that mediate social bonding, even though we can anticipate that the cingulate cortex, septal area, bed nucleus of the stria terminalis, preoptic area, dorsomedial thalamus, and periaqueductal gray (PAG) will be important—namely, all of the areas that mediate feelings of separation distress. Also, in animals that utilize olfactory cues in the establishment of social attachments,

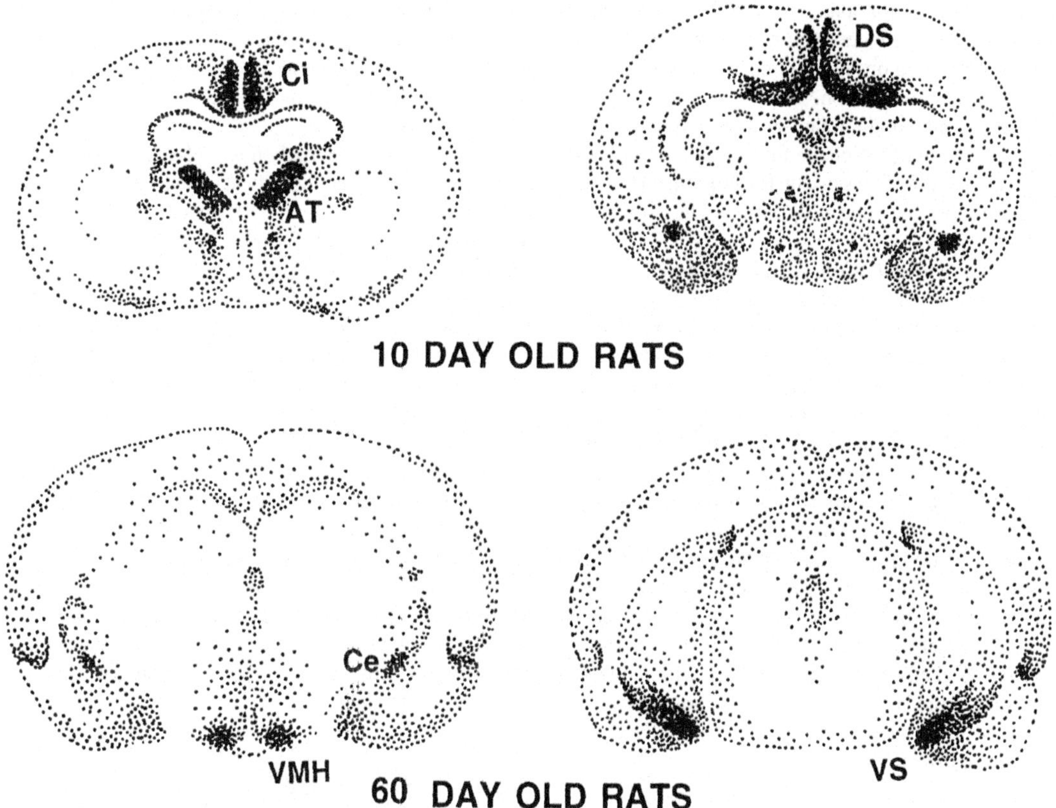

Figure 14.10. Artist's rendition of the redistribution in the density of oxytocin receptors in the rat brain during infancy (top two figures) and maturity (bottom two). It is evident that in the infant, very high receptor densities are present in the cingulate cortex, the anterior thalamus, and the dorsal hippocampal/subicular region. These areas of the brain probably control infantile emotions such as separation distress and primary social bonding. On the other hand, in adult female rats, the densities are highest in the ventromedial hypothalamus and the ventral hippocampal/subicular region. These areas probably mediate female sexual receptivity and memory processes related to sociosexual issues. (Adapted from Shapiro & Insel, 1989; see n. 50.)

including sheep and rodents, the olfactory bulbs play a role. Indeed, the release of norepinephrine in the bulbs is an essential component for solidifying social memories in such creatures.[55]

During the past decade, there has been considerable progress in identifying the brain mechanisms of imprinting in birds. Key areas, such as the intermediate part of the hyperstriatum ventrale (IMHV) and lateral forebrain, are rich in opioid receptors. Lesions of the IMHV have been most extensively studied and found to reduce both the acquisition and retention of imprinting.[56] Likewise, the IMHV exhibits a variety of changes as a function of imprinting, including increases in synaptic density and elevated glutamate binding.[57] It is not clear what is the mammalian homolog of the IMHV, but it may well be the cingulate cortex.

Brain opioids do not appear to be essential for the development of simple imprinting responses (the mere act of following objects). When young domestic chicks are given high doses of naltrexone, an opiate receptor antagonist, during formal imprinting trials, they do not exhibit a diminution of subsequent following responses. Indeed, such animals appear to be more eager than usual to follow the imprinting stimulus, even though they vocalize more, as if they are not getting as much satisfaction from the interaction.[58] In other words, although the birds appear to become cognitively imprinted in the absence of opioids, their sense of security is not as great as one would normally expect. Thus, it is noteworthy that the fine discriminative aspects of imprinting are impaired by opioid blockade.[59] In other words, opioid activity may be important in the establishment of social choices in the same way that it appears important for gustatory choices (see Figure 9.4). However, if we give moderate doses of opiates to animals that have been imprinted, they no longer exhibit a vigorous following response, affirming once more that low opioid activity increases social motivation.[60]

From the mammalian data on oxytocin and social bonding, one might anticipate that the avian homolog, vasotocin, would be important for bonding. Unfortunately, support for such a hypothesis has remained elusive.[61]

In sum, the most reasonable supposition at present is that social bonding ultimately involves the ability of young organisms to experience separation distress when isolated from social support systems and to experience neurochemically mediated comfort when social contacts are reestablished. In addition to answering basic science questions of considerable importance, the analysis of the biological substrates of social processes in animals has important ramifications for our understanding and treatment of various psychiatric disorders. Although all such disorders are strongly influenced by social variables, some, such as panic attacks, depression, and early childhood autism, seem especially closely connected to the brain dynamics that underlie social emotions. Each of these will be briefly discussed in the next three sections, but first I will explain why we need to distinguish the PANIC system from that which mediates FEAR.

Neurochemical Distinctions between Separation-Distress and Fear Processes in the Brain

An issue raised in Chapter 11 deserves to be reemphasized here—namely, how we can objectively distinguish between the PANIC and FEAR systems of the brain. As indicated by brain stimulation studies, the systems have different neuroanatomies, even though there is considerable overlap and probably interaction in certain parts of the brain, especially lower areas such as the PAG of the mesencephalon. We may even be able to intuit some of the functional interactions from introspective experiences—for instance, we can easily develop anticipatory anxiety in response to situations that will provoke intense feelings of separation. Likewise, some parents find it anxiety-provoking to visit the graves of children who have died. Some children find it extremely anxiety-provoking to be separated from their parents, in situations as simple as going to school for the first time, a reaction that goes by the designation *school phobia*.[62]

Thus, separation distress may promote activity in fear circuits, but behavioral data suggest that the converse does not occur. For instance, the presentation of fearful stimuli tends to reduce the frequency of separation calls,[63] presumably because it would be maladaptive for young animals to reveal their locations when predators are nearby. Also, as we will see later, anticipatory anxiety and panic attacks appear to be generated by distinct neural systems; the assumption here is that much of the former emerges from the FEAR system and much of the latter from the separation-distress or PANIC system.

Some puzzling neurochemical effects may also be clarified by distinguishing between the two systems. For instance, the neuropeptide CRF appears to participate in both FEAR and PANIC processes. Thus, while CRF placed into the brain increases DVs dramatically in young chicks and modestly in young primates, the same manipulation reduces DVs in guinea pigs.[64] This difference could be explained by the fact that CRF in the first two species has stronger effects on the PANIC system, while in the latter it has stronger effects on the FEAR system.

Pharmacologically, we can also distinguish these systems by noting that opiates are very effective in reducing separation distress but not fearful behaviors.[65] Conversely, benzodiazepines are quite effective in reducing fear behaviors but not as effective in reducing separation calls.[66] As we will see at the end of this chapter, similar patterns of results have been observed with the different drugs used to treat generalized anxiety disorders and panic attacks.

Separation Systems and the Origin of Panic Attacks

The selection of the term PANIC for the brain system that mediates separation distress was originally premised on the hypothesis that the emotional problem known as panic attacks may emerge from precipitous arousal of the separation-distress system. This hypothesis was based on several relationships between the two responses: People who suffer from repeated panic attacks typically have had childhood histories characterized by separation anxiety problems.[67] During separation distress as well as during panic attacks, the victims feel as if their center of comfort and stability has been abruptly removed, leading to active solicitation of help and social support. Both are commonly accompanied by such autonomic symptoms as a feeling of weakness, difficulty in getting one's breath, and a feeling of having a lump in the throat.[68] Perhaps most strikingly, the type of medication that was first found to be beneficial for panic attacks,[69] the tricyclic antidepressant imipramine, was also the first drug that was found to exert a substantial ameliorative effect on separation-distress vocalizations in a variety of species, including primates and dogs.[70] Although this by no means proves that these two types of emotional expression emerge from the same system, the pharmacological analysis of panic attacks clearly indicates that the disorder is not simply a variant of fearful, anticipatory anxiety.

Careful work by the psychiatrist Donald Klein in the early 1960s indicated that the newly discovered benzodiazepine-type antianxiety agents such as chlordiazepoxide (Librium®) and diazepam (Valium®) had little beneficial effect on the incidence of panic attacks. Since the tricyclic antidepressant imipramine had just been discovered, Klein proceeded to evaluate it as well. Even though patients first claimed that imipramine had no beneficial effect, in fact they complained of panic attacks much less often than they had prior to taking the drug.[71] When the incidence of panic attacks was actually counted, it was clear that they had markedly diminished during medication. Apparently the patients had not noticed their improvement because the drug did not diminish the anticipatory anxiety associated with the disorder—namely, the fear that an attack might be forthcoming. While the antianxiety agents tested had diminished anticipatory anxiety, they did not diminish the frequency or intensity of the panic attacks themselves.

Subsequent work has found that children who suffered from "school phobias" could also be helped with tricyclics.[72] Such children seem to be seriously disturbed by the prospect of separation when they first have to leave home to enter the school system, but when given low doses of imipramine they feel more confident, presumably in part because the underlying arousal of the PANIC system is diminished through the facilitation of brain serotonin activity at synapses that modulate separation-distress responses. Of course, it remains to be clearly demonstrated that this, in fact, is the case in humans, but facilitation of serotonin activity is quite effective in reducing DVs in animals.[73] More recent work has indicated that the new generation of selective serotonin reuptake inhibitor (SSRI) antidepressants are also quite effective in controlling panic, as are some of the more potent modern benzodiazepines such as alprazolam.[74] In general, these lines of evidence suggest that the arousal of separation-distress circuitry may promote the incidence of panic attacks.

Alternative views are, of course, possible. For instance, Klein has recently suggested that panic attacks arise from precipitous arousal of a suffocation alarm mechanism in the brain stem.[75] It may well be that this primitive self-defense system is, in fact, functionally coupled to arousal of the PANIC system. A common denominator of both is that they are closely linked to respiratory and audiovocal dynamics, and under both emotional states one feels in desperate need of immediate aid.

There are also milder forms of separation distress that can lead to social phobias, such as a chronic feeling of insecurity when one is interacting with others. Phenelzine, a monoamine oxidase (MAO) inhibitor, has been found to have remarkable efficacy in reducing such symptoms.[76] Recently other serotonin-facilitating drugs that reduce separation distress, such as fluoxetine (i.e., better known as Prozac®), have been touted to increase social confidence.[77]

Psychiatric Implications: On the Nature of Social Loss and Depression

Chronic arousal of the PANIC system may have long-term psychiatric consequences. The persistent stress of social isolation, as indicated by overresponsiveness of the pituitary adrenal system (see Figure 6.9),[78] may eventually contribute to the despair and depression that commonly follow social loss and long-term separation.[79] As Harry Harlow's well-known research demonstrated,[80] isolated rhesus monkey babies will seek out any comfort they can find, including inanimate "terry-cloth mothers," in preference to hard wire ones that provide only nourishment. When this type of social isolation was sustained for an excessive period, the animals exhibited lifelong problems in social adjustment.[81] Females that had been reared in isolation were poor and abusive mothers, especially in response to their firstborn infants. Subsequent offspring typically received better treatment, apparently because of the beneficial effects of previous learning. In general these motherless mothers were rather timid and emotionally overexcitable, exhibiting behavior patterns resembling a severe form of insecure attachment in human children.

No type of conventional "therapy" administered to such animals provided any substantive long-lasting assistance in restoring normal social functions. The most effective treatment was exposure to much younger monkeys, apparently because they provoked safe and playful social interactions that drew the isolates out of their self-centered misery.[82] In this context, it is noteworthy that dogs made excellent surrogate mothers for isolated monkeys, which fared much better than those that did not have a cross-species pet-mom. This highlights why pets can be so important in promoting mental health and emotional equilibrium in humans; it is much better to have a warm furry or feathered friend to interact with than no one at all.[83] Clearly, practically all mammals need important others in their lives to maintain emotional equilibrium.

It is well documented that the major life factor in humans that precipitates depression is social loss.[84] The genesis of many forms of depression can be linked to the neurobiological nature of the primal-loss experience—the despair of children who have been irreparably separated from their parents. Many believe that we will be able to understand the sources of depression when we understand the cascade of central neurological changes that arise from the successive emotions aroused by social separation—from active protest (crying) to the eventual despair response (depression).[85] Although animal models for evaluating such processes have been perfected, few neurochemical analyses of the associated brain changes have been conducted.[86]

It is generally thought that there may be some evolutionary use for young organisms to exhibit a depressive response to separation after the initial protest response. After a period of intense vocalization, which could help parents find their lost offspring, it might be energetically adaptive to regress into a behaviorally inhibited despair phase in order to conserve bodily resources. Such a depressive state would help conserve limited energy resources and discourage the helpless organism from wandering even farther from safety. Silence would, of course, also minimize detection by predators. In other words, if initial protest did not achieve reunion, a silent despair response might still optimize the likelihood that parents would eventually find their lost offspring alive. No doubt the separation call returns in a periodic manner during the circadian cycle, but this issue remains unanalyzed.

In any case, the cascade of events during the initial protest phase of separation appears to establish the brain conditions for the subsequent despair phase. This includes activation of the brain CRF system along with the pituitary adrenal stress response,[87] followed by a depletion of brain norepinephrine, serotonin, and certain dopamine reserves.[88] Indeed, depressive symptoms in animals and humans can be evoked experimentally by establishing these types of physiological changes in the body.[89] For instance, prolonged administration of CRF, along with depletion of the biogenic amines, can promote depressive responses.[90] We do not yet know precisely how this ultimately leads to the persistent psychological changes that characterize clinical depression, but medications that counteract these changes tend to have antidepressant effects. For instance, all antidepressants facilitate synaptic activity of biogenic amine systems,[91] whether it is by blockade of synaptic reuptake of the transmitters, as achieved by the tricyclic antidepressants and SSRIs, or by inhibition of degradation, as produced by MAO inhibitors.[92]

In the early days of psychopharmacology, even morphine was used as an antidepressant,[93] but this practice diminished with the advent of more effective medications. Presumably, future drugs that inhibit brain CRF and promote oxytocin activity should have new and useful profiles of antidepressant activity. Of course, environmental and cognitive therapies can also help, perhaps partly by providing the social support that depressed individuals need. In fact, perhaps the most effective nonphysiological maneuver for alleviation of depression is to provide increased social support. After young animals exhibit depressive responses to isolation, social contact is sometimes sufficient to cure them.[94]

In sum, even though early investigators did not believe in the existence of intrinsic social processes within the brain, it now seems likely that a great deal of higher brain organization evolved in the service of promoting social behaviors and sustaining feelings of social homeostasis.[95] Much more work along these lines needs to be conducted before the puzzle of the social brain is solved, but progress will have profound implications for the development of new treatments for various psychiatric disorders, including the most devastating ones, such as early childhood autism.

Additional Psychiatric Implications: Autism and Brain Socioemotional Systems

Early childhood autism is characterized by severe failures in socialization, communication, and imagination. As Leo Kanner said in his seminal 1943 paper, autistic children "have come into the world with an innate inability to form the usual, biologically provided affective contact with people."[96] A current theoretical perspective is that these children do not develop a "theory of mind," which refers to the ability of most children past the age of 2 to begin recognizing the types of thoughts and feelings that go on in the minds of others.[97] Obviously, the appreciation of these thoughts can become highly complex, and often delusional, in adults.

The existence of this syndrome affords investigators a unique opportunity to study the workings of social emotional systems in human beings. After a long period in which many claimed that the disorder arose from faulty parenting, virtually all investigators now agree that autism is a neurobiological disorder,[98] which probably reflects some type of dysfunction in normal neural development originating in the second trimester of pregnancy, when primitive brain stem and limbic circuits are laid down in the developing brain.[99] Exactly what goes wrong during the development of an autistic brain is not yet known precisely, but a large number of brain changes have been documented in these children.[100]

In addition to a variety of gross brain abnormalities, such as an undersized cerebellum and brain stem, and a larger than normal cerebrum, significant abnormalities have recently been described at the fine structural level. Autistic children have too many densely packed small neurons within parts of the limbic system,[101] suggesting that selective cell death, a natural process of the developing brain called *apoptosis*, has not progressed normally.[102] This also means that the neurons do not interconnect with the rest of the brain as well as in normal children, which all goes to suggest that a biochemical program for neuronal development has malfunctioned. It is presently impossible to correct such a wiring problem of the brain.

Without prenatal detection of autism, it will be impossible to correct such deficits even with new maneuvers such as the administration of appropriate neural growth factors (see Chapter 6). At the time most children are diagnosed, at around 2 years of age, neuronal development has progressed to an irreversible point. Still, many affected children do exhibit some functional improvements following the readjustment of brain chemical imbalances.[103] Since there are so many abnormalities in autism, related to deficits in communication, socialization, and imagination (known as the "autistic triad"), no single medication is likely to help all children. Indeed, no drug is yet medically approved for the treatment of autistic disorders, and much research work remains at a hit-or-miss level. However, some lines of work are emerging from a careful consideration of the many potential underlying causes.[104]

For instance, numerous similarities have been noted between the behavior of young animals with medial temporal lobe damage as well as those treated with opiates and the symptoms of children diagnosed with autism.[105] Both are characterized by pain insensitivity and deficits in communication, play, and curiosity. For instance, opiate-treated animals, like autistic children, do not exhibit a high desire for social companionship; rather, they exhibit a pervasive reduction in social responsivity, with the exception of rough-and-tumble play, which, as we will see in the next chapter, can be increased by low doses of opiates at least in rats. Indeed, the motivation for rough-and-tumble activity is practically the only social desire that autistic kids exhibit at a relatively high level, but not with the reciprocating give-and-take and fantasy structures of normal childhood play.

Young animals chronically treated with opiates also exhibit a pervasive stunting of development in all realms, from growth and bodily maturation to the onset of various behavioral abilities.[106] It is now generally agreed that opiates given during early development can regulate growth.[107] This raises the possibility that autistic children may have been exposed to excessive levels of endogenous opioids, or related molecules, during early development. Moreover, they may continue to experience excessive opioid activity within certain circuits of their brains as they mature. This could explain their pain insensitivity and consequent tendency to exhibit self-injurious behavior, as well as many other symptoms ranging from stereotypies to social aloofness.[108] Because of these considerations, it has been suggested that some benefits may be brought to these children by the administration of opiate receptor blocking agents such as naltrexone.[109]

Although tests of this hypothesis have yielded mixed clinical results, the lives of about half of all autistic children can be improved with the judicious use of this medication. Moderate doses of naltrexone can reduce some of the active symptoms of autism such as overactivity, stereotypies, and self-injurious behaviors, and in low infrequent doses, it can promote social activities. Many investigators have reported positive signs such as increased social initiative and interaction, heightened desires to communicate and cooperate with others, and increases in attention, curiosity, and social interchange, often accompanied by a better mood.[110] Most of these benefits reflect a general normalization of day-to-day living. Although naltrexone does not produce improvements in all children, nor can it be deemed anything close to a cure, the benefits are often substantial enough that parents choose to keep their children on the medication for the long term. Family life is generally less stressful and more cheerful. Although there is presently no way to predict which children will be helped, presumably it will be those who have high circulating levels of opioids in the brain, a condition that has been demonstrated in about half of all autistic children who have been tested.[111]

Although naltrexone is only a marginally beneficial medicine, it highlights a coherent theoretical strategy for developing new and better agents: Substances that increase social motivation in animal studies, as indicated by increased vocalizations and gregariousness, may be beneficial in these children. One could also focus on other symptoms, such as the highly irregular sleep patterns found in many autistic children, suggesting that natural sleep-promoting agents such as melatonin might be beneficial (see Chapter 7). Indeed, melatonin has recently proved to be an effective treatment for developmentally delayed children, with improvements seeming to extend to domains other than sleep.[112] However, this could be an indirect effect of the medication. Perhaps the stabilization of sleep rhythms allows the restorative effects of sleep to provide widespread benefits in many realms of brain functioning. Investigators are presently also looking into the potential roles of oxytocin and serotonin in the genesis of the disorder.

It should also be noted that there is a related genetic disorder, Williams syndrome, whose symptoms are just the opposite of those of autism.[113] Children with this syndrome tend to have a characteristically elfish facial appearance and a sweet social disposition. They are extremely friendly, socially outgoing, and can chatter on smoothly as if at a stimulating cocktail party, but there is comparatively modest propositional content in their speech. Nothing substantive is known about this syndrome at the neural level, but it almost appears to be the mirror image of autism. They love to socialize. We might surmise that children with Williams syndrome have highly responsive social interaction systems that are poorly connected to cognitive analyzers. Clearly, we will need to know more about the social circuits of the mammalian brain before we can understand these perplexing disorders. Indeed, the manifestations of these emotional systems in real life are remarkably diverse.

Conclusions and Future Prospects

Although many psychologists study and speak of the importance of attachment processes for human personality development, the critical information about these mechanisms has come from brain research on animal models. Once we understand the underlying brain processes in other animals, we may be able to intervene in such processes in humans. We may be able to help mothers who are having difficulty bonding to their children, perhaps because of postpartum depressions or psychoses, or simply for the lack of neural resilience within their bonding systems. It is possible that certain manipulations of brain opioid or oxytocin systems would facilitate bonding even among relative strangers, such as occurs during the social reconstruction that typically transpires in broken families following divorce.[114] Of course, these are far-fetched possibilities, and they may be unrealistic options within our current social milieu. As a society, we still have great difficulty in coming to terms with the neurochemical nature of the human mind. However, this type of transformation in thinking has already transpired in biological psychiatry.

The emotional distress that accompanies major psychiatric disorders is probably more closely linked to the changing dynamics of underlying emotional systems than to the cognitive systems in which we most commonly see the symptoms. However, the separation-distress system poses a new challenge for psychiatry. It seems evident that depression and panic attacks are most common in individuals who have had a history of separation anxiety, while autistic children appear to have a primary deficit in the ability to experience social emotions and to perceive the meaning of such emotional dynamics in others. This suggests that all these disorders are at least partly modulated by separation-distress mechanisms of the brain.

Although many investigators now accept that the primary deficits in these disorders must be sought in neurobiological imbalances rather than simply in social dynamics, the recognition of separation-distress systems in the creation of affective turmoil is not yet well recognized. An understanding of this emotional system takes us to the very heart of what it means to be a socially sensitive and deeply caring human being. Also, this type of knowledge may eventually help clarify the most noble human aspirations, namely, the desire to help others—in a word, what it means to be altruistic as opposed to selfish.[115]

AFTERTHOUGHT: Music and Chills

Might transient arousals of our ancient separation-distress response systems be felt during certain aesthetic experiences? I believe one of the most intriguing manifestations of separation distress in the human brain may reflect a powerful response many of us have to certain types of music. It is widely recognized that music is the language of emotions. It is one of the few ways that humans can allow the external world *voluntary* access to their emotional systems on a very regular basis. Most of us listen to music for the emotional richness it adds to our lives. We even love to hear sad songs—especially bittersweet songs of unrequited love and loss. A common physical experience that people report when listening to such moving music, especially melancholy songs of lost love and longing, as well as patriotic pride from music that commemorates lost warriors, is a shiver up and down the spine, which often spreads down the arms and legs, and, indeed, all over the body.[116] To the best of our knowledge, this response reflects a mixture of vasoconstriction, local skin contractions caused by piloerection, and perhaps changes in evaporative cooling at the skin surface. Such effects can be objectively measured as a galvanic skin response (GSR), which is a general yardstick of skin resistance. Of course, there is great variability in the incidence of this response. Some people rarely recognize such feelings in their lives, while others, probably the more social ones, delight in them frequently. For many years, I have sought to understand this intriguing phenomenon. Here I will summarize the insights I've obtained, as described in detail elsewhere.[117]

I will refer to this shivery-tingly experience by the term *chills*, although many, especially males, tend to use the term *thrills*. I prefer the label *chills* because females use it predominantly, and it is clear that females, as a population, exhibit this response more frequently than males. There are many exceptions, of course. I, for one, am so sensitized that I can have the experience on a regular basis just thinking about events. Females typically recognize that sad music is more likely to produce this chill phenomenon than happy pieces, while males more commonly suggest that happy music is the cause. However, when one actually conducts an experimental analysis, it is clear that sad music does in fact produce more chills than does happy music, even in males. Conversely, those pieces of music that produce more chills are typically rated as sad rather than happy by listeners. People tend to have many more chills to pieces they themselves have selected, which may reflect the rich networks of associations people have to music they have enjoyed often. What is the underlying meaning of this emotional phenomenon?

An intriguing possibility is that a major component of the poignant feelings that accompany sad music are sounds that may acoustically resemble separation DVs—the primal cry of being lost or in despair. In other words, a high-pitched, sustained crescendo capable of piercing the "soul" seems to be an ideal stimulus for evoking chills. A single instrument, like a cello or trumpet, emerging from a soft orchestral background is equally provocative. Thus, the chills we experience during music may represent the natural tendency of our brain emotional systems, especially those that are tuned to the perception of social loss, to react with an appropriate homeostatic thermal response. When we are lost, we feel cold—not only physically but also as a neurosymbolic response to social separation. As mentioned earlier, the roots of the social motivational system may be strongly linked to thermoregulatory systems of the brain (Figure 14.1). Thus, when we hear the sound of someone who is lost, especially if it is our child, we also feel cold. This may be nature's way of promoting reunion. In other words, the experience of separation establishes an internal feeling of thermoregulatory discomfort that can be alleviated by the warmth of reunion.

In music that provokes chills, the wistful sense of loss and the possibility of reunion are profoundly blended in the dynamics of sound. Thus, there may be no better stimulus for chills than a sustained note of grief sung by a soprano or played on a violin. This audiovocal experience speaks to us of our humanness and our profound relatedness to other people and the rest of nature. Since naloxone can reduce the incidence of chills, we can conclude that the chill response to music is partly controlled by endogenous opioids.[118] Avram Goldstein, the pharmacologist who originally discovered the opiate receptor and the powerful opioids ß-endorphin and dynorphin, interpreted this finding to reflect the fact that release of brain opioids may produce chills (or "thrills," as he referred to them). From the present perspective, it seems more likely that opioid blockade reduces chills because one no longer experiences the rapid decline in opioid activity that is produced during the perceptually induced affective experience of social loss, an experience that, in the human mind, is always combined with the possibility of redemption—being found and cared for when one is lost. The study of music will have profound consequences for understanding the psychology and neurobiology of human emotions.[119]

Suggested Readings

Bowlby, J. (1973). *Attachment and loss*. Vol. 2, *Separation: Anxiety and anger*. New York: Basic Books.

Hess, E. H. (1973). *Imprinting: Early experience and the developmental psychobiology of attachment*. New York: Van Nostrand.

Horn, G. (1985). *Memory, imprinting, and the brain*. Oxford: Clarendon Press.

Insel, T. R. (1992). Oxytocin—a neuropeptide for affiliation: Evidence from behavioral, receptor autoradiographic, and comparative studies. *Psychoneuroendocrinol*. 17:3–35.

Newman, J. D. (ed.) (1988). *The physiological control of mammalian vocalization*. New York: Plenum Press.

Olivier, B., Mos, J., & Slangen, J. L. (eds.) (1991). *Animal models in psychopharmacology*. Basel: Birkhäuser Verlag.

Panksepp, J. (1981). Brain opioids: A neurochemical substrate for narcotic and social dependence. In *Theory in psychopharmacology*, vol. 1 (S. J. Cooper, ed.), pp. 149–175. New York: Academic Press.

Panksepp, J., Newman, J., & Insel, T. R. (1992). Critical conceptual issues in the analysis of separation distress systems of the brain. In *International review of the studies of emotion*, vol. 2 (K. T. Strongman, ed.), pp. 51–72. Chichester, U.K.: Wiley.

Reite, M., & Fields, T. (eds.) (1985). *The psychobiology of attachment and separation*. New York: Academic Press.

Zahn-Waxler, C., Cummings, E. M., & Iannotti, R. (eds.) (1986). *Altruism and aggression: Biological and social origins*. New York: Cambridge Univ. Press.

15

Rough-and-Tumble Play

The Brain Sources of Joy

When children play, they exercise their senses, their intellect, their emotions, their imagination—keenly and energetically. . . . To play is to explore, to discover and to experiment. Playing helps children develop ideas and gain experience. It gives them a wealth of knowledge and information about the world in which they live—and about themselves. So to play is also to learn. Play is fun for children. But it's much more than that—it's good for them, and it's necessary. . . . Play gives children the opportunity to develop and use the many talents they were born with.

Instruction sheet in Lego® toys (1985)

CENTRAL THEME

When children are asked what they like to do more than anything else, the most common answer is "to play!" It brings them great joy. And roughhousing play is the most fun of all, even though most investigators recognize other types such as "object play" and "fantasy play." Although thousands of papers have been written on the topic, play is still considered a frivolous area of inquiry among most neuroscientists. Only recently have some become interested in the underlying brain issues. Now increasing numbers of investigators are beginning to realize that an understanding of play may reveal some major secrets of the brain and yield important insights into certain childhood psychiatric problems such as autism and attention deficit disorders (or hyperkinesis, as it used to be known). It is now certain that the brain does contain distinct neural systems devoted to the generation of roughhousing or rough-and-tumble (RAT) play. Indeed, one of the best species for systematic study of this behavior is the laboratory rat, and practically all the work summarized here is based on such play in rats. Although our knowledge about the underlying PLAY systems remains rudimentary, RAT play appears to be intimately linked to somatosensory information processing within the midbrain, thalamus, and cortex. Certain synaptic chemistries are especially effective in arousing play (e.g., acetylcholine, glutamate, and opioids), while others reduce playful impulses (e.g., serotonin, norepinephrine, and GABA), but neuropharmacological studies tell us little about the adaptive function(s) of play. There is an abundant theoretical literature regarding these functions, comparable to that found in dream research, but relevant data are decidedly scarce. The description from a leaflet in a box of Lego® toys says it all. Now it is necessary to judge the various possibilities with rigorously conducted experiments. Fortunately, roughhousing PLAY systems appear to be conserved in the brains of many mammalian species, and we should be able to obtain a credible answer to the functional questions, even for humans, by carefully analyzing animal models. We anticipate that play will be found to have many beneficial effects for both brain and body, including the facilitation of certain kinds of learning and various physical skills. Most important, play may allow young animals to be effectively assimilated into the structures of their society. This requires knowing who they can bully, and who can bully them. One must also identify individuals with whom one can develop cooperative relationships, and those whom one should avoid. Play probably allows animals to develop effective courting skills and parenting skills, as well as increasing their effectiveness in various aspects of aggression, including knowledge about how to accept defeat gracefully. It seems that most of the basic emotional systems may be recruited at one time or another during the course of play, and in higher organisms, play may encourage organisms to test the perimeters of their knowledge. In short, the brain's PLAY networks may help stitch individuals into the social fabric that is the staging ground for their lives. Is it any wonder, then, that play is such fun—perhaps one of the major brain sources of joy? It is sad that play research has not been of greater interest for neuroscientists, but perhaps that is because they are having great fun working on the minutest details of the most trifling problems (or so it may seem to outsiders). However, it is often there, among the fine details of nature, that scientists find startling things that can move heaven and earth. This is what Einstein did when he imagined what it would be like to ride a beam of light, and he remained mentally young and playful throughout his life. Perhaps the modern search for the mythological "fountain of youth" should focus as much on the neurobiological nature of mental youthfulness and play as on ways to extend longevity.

Conceptual Background for the Neural Sources of Ludic Urges

A great deal of joy arises from the arousal of play circuits within the brain. Although this is a reasonable assertion, it can only be a supposition until the identity of play circuits has been more completely revealed by brain research. That play is a primary emotional function of the mammalian brain was not recognized until recently, but now the existence of such brain systems is a certainty. For instance, juvenile rats will exhibit roughhousing or RAT ludic behaviors (from *ludare*, meaning "to play") even if they have been prevented from having any prior play experiences during earlier phases of development. Just as most young birds fly when the time is ripe, so do young mammals play when they have come of age. Young rats start to play around 17 days of age, and if denied social interaction throughout the early phases of psychosocial development (e.g., from 15 to 25 days of age), they play vigorously as soon as they are given their very first opportunity.[1]

Thus, the impulse for RAT play is created not from past experiences but from the spontaneous neural urges within the brain. Of course, a great deal of learning probably occurs during the course of roughhousing play, but this is ultimately the result of spontaneously active PLAY impulses within specific circuits of the brain, some of them in ancient parts of the thalamus, which coax young organisms to interact in ludic ways on the field of competition. It may well be that various neuronal growth factors are recruited during play (see Chapter 6), but evidence at such molecular levels of analysis remains nonexistent.

Although we presently have little detailed knowledge about the underlying brain mechanisms of play, rigorous psychobiological experiments are finally being conducted. We now have the empirical and conceptual tools to identify the primal circuits that lead animals to play. This work may eventually yield a neural understanding of what it means for humans to experience joy, or at least one of the most intense forms of joy. This work will also eventually reveal the true adaptive nature of play, but for the time being our ignorance remains vast, especially since it is hidden by an abundance of compelling theories propounded liberally by psychologists and others, without sufficient evidence.

Although play reflects genetically ingrained ludic impulses of the nervous system, it requires the right environment for full expression. For instance, fear and hunger can temporarily eliminate play.[2] In most mammals, play emerges initially within the warm and supportive secure base of the home environment, where parental involvement is abundant. Jane Goodall described the sequence of events as play first unfolds in chimpanzees: "A chimpanzee infant has his first experience of social play from his mother as, very gently, she tickles him with her fingers or with little nibbling, nuzzling movements of her jaws. Initially these bouts are brief, but by the time the infant is six months old and begins to respond to her with play face and laughing, the bouts become longer. Mother-offspring play is common throughout infancy, and some females frequently play with juveniles, adolescents, or even adult offspring."[3] The role of the mother in guiding the play and initial social interactions of young children is evident in humans, and such trends are evident even in rats.[4] In many species, fathers seem less playful and less socially tolerant than mothers, but humans *may* be an exception, perhaps partially because of cognitive mediation. In any event, it is now clear that the most vigorous play occurs in the context of preexisting social bonds. As discussed in the previous chapter, it is not unusual in nature for social bonds to be stronger between infants and their mothers than their fathers, who all too commonly exhibit little enthusiasm for nurturance.

Thus, contrary to conventional wisdom, it may be that females of most species remain more playful than males (at least in friendly, nonharmful ways) as they approach adulthood. As we will see, the prevailing notion that males intrinsically have stronger play tendencies[5] is certainly not justified for rats, and we should doubt it for other species until *well-controlled* studies have been conducted. The larger size and stronger competitive/aggressive urges of males may make their play rougher, so that social reinforcement of victory makes them appear more playful during the later stages of juvenile life. However, this difference may reflect the drive to attain dominance (which may, of course, become integrally associated with PLAY circuits), rather than elevated neural impulses for vigorous and joyful social interaction.

The stronger urge for social dominance in males (which is only one component of RAT play) may have incorrectly led to the widespread supposition that roughhousing play impulses are more intense in males than in females. For instance, in humans, the apparent heightened male enthusiasm for rough sports may be due as much to their biologically and socially based "power needs" as to any intrinsic differences in the arousability of their basic PLAY circuits. This is affirmed by the fact that the recent liberalization of sports policies in America has led to a stupendous growth in female participation in competitive sports. In any event, the extent to which human enjoyment of sports emerges from activities of primal PLAY circuits will be an important (but yet unresolved) question for us to consider.

Overview of the Experimental Analysis and Sources of Play

In most primates, prior social isolation has a devastating effect on the urge to play. After several days of isolation, young monkeys and chimps become despondent and are likely to exhibit relatively little play when reunited.[6] Apparently, their basic needs for social warmth, support, and affiliation must be fulfilled first; only when confidence has been restored does carefree playfulness return.[7] Laboratory rats, on the other hand, deviate markedly from this general pattern and thereby provide a useful model for the systematic analysis of play mechanisms within the brain. Laboratory rats show a greater emotional equanimity in coping with social isolation as compared to many other mammals (see Figure 2.1). Also, as emphasized in the previous chapter, the social-bonding mechanisms in laboratory rodents are comparatively weak. Perhaps for this reason, isolation housing does not readily produce obvious depressive responses in laboratory rats and mice.[8] Thus we can take advantage of social-deprivation variables to control levels of playfulness. Prior social isolation systematically increases roughhousing play in juvenile rats, while social satiation systematically reduces it (Figure 15.1).[9]

The facilitation of play in rats by prior isolation is due not simply to social deprivation itself but to the specific effects of play deprivation. If one houses animals together in the tight confinement of a "jungle gym" type of living environment where they cannot readily roughhouse, they show abundant play in an open play arena. Likewise, if one houses juvenile rats with adult animals that are not very playful, they will play with other juveniles as intensely as if they had just emerged from total isolation.[10] In any event, with the use of prior social deprivation, RAT play can be analyzed efficiently in the laboratory. The systematic nature of the results again affirms that the urge to play is an intrinsic function of the mammalian nervous system.[11]

Although there is substantial diversity in the specific play patterns exhibited by different mammalian species, the evolutionary roots probably go back to an ancient PLAY circuitry shared by all mammals in essentially homologous fashion. It is also possible that creatures other than mammals (especially birds) exhibit social play, but avian play is less predictable and hence harder to study.[12] Accordingly, the present discussion will be restricted to mammals, although the evolutionary roots may well go back to an era predating the divergence of mammalian and avian lines more than a hundred million years ago (see Appendix A). Once we understand the

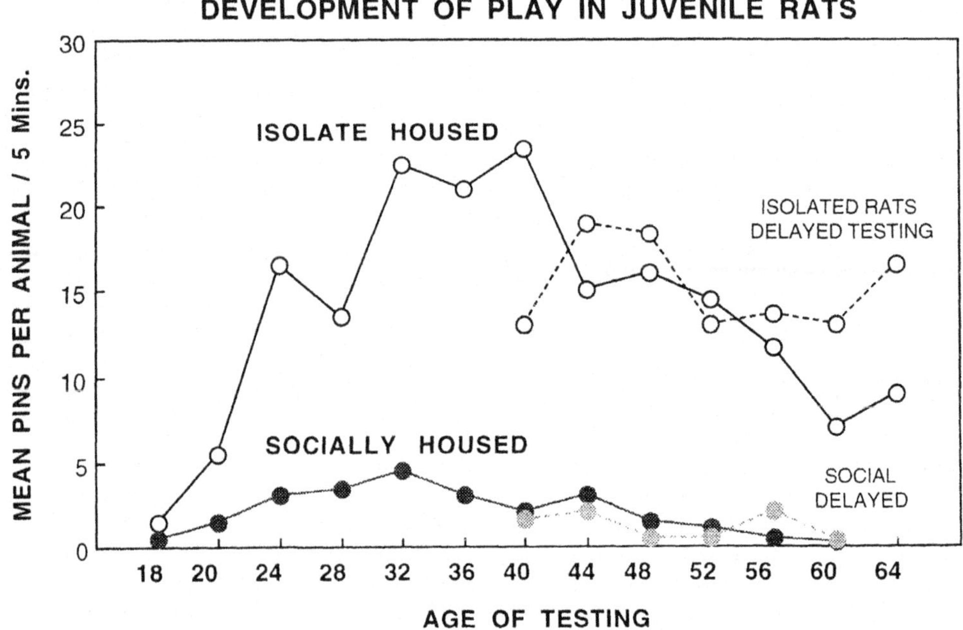

Figure 15.1. Ontogeny of play in socially isolated and socially housed laboratory rats. (Adapted from Panksepp, 1981; see n. 18). The pinning measure is depicted in Figure 15.2.

neural circuitry of mammalian play, it should be easier to determine whether birds have homologous brain mechanisms, or whether their seemingly playful behaviors emerge from different types of neural systems.

Before discussing the most basic form of play—namely, roughhousing play—it should again be emphasized that several distinct forms are widely recognized in human research. Human play has been divided by social and developmental psychologists into exploratory/sensorimotor play, relational/functional play, constructive play, dramatic/symbolic play, and games-with-rules play, as well as RAT play, of course.[13] This last form, rough-and-tumble play, is presently easiest to study in animal models, but except for a few outstanding pieces of work, it has received the least attention in human research.[14] This is understandable, for roughhousing is boisterous and often viewed as disruptive and potentially dangerous by adults. Of course, kids love it (it brings them joy), and animals readily learn instrumental responses to indulge in it.[15] This is the main form of play that other mammals exhibit, and it remains possible that the relatively solitary motor play of many herbivorous animals, such as running, jumping, prancing, and rolling, emerges from the same basic PLAY urges that control roughhousing play between young animals. Unfortunately, there is no neurological evidence yet that allows definitive conclusions.

Although human play has been extensively taxonomized, it is still worth contemplating to what extent the various forms are merely higher elaborations (culturally derived, as well as higher neuroevolutionary variants) on a single primal theme: Are there multiple executive circuits for play in the human brain, or do they all reflect manifestations of a single underlying PLAY system of the mammalian brain? Until demonstrated otherwise, we should be parsimonious and subscribe to the single command-circuit alternative.

Just as each basic mammalian emotion can be expressed in many ways in human cultures—including dance, drama, music, and other arts—arousal of a single basic ludic circuit could add "fun" to the diversity of playful activities. In other words, PLAY impulses that are processed through the higher cognitive networks of the human cortex (i.e., via social constructions) may result in many seemingly distinct forms of human play. The common denominator for all, however, may arise from basic neuronal systems that were originally designed to generate RAT ludicity. Indeed, it is a testable proposition: Once we unravel the details of RAT PLAY circuits, their role in other forms of play can be evaluated. Accordingly, let us briefly entertain ways in which play diversity in humans may emerge from the "simplicity" of a single system.

Perhaps, in humans, the source energy for roughhousing play can be channeled voluntarily into a large variety of distinct activities. At times humans simulate playfulness and thereby attempt to evoke ludic feelings indirectly through pretenses. For instance, children like to stage various skits and shows, but as they attempt to perform seriously, all too often they simply end up giggling in glee. Perhaps the culturally sanctioned playful expressions, such as dancing, remain emotionally hollow until the ancient circuits of playfulness—affectively characterized by "lightness," "joy," and "flow"—are recruited?

Through their attempts to voluntarily activate the natural ludic mechanisms of the brain, humans may achieve totally new forms of playfulness (including various games, toys, and dramatic and linguistic devices). In this context, it should be remembered that each basic emotional system can energize a number of distinct behavioral options, and perhaps PLAY systems help generate a diversity of emotional behaviors upon which learning can operate. It must also be noted that playfulness in humans can eventually be expressed in symbolic ways, which may be largely linguistic, such as puns, joking, and verbal jibes, that lead to a great deal of mirth and laughter.

A discussion of the functions of play will be reserved for a later section, but here I will anticipate the main conclusion. PLAY circuitry allows other emotional operating systems, especially social ones, to be exercised in the relative safety of one's home environment. Play may help animals project their behavioral potentials joyously to the very perimeter of their knowledge and social realities, to a point where true emotional states begin to intervene. Thus, in the midst of play, an animal may gradually reach a point where true anger, fear, separation distress, or sexuality is aroused. When the animal encounters one of these emotional states, the playful mood may subside, as the organism begins to process its predicaments and options in more realistic and unidimensional emotional terms. In human children this may often consist of running to mother in tears, with complaints about the injustices they have encountered to see what type of social support and understanding (i.e., kin investment) they might be able to muster.

Finally, as will be discussed more fully later in this chapter, play and exploratory systems (i.e., of the type discussed in Chapter 8) appear to be distinct in the brain. Although these concepts are often combined in human research,[16] as if they reflected synergistic processes, they appear to be independent and at times mutually exclusive. For instance, psychostimulants such as amphetamines, which invigorate exploratory activities, markedly reduce play behaviors.[17] Indeed, when placed in new environments, animals typically exhibit strong exploratory activity with little tendency to play until they have familiarized themselves with the new surroundings.

In sum, we now have highly effective laboratory procedures to analyze the neural substrates of RAT play. A straightforward experimental approach will surely yield more important insights into the nature of this phenomenon than any armchair theorizing of the type highlighted in the description of children's play at the beginning of this chapter.

A Description of Rough-and-Tumble Play

It is difficult to capture the dynamic image of real-life play in words. But the overall impression given by practically all mammals is a flurry of dynamic, carefree rambunctiousness. In rats, one sees rapid spurts of activity, toward and away from a play partner. Sometimes one animal "bowls" the other animal over, which leads to a flurry of playful chasing. In turns, the animals pursue each other, with rapid pivoting and role reversals. Animals often pounce on each other's backs as if they are soliciting vigorous interaction; these "dorsal contacts" can be easily quantified and have been commonly used as an explicit measure of play solicitations (Figure 15.2). Sometimes the dorsal contacts do not yield reciprocation, instead ending up as prolonged bouts of dorsal grooming. At other times, the recipient of play solicitations responds by either running away or twisting laterally; an apparent bout of wrestling ensues, in which one animal winds up on its back with the other animal on top. This "pinning" posture can also be easily quantified (Figure 15.2) and is the clearest measure of the consummatory aspects of play. If animals are allowed to play on an activity platform, one can also obtain an overall measure of RAT activity. There are surely many other ways to monitor play, and each of these measures can be subcategorized. For instance, most pins are of short duration, occurring in the midst of ongoing "wrestling" matches, while others are more prolonged, often signaling the end of a play bout. Dorsal contacts can be strong or sustained, or made passingly as one animal bounds leapfrog-style off another. The precise details of play episodes vary widely among different mammalian species, but the general flavor remains the same—one of joyful social exchange with a strong competitive edge. It may come as a surprise to some, but young rats given no other ludic outlets love to be tickled by and play with a frisky human hand.

RAT play in most species exhibits a characteristic developmental time course, with the amount of play increasing during the early juvenile period, remaining stable through youth, and diminishing as animals go through puberty (see Figure 2.1).[18] We presently know essentially nothing about the neurobiological factors that control this inverted U-shaped developmental function. Presumably it is related to aspects of brain maturation, as well as neurochemical shifts that occur during development.[19]

Play dominance clearly emerges if two rats are allowed to play together repeatedly.[20] After several play episodes, one rat typically tends to become the "winner," in that it ends up on top more often during pins. On the average, the split is that the winner ends up on top about 70% of the time, while the "loser" achieves less success, but the continuation of play appears to require reciprocity and the stronger partner's willingness to handicap itself. If one animal becomes a "bully" and aspires to end up on top all the time, playful activity gradually diminishes and the less successful animal begins to ignore the winner. There are reasons to believe that similar dynamics are present in human verbal play, which is a common way for folks to get to know each other and to best each other.

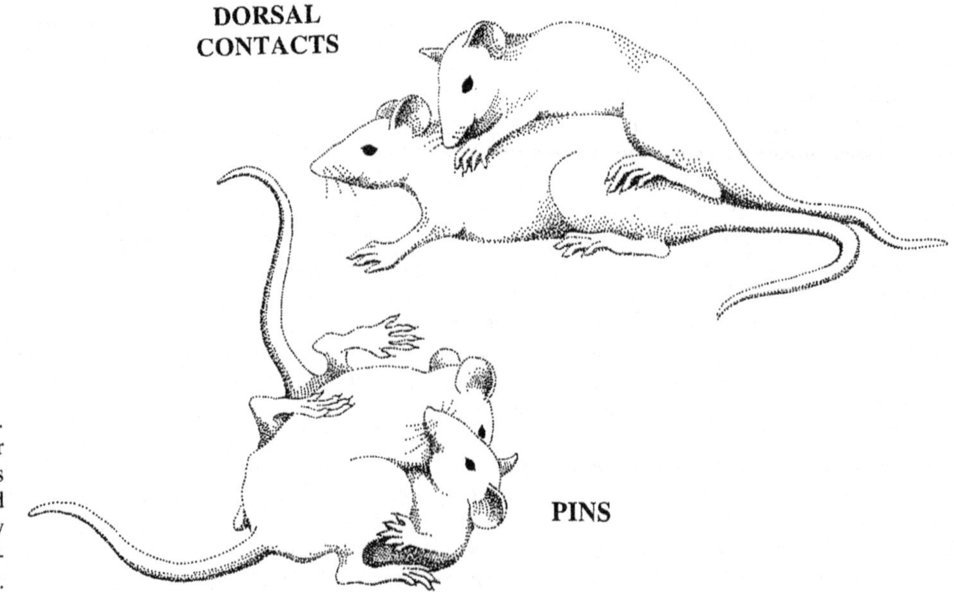

Figure 15.2. Two major play postures that are used to quantify rough-and-tumble play.

As might be expected, body weight is an important factor in dictating which animal of a pair becomes the winner, as is neurochemical activity.[21] With regard to weight, approximately a 10% weight advantage, just like in human boxing and wrestling, is sufficient to give a statistical edge to the heavier combatant (we are here ignoring the more complex issue of physical strength, not to mention psychological "strength," which as we will see is partly opioid-mediated). Neurochemically, if one animal of a play pair is given a small dose of an opiate agonist such as morphine and the other is given a small dose of an opiate antagonist such as naloxone, all other things being equal, the animal receiving morphine always becomes the winner (Figure 15.3). A similar effect is seen in vehicle-treated rats pitted against naloxone-treated ones, but a morphine-treated animal does not invariably win against controls.[22] These effects suggest that brain opioids control social emotionality, so that without brain opioids an animal tends to feel psychologically weaker, causing it to lose because it is more prone to experience negative feelings such as separation distress, as discussed in the previous chapter. To the contrary, control animals as well as morphine-treated ones may prevail because they experience heightened social confidence, a feeling of psychological strength that presumably emerges from the neurochemical correlates of social bonding.

Of course, there are alternative explanations for these effects, as there are for all the findings of science (see Figure 2.3). For instance, opiate receptor antagonists may reduce or eliminate the opioid-mediated reinforcing pleasure of social interaction, while opiate agonists enhance such forms of reinforcement. Also, it is possible that the opiate antagonists make some playful blows more painful, while morphine dulls those play-reducing sensations. Surely, if the scrapes of life become less painful, animals should play more. In any event, the play-dominance effects of opioid manipulations are remarkably clear-cut in animals that begin receiving these agents at the outset of their mutual play experiences (Figure 15.3). The fact that it takes some time for the full manifestation of the effects suggests that social learning promotes the emergence of the dominance asymmetry. However, if social dominance has already transpired prior to the neurochemical manipulations, play-dominance patterns do not shift readily. Indeed, past social learning is a powerful force in all social encounters. On the basis of this simple fact, one must again wonder whether some of the effects that have been widely disseminated in the literature, such as the oft-reported sex differences in play whereby males supposedly exhibit more RAT play than females, merely reflect assertiveness biases that have emerged from prior social learning based on body weight and strength asymmetries between the sexes. Persuasive data are presently not available on this issue.

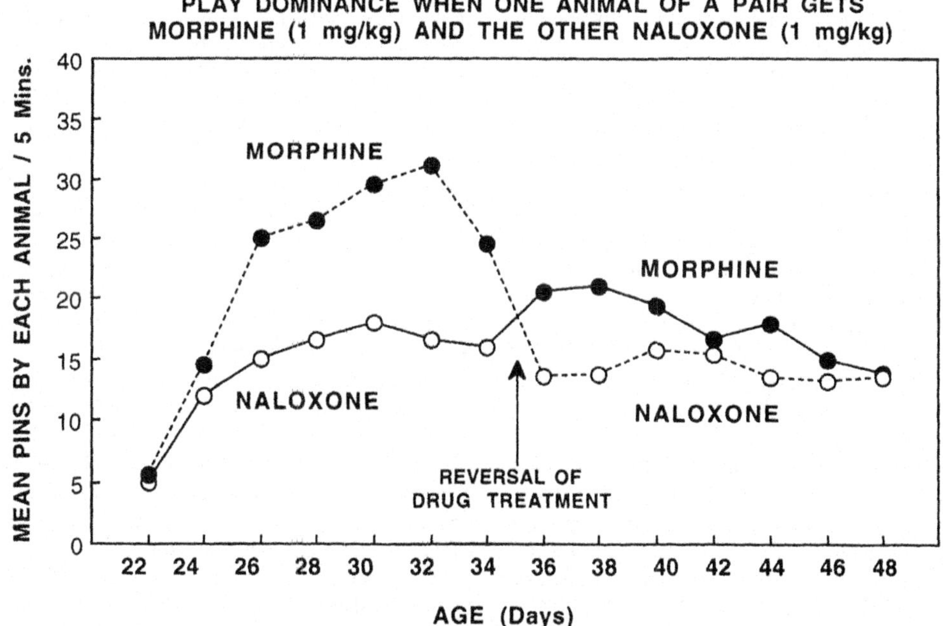

Figure 15.3. Pinning on successive days, with one animal getting naloxone (1 mg/kg) and the other getting morphine at the same dose. After seven days, drug conditions were reversed. (Adapted from Panksepp et al., 1985; see n. 22.)

Play and Aggression

RAT play in animals is often called *play-fighting*, and some believe it is little more than the juvenile expression of certain types of aggressive activity—for instance, intermale aggression. Although RAT play often has the outward behavioral hallmarks of aggressive fighting, a formal behavioral analysis indicates that the behavioral sequences exhibited during real fighting and play are remarkably different.[23] Resemblances between the two are only superficial. For instance, serious aggressive postures are rarely seen in play-fighting. In a real fight, rats often exhibit boxing, consisting of standing on their hind paws and paddling each other with their front paws, as well as laterally directed aggressive postures called "side-prancing," commonly accompanied by piloerection. These postures essentially never occur during social play. Sometimes play does end up in real fighting, but then the signs of behavioral rambunctiousness (frantic hopping, darting, and pouncing) immediately cease.[24] A behavioral tension emerges as RAGE and FEAR systems are presumably activated.

Moreover, true aggression and play follow different rules and are differentially sensitive to a variety of experimental manipulations: (1) In real intermale dominance fights, all other things being equal, the resident animal is invariably the winner if the behavioral test is conducted in the home territory of one of the animals. This is not the case during play-fighting.[25] (2) During play there are no *sustained* defensive postures in which one animal lies on its back while the other sustains a menacing top position for extended periods (i.e., thus, pins during play move along more gracefully and rapidly). (3) Play-fighting is a positive reward for both participants. The winners and the losers of previous play fights readily learn instrumental tasks, such as making an appropriate choice in a T-maze, in order to gain the opportunity to play together again, and they both run toward the opportunity to play with equal speed. The only difference is that the winners barge quickly into the play box, while the so-called losers are a bit more hesitant in making their entry into the play arena.[26] (4) Testosterone, which is quite powerful in promoting aggressive dominance, has relatively little effect except that in some pairs it reduces play-fighting.[27] In animals that exhibit reductions in play following several days of testosterone treatment, it seems that the play bouts quickly become too aggressive. When this occurs, the behavior loses its "carefree" quality, and overall playfulness becomes inhibited. (5) Highly specific antiaggressive drugs such as fluprazine and eltoprazine, which can markedly reduce various forms of fighting (see Chapter 10), do not clearly reduce play and in some instances appear to increase playful interactions.[28]

Although there are bound to be continuities between the skills learned during play-fighting and eventual adult dominance abilities, there is presently no clear evidence for powerful continuities in the executive brain mechanisms of roughhousing play and adult forms of aggression. The two seem to have distinct motivational substrates, although it remains possible that the play circuits of juvenile stages of development may take on a more adultlike luster as animals mature. Similarly, in humans, we see childhood play fading into ritualized dominance sports such as football or basketball.

It is unlikely that professional football or other sports require the participation of PLAY circuits in adult humans, but the quality of performance is probably increased when such circuits are aroused. On the other hand, it is possible that few spectators would consider professional sports to be fun were it not for the existence of PLAY circuits in their brains that are vicariously aroused by observation of play activities in others. Professional wrestling may be especially attractive to certain audiences because its choreography closely resembles the instinctual expressions of RAT play in humans.

Another dimension of sports that deserves attention is the possibility that it is an institutionalized way to dissipate intermale aggressive energies that might otherwise cause chaos in peaceful societies. Keeping "warrior energies" constrained within the guise of playfulness may help reduce the level of violence in peacetime. Indeed institutionalized forms of play, such as professional sports, have become big business around the world. This development casts a new and sometimes dark shadow over the spontaneous expressions of emotionality that should characterize the playing field.

Although there is still a great deal of joy and despair among those participating in professional sports, with spectators being overcome by waves of positive and negative emotions as the fortunes of their teams wax and wane, the new economic dimensions of professional sports have made us realize that in humans, games are simply no longer what evolution meant them to be. Instead of exercising various skills and having a good time, institutionalized play has become the arena for demonstrating one's acquired and aggressive skills. Although I do not dwell on such issues in this book, it is obvious that cultural forces in human societies have the ability to change emotional forces into new entities, both beautiful and horrific.

In sum, it seems evident that PLAY circuits are largely independent of aggression circuits, even though during development they may eventually contribute to the intermale types of aggression that were highlighted in Chapter 10. It is certainly possible that PLAY systems contribute to social dominance urges, which may help explain our love of rough professional sports, where such issues are paramount in the minds of players and spectators alike. Also, since sports provide the opportunity for expressions of symbolic dominance, it is little wonder that they are accorded such high esteem in our society, even by administrators of so many universities.

The Varieties of Play and Laughter, Especially in Humans

Humans are a uniquely playful species. This may be due in part to the fact that we are neotenous creatures who benefit from a much longer childhood than other species. For instance, our childhood and adolescence constitute about 20% of our life span, which is comparable to other great apes. However, the corresponding proportion for other primates is generally less than 10%; in dogs, cats, and rats, it typically approaches 5%. Another feature that adds to the complexity of our playfulness is the simple fact that our play instincts are modified so markedly by our cognitively focused higher brain areas. Although cortical processes surely add a great deal of diversity to our playful behaviors, especially as we develop, it is unlikely that the primal brain "energy" for playfulness emerges from those higher brain functions. These energies probably emerge from the same ancient executive systems that govern RAT play in other species. As those primitive playful impulses percolate through the brain, they assume new forms ranging from slapstick humor to cognitive mirth. Indeed, the hallmark of PLAY circuitry in action for humans is laughter, a projectile respiratory movement with no apparent function, except perhaps to signal to others one's social mood and sense of carefree camaraderie.[29] Some believe laughter is uniquely human, but we would doubt this proposition.

Ethologists have long distinguished two general types of happy or friendly faces: the social smile and laughter. The smile, with its prominent baring of teeth, probably harks back to ancient mammalian threat displays.[30] For instance, many creatures exhibit bare-toothed hissing in response to potential threats. In a social context, this may communicate that one possesses quite a dangerous set of teeth and is potentially willing to use them. No doubt, the probable evolutionary adaptation behind the display is that the potentially tense situation will require no further action if one smiles. The human smile may have evolved from such preexisting old parts to communicate that one is basically friendly but quite capable of dealing with any difficulties that may arise. Laughter, on the other hand, seems to have emerged largely from a different brain system; as some have cogently argued, it may emerge from PLAY motivation.

In children, laughter occurs most commonly in playful situations. Indeed, an openmouthed display characterizes the most intense forms of human laughter, and similar gestures are used as signals for play readiness in other species such as chimpanzees and dogs. Also, the rhythm of laughter has an outward resemblance to the rhythmic kicking and thrashing commonly seen in the roughhousing play of many mammals. Although we commonly associate the presence of laughter with the punch line of a joke, making it functionally similar to the pin position that is the terminal component of a RAT play episode, laughter certainly does not require much cognitive complexity. Physical tickling is one of the easiest ways to provoke laugher in young children; indeed, this response can be induced in infants within the first half year of life, even though it appears to be preceded by a period in which there is a strong tendency to smile in response to social interaction, starting at about 4 months of age.[31] A cyclical pattern, resembling laughter, with respiratory panting and grunting vocalizations can also be induced in chimpanzees and gorillas by tickling, and we have recently discovered a seemingly homologous process in young rats.

To evaluate whether rats laugh, we took a simple tickling approach. Listening in to the ultrasonic frequency range at which rats communicate, we rapidly found that friendly tickling induced very high-frequency chirping at about 50 KHz. This response could be provoked more effectively when the tickling occurred at the nape of the neck, where animals normally solicit play, than on the rump, and full body tickling was most effective of all (Figure 15.4). Animals that had been deprived of social contact from weaning at 24 days of age through puberty exhibited more chirping to tickling than littermates that had been allowed two play sessions each day through this interval. Also, the amount of playfulness in these animals correlated highly with the amount of tickling-induced "laughter," but while play declined with age, tickling effects did not (Figure 15.4). Tickling was a positive incentive for our animals: They would seek out this kind of stimulation and would rapidly begin to chirp to cues associated with tickling. If this vocalization pattern is truly homologous to basic human laughter, we may come to understand human joy by studying the circuits that generate such vocalization in rats.[32]

Apparently, laughter is not learned by imitation, since blind and deaf children laugh readily.[33] The ability to laugh precedes one's ability to comprehend the point of a joke; a great deal of children's laughter typically occurs in free play situations rather than in response to verbal jests. It is reasonable to suppose that the sources of human laughter go back to ancient social engagement systems that first mediated mammalian playfulness.

Laughter may now be one signal for victory within playful social encounters as the philosopher Thomas Hobbes argues,[34] just as being in the top position during pinning in RAT play is the preferred physical position (Figures 15.2 and 15.3). Indeed, this is the dark side of laughter, for it often occurs in response to seeing others hurt, humiliated, or embarrassed, and it indicates a recognition of the victim's slapstick predicament coupled with the feeling that one has been psychologically luckier and perhaps even smarter than the poor sod who is the brunt of some misfortune. In competitive playful encounters in humans, laughter is invariably exhibited more by victors than by losers. Likewise, the perpetrator of a practical joke is much more likely to

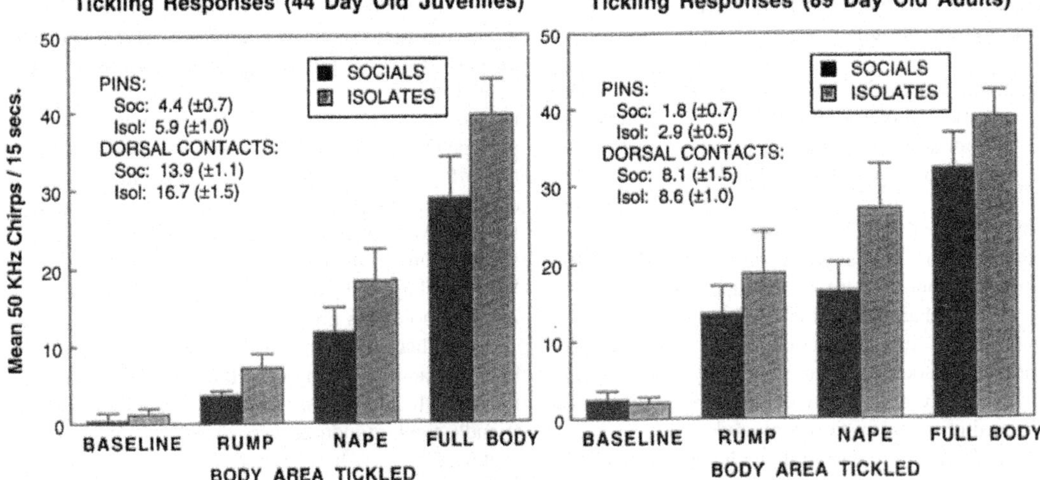

Figure 15.4. Mean (±SEM) levels of chirping in 44- and 89-day-old rats as a function of social history and the area of the body tickled. The animals had been weaned and individually housed at 24 days of age, and half the animals (socials) had received two 0.5-hour play sessions each day through puberty (50 days of age), while the others (isolates) had no opportunities for social interaction. Testing occurred in both groups following 48 hours without social interaction. Pinning and dorsal contacts during a 2-minute play session on an adjacent day are also provided. (Unpublished data, Panksepp & Burgdorf, 1997.)

laugh than the recipient. Groups of humans also often laugh together (it is infectious); this may help cement group solidarity, which is another popular view of the function of laughter.

Neurologically, laughter emerges from primitive subcortical areas of the brain as indicated by the types of brain damage that are correlated with pathological laughter. One disease process that can release impulsive laughter is amylotrophic lateral sclerosis (ALS), a demyelinating disease that affects the brain stem. Another is gelastic epilepsy, which is accompanied by bouts of laughter. Individuals with such a brain disorder can exhibit strong motor components of mirth without any accompanying experience of happiness. Although the victims of such disease processes look happy when they are spontaneously smiling and laughing, they often report no associated positive affect.[35] Most interestingly, such individuals typically exhibit pathological crying during earlier phases of the disease, again without any accompanying feeling of sadness. Not only does the onset of pathological crying typically precede the onset of laughter during the development of ALS, but the crying seems to emerge from lower levels of the neuroaxis than does the laughter.[36]

The apparent neural relationship between these two motor displays suggests that laughter and crying are intimately related in the brain, although the ability to cry appears to have preceded the ability to laugh in brain evolution. In other words, separation-distress mechanisms, and social-bonding ones, may have been essential prerequisites for the evolution of laughter. From this, one might suppose that the evolution of the social bond, and the consequent ability to cry, may also have been social prerequisites for the evolution of play. If so, we might suppose that both play and laughter still serve social-bonding functions, thereby helping to discriminate friends and family from strangers. Indeed, reunion "rituals" in chimpanzees, especially after long separations, are typically characterized by a lot of hooting, howling, and touching.[37] Also, in this context, it should be recalled that the preeminent sensory system, which both provides comfort after separation and most readily provokes play, is touch. Thus, in evolution, the pleasure of touch may have established a neural framework for the emergence of play.

Of course, in humans, play impulses can be manifested in many ways. As individuals mature, a great deal of human play may come to be focused on verbal interchange. The persistent verbal repartee that often characterizes nonserious interactions, such as teasing (e.g., when humans "rib" each other), seems to have the outward characteristics of dorsal contacts and pinning. One tries to arouse the other individual with some provocation, at times even sharp and biting comments; then, if others respond, there is often a desire to "sock it to them" with an especially clever response. If successful, this tends to yield peals of laughter among the young and chuckles among the elderly. This type of repartee may be repeated many times, with each individual trying to best the other—to be cleverest—until it is clear that one is prevailing or until each is satisfied that he or she is a match for the other. Presumably, when that happens, the individuals have a high potential to establish a special respect and friendship. If one verbally "pins" the other too insistently, the relationship will probably be different, with a much greater sense of dominance and submission asymmetries, which may decisively guide future interactions. Perhaps this is one reason most humans are better talkers than listeners—humans are more likely to feel that they have prevailed if they sustain a high level of output instead of "wasting" time attending to inputs.

Such bonding and social-stratification functions of play and laughter are also especially evident in institutionalized sports. Perhaps for similar reasons, our culture has formalized "roasting" as a special occasion for individuals to exhibit their well-honed playfulness and dominance skills toward people they like. Apparently, the manifestations of PLAY circuitry have permeated human cultures and, perhaps, a great deal of higher brain organization.

Obviously, it would be presumptuous to reduce human playfulness to the operation of a single primitive system that controls RAT play in other animals. Too many layers of neural complexity have been added to the original PLAY instigation systems. In a hierarchically controlled structure like the brain (see Figure 2.2), each level of control has some consequences for the form of the final output. To use an analogy from physics, evidence about the basic emotional systems resembles our general knowledge of atomic structure, which constrains but does not readily allow us to predict the complexity of molecules and man-made materials that can be constructed from those basic structures. However, as we accept the complex reality of playfulness and other emotions in humans and their societies, an adequate analysis of the lower levels that we share with animals is essential for a satisfactory understanding of the complex manifestations that the higher levels permit. Thus, I will assume that the neural mechanisms of RAT play will ultimately prove illuminating for understanding play and joy in humans. It may also help us better understand certain childhood problems such as autism and attention deficit, hyperactivity disorders (ADHDs).[38] In any event, it is remarkable that the existence of this brain system has not yet been generally accepted in either neuroscience or psychology.

The Somatosensory Control of Play

Since RAT play ultimately emerges from powerful endogenous neural activities of the brain that interact with many forms of learning, it is especially difficult to study comprehensively. The motor features of RAT play are so complex that it is hard to imagine how one might trace the source mechanisms in a systematic manner. One approach is to consider that play is a socially contagious process. When playful urges arise in one animal, they seem to "infect" other animals via some type of sensory-perceptual influence. Accordingly, a reasonable question to ask would be: Which sensory systems are most important for social play? Studies that have selectively eliminated individual sensory influences clearly indicate that, at least in rats, neither vision nor olfactory senses (including vibrissae) are necessary for the generation of normal play. One can eliminate any one of these senses without reducing the overall *amount* of RAT play, even though the exact patterning of play has not yet been carefully analyzed in such animals. The auditory system contributes positively to play to some extent, since deafened animals play slightly less, and rats do emit many 50-KHz laughter-type chirps both during play and in anticipation of play.[39] However, the premier sensory system that helps instigate and sustain normal play is touch.

Indeed, certain parts of the body surface are more sensitive to play-instigation signals than others. This has been established by anesthetizing various zones of the body (Figure 15.5). Local anesthetization of the neck and shoulder area is highly effective in reducing the level of playful pinning in young rats, even though the motivation for play, as measured by dorsal contacts, is not reduced.[40] A substantially smaller effect on pinning is obtained if the anesthetic is applied to the rump, and no effect is evident if it is applied to either rostral or caudal areas of the animal's ventral surface, or when it is injected systemically. These findings correspond nicely to the tickling results summarized in Figure 15.4. This suggests that rats have specialized skin zones that send play signals into the nervous system when they are touched. In other words, mammals appear to have "play skin," or "tickle skin," with specialized receptors sending information to specific parts of the brain that communicate playful intentions between animals. Obviously, humans also have tickle skin. It is situated at the back of the neck and around the rib cage, where it is easiest to tickle young children and get them into a playful mood.

In rats the homologous play skin of the body seems to be on the rostral dorsal surface of the body, where most play solicitations (i.e., dorsal contacts) are directed. This is not the only target of play solicitation in rats, but PLAY circuitry of the brain does appear to receive especially potent somatosensory inputs from certain body zones. This helps answer the question that has perplexed so many children: Why can't I tickle myself? Apparently, the system is tuned to the perception of social stimulation partially by being sensitive to unpredictability. The underlying neural systems are designed so that one cannot easily be his or her own social partner or play companion. Tickling requires other selves to arouse playfulness. Thus, the ability to identify and perceive play partners is not a mere sensory phenomenon but a powerful, ingrained central

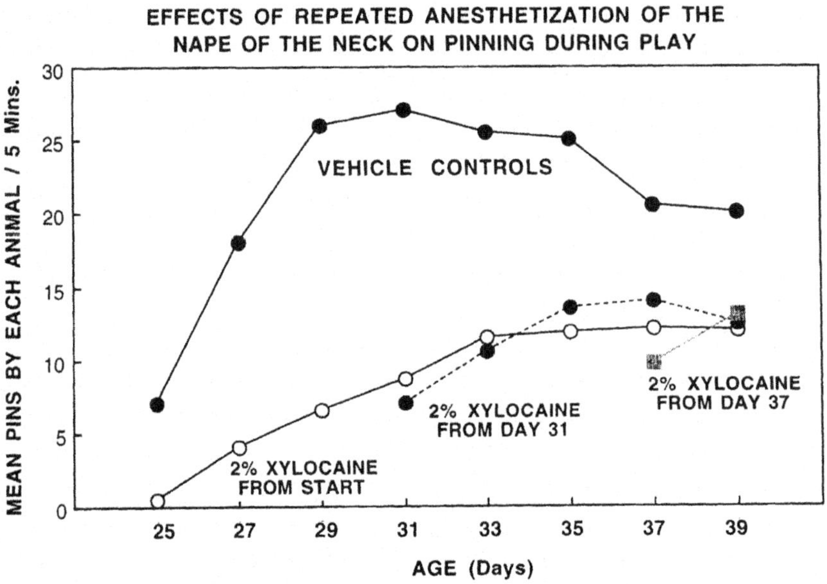

Figure 15.5. Play as a function of age in animals treated at the nape of the neck with xylocaine after 25, 31, and 37 days of life. The reduction of play exhibited no clear tolerance, suggesting that without appropriate somatosensory input, the consummatory aspects of play are seriously compromised. (Adapted from Siviy & Panksepp, 1987; see n. 40.)

nervous system concept (one that may have gone awry in autism).

Apparently, the broadly ramifying PLAY system of the brain can instigate rapid forms of learning. For instance, with some experience and the right ludic attitude, one can "tickle" a young child simply by wiggling a finger in midair or by intoning a "coochi-coochi-coo." Young rats also exhibit rapid conditioning to the cues associated with tickling. Presumably, this is because such rapidly learned play signals can generate the internal interpretation that one has a playful companion. Indeed, if a child is already in a playful mood, it is sometimes sufficient for them to simply look at another person to trigger laughter and playfulness. Indeed, children get into patterns of uncontrollable laughter rather easily, especially when sharing special mental games during culturally pretentious events—formal dinner tables and classrooms, where the abiding adult expectation is that ludic impulses should be controlled. In such circumstances, children's mutual "knowing" glances can generate great hilarity, often in an inverse relation to the level of self control that adults are expecting from them. This tendency indicates that, in humans, the visual system rapidly learns the patterns of behavior that are especially playful. Whether the visual system can generate playfulness without any prior participation of touch during earlier phases of development is unknown. At least in rats, vision is not essential; blind animals play with undiminished vigor.[41]

In sum, the existence of PLAY circuits in the brain probably explains the phenomenon of tickling and highlights the fact that the analysis of somatosensory stimulation of play skin may be a key to understanding the neural processes of PLAY systems. Parenthetically, it should be noted that the apparent expansion of play skin on the body surface when one is in a playful mood highlights a key property of an emotional system—namely, its ability to modify sensory and perceptual sensitivities that are relevant for the emotional behavior being exhibited.

It should be emphasized that anesthetization of the body surface (Figure 15.4) only reduces the animal's ability to perceive proximal play signals, which leads just to a reduction in pinning. It does not reduce the apparent desire to play, since the reduced pinning is not accompanied by a decrease in the emission of dorsal contacts, although it apparently results from diminished appreciation of such contacts. In other words, the anesthetized animal still exhibits normal play-solicitation tendencies. The basic desire to play is not dependent on sensory inputs. It is an endogenous urge of the brain.

The Neuroanatomy of Play

Analysis of the somatosensory projection systems of the brain yields a coherent way to address the neuroanatomy of play systems. Since anesthetization of the dorsal body surface can reduce pinning, it is not surprising that similar effects can be obtained by lesioning the ascending somatosensory projection circuits from the spinal cord such as the spinothalamic tract.[42] However, this is also not a result of diminished play motivation, since such animals exhibit a normal desire to play. Only when somatosensory information enters the thalamic projection areas do we begin to get more specific motivational effects.[43] At that level, somatosensory information diverges into the *specific thalamic projection areas* of the ventrobasal nuclei that project discriminative information up to the parietal cortex and into *nonspecific reticular nuclei,* such as the parafascicular complex and posterior thalamic nuclei, that seem to elaborate a ludic motivational state within the animal. In other words, bilateral damage of the nonspecific reticular nuclei yields what appear to be specific play effects. Following such damage, pinning and dorsal contacts are both reduced, and the lesioned animals are no longer motivated to play. This effect is specific, since other relatively complex motivated behaviors, such as food seeking (foraging), are not diminished. This suggests that the parafascicular and posterior thalamic nuclei do specifically mediate play urges.

The parafascicular area is also thought to participate in pain perception because it contains neurons that respond to pinpricks and comparable noxious stimuli.[44] It may be, however, that these stimuli are closer to nipping or tickling ones than to painful ones. In this context, it is worth recalling that in humans, intense tickling is almost unbearable. Dorsal contacts may generate stimulus effects resembling the types of provocative stimuli that are especially effective in activating neurons in this brain area. It is of considerable import that human laughter systems have also been associated with these brain zones.[45]

Obviously, play recruits many brain abilities concurrently, and it is to be expected that many neural circuits are called into action during RAT play. There are bound to be powerful influences from the vestibular, cerebellar, and basal ganglia systems that control movement. However, little is known about the ludic functions of these brain areas, since extensive damage to them compromises virtually all of the animal's complex motor abilities. For instance, in some early unpublished work, we inflicted extensive bilateral damage to the caudate-putamen nuclei of several young rats; their play was abolished, but so was their appetite, curiosity, and desire to exhibit simple locomotor acts. They had to be sacrificed, since they were incapable of taking care of themselves. Obviously, that line of research could not have provided convincing evidence for the role of those brain areas in play. Large lesions in other areas, such as cerebellum, temporal lobe/amygdala and lateral hypothalamus, also markedly reduce play, but again, the overall behavioral competence of the animal is so impaired that it precludes any interpretation with respect to specific play circuitries. Smaller lesions are generally more interpretable, and early anectodal observations suggest that play circuitry is not heavily concentrated in the amygdala or temporal lobes. For instance, monkeys exhibiting the Klüver-Bucy syndrome, although emotionally placid and socially deranged, were "always eager to engage in playful activities with the experimenter."[46] Likewise, the comparable initial experiment with cats reported that the lesioned subjects exhibited augmentation of pleasure reactions and were generally playful, docile, and friendly.[47]

It is worth emphasizing that the neocortex is not essential for play.[48] Even though decortication, such as that depicted in Figure 15.6, can reduce pinning behavior to about half of control levels, those effects are not due to a reduced playfulness, since play solicitations and overall roughhousing, as monitored by direct activity measures, remain intact.[49] The reduced levels of pinning appear to be due to the animal's reduced willingness to respond to play solicitations by rolling over on its back. This may again reflect a heightened level of somatosensory and social insensitivity.

Contrary to the observations of other investigators, in our experience, massive lesions of the cingulate cortex also have little effect on the play of rats. Substantial increases in play can be produced with large frontal lesions[50] as well as septal ones, suggesting that those brain areas participate in the developmental processes that normally diminish play as animals mature. Other lesions may arouse emotional states that are incompatible with play. For example, VMH lesions, which make animals pathologically aggressive (see Chapter 10), will markedly reduce play.[51]

Clearly, the study of play circuitry remains in its infancy, and new techniques are needed to identify the relevant brain systems. One of the most promising techniques would be to analyze early gene markers of neuronal activity, such as *cfos* expression, described in Chapter 5. Using this approach, it becomes evident that wide fields of cells in the higher brain stem and telencephalon are activated during RAT play. This seems to be a common feature of all emotional processes—vast areas of the brain are aroused during each emotional state. As is evident in Figure 15.7, play elevates *cfos* expression in such medial thalamic areas as the parafascicular, in the hippocampus, and in many higher-brain areas, especially the somatosensory cortex.[52] Thus, even though decortication does not eliminate play motivation, it seems clear that play has powerful effects on the cortex. In other words, one of the adaptive functions of juvenile play may involve programming various cortical functions. In a sense, the cortex may be the playground of the mind, and PLAY circuits may be a major coordinator of activities on that field of play. Unfortunately, aside from such data as are summarized in Figure 15.6, there is presently no compelling evidence to support such a contention. A similarly unsatisfactory level of closure on key issues exists at the neurochemical level.

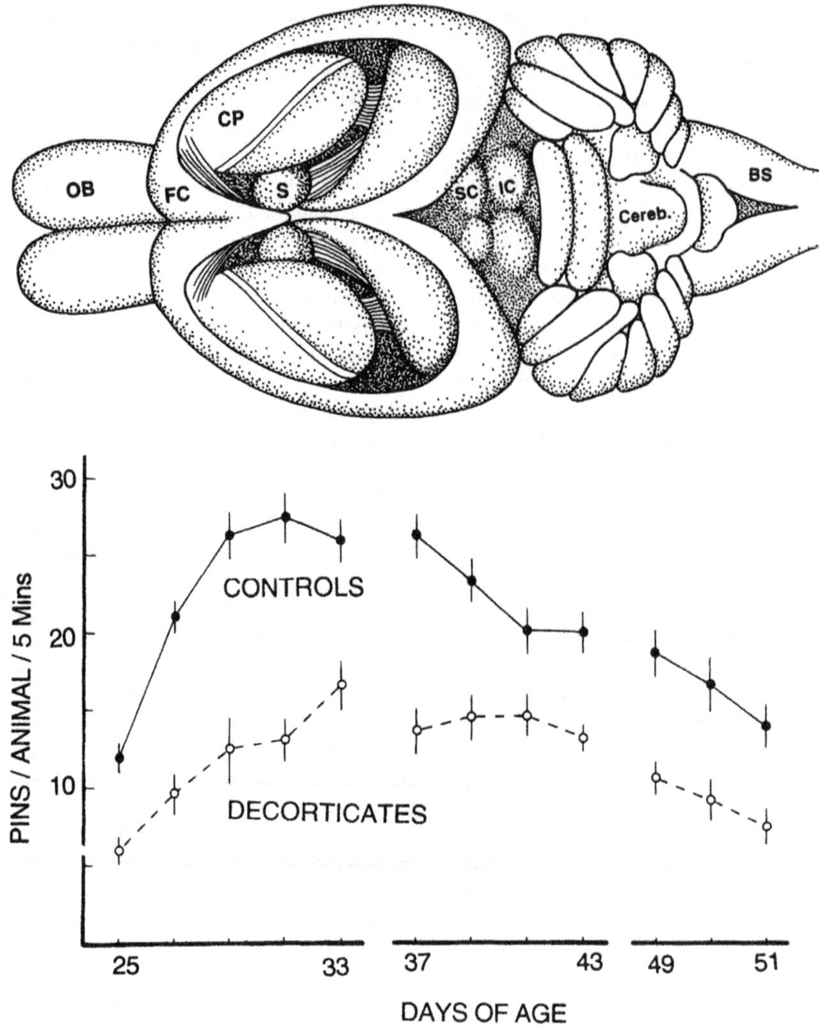

Figure 15.6. Play as a function of development in decorticate and control animals. (According to Panksepp et al., 1994; see n. 49.) The anatomical drawing depicts the appearance of the brain following the neonatal decortication, with many of the structures clearly visible that were described in Chapter 4, especially the hippocampus (HC), the caudate nucleus (CN), and the septal area (S).

The Neurochemistry of Play

It is remarkably easy to inhibit play using pharmacological manipulations, but it is very difficult to determine whether the effects reflect specific changes in the underlying regulatory mechanisms or merely the generally disruptive psychological and behavioral effects that many psychoactive drugs produce. Likewise, a great number of environmental manipulations can reduce play—including all events that evoke negative emotional states such as fear, anger, and separation distress. In addition, hunger is a powerful inhibitor of play,[53] as are many other bodily imbalances, including, of course, illness. In short, play is both a robust and a fragile phenomenon. When animals are healthy and feel good, play is an appealing psychobehavioral option. When they feel bad, it is not. Presumably many of these negative factors will have neurochemical underpinnings, and if we arouse them in a play context, play will be reduced (see Figure 1.1). Unfortunately, such manipulations do not measure the normal processes whereby an individual attains play satiety (i.e., reaches a healthy state of having played enough). Because of such specificity problems, which beset all behavioral experiments to some extent, it will be difficult to sort out those manipulations that reduce play because of physiologically important PLAY regulatory effects from those that reduce play for many other reasons.

One reasonable criterion for establishing that certain neurochemical systems have specific effects on play is to demonstrate that drugs that facilitate and inhibit neural transmission in a given system have opposite effects on play. With this criterion in mind, there is presently considerable evidence that opioids specifically modulate play. Low doses of morphine can increase play, and opiate antagonists can reduce play (even though, as highlighted in the previous chapter, these same manipulations decrease and increase the desire for social interaction, respectively).[54] Presumably, the reduction in play following opiate antagonists is a result of reduced activity and heightened negative emotionality, such as might be produced by mild arousal of separation-distress circuits. If the latter is the main cause, one would expect opioid blockade (at doses that normally reduce play) to increase play solicitation in animals that feel very secure about their social situation. Indeed, when tested against a totally nonthreatening, nonreciprocating partner who has been made unplayful via administration of cholinergic blocking agents such as scopolamine, animals treated with naloxone gradually begin to exhibit heightened play solicitations.[55]

In addition, as previously mentioned, play-dominance studies suggest that brain opioids may increase feelings of "social strength"; hence, animals treated with opiate antagonists are consistently submissive to normal control animals as well as those treated with low doses of morphine (Figure 15.3). Indirect evidence (from in vivo subtractive autoradiography studies)[56] suggests that there is widespread release of opioids in the nervous system during play, especially in such brain areas as the medial preoptic area, where circuitries for sexual and maternal behaviors are situated.[57] Of course,

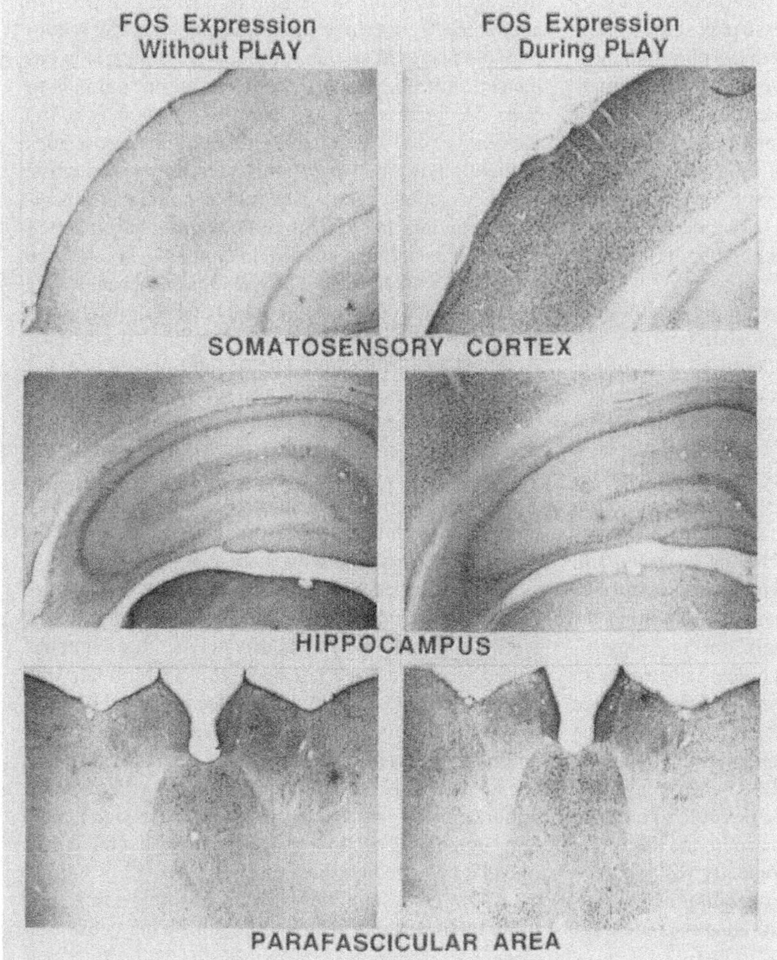

Figure 15.7. Photomicrographs depicting Fos protein labeling in parietal cortex, hippocampus, and dorsomedial/parafascicular thalamus of rats that had played for half an hour and those that had been placed into the play chamber alone. Each dark dot represents a neuron that is expressing the neuronal activity marker cFos. I thank Steve Siviy (1997) for sharing these data; see n. 52.)

to facilitate play, opiate doses must be kept low. Higher doses of opioids reduce all social behaviors including play, and very high doses of opiates reduce all behaviors and induce a catatonic immobility. In any event, we can conclude that modest brain opioid arousal promotes play, and ongoing play promotes opioid release, which may serve to gradually bring the play episode to an end. However, opioids are surely not the only factor mediating play motivation, for it is not possible to restore playfulness in older rats or younger rats that are satiated with play by administration of low doses of opiate agonists or antagonists.

Many other neurochemical systems that have been studied also appear to have specific effects on play.[58] For instance, the muscarinic cholinergic receptor system appears to promote play; blockade of cholinergic activity with scopolamine or atropine markedly reduces play. Unfortunately, no one has yet been able to enhance play by activation of the cholinergic system. This may be partly because of the opposite roles of the nicotinic and muscarinic receptor components. Nicotinic receptor agonists reduce play, and antagonists mildly increase play.[59] Activation of serotonergic and noradrenergic systems also reduces play, while receptor blockade of certain of these systems can increase play somewhat.[60] Conversely, dopamine blockade reduces play, and most agonists do the same, which may indicate that animals need normal levels of synaptic dopamine activity in order to play. A comprehensive analysis of the many receptor subtypes within these biogenic amine systems should provide further clarity about their precise contributions.[61] Of course, all of these chemical systems participate in the control of a large number of brain and behavioral processes.

There may well be highly specific play-promoting neurochemicals in the brain, perhaps neuropeptides, but no such substance has yet been identified. Part of the problem in searching for relevant evidence is that virtually all of the neuropeptides must be administered directly into the brain, and we really do not know enough about play circuitry (especially about the relevant synaptic fields) to place the substances into the appropriate areas. However, we have evaluated the effects of a few neuropeptides, including oxytocin and CRF, both of which reduce play, while vasopressin does not appear to affect play.[62] We are still searching for that neurochemical system that will "turn on" playfulness in animals that are not psychologically ready to play, but this has proved to be a very difficult task (see the "Afterthought" of this chapter). It may require just the right combination of many manipulations. The fact that social deprivation increases the desire to play (Figure 15.1) suggests that it should be possible to produce such a state artificially. Only when someone has found a way to turn on play pharmacologically will we have achieved a profound neural understanding of playfulness, but even that may not reveal its adaptive functions.

The Functions of Play

The possible functions of play have been discussed extensively,[63] and the proposed ideas are remarkably wide-ranging. Suggestions fall into two categories: social and nonsocial. Among the first are the learning of various competitive and noncompetitive social skills, ranging from behaviors that facilitate social bonding and social cooperation to those that promote social rank and leadership, as well as the ability to communicate effectively. Among the potential nonsocial functions are the ability of play to increase physical fitness, cognitive abilities, skillful tool use, and the ability to innovate. Innovation can range from very generalized cognitive skills such as the ability to think creatively in a wide range of situations to very specific aptitudes such as learning to hunt among young predators and predator-avoidance skills in prey species. The collective wisdom is well summarized in the instruction sheet to Lego® toys that was quoted earlier. Unfortunately, there is no substantial scientific database for any of these ideas.

One could also propose a variety of additional fitness-promoting effects of RAT play, such as inoculation against social stress in future adult competitive encounters[64] or perhaps the facilitation of social attractiveness and skill so that reproductive potential is enhanced. Indeed, perhaps play even allows animals to hone deceptive skills, and thus in humans may refine the ability to create false impressions. It almost goes without saying that play must increase reproductive fitness in some way, but it should be noted that sexual-type behaviors are very infrequent during the course of RAT play in animals. Indeed, in unpublished work, we have been unable to find any evidence that male rats that had been socially deprived during the entire juvenile period (21 to 45 days of life) exhibited any deficiency at maturity in the latency and onset of sexual behaviors toward a hormonally primed female. However, if placed into a competitive situation, play-experienced animals were more effective in thwarting the advances of play-deprived animals than vice versa. Also, we have found that animals like to spend slightly more time with conspecifics that have had abundant play experiences than with those that have not.[65]

The best-documented beneficial effect of play discussed in the rodent behavioral literature is a mild increase in problem-solving ability in rats,[66] but in unpublished work we have not been able to replicate this effect. Other reported effects are decreased habituation to novelty in animals that have not experienced normal amounts of juvenile play and increased fearfulness in social situations.[67] Also, animals that have had much opportunity to play appear to be more effective in certain competitive encounters later in life,[68] but more data must be collected on these issues.

Although systematic work on this question is still in its infancy, there seems to be a growing consensus that play is not superfluous, and that some distinct adaptive function should be demonstrable in a reasonably rigorous fashion. The issue of play functions in humans is muddied by the great variety of distinct forms of activities that are labeled as play, especially activities such as board games, where a great deal of previous learning is essential for the "play" to proceed. Indeed, it is generally believed that children learn more rapidly when they have fun, but the whole concept of play as it relates to educational ends remains murky.

By attempting to intentionally and formally recruit playfulness for educational ends, humans probably exercise many cortical potentials independently of PLAY-related functions. One is led to wonder to what extent the literature that has evaluated the role of play in facilitating learning and development of social competencies has simply evaluated the power of positive social interactions to facilitate desired educational goals.[69] It does seem that many of the supposed benefits of play that have been revealed by formal investigation simply reflect the beneficial effects of other types of social activities and supplemental tutoring.[70] There is presently no assurance that the many play interventions that have been studied in laboratory settings do in fact arouse primary-process PLAY circuits intensely. Of course, it remains very attractive to assume that the consequences of playful activities are beneficial for learning, but unfortunately, there are no robust and credible demonstrations of this in either humans or animals.[71] Once we have a clear understanding of basic PLAY circuits in the mammalian brain, it may be possible to monitor the development of behavioral and social competence in animals deprived specifically of normal activity in those circuits. Such experiments may be able to yield some definitive data.

Play and Dreaming

One straightforward perspective is that during play all of the natural (unconditional) emotional-behavioral potentials of the brain can be exercised. However, in addition to the relatively obvious functional hypotheses summarized here, only a few of which have even modest empirical support, it is to be expected that play may also be important in the functional control of brain organization. One molecular view might be that play promotes certain types of neuronal growth. A higher-level view is that play may serve to exercise and extend the range of behavioral options under the executive control of inborn emotional systems.[72] In fact, play may be the waking functional counterpart of dreaming.

As discussed in Chapter 7, a key function of rapid eye movement (REM) sleep may be to promote the processing of information that is especially important for complex emotional integration. PLAY systems may serve a similar function during waking. Since one of the characteristics of play is that many types of emotional behaviors are exhibited in the context of nonserious interactions, it is reasonable to hypothesize that play exercises the behavioral potentials of emotional circuits (Figure 15.8). According to this view, play may serve a function that is orthogonal to that of REM sleep: Namely, REM may exercise the potentials for organizing affective information in emotional circuits, while play exercises the emotive behavioral potentials of these same circuits in the relative emotional safety of a positive affective state. In other words, dreaming and play may have synergistic functions—providing special opportunities for exercising the psychobehavioral potentials of emotional operating systems within socially supportive environments. Thus, there could be as many behavioral variants of play as there are primary emotional systems within the brain.

A relationship between REM and PLAY processes is suggested by the fact that both are under strong cholinergic control. If there is, in fact, a neural continuity between REM and PLAY impulses, one might expect that

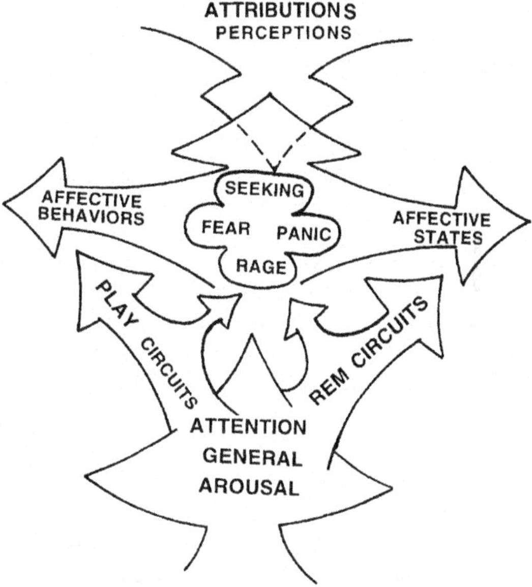

Figure 15.8. Emotional circuits are embedded in multiple convergent control processes such as startle, REM, and play circuits. REM may preferentially influence the higher affective consequences of emotive circuits, thereby helping process information that was collected during waking through the auspices of the various basic emotional circuits (see Chapter 7). Play may preferentially access the motor subroutines that are normally accessed by emotional circuits, thereby providing exercise and practice of instinctual motor patterns that are essential for competent emotive behavior patterns. (Adapted from Panksepp, 1986; see n. 72.)

RAT play may be characterized by unique EEG signals—for instance, large spikes during play jumpiness, which may resemble the PGO spikes of REM (see Chapter 7)—but this has never been evaluated. Also, since norepinephrine and serotonin neurons are silenced during REM, it is of interest that modest pharmacological reduction of activity in these two systems can modestly increase play.

Obviously, play will provide food for thought to scientists for a long time to come. Indeed, perhaps play provides "food for thought" for the brain, as recurring patterns become especially well consolidated into new habits during dreams. It will be interesting to determine to what extent preceding play periods affect subsequent REM periods, and how REM deprivation affects the information that is processed in the midst of play (e.g., whether play dominance, such as summarized in Figures 15.2 and 15.3, emerges without subsequent REM).

From this perspective, it would also seem likely that play may have direct trophic effects on neuronal and synaptic growth in many brain systems. Although the evidence is modest, environmental enrichment, including social dimensions, has been well studied in lab animals,[73] and there is some evidence that the observed social effects are due to RAT play. Neuronal effects of social enrichment (such as increased brain RNA and heavier cortices) can be observed after as little as 10 minutes of exposure for four days during sensitive periods of juvenile development.[74] Another basic hypothesis concerning play that deserves more experimental attention is the possibility that play is a "neuro-tonic" that can have antistress, health-promoting effects. We have evaluated this possibility via analysis of corticosterone secretion to mild stress in play-experienced versus nonexperienced animals. Unfortunately, we found no evidence to support the hypothesis that RAT play can regulate other stress responses.[75] Still, I believe more work along these lines will yield positive findings.

Distinctions between Play and Exploration

One psychobehavioral dimension that deserves special attention in future work is the role of SEEKING circuits in playful activities.[76] It has been quite common in the human literature to combine play and exploratory activities under the same rubric.[77] This is more problematic than is commonly realized. The mammalian brain probably contains distinct circuits for arousal of roughhousing types of social interactions and others for the arousal of exploratory and investigatory activities. These circuits may not always operate in synergistic ways. For instance, one highly effective way to reduce RAT play in animals as well as in humans (as indicated by the observation of "hyperkinetic" children) is to administer psychostimulants such as amphetamines, which concurrently increase attention and investigatory activities.[78] Such data raise the possibility that activities in PLAY and SEEKING systems may typically be antagonistic rather than synergistic.

Since the exploratory urge seems to be triggered to a substantial extent by brain dopamine activity,[79] it has been of some interest to determine whether dopamine systems are aroused during the course of RAT social play. To evaluate this, we once placed small amounts of the dopamine neurotoxin 6-hydroxydopamine into the nucleus accumbens at doses that did not debilitate the animal, but no clear effects on play were observed.[80] However, others have found some reduction in play from placing this same toxin into the dorsal striatum.[81] In more recent work, we measured the levels of forebrain dopamine and 3.4-dihydroxyphenylacetic acid (DOPAC), the metabolite that is commonly taken to reflect impulse flow in dopamine systems of the brain. Twenty minutes of RAT play led to an apparent increase of utilization of dopamine in the brain.[82] This result suggests that certain dopamine neurons are especially active during play, which is not surprising from the perspective that brain dopamine controls psychomotor arousal related to the perception of positive incentives (see Chapter 8). However, a determination of whether the same populations of dopamine neurons are active during the various forms of play and exploration will require a finer analysis of neural changes than has yet been achieved.

At present, it seems reasonable to provisionally conclude that basic exploratory and PLAY circuits in the brain are distinct, and that they normally operate antagonistically. However, we should remain open to the possibility that vigorous activity of the SEEKING system is a source process for what is typically called *object* or *manipulative play*. Because of concerns such as these, it will be difficult to determine to what extent the massive child development literature on the effects of "play" on psychological development reflects the functions of brain systems that control roughhousing play, as opposed to those that control exploration. These distinct psychobehavioral processes should not be placed under the same verbal construct.

There is presently an urgent need to determine what contributions to child development are in fact exerted by the PLAY circuits of the brain. Since roughhousing play cannot be readily studied in long-term and controlled experiments in human children, the use of animal models will be essential for adjudicating critical issues. Even more important, since this emotional system may be subject to pathologies, just like all the other emotional systems, it is worth considering how knowledge about the underlying circuits may relate to psychiatric disorders.

Play Disorders: Mania, Impulse Control Disorders, and Hyperkinesis

Since the PLAY circuitry of the brain appears to represent a fundamental emotional system, it is to be expected that there may be psychiatric disorders related to overarousal and underarousal of the system. Underarousal may well be related to certain types of depression and melancholic responses. Overarousal may be related to various manic symptoms, hyperkinetic or attention deficit disorders, and perhaps even Tourette's syndrome and other impulse-control disorders.[83] At present, there is no direct evidence for such assertions, but the symptoms of mania—expansiveness, unrealistic optimism, excessive happiness, and grandiosity—are the types of psychological symptoms one might expect from a highly playful brain.

Attention deficit hyperactivity disorders (ADHD) and impulse-control disorders are due in part to underarousal of cortical functions.[84] If we accept that heightened cortical activity can inhibit playfulness, it might well be that many children diagnosed with ADHD may, in fact, be exhibiting heightened play tendencies. Their hyperactivity, impulsiveness, and rapid shifting from one activity to another may be partly due to their unconstrained and unfocused playful tendencies. Indeed, the medications that are used to treat the disorder—psychostimulants such as methylphenidate (i.e., Ritalin®) and amphetamines—are all very effective in reducing playfulness in animals.[85] Moreover, parents of hyperkinetic children often complain that one of the undesirable side effects of such medications is the reduced playfulness of their children.[86] Obviously, parents value these childlike characteristics and are typically disturbed when the children's natural playfulness is pharmacologically diminished.

If at least part of ADHD is caused by excessive playfulness, it becomes a profound societal issue whether it is ethical to drug children for such traits (for more on this question see "Afterthought," Chapter 16). Obviously, it is essential to maintain attention to academic matters in the classroom, but is it appropriate to induce compliance in children through pharmacological means? At the very least, more benign interventions should be attempted first, such as provision of abundant RAT activity early in the morning prior to classes. This is especially important in light of the possibility that such drugs can produce long-lasting changes in the responsivity of brain catecholamine systems, as is seen in the psychostimulant-induced sensitization phenomenon (see "Afterthought," Chapter 8).

Finally, it is worth considering that Tourette's syndrome, with its bizarre nervous impulses—which lead to tics and sudden verbal expletives, commonly including "forbidden" expression such as curses and slurs[87]—may represent aberrant play impulses, or components of play impulses, circulating without restraint within the nervous system. Although this may seem far-fetched, pharmacological evidence provides some support for the hypothesis. Dopamine blocking agents, which presently are most effective in bringing Tourette's symptoms under control,[88] are also very effective in reducing playfulness in animals.[89]

Although these connections are highly speculative, if we keep our minds open to such possibilities, we may achieve a better understanding of both the nature of play and other perplexing disorders of childhood. In this context, it might be noted that autistic children typically like RAT play; if this is essentially the only type of social activity a child seems to favor, it is taken to be consistent with the diagnosis of autism.[90] This is also consistent with the idea that such children may have slightly excessive opioid activity, a brain chemical state that is compatible with abundant RAT play in animals (see Figure 15.3).

One thing is certain: During play, animals are especially prone to behave in flexible and creative ways. Thus, it is not surprising that play interventions have been used in educational and therapeutic settings (i.e., play therapy) to facilitate more efficient acquisition of new information and behavioral change. However, since play is fun, it could also be used more effectively as a reinforcer for desired behavioral change. To what extent would children be willing to discipline themselves with academic tasks if the availability of roughhousing play were made contingent on good academic performance? The benefits, for both classroom discipline and educational progress, might be enhanced if the availability of roughhousing was used to systematically reward scholarly achievement. But this would require us to begin viewing this ancient evolutionary brain function as a potentially desirable activity, rather than a disruptive force whose energies need to be suppressed or dissipated on the playground after the earnest business of education has been completed.

It is worth considering whether it might be possible to develop maneuvers to reduce disruptive RAT play impulses in the classroom, while utilizing opportunities to release those impulses as a reward for scholarly achievement. This approach is used by some high schools and colleges to increase the probability that athletes also become scholars, but it needs to be implemented in the earlier grades. Of course, the bottom line is that play is such fun. If we were able to make the process of learning more playful, the whole enterprise of education might become easier. The computer revolution now allows us to pursue such joyous modes of cultural development.

AFTERTHOUGHT: Future Research and the Search for Ludic Cocktails and Fountains of Youth

In addition to the many hypotheses that have been generated concerning the possible adaptive functions of play—ranging from the idea that play promotes muscular development to the possibility that play promotes the generation of new ideas—there are other provocative alternatives. For instance, it could still be the case that a major adaptive function of play is simply the generation of a powerful positive emotional state. This could have direct health benefits by establishing a certain type of neurohumoral tone in the brain and body, which may promote more vigorous immunological patterns and other beneficial physiological responses. There are instances in the literature of prominent individuals claiming they have experienced remarkable medical benefits in the midst of serious illnesses by sustaining playful attitudes accompanied by abundant laughter.[91]

In a sense, play is an index of youthful health. From this vantage, the search for play transmitters can be thought of as a modern version of the search for the fountain of youth. It is the PLAY instinct that, more than any other, uniquely characterizes the joy of youth. Presumably there are brain chemistries, or combinations of chemistries, that can vigorously promote playfulness, but they have not yet been found. One way to discover them would be to identify neurochemical influences that gradually lead to the diminution of play as organisms grow older. The period of childhood has been greatly extended in humans and other great apes compared with other mammals, perhaps via genetic regulatory influences that have promoted playful "neoteny."[92] Indeed, we humans have the longest childhood of any creature on the face of the earth. One influence that might be irreversible is the maturation of the neocortex, which may tend to inhibit RAT ludic activities or at least channel those energies in different, more symbolic, directions.

Another way to understand playfulness might be to consider why playful impulses tend to return during adulthood, when one has offspring of one's own. Generally, parents seem to be more playful than nonparents, and it is reasonable to suppose that this tendency is promoted by neurobiological vectors in addition to the obvious cultural ones. In this context, it is worth reemphasizing that motherhood promotes specific neurochemical changes in the brain. For instance, oxytocin gene expression is increased, which certainly helps promote parenting behavior.[93] Perhaps this same neurochemical change promotes playfulness. For this reason, we evaluated the effects of intraventricular injections of oxytocin on play, but, as already noted, we only observed reductions in play. Vasopressin did seem to increase play slightly, but the results were not definitive. Thus, we presently only have hypotheses regarding which changes during parenthood may promote playfulness. Although we have an abundance of neuropharmacological data suggesting a variety of inhibitory influences on play circuitry,[94] we presently have no way to markedly increase playfulness in a nonplayful mature animal, except by play deprivation.

Over a decade ago, we took some of the more suggestive items from the list of available pharmacological manipulations that seemed to mildly promote play to see if we could generate some combinations that would facilitate play in a vigorous fashion. We were hoping to find a "ludic cocktail." The items selected included the opiate receptor agonist morphine, the serotonin receptor antagonist methysergide, and the dopamine receptor agonist apomorphine, each of which, given at low doses, had exhibited some tendency to increase play. These drugs were given in all possible permutations (a single drug, or two or three drugs concurrently), using various levels of social deprivation that should have allowed one to see both increases and decreases in play. These efforts were eminently unsuccessful. No combination of drugs seemed to clearly potentiate play, and each of the agents alone was, at best, marginally effective. However, we have recently had some modest success with cannabis-like molecules.

It remains possible that age-related decrements in play emerge from a diminished vigor of the underlying play circuits rather than a diminished availability of "play transmitters." If this is the case, it will be unlikely that a "ludic cocktail" can ever be generated, and the search for this "fountain of youth" will be as unproductive as the ones that have gone before. However, many lines of inquiry remain to be pursued.

Indeed, the pursuit of the neurochemical fountain of youth is becoming an active area of inquiry. Already, a series of agents have been found to exert powerful effects on longevity. I will discuss only one here—the antidepressant monoamine oxidase inhibitor deprenyl, which can selectively increase dopamine availability in the brain.[95] In fact, deprenyl is highly effective in reducing the symptoms of Parkinson's disease[96] and also provides neuroprotection against the progressive degeneration of dopamine systems that occurs with aging.[97] The vigor of brain dopamine declines markedly in most individuals after the age of 50, and most would become parkinsonian if they lived long enough.[98] Deprenyl, given daily in low doses, reduces this decline and seems to promote youthful vitality: It extends the maximal life span in animals by almost 30%, and male animals that have become sexually sluggish tend to regain their lustiness.[99]

It will be interesting to see how such agents influence the ontogeny and dynamics of play throughout juvenile and adult development. One would think that agents that can maintain psychological vitality would also tend to increase playfulness. Indeed, we should also consider the reciprocal idea—whether playful social companionship may actually extend life span. It is disconcerting how little work is presently being devoted to trying to understand the underlying mechanisms and the adaptive nature of this and other fundamental emotional processes of the mammalian brain.

Suggested Readings

Aldis, O. (1975). *Play fighting*. New York: Academic Press.

Fagen, R. (1981). *Animal play behavior*. New York: Oxford Univ. Press.

Groos, K. (1898). *The play of animals*. New York: Appleton.

Joubert, L. (1579/1980). *Treatise on laughter* (translated and annotated by Gregory David de Racher). Birmingham: Univ. of Alabama Press.

MacDonald, K. (ed.) (1993). *Parent-child play: Descriptions and implications.* Albany: State Univ. of New York Press.

Panksepp, J. , Siviy, S. , & Normansell, L. (1984). The psychobiology of play: Theoretical and methodological perspectives. *Neurosci. Biobehav. Revs.* 8:465–492.

Smith, E. O. (ed.) (1978). *Social play in primates.* New York: Academic Press.

Smith, P. K. (1982). Does play matter? Functional and evolutionary aspects of animal and human play. *Behav. Brain Res.* 5:139–184.

Smith, P. K. (ed.) (1984). *Play in animals and humans.* London: Blackwell.

Symonds, D. (1978). *Play and aggression: A study of rhesus monkeys.* New York: Columbia Univ. Press.

16

Emotions, the Higher Cerebral Processes, and the SELF

Some Are Born to Sweet Delight, Some Are Born to Endless Night

The mind of man seems so far removed from anything known in other animals and the animal mind seems so inaccessible to us that those who approach the problem from this side seem prone to seek a way out through metaphysics or mysticism, though relief of this sort is obtained only at the expense of profound narcosis of critical and scientific method.

C. Judson Herrick, *Neurological Foundations of Animal Behavior* (1924)

CENTRAL THEME

Although primal emotional feelings arise from the subcortical systems of the animal brain, their consequences ramify widely within the unique conscious abilities of the human mind, as well as the social fabric of our cultures. For 15 chapters I have focused on the former, but now I will turn to the latter. The critical issue that I have avoided until now is the nature of consciousness and the self. Emotional feelings cannot be fully understood without understanding these matters. Do animals have a spontaneous sense of themselves as active creatures in the world? Descartes suggested that animals, unlike humans, did not have a sentient self—that they were closer to reflex automatons than feeling creatures. Many scholars have recently chosen to disagree with this cold view of animal nature, but to be scientifically useful such alternative perspectives need to probe the neuroevolutionary roots of consciousness. I have constructed a brain perspective that acknowledges the existence of internal feelings in other animals. The indirect evidence seems overwhelming that other mammals do have basic forms of affective consciousness, not unlike our own (which is not meant to imply that they can have the same cognitive contents in their consciousness as we have in ours). All mammals appear to experience pain, anger, fear, and many other raw feelings, but they do not seem able to cognitively reflect upon such feelings as we do. They do not appear to extend feelings in time, as we can with our rich imaginations. If the existence of such feelings is not an illusion but a substantive part of nature, we cannot understand their brains, or ours for that matter, without fully confronting the neural nature of that undefinable attribute of mind that we commonly call our sense of self, our ego—the feeling of "will" or "I-ness" by which we come to represent ourselves and our self-interests within the world. Here I will develop the idea that a neural principle of self-representation emerged early in brain evolution, and that it became rooted first in brain areas as low as those situated in ancient midbrain regions where primitive neural systems for motor maps (i.e., body schema), sensory maps (world schema), and emotional maps (value schema) first intermixed. Although this neuropsychic function emerged early in brain evolution, it did not remain primitive. It continued to evolve as brains became increasingly encephalized, which allows us more behavioral flexibility and the ability to have complex thoughts and internal images. Thus, with the evolution of higher brain functions in humans (such as the ability to reflect on our own reflections, as commonly occurs in writing and reading, not to mention our penchant for narcissistic gazing into mirrors), a multidimensional conscious sense of self came to be greatly expanded in the human brain/mind. Although higher forms of human consciousness (namely, awareness of events and our role in them) surely emerge from the cortex and higher reaches of the limbic system, they are not independent of the lower reaches of the brain, which generate our basic emotions, feelings, and other instinctual tendencies. Although our higher cerebral functions have led to the great achievements of humankind, including the construction of civilizations via cultural evolution, they have also generated the illusory half-truth that humans are rational creatures above all else. Despite the appeal of this rational fallacy, our higher brain areas are not immune to the subcortical influences we share with other creatures. Of course, the interchange between cognitive and emotional processes is one of reciprocal control, but the flow of traffic remains balanced only in nonstressful circumstances. In emotional turmoil, the upward influences of subcortical emotional circuits on the higher reaches of the brain are stronger than the top-down controls. Although humans can strengthen and empower the downward controls through emotional education and self-mastery, few can ride the whirlwind of unbridled emotions with great skill.

Appraisals and Higher Brain Mechanisms in Emotions

For every investigator studying the brain substrates of emotions, there are dozens focusing on sociocultural issues. Because of the massive development of the human cortex, many investigators presently see human emotionality as being constituted largely from higher appraisal functions of the human mind that evaluate various situational complexities—ranging from the subtleties of perceptual interpretations to the many intricacies of learning and planning strategies. The human cognitive apparatus dwells easily on the various emotional issues that the world offers for our consideration. By examining the higher sociocultural perspectives, we can pursue many issues that cannot be tackled thoroughly at the neurological level. For instance, many human emotions—from avarice to xenophobia—are almost impossible to study in the brain even with modern brain-imaging technologies, not to mention in animal models.

We humans can experience guilt, shame, embarrassment, jealousy, hate, and contempt, as well as pride and loyalty. However, in some yet undetermined manner, these secondary, cognitive-type emotions may also be linked critically to the more primitive affective substrates that we have discussed so far. Perhaps they emerge largely from social-labeling processes, whereby we experience slightly differing patterns of primitive feelings in various social contexts and come to accept them as distinct entities. Perhaps they reflect intermixtures of several basic emotions, even though no one has yet specified the proportions in the various recipes. However, they may also reflect newly evolved neural functions that have developed within the higher areas of the human brain. Perhaps human brain evolution yielded some totally new forms of affective-cognitive feelings, making us the complex creatures of history and culture that we are. No one really knows for sure, but it seems unlikely that those affective proclivities will ever be clarified at a neurological level, at least until the more primal passions are understood. I do not believe that distinct neurochemical systems will ever be found for such higher feelings, even though they may certainly have emerged from the evolutionary engraving of some additional paths of emotional epistemology within our general-purpose cerebral functions.

It is reasonable to view the evolution of higher cortical processes as a way for nature to provide ever more effective ways for organisms to cope with their intrinsic biological values—to seek resources and reproduce more effectively and to find better ways to avoid dangers. Once special-purpose mechanisms, such as the emotional systems we have discussed, became less adaptive, evolution created ever more sophisticated general-purpose learning mechanisms to provide systems that could cope with the increasing variability of animate nature. The higher reaches of the human brain now contain layers of complexity of such proportions that some investigators find it difficult to accept that many of our psychological processes are still controlled by the basic systems that have been the focus of this book. Such a view, I believe, ignores the evidence. Still, the intricacies of our cerebral abilities pose many conceptual dilemmas for our minds. Our lives, our values, and our aspirations are remarkably complex.

When the mushrooming of the cortex *opened* up the relatively *closed* circuits of our old mammalian and reptilian brains, we started to entertain alternatives of our own rather than of nature's making. We can choose to enjoy fear. We can choose to make art out of our loneliness. We can even exert some degree of control over our sexual orientations. Most other animals have no such options. Affectively, we can choose to be angels or devils, and we can construct and deconstruct ideas at will. We can choose to present ourselves in ways that are different from the ways we truly feel. We can be warm or acerbic, supportive or sarcastic at will. Animals cannot. These are options that the blossoming of the human cerebral mantle now offers for our consideration.

I believe the basic emotional messages that have been summarized here will still be quite clear and evident in any population analysis of human values and behaviors, but they will always be embedded in innumerable complexities that characterize human life. We rarely see human emotional systems in action except as they are refracted through higher cerebral mechanisms. However, we can still see the underlying brain structures and functions reasonably clearly through animal brain research. These lower levels of understanding are essential for clarifying the foundations of our higher thoughts, feelings, and actions. Affective neuroscience aspires to provide answers to such questions, but to do so with any sense of completeness, we must now probe deeper into the very nature of affective consciousness. Only when we begin to understand how primitive subjective feelings are created within the brain will we be able to understand the nature of the values that are stitched together by our more recently evolved cognitive apparatus.

A Prospectus

Thus, this book ends where many books on emotions begin—with a consideration of emotions in conscious experience. But even here I will need to go below the surface glimmer of experience to the deeper causal issues. Because there is less substantive knowledge at this level, this chapter must be more speculative than the rest. To shed new light on the "hard questions" concerning human and animal consciousness,[1] namely, to clarify the brain sources of subjective experience, we must be willing to entertain novel ideas that will lead to new lines of research. Only when there are substantive, testable conjectures on the table will we be able to crawl toward a causal neurodynamic resolution of the mind-body problem (see Appendix C). In pursuing such a path, there will be inevitable mistakes, but hopefully they can be corrected through successive empirical approximations.

By appreciating how the brain is organized, we may gradually outgrow the illusory sense that we are creatures of two distinct realms, of mind and matter, and come to monistically accept that we are simply ultracomplex creatures of the world—with complex feelings, thoughts, and motor abilities that have arisen from the dynamic interaction of our brains with environments, both past and present. So far, I have focused more on the aspects of emotionality that evolved from ancestral challenges of such importance that they became genetically coded into the circuits of the brains we inherit. These ancient structures now constitute the neural substrates from which our primary-process affective consciousness—our "raw feels"—arise. The power of these systems was presumably pulled along during the subsequent mushrooming of the cerebral mass. It is likely that our more subtle feelings are a consequence of this neural expansion, but it is unlikely that those feelings could exist without the basic neural scaffolding we have so far explored.

An image that can serve us well here is that of a tree: Most full-grown trees have a remarkable canopy of branches and leaves that interact dynamically with the environment. However, the spreading branches cannot function or survive without the nourishment and support they receive from the roots and trunk. We may appreciate the tree for its spreading leaves, but our understanding must begin with the seed, the roots, and the emerging trunk. The same metaphor applies to the many neuronal "trees" that mediate emotions. It is certainly likely that the dynamic changes in our moods and feelings can arise from the perceptual capacities of our cerebral canopies, but all that could not exist without the emotional trunk lines.

In any event, the precise manner in which subjective experiences of primitive emotional feelings emerge from neural interactions remains a mystery, but because of the neuroscience revolution, it is fast becoming a scientifically workable problem. An understanding of such fundamental issues as primitive forms of consciousness will prepare us to address the nature of the more recent forms (see Figure 2.6), such as our ability to conjure images and to think about our perceptions and feelings. In other words, the more recent forms of consciousness may be linked critically to the rich neural "soil" that originally allowed our mammalian ancestors to experience primary-process affective states.

Trying to analyze consciousness coherently is difficult enough when we just consider the human mind, to which we have some introspective access, but the enterprise becomes increasingly treacherous when we try to understand the animal mind. However, from a formal scientific/experimental perspective, it should be no more difficult to understand the basic conscious abilities of other animals than our own. Indeed, it is possible that a careful study of animal behavior may take us to valid general principles more quickly than the study of the complex behaviors of humans. Obviously, we can only proceed experimentally if we accept objective animal and human behaviors as accurate indices of inner states (see Figure 2.3). It is unlikely that human verbal reports will provide the *only* inroad to the analysis of conscious experience. Our exquisite ability to transcribe experience into verbal symbols may be a lens that distorts reality as readily as it reveals it. Evolutionarily, the brain mechanisms for language were designed for social interactions, not for the conduct of science (see Appendix B).

Indeed, words give us a special ability to deceive each other. There are many reasons to believe that animal behavior will lie to us less than human words. This dilemma is especially acute when it comes to our hidden feelings that we normally share only through complex personal and cultural display rules. In addition, it now appears that our two cerebral hemispheres have such different cognitive and emotional perspectives on the world that the linguistic approach may delude us as readily as inform. Medical research in which the nonspeaking right hemisphere has been selectively anesthetized indicates that people express very different feelings when their whole brain is operating than when just the left hemisphere is voicing its views.[2] In short, our left hemisphere—the one that typically speaks to others—may be more adept at lying and constructing a social masquerade rather than revealing deep, intimate emotional secrets. If this is so, an indeterminate amount of information that has been collected with questionnaires and other linguistic output devices may be tainted by social-desirability factors, making the data next to useless for resolving basic issues. However, if we accept the reality of the psychological forces that have been long accepted in folk psychology—our ability to feel happy, sad, mad, and scared—and include a careful study of comparable emotional behaviors in animals and their brain substrates, the issue of affective consciousness should be resolvable.

Although emotionality has typically been deemed among the most difficult psychological issues to tackle scientifically, contrary to a traditional assumption of cognitive psychology,[3] the basic emotions we share with other animals may actually be easier to understand in neural terms than are their cognitive representations. As emphasized throughout this book, a consideration of the relevant details in the animal brain may offer an especially robust empirical way to shed definitive light on the neural nature of such forms of consciousness in humans. Moreover, affective feelings are clearly very important forms of consciousness to understand in their own right. Such knowledge has the real potential to improve human existence (by the development of new medications for psychiatric problems) and to reveal the fundamental nature of our core values. It follows that such knowledge should also have profound implications for scientific psychology—one that is not simply an experimental discipline describing surface appearances but also based on a causal, neurobiological understanding of fundamental principles.

If we could come to understand affective experience in neural terms, it could provide the fragmented discipline of psychology with a new unity that often appears unimaginable.[4] At present, there is still one enormous missing piece in scientific psychology. Clearly, we are not just behavioral creatures, as one old school of psychology, by no means dead, continues to assert. Nor are we merely mental creatures, as the prevailing cognitive paradigms would have us believe. We are also deeply feeling and deeply biological creatures who possess values handed down to us not simply through our sociocultural environments but also by the genetic heritage derived from our ancestral past. It is this last dimension, so lacking in modern psychology until quite recently, that has the strength to serve as a foundation for many higher concepts.

We are ultimately creatures whose capacity to feel is based on inherited brain representations of times past. Although the *details* of each individual's mental and behavioral life are constructed by living in the here-and-now world, our values remain critically linked to those encoded in our ancient modes of affective consciousness. Just as most people have always believed, our thoughts and actions are probably guided by our internal feelings—feelings that initially, in our youth, were completely biological and affective but which, through innumerable sensory-perceptual interactions with our environments, become inextricably mixed with learning and world events.

Once we accept the need for such deep evolutionary views, we will eventually have to come to terms with many unconventional premises. For instance, in this chapter I will argue that human and animal affective consciousness is based fundamentally on motor processes that generate self-consciousness by being closely linked to body image representations. I will try to show how an acceptance of such a seemingly incorrect premise—that the fundamental nature of consciousness is constructed as much from motor as from sensory processes—may help us resolve some key conceptual sticking points concerning the nature of consciousness, such as its apparent psychological coherence and unity (i.e., or the "binding problem," as it is traditionally called). Consciousness is not simply a sensory-perceptual affair, a matter of mental imagery, as the contents of our mind would have us believe. It is deeply enmeshed with the brain mechanisms that automatically promote various forms of action readiness. If this nontraditional view is on the right track, it may allow us to come to terms with our deepest nature in a nondualistic way.

If one accepts the importance of consciousness in understanding many psychological issues, the ultimate questions are: How can a brain feel its ancestral emotions and motivations? How are the intrinsic emotional processes generated by brain tissue and intermixed with representations of specific life activities? And how can we construct a third-person consensual science that is intimately linked to first-person subjective experiences?

On the Nature of Affective Consciousness

So far I have argued that the fundamental executive substrates for a large number of affective processes are coded into mammalian brains as a birthright—as cross-species, genetically provided neural functions that are experientially refined through maturation within the developing functional architecture of the brain. The basic emotional systems serve adaptive functions that emerged during the evolutionary history of mammals. They help organize and integrate physiological, behavioral, and psychological changes in the organism to yield various forms of action readiness. The emergence of emotional circuits, and hence emotional states, provided powerful brain attractors for synchronizing various neural events so as to coordinate specific cognitive and behavioral tendencies in response to archetypal survival problems: to approach when SEEKING, to escape from FEAR, to attack when in RAGE, to seek social support and nurturance when in PANIC, to enjoy PLAY and LUST and dominance, and so forth. Each of these systems is affectively valenced, yielding feelings that are either positive or negative, desirable or undesirable, but there are probably several distinct forms of each of these general types of affective experiences. Considerable evolutionary diversity has been added by species-typical specializations in higher brain areas as well as lower sensory and motor systems, but as we have seen, the basic affective value systems, deep within ancient recesses of the brain, appear to be reasonably well conserved across mammalian species.

These systems provide a solid foundation of biological values for the emergence of more complex abilities. Without a consideration of the types of underlying brain functions, it will probably be impossible to provide definitive *inclusion* and *exclusion criteria* for what constitutes the various emotional processes and how one emotional process might be distinguished from another. Such issues are solvable, in principle, when one begins to anchor his or her thinking about basic issues in neural terms. The ultimate inclusion and exclusion criteria for basic emotional processes must be found within the intrinsic potentials of the brain as opposed to the peripheral physiological and expressive changes of the body. Obviously, they cannot be based simply on our "feelings" or on psychological appraisal processes. For instance, the inclusion criteria for one type of fear are the properties of a specific neural circuit that extends from the lateral and central amygdaloid areas to the central/periventricular gray (see Figure 11.1) The exclusion criteria are the properties of many other nearby emotional and motivational systems. Furthermore, the properties of these brain systems can, I believe, be linked credibly to our deepest human concerns.[5]

Affective neuroscience seeks to provide conceptual bridges that can link our understanding of basic neural circuits for the emotions with straightforward *cognitive* and *folk-psychological* views of the human mind and, most important, its emotional disorders. This interdisciplinary approach would have little chance of working were it not for the simple fact that we humans do have some introspective-linguistic access to our subjective feelings.[6] Because of that small psychological window, and because the key emotional circuits are conserved in the brains of all mammals, the two can be linked in such a way that we can finally understand the neurobiological underpinnings of our human feelings. Conversely, and equally important, our introspective access to primitive feelings may also provide a credible scientific view, albeit indirect, on the minds of other animals.[7] This conceptual bridge can yield clear empirical predictions in both directions, from animal to human and from human to animal, and it can serve as an intellectual highway for productive commerce between the psychosocial and neurobiological sciences, at least as far as the basic, genetically dictated foundations of our natures are concerned.

The present era is an opportune time for such views: Brain research, because of its abundant factual riches, is finally ready to deal with some subtle integrative issues. Also, there is now increasing agreement that humans do have some universal psychological traits,[8] a possibility that was long viewed skeptically because no unambiguous methodologies existed to resolve the inevitable debates. Until recently, the most compelling evidence came from studies of identical twins separated at birth and cross-cultural ethological analyses of behavior patterns, such as facial, vocal, postural, and other behavioral expressions.[9] Now, however, there is an additional and remarkably robust strategy: the comparative neurological study of homologous psychobehavioral functions across mammalian species. Our neuroscientific knowledge allows us to probe below the surface details, to recognize the deep emotional and motivational homologies that guide animals in the use of their different toolboxes of sensory and motor skills. For instance, there is little doubt that the 24-hour biological clock of the suprachiasmatic nucleus guides the distribution of behaviors in all vertebrate species, or that the neuronal regulators of sleep are conserved in essentially all mammals, or that our urges to eat, drink, and make merry (i.e., play) are strikingly similar.

Currently, an increasing number of psychologists and other social scientists are beginning to develop an enthusiasm for the brain sciences, largely because of the great advances in clinical psychopharmacology and the spectacular advances in our ability to image brain functions in humans. Still, we should recognize that detailed animal brain research will be essential for us to make progress on the details of every one of the mechanistic issues. Such work has the best chance of filling in anatomical, neurophysiological, and neurochemical details for the basic psychological concepts derived from higher levels of analysis.[10] Indeed, for those who believe the new brain-imaging technologies will soon answer all the important brain questions, I simply note, once more, that they are not terribly precise in highlighting many of the subcortical neural circuits and chemistries involved in governing basic psychological processes, partly because multiple interacting systems are so incredibly tightly intermeshed in the brain stem.[11]

In any event, because of the many emotional homologies that have been revealed across species, we must also now seriously consider that other animals possess a conscious appreciation, rudimentary though it may be, of their own personal circumstances in the world. Of course, a great deal of their perceptual consciousness as well as ours is sensory, but there are good reasons to conclude that they also can feel internal affective states in ways that are not remote from our own. A rabbit trying to evade a mountain lion may subjectively experience an emotional state of fear embedded within a cognitive context of having perceived and identified a threat, and it may have some automatized awareness of its behavioral options. The rabbit's consciousness is surely much more tightly constrained to the present than is ours because of the animal's comparatively modest frontal lobes. When a rabbit is in the midst of danger, it probably has little thought about the past and future. It is dealing with its present circumstances on a moment-to-moment basis. It is precisely those here-and-now states of consciousness that we must seek to understand before we can grasp how they come to be extended in time, as they are within the human mind through our frontal cortical time-extending and planning abilities.[12]

I will propose a conceptual scheme of how the brain may generate subjective feelings through the neural mechanisms of self-representation at a primitive motor and sensory level. As I have reflected on the current, rapidly expanding literature on the nature of consciousness, it seems that this view is still a novel one. It may also be closer to the truth than many of the others, or as remote as any of them. The only thing we can be confident about with regard to this difficult topic is that our doubts must still outweigh certainties, and that our ideas should be cast in ways that can lead to empirical tests.

We should also recognize that many dedicated investigators remain doubtful that there can be any credible science of consciousness. Many psychologists, neuroscientists, and philosophers believe that the transmogrification of brain processes into subjective experience may be inexplicable on the basis of first principles: There is simply no way to understand mental states that we all experience firsthand by applying the consensual observational approaches of our third-person scientific methodologies. Such concerns are profound and appropriate, and they can only be skirted by the development of new and indirect strategies such as the one advocated throughout this text. If one assumes or can demonstrate that the affective neuroscience approach simply cannot work, then the task is, most assuredly, undoable at least for emotional consciousness. I believe the skeptical views are wrong and counterproductive; the powerful lessons of 20th century particle physics suggest that a comparable highly theoretical but empirically constrained strategy might succeed in psychology and neuroscience. Only because of the advances in behavioral brain research is this matter now an empirical issue that must be resolved on the basis of the predictions that can be made.

A growing number of investigators[13] believe that the solution to the mind-body problem—namely, the *fundamental* nature of consciousness—can emerge only when we begin to theoretically blend "first-person" insights concerning primitive states of consciousness that we humans share with the other animals with "third-person" empirical observations that can be made in the behavioral brain research laboratory. I believe that if we deploy the full flexibility of empiricially guided theoretical inference (i.e., the so-called hypothetico-deductive method of traditional science), there is no unbridgeable chasm between the nature of subjective experience and relevant brain and behavioral facts that can be gathered through traditional scientific modes of inquiry. Before I proceed into the center of the hornet's nest of primary-process consciousness, let me dwell briefly on a few examples of the problems that arise when we begin to address such ephemeral matters scientifically.

Common Mistakes in Conceptualizing Psychological Functions in the Brain

In our continuing quest to reveal the natural order of brain processes (or, as the popular saying goes, "trying to carve nature at its joints"), will the search for affective consciousness in the brain of other mammals help reveal human realities, or will it take us down a misguided path of postulating brain functions that do not exist? Many examples of such mistakes come to mind from the history of the physical sciences—including "the ether," a nonexistent substance that was postulated to transport light in space, and "phlogiston," which was thought to do the same for heat. The history of functional brain research, rooted as it is in the phrenological tradition of postulating organs for mental faculties, still makes many of us shudder with shame for some of the gross oversimplifications of our predecessors.[14] Such mistakes remind us of the empty concepts that litter the history of science. Such "empty categories" and "block diagrams" are even easier to create in the psychological sciences, partly because of the complexity of the matters we seek to understand and partly because of the social nature of language, which, from an evolutionary vantage, was surely not designed for scientific discourse (see Appendix B). In any event, serious investigators of the brain are loathe to contribute more verbal rubbish to existing confusions so they are prone to remain silent on such matters.

Let me share one minor but instructive example of a conceptual mistake that has assumed the status of accepted fact in the popular imagination—the observation of "sexual cannibalism" in certain insects. On occasion, female praying mantises have been observed to consume the head parts of males that have pounced on them with copulatory intent (all presumably done unconsciously, of course). A functional evolutionary story has been generated that this type of "sexual cannibalism" emerged to release the natural sexual reserves of the male. By removing higher sources of inhibition, the female supposedly promotes (unconsciously again) unbridled copulation in her headless suitor. This type of beheading has been widely assumed to be an evolved behavioral strategy that helps ensure reproductive success.

Many even believe that evolution coaxed the male to offer his life (or, more accurately, his bodily energy) to help assure the female's ability to rear the next generation successfully. Are such tendencies toward "self-sacrifice" and "sexual cannibalism" real *sexual* repertoires of male and female mantises, or simply a myth created by scientists awed by the predatory rapaciousness of these creatures? Careful evaluation of the evidence now suggests that mantises are simply very predatory creatures and that cannibalistic tendencies are amplified by limitations imposed on their opportunity to hunt in captivity. Perhaps only because of certain experimental procedures (i.e., the use of isolation housing that precludes predation) do sexually eager males unwittingly come to gratify the female in more ways than one. There may, in fact, be no evolutionary connection between the two acts. The females merely grasp their opportunity to express predatory urges when males are copulating close at fang.[15] Thus, there may be no neural mechanism for sexual cannibalism or self-sacrifice within the nervous systems of female and male praying mantises.

It is certainly possible that other animals, despite their many emotional behaviors, have no internal experience of any ongoing emotional states. As asserted by René Descartes, who formally introduced dualism into our sciences almost 400 years ago, the other animals of the world may be more akin to reflexive robots than to the feeling creatures some of us believe them to be.[16] If this is so, a search for mechanisms of affective consciousness in the animal brain will be futile. However, it does *seem* self-evident to most observers that animals experience emotional states. Not only is this apparent in their outward behaviors, but it has now repeatedly been indexed by their motivation to exhibit various conditioned approach and avoidance behaviors. Other compelling lines of evidence come from psychopharmacology, where behavioral changes in animals can predict human clinical and subjective responses, and from brain stimulation studies, where the subjective responses of humans and the corresponding behavioral responses of animals are remarkably similar. Indeed, on a related topic, formal analysis of rat behavior has led to the conclusion that such creatures do exhibit some true intentionality.[17]

Hence, it seems likely that the pursuit of the underlying mechanisms of affective consciousness in the animal brain may help reveal the nature of homologous processes in the human brain/mind. If so, the eventual knowledge we may achieve by pursuing this path of reasoning may be more worthwhile than the rather sterile views promoted by the strict paths of logical positivism and skepticism (i.e., that only the consensual evidence arising from our visual system is to be believed in science). Instead, we should come to respect a new and more powerful criterion: Our ability to predict new observations should serve as the only credibility discriminator for various competing lines of thought.

A Rapprochement between Logical Positivism and Folk Psychology

It is obvious that the concepts we choose to guide our experimental inquiries must be as flexible and profound as the functional processes that actually exist in nature. The recent neuroscience revolution has finally provided the necessary tools and findings for a major rapprochement between the internally situated emotional powers long recognized in folk psychology and the subcortical neural controls that can be detailed through animal brain research. We can finally seek the neurobiological wellsprings, albeit not the diverse cultural consequences, of human emotionality by studying the neural mechanisms for affective experiences in other animals. Their emotions will surely not resemble the cognitively detailed and emotionally subtle experiences that fill our minds. But they may resemble the deeply felt, visceral emotions of children, which some adults again experience when they succumb to psychiatric disorders.

So how shall we ever understand how felt experience actually emerges from brain matter? Let me suggest a new brain process—one that is not as controversial in developmental psychology as it is in neuroscience: To really understand the basic affective states of consciousness, we may have to understand the primal nature of "the self." We need to fathom how humans and animals naturally come to experience themselves as active, feeling creatures in the world. To do so, we must learn to conceptualize subtle brain processes such as "the self" in neuroscientific terms. Such a neural entity, in its primordial form, may constitute the preconscious foundations for all other forms of consciousness—it may be the essential object of mature consciousness without which higher levels of consciousness could never have emerged. However, before I tackle this thorny issue, let me first dwell on several "higher types" of conscious awareness of which the human brain/mind is capable. This may ease our difficult journey into this central mystery of the animal mind—the nature of primary-process affective consciousness.

Obviously, within the human cortex, there is not just a single form of consciousness but various types of awareness, as indicated by changes that can result from damage to specific parts of the brain. The higher levels of consciousness give us awareness of the almost infinite regress of self-reflection: We can be conscious of being conscious of being conscious, and so on.[18] An initial consideration of these levels may help us distinguish the lower forms of consciousness. That will help us understand how emotional feelings are actually encoded within the intrinsic potentials of brain dynamics.

Higher Levels of Human Consciousness

There is great appeal in trying to find the keys to conscious activities within the higher sensory-perceptual reaches of the human brain. However, the functions of most higher brain areas may be more closely related to the neural computations required for specific skills—namely, the various "tools of consciousness"—as opposed to the construction of primary-process consciousness itself. For instance, although we are getting close to understanding the conscious experience of vision, few are tempted to argue that elimination of visual abilities or any other single sensory system markedly impairs primary-process consciousness.[19]

The most discrete disruptions of perceptual awareness occur as a result of various forms of cortical damage. One of the most striking is the loss of consciously appreciated vision following damage to the occipital cortex. Although individuals with these impairments report being completely blind, they can accurately identify the locations of moving objects in their visual fields. This "blindsight" has perplexed students of consciousness, for it highlights how wrong our conscious understanding of our behavioral abilities can be. It seems likely that blindsight is mediated by our ancient frog-type visual abilities, seated in the superior colliculi of the midbrain. That ancient visual system allows all animals to identify *where* objects are in visual space without being able to decode *what* they are. Our higher levels of conscious awareness are no longer well tuned to movement information in the absence of object information. Such blindsight leaves only a vague feeling of something having happened.[20]

Comparable types of effects have been found with the loss of face-recognition abilities, or *prosapagnosia*, following damage to the bottom surface of the temporal lobes and the neglect of personal space following damage to the parietal lobe, especially when these forms of damage are situated in the right hemisphere. Such *agnosias* clearly tell us how important specific types of cortical information are for constructing a detailed awareness of our world. Not only are afflicted individuals still able to identify others by their tone of voice and by the clothes they wear, they can still process incoming facial information at a preconscious level. For instance, people with prosapagnosia still selectively exhibit galvanic skin responses to familiar faces, indicating that their autonomic nervous systems remain in touch with the facial features of the people they have known.[21] We do not know whether this type of autonomic information is simply unable to be represented in consciousness, or whether it has come to be neglected during development because of the power of the more salient types of visual information—namely, it became a "preconscious" ability. I would assume that the latter is true, and that such alternative channels of information can be made more salient within affective consciousness through emotional education (i.e., by training people to get in closer touch with their feelings).

Phenomena such as blindsight and prosapagnosia highlight how powerfully preconscious perceptual processes may control our behavior. Such findings have generally led to the widespread view that the contents of consciousness are mediated by very specific neocortical functions. As a consequence, it is now commonly believed that most subcortical processes operate unconsciously. However, this is far from true. By comparison to cortical damage, very small lesions of subcortical areas can severely compromise human consciousness, and electrical and chemical stimulation at many subcortical sites can have effects on affective consciousness that cannot be matched by any form of cortical stimulation.[22] Still, because of such examples, we should obviously remain cautious in trying to understand conscious awareness in animals by simply interpreting their outward behaviors. Special behavioral assays need to be conducted before such conclusions are warranted. When we do use procedures such as conditioned place preference and avoidance, a mass of data from animals as well as humans suggests that the fundamental sources for affective and intentional consciousness are subcortical, but they are also represented in higher regions.

Split-Brain Data and the Subcortical Sources of Consciousness

A subcortical location for the essential mechanisms of consciousness can be derived from the many fascinating studies of "split-brain" individuals in whom the corpus callosum has been severed, eliminating the main communication channels between the two cerebral hemispheres. Although such data are more commonly used to argue that human conscious awareness is cortically elaborated, the continued unity of primary-process consciousness and a primal form of behavioral intentionality following the splitting of the human brain are also striking.

Although each hemisphere can have independent realms of perceptual awareness, cogitate independently, and have distinct emotional communication styles, careful behavioral observation of split-brain individuals yields an additional overriding conclusion: Despite massive hemispheric disconnection, the deep and essential coherence of each person's personality and his or her sense of unity appears to remain intact. Most forms of intentionality and deep emotional feelings are not split in any obvious way by a parting of the hemispheres. Only the cognitive interpretations of specific events are affected. For instance, when one side of the brain is exposed to a sexually arousing visual stimulus, the other side feels the arousal but is not able to interpret the precipitating event correctly and often dissembles and rationalizes.[23] The unity of an underlying form of consciousness in split-brain individuals, perhaps their fundamental sense of self, is affirmed by the fact that the disconnected hemispheres can no more easily execute two cognitive tasks simultaneously than can the brains of normal individuals.[24] The inability to distribute attention simultaneously to two tasks is a characteristic feature of a unified consciousness in neurologically intact individuals. In split-brain people, a central workshop of consciousness,[25] which simultaneously influences both hemispheres, continues to limit distribution of attentional resources.

Only with special procedures can we demonstrate distinct types of cognitive and affective styles, as well as perceptions and information-processing strengths within each hemisphere.[26] To put it simply, the left hemisphere is generally more socially communicative and seemingly happier than the right hemisphere, while the right side is more reserved and prone to feel intense negative emotions and to become depressed.[27] Even though it is clear that the right and left hemispheres have different affective styles, this does not mean that the affect they help weave can be generated without subcortical inputs. It is possible that the distinct affective abilities of the hemispheres arise from how they handle ascending emotional messages from subcortical circuits. This possibility has been explored in some detail.[28] It is also noteworthy that in day-to-day activities, the longitudinally severed hemispheres of split-brain people rarely meddle with each other's affairs. For instance, when a split-brain individual dives into a swimming pool, there are no behavioral signs, such as one side of the body flailing, to suggest that half of the brain has been taken by surprise. Thus, the most impressive message is that despite a massive division of the major toolboxes of human consciousness, split-brain individuals still operate as coherent wholes in the affective, intentional, and motor conduct of their daily lives. Thus, the foundations for our subjectively experienced core of being must lie deeper within the brain than the cerebral hemispheres. Indeed, there are many subcortical channels for interhemispheric communication of information that could sustain coherence between the two hemispheres.

A similar conclusion is evident from the study of animals that have been decorticated early in life: They sustain a remarkably strong level of behavioral coherence and spontaneity. Indeed, as mentioned in the previous chapter, college students asked to observe two animals, one normal and one decorticate, typically mistake one for the other. This arises from the fact that decorticates are generally more active, while the normal animals appear more timid. Students tend to believe that the energized affective behavior is an indication of normality. The ability of such decorticate animals to compete effectively with normal animals during bouts of rough-and-tumble play is further testimony to the likelihood that internal self-coherence is subcortically organized.[29]

Such diverse lines of evidence, taken together, suggest that the essential "core of being" is subcortical. In my estimation, it was first elaborated in brain evolution within central motor–type regions of the midbrain—in periventricular and surrounding areas of the midbrain and diencephalon that are richly connected with higher limbic and paleocortical zones. These brain areas appear to be the most likely sources for the primal neural mechanisms that generate affective states of consciousness. It will be argued that those primordial circuits may elaborate a fundamental sense of "self" within the brain. Although this is not a very skilled and intelligent self and its pervasive influence may often seem preconscious (especially when higher forms of consciousness have matured during ontogenetic development), it ultimately allows animals to develop into the intentional, volitional, and cognitively selective creatures that they are.[30] It may do this in part by providing a basic body image that can control primitive attentional and intentional focus. I will assume that such archaic brain functions provide a fundamental reference point for the development of more sophisticated levels of competence throughout the rest of the nervous system.

If, as John Milton suggested, "The child is father of the man," a primordial sense of self may ultimately be mother to all higher forms of consciousness. This is not to imply that higher forms of conscious awareness do not require higher brain mechanisms, only that the elaboration of conscious abilities in the brain germinates and sprouts from a primal neural field that intrinsically represents a basic body image within the brain stem. This mechanism is shared by all mammals, and it is presumably grounded in various intrinsic circuits that exhibit spontaneous types of oscillatory activity. Because of the different paths of cortical evolution in different species, and distinct forms of higher epigenetically derived paths of cognitive development among different individuals of a species, these primal mechanisms come to be manifested in many ways. To simplify my analysis, I will focus, once more, on essential evolutionary sources rather than on their ultimate manifestations.

Obviously, humans can have contents within their conscious awareness that other animals never have, and vice versa. Simply consider the importance of language for the temporal extension and deepening of human thought, the sophisticated olfactory abilities of the rat and the ability of bats to represent the world in auditory coordinates. It is as unlikely that classical speech areas of the brain mediate the elemental infrastructure of primary-process consciousness in humans as it is that the auditory cortex or olfactory bulbs do so for bats and rats. Many of us know individuals with left hemisphere strokes who in most realms act as do unimpaired individuals, even though they can no longer use language effectively. In short, one can damage many higher parts of the brain, eliminating specific cognitive abilities, but the organism's internally sustained neural representation of itself as a coherent creature remains intact. Likewise, following damage to higher motor areas, people can be paralyzed while sustaining the internal experience that they are not. Just ask a hemiplegic person, paralyzed on one side because of a stroke to the opposite side of the brain. Such individuals typically retain the internal feeling that they can still move the impaired limb. This is a motor counterpart to the common feeling of amputees that they still have their missing body parts (i.e., the experience of "phantom limbs").[31]

In sum, following many forms of higher brain damage, an individual's "center of being" or "sense of self" appears to be intact. Is there, in fact, such a center of being within the brain, or is it a mere mythical entity?

No one knows for sure, but here I will develop the position, probably uncontroversial to most neuroscientists, that a variety of key processes centered in the ancient circuits of the brain stem are absolutely essential for the creation of consciousness within the brain. For instance, there is general agreement that the extended ascending reticular activating system, including thalamic reticular nuclei, is necessary for normal waking and attentional activities.[32] However, I think we have almost totally ignored one of the ancient foundation processes—a neurosymbolic affective representation of I-ness or "the self" that may be critically linked to a primitive motor representation within the brain stem. It is easy to overlook this motor foundation for consciousness when we are continually entranced by the seemingly endless forms of sensory-perceptual awareness. However, I would suggest that the self-referential coherence provided by ancient and stable motor coordinates may be the very foundation for the unity of all higher forms of consciousness.

A Proposal concerning the Fundamentally Affective Nature of Primal Consciousness

No matter how one views it, discussions of consciousness resemble the heads of Hydra—from each severed observer, many others can sprout. To use this slightly mixed metaphor, each observer gazes at the others, wondering if there is some more powerful observer who can see all the rest, leaving all to ponder the infinite regress of who is observing the observer, and so forth. Is there a primal monitoring function within the brain, one that observes but is not observed? Many, including myself, believe there is no such entity.[33] In anticipation of the main point of this chapter, I will suggest just the reverse—that there is a coherent foundational process, or "self-representation," that does not observe in the conventional sense but is observed or at least strongly "intermeshed" with various higher perceptual processes. In other words, the self-schema provides input into many sensory analyzers, and it is also strongly influenced by the primal emotional circuits discussed in the previous chapters. These interactions may constitute affective consciousness. This foundation process—the primordial self-schema—was first laid out in stable motor coordinates within the brain stem. It not only helps guide many higher perceptual processes, by promoting attentional focus and perceptual sensitivity, but also may provide a fundamental stability for the psychological "binding" that is characteristic of our perceptual field. Presumably, this foundation process is not *directly* influenced by higher contents of consciousness, although it may be strongly and automatically modified by various other influences—by conditioned emotional "triggers," by meditation, by music, dance, and probably a variety of other rhythmic sensory-motor inputs and activities.

To facilitate discussion, I shall henceforth refer to this "it" as the SELF—a Simple Ego-type Life Form—deep within the brain. At present, our knowledge about this brain function is so rudimentary that we can only generate "best guesses" as to its nature. I will advance one proposal with some confidence, since it squares with known facts and yields testable hypotheses. I will advocate the view that the SELF first arises during early development from a coherently organized motor process in the midbrain, even though it surely comes to be rerepresented in widely distributed ways through higher regions of the brain as a function of neural and psychological maturation. Not only does this archaic SELF-representation network control motor tone and some simple orienting responses, its intrinsic rhythms can be transiently modulated by a wide array of regulatory inputs, and it is highly interactive with all the basic emotional circuits discussed in this book. Feelings may emerge when *endogenous sensory* and *emotional systems* within the brain that receive direct inputs from the outside world as well as the neurodynamics of the SELF begin to reverberate with each other's changing neuronal firing rhythms.

By directly modifying the intrinsic neurodynamics of the SELF, emotional circuits establish the conditions by which the essential neural conditions for affective consciousness are created. Here I will argue that the changing neurodynamics of the extended representation of SELF networks are essential for generating subjective emotional feelings in all mammalian brains. Thereby, the neurodynamic ripples of various affective codes may spread widely through the brain. The interaction of these neurodynamics with the sensory analyzers of the thalamus and cortex and the motor systems they regulate allows organisms the possibility of various species-typical modes of emotional SELF-expression and SELF-regulation. The ensuing affective states may be the internally experienced regulatory value signals around which much of animal behavioral and cognitive activity revolves. Organisms aspire to maximize certain states of the system and to minimize others.

Considering this possibility, I would argue that basic affective states, which initially arise from the changing neurodynamics of a SELF-representation mechanism, may provide an essential psychic scaffolding for all other forms of consciousness. Thus, a primitive affective awareness may have been an evolutionary prerequisite for the emergence of perceptual-cognitive awareness. If so, computational and sensory-perceptual approaches to consciousness must take affective bodily representations into account if their higher extrapolations are to be correct. From such a vantage, Descartes's faith in his assertion "I think, therefore I am" may be superseded by a more primitive affirmation that is part of the genetic makeup of all mammals: "I feel, therefore I am."[34]

Evolutionary Relations between Primary-Process and Secondary Forms of Consciousness

To get at the root of primary-process consciousness empirically, one will surely need to distinguish between the varieties and sources of distinct conscious abilities in different species and the shared neural foundations across species. For instance, other animals obviously do not have linguistic consciousness, although they no doubt have some complex ideas that emerge from the association cortices that eventually led to the evolution of linguistic abilities in humans. The emergence of a multimodal association cortex capable of constructing ideas by intermixing information from various senses surely preceded the ability of such tissues to represent those ideas in concrete symbols such as grunts and eventually words.[35] Thus, while the mental activity that emerges from multimodal association cortex in humans can now focus on the detailed meanings of words, the integration of information in similar brain regions of other animals may create comparatively simple holistic perceptions and appraisals. For instance, the apparent sound or smell of a predator at a certain location means that danger may be nearby, perhaps leading to the automatic evocation of wariness—fearful internal feelings and images of potential predators along with some simple strategies to avoid them. In other words, the cognitive and affective contents of consciousness may become inextricably intertwined within the highest forms of neural symbolization that can be created by the animal's cortex.

Presumably, some of the neural connections that instantiate such internal images arise from neural computations that occur in rapid eye movement (REM) sleep (see Chapter 7). Unfortunately, such cognitive issues are horrendously difficult to analyze neuroscientifically. Short of someone identifying neurophysiological or chemical markers for the animal's internal representations, such issues are scientifically unworkable.[36] Such difficulties help highlight why the study of spatiotemporal abilities, as opposed to internal images, is such a popular topic of study in the field of animal cognitions. It is comparatively easy to determine how animals use cognitive strategies with reference to measurable events in the outside world.[37] Although the various brain-imaging technologies are now providing a glimmer of the higher cognitive-emotional interactions in human brains, it would be premature to conclude that these representations actually reflect the fundamental affective substrates in action.[38] Most of the affect-related brain changes observed so far may be more closely aligned with the cognitive contents of different affective states rather than with the primary-process affective states themselves. The types of work that are needed to reveal the latter are direct chemical and electrical stimulation procedures that arouse emotional states unconditionally—work that is best done in animals.

Conceptualizations of SELF-Consciousness

For the present purposes, primary-process consciousness will not be conceptualized simply as the "awareness of external events in the world" but rather as *that ineffable feeling of experiencing oneself as an active agent in the perceived events of the world.* Such a primitive SELF-representation presumably consists of an intrinsically reverberating neural network linked to basic body tone and gross axial movement generators. It may provide a coherent matrix in which a variety of sensory stimuli become hedonically valenced. In other words, primary-process consciousness is probably rooted in fairly low-level brain circuits that first represented the body as an intrinsic and coherent whole. When other incoming stimuli, both internal and external, interact with this body schema and establish new kinds of reafferent reverberations,[39] the potential for an internal state of affective awareness is created. Obviously, for such an entity to have adaptive value, it must be able to control certain basic motor and attentional processes.[40]

This type of analysis suggests that the brain substrate of "the SELF," and hence primary-process consciousness, has certain explicit attributes. Contrary to some traditional religious and philosophical thought on the matter (i.e., concerning the nature of the soul), the SELF has concrete neuroanatomical, neurochemical, and neurophysiological characteristics. First, it should be ancient in brain evolution and hence situated near the core of the brain. Also, one would expect that it would be richly connected to the rest of the brain, both higher and lower areas, presumably more richly than any other area of the brain stem.[41] It would be highly multimodal, allowing for rerepresentation at many levels of the neuroaxis during ontogenetic development. With the emergence of such rerepresentations, a variety of recursive observers and observers of observers seems to emerge within the maturing fabric of the brain. Presumably such higher SELF reverberations would typically operate in coordinated fashion with the lower substrates, but the possibility of semi-independent action may also emerge.

According to such a view, emotional feelings, as well as the unique character of various emotional behaviors, may arise from the ways in which the basic emotional command circuits modulate neuronal reverberations or resonances within these extended representations of the SELF. FEAR circuits may push the SELF-schema into an "up-tight," shivery state of tension. RAGE circuits may pressure it into an invigorated cycle of forceful actions, and so on. These changes in the ongoing neurodynamics of the SELF would set the stage for a variety of discrete emotional behaviors and mood-congruent forms of information processing. It would also establish a homeostatic "set point" or "settling point" (see Chapter 8) whereby various emotional self-regulatory strategies could be established.

In sharing this viewpoint about the sources of consciousness, I am affirming a truism of 20th century behavioral science: Evolution can mold brain functions only by inducing changes that modify the efficacy of behaviors. Affective representations promote certain classes of behavior patterns, and with the additional evolution of various highly differentiated sensory and motor tools, affective states may increasingly provide an internal reference point for more complex abilities. Thus, in complex organisms such as human adults, affective feelings may arise from a build-up of reverberations in the extending SELF-schema, which is experienced as a mounting sense of "force" or "pressure" to behave in a certain way. With psychological development, organisms may develop a variety of counterregulatory strategies, ranging from various cognitive-perceptual reorientations to the withholding of behavior patterns. In other words, since the basic emotions provide fairly simpleminded solutions to problems, it would be adaptive for organisms to be able to generate alternative plans. Still, such newly evolved brain abilities may continue to be referenced to the affectively experienced neurodynamic status of the primal SELF. To put it quite simply: Animals may adjust their behaviors by the way the behaviors make them feel.

We cannot be confident of the predominant anatomical source of the primal SELF in the brain, but two areas recommend themselves—the deep cerebellar nuclei, which receive a great deal of primitive sensory and emotional information and control body movements, especially those guided by sensory feedback, and the centromedial areas of the midbrain, including the deep layers of the colliculi and the periventricular gray, which do the same. Many believe these areas are too low in the neuroaxis to create consciously perceived affect, but this is certainly not so during infancy and early childhood. Because removal of the cerebellum does not severely compromise consciousness, I favor the option that the centromedial zones of the midbrain are the very epicenter of the primordial SELF (see Figure 16.1).[42]

A SELF-Referencing Mechanism in the Brain: A Foundation for Primary-Process Affective Consciousness?

Recently, and without much data to bear on the issue, it has become fashionable to question the existence of central agencies within the brain that permit conscious awareness. Many claim that there is no coherent neural referent for the pronoun "I." Contrary to that trend, I would advocate the position that such a central processor (albeit perhaps not an observer) does exist within the "Cartesian theater"—a current philosophical catchphrase for the neural work space of consciousness within the brain.[43] Thus, a key element in the present conception of primary-process consciousness is the SELF—an ancient neural process for the generation of spontaneous emotional actions that *is observed* within the Cartesian theater by a series of more recently evolved "monitors" or sensory-perceptul processors. It is assumed that with the aid of such a primal SELF-referencing mechanism, deviations from a resting state came to be represented as states of action readiness and as affective feelings. Further, this central faculty may have served as a critical neural vector for the evolution of a variety of higher forms of consciousness that humans spill out so casually with phrases such as "I felt this" and "I felt that."

As already mentioned, traditional contemplations about the nature of conscious awareness have led thinkers to envision an infinite regress of sensory homunculi observing each other ad infinitum. It is obviously quite difficult to contemplate how an ultimate observer could ever have evolved. The existence of an archaic SELF-network, especially one that is referenced in motor coordinates, can help solve this dilemma and others as well: All higher monitors are entranced by a central process that itself does not observe but exists in the very center of the Cartesian theater as the primordial neurosymbolic representation of the core of each individual existence. The SELF does not have thoughts or clearly defined perceptions, but it does help elaborate primitive feelings, and it serves as an anchor that stabilizes or "binds" many other brain processes.

At a practical neurobiological level, the postulated existence of a primitive motor-action homunculus that is the primal representation of the SELF allows us to envision ways in which primary-process consciousness can begin to be empirically studied. In its essential state, I assume the SELF provides the first executive mechanism for behavioral coherence and bodily awareness. In neural representational terms, the SELF may be topographically like a body of quite primordial shape. Perhaps an image of a stingray may serve as an approximate metaphor here. While it is reasonable to assume that the SELF is not unchanging but becomes more sophisticated in the course of both ontogeny and phylogeny, this is more likely due to the addition of new layers of neural control as opposed to a reshaping of the original form.

The intrinsic neurodynamics of the archaic SELF may be a primary influence in guiding the neurodevelopmental maturation of higher levels of consciousness, perhaps through various iterative bootstrapping processes, whereby closely interconnected brain areas begin to resonate with the inherent neurodynamics of the lower substrates. Also, the existence of use-dependent neuronal growth factors (see Chapter 6), which guide the development of certain patterns of brain interconnectivities, may contribute to the neuronal maturation of the SELF through higher regions of the neuroaxis. Such spreading epigenetic interactions may help make certain higher brain circuits more permeable to lower influences, leading to a sense of SELF and a feeling of internal coherence or discoherence that are represented ever more widely in the brain as organisms develop and mature. Thus the developmental reflections of the SELF may eventually come to reside in many brain areas, in individualized ways, thereby providing higher brain circuits a concrete value focus for their complex deliberations about the external world. Presumably this immigration would at least initially be controlled by the richness of intrinsic, genetically and epigenetically guided connectivities of the basic SELF circuits with higher brain areas.[44]

This, I believe, is the type of primitive but developmentally flexible and intrinsically dynamic substrate of consciousness that we should be seeking deep within the brain stem—not the final observer, not the ultimate perceptual monitor in the Cartesian theater, but a spontaneously active "stage manager" that helps create a neuropsychic focus of existence for a multitude of higher observers that emerge as the SELF-process migrates through higher regions of the brain, especially the frontal, temporal, and cingulate regions of the cortex.[45] Thus, fully developed consciousness is reflected in hierarchical but recursive sets of neural processors, all still rooted in some primal aspects of SELF ontogenesis.

I will now elaborate the idea that the primary template or "seed" of the SELF process, and hence the roots of primary-process consciousness, reside deep within medial zones of the brain stem. In one sense this is an uncontroversial issue, since the reticular formation of the brain stem, with extensions into the thalamus and hypothalamus, has long been considered an essential substrate for conscious, attentional activities (see Chapter 7). However, in another sense, what I suggest here is significantly different from, albeit complementary with, that view. Rather than focusing on the basic waking and attentional systems of the ascending reticular activating system (ARAS), which certainly allow higher brain areas to work efficiently, I will now develop the idea that the deep layers of the colliculi and underlying circuits of the periaqueductal gray (PAG) are the neuroanatomical focus of the intrinsic motor SELF (Figure 16.1).

A remarkable amount of neuropsychological and neurobehavioral evidence is consistent with such a possibility. The deeper layers of the colliculi constitute a basic motor mapping system of the body, which interacts not only with visual, auditory, vestibular, and somatosensory sytems but also with nearby emotional circuits of the PAG. The PAG elaborates a different, visceral-type map of the body along with basic neural representations of pain, fear, anger, separation distress, sexual, and maternal behavior systems (as summarized throughout this text). Adjacent to the PAG is the mesencephalic locomotor region, which is capable of instigating neural patterns that would have to be an essential substrate for setting up various coherent action tendencies.[46] If one had to select between these functions (the motor or sensory zones of the tectum) as the very focus of the SELF process, I am inclined to envision the motor map as being more central to the SELF than the incoming somatosensory processes. This is based partly on evolutionary considerations: A level of motor coherence had to exist before there would be utility for sensory guidance. Neurophysiological evidence also indicates that the somatomotor, eye-movement map that borders the PAG is intrinsically a more stable tectal circuit than are the overlying sensory maps of the superior colliculi. While the superficial layers of the su-

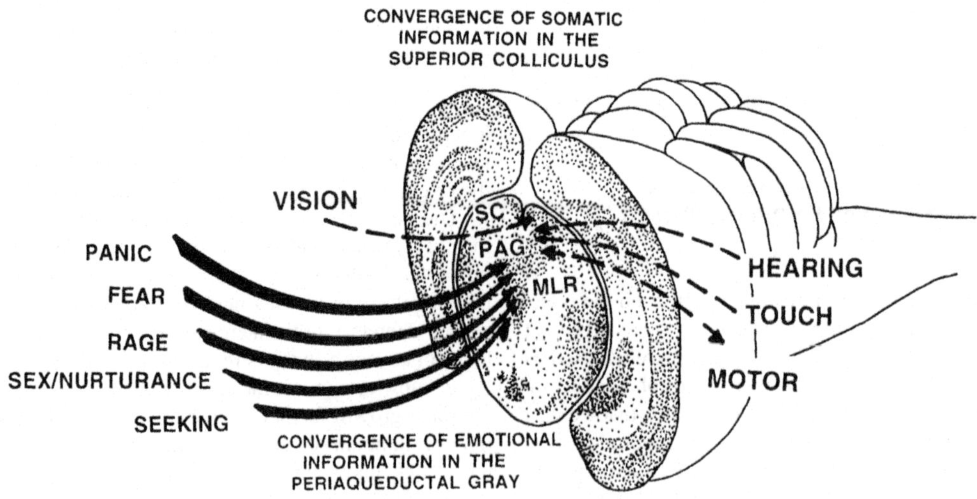

Figure 16.1. Overview of mesencephalic organization of convergent somatic and emotional processes in the interface area of the periaqueductal gray (PAG) and the superior colliculi (SC) of the tectum. The adjacent mesencephalic locomotor region (MLR) can generate coherent forward locomotion.

perior colliculi flexibly harvest information about the location of visual stimuli, the underlying motor system generates appropriate orienting movements using what appears to be a remarkably stable set of action coordinates. In other words, the sensory maps of the tectum appear to shift markedly in reference to stable motor coordinates when the motor map initiates specific actions.[47] I take this stability of the somatomotor system to indicate that it has primacy in the evolution of the psychobehavioral coherence that this system spontaneously generates. In addition, the underlying PAG tissues, which contain representations of all emotional processes, may constitute an even deeper and more primitive visceral SELF. To keep things relatively simple, for the present purposes the somatic and visceral components will be considered as an interactive unity.

The mesencephalic roots of the SELF, through its many neural connections with higher brain areas, help us envision, albeit dimly, the emergence of higher forms of self-consciousness. The deep tectal and underlying PAG zones are more richly connected with frontal motor areas, where plans and intentions are generated, than with posterior sensory areas, where perceptions are constructed. Again, in selecting one or the other of these large cortical regions of the brain—sensory or motor—as being more closely linked with primal consciousness, the frontal cortex clearly has a great deal to commend it. To establish behavioral priorities in time, the frontal cortex needs to *actively* retrieve perceptual information from sensory cortices. It is also significant that more powerful personality changes result from frontal cortical damage than from comparable damage to posterior sensory areas.[48]

It should be recalled that the frontal areas are the motor association or planning cortex. Thus, even though the exteroceptive contents of consciousness are obviously created by sensory zones, those zones must send massive outputs into the motor areas in order for coherent behavior to occur. I suspect this has led many thinkers to mistake sensory awareness for consciousness itself, as opposed to the toolbox of consciousness that it really is. In sum, I would suggest that a careful consideration of all issues indicates that primary-process affective and intentional consciousness is more critically linked to motor than to sensory cortices. This is not to deny the importance of sensory-perceptual processes in the guidance of behavior, but to make a distinction between the essential foundations of consciousness and the contents of consciousness. The contents of consciousness (which I would consider a secondary or derivative form of consciousness) are obviously created from the various sensory-perceptual processes—visual, auditory, somatosensory, olfactory, gustatory, vestibular, and kinesthetic—to which may be added the various thinking and cognitive operations that allow these systems to be interrelated. I assume that primary-process consciousness is more than that, and it resides in the intrinsic action-readiness of the system. I assume the action-readiness system provides a massive stability for the perceptual apparatus, and that it is essential for the retrieval of information from those toolboxes of consciousness. Changes in the neural activities of primary-process SELF-schema, I assume, constitute the changing nature of affective consciousness.

A Putative Neuroanatomical Roots for Primary-Process Consciousness

The massive and unparalleled convergence of information onto a simple and ancient body representation makes the centromedial areas of the midbrain an excellent candidate for the basic integrative framework that provided a neural scaffolding for a primitive neurodynamic of emotional SELF-awareness. As mentioned, this may have been achieved by the ability of the SELF-map to establish a characteristic resting tone within the somatic and visceral musculatures. The establishment of such a tone throughout the body and brain, along with a variety of reafferent processes, may have provided each organism with the feeling of individuality—of "I-ness." Upward influences into higher parts of the brain may have been achieved through the control of certain neural rhythms (e.g., delta, theta, alpha, beta, and gamma) that appear to have general properties in the control of exteroceptive information processing.[49]

This postulated SELF-schema presumably can trigger basic forms of bodily orientation and promote the extraction of values from the interaction of the internal milieu with environmental incentive stimuli. It may not be exceedingly difficult to imagine how such a system might generate intrinsic biological meaning structures within the organism. For instance, brain hormone detectors that instigate sexual urges may do so partly by promoting a natural copulatory LUST-type neurorhythm within the SELF-schema. This rhythm would reverberate through the body and, at a cultural level, find representation in the varieties of dance. Hence, certain types of music, such as the pulsing rhythms of rock and roll, may help simulate a sexual neural reverberation in the brain, promoting energetic forms of dance with strong pelvic movements. Other rhythms may promote the expression of other affects that can be expressed in dance, or simply felt. For instance, the "chills" discussed in the "Afterthought" of Chapter 14 may reflect a local sound-induced isolation-type change within the neural representation of the primal SELF. If various emotional and regulatory inputs modulate the SELF-schema in distinct ways (each with a characteristic neurodynamic and neurochemical signature), the internal result may be a large number of subjectively experienced feeling states.

Although one might fault this schema by noting its failure to specify the exact manner in which subjective experience emerges from neurodynamics, that shortcoming may reflect our human inability to verbally symbolize the operations of complex, intrinsically active neural systems in action. At such levels of ultracomplexity, where our human imagination does not reach, we have to rely on the power of predictions. For instance, from the preceding analyses, I would suggest that the emotional power of music may arise from auditory inputs from the inferior colliculi invading the underlying emotional circuits of the PAG. Also, if this hypothesis is essentially correct, extensive damage to the PAG should have disastrous effects on all forms of conscious activity, while more modest damage should dampen many affective tendencies.

Indeed, extensive PAG damage does produce a spectacular deterioration of all conscious activities, but to achieve that, the damage must extend along the whole length of the PAG. For instance, early studies in which lesioning electrodes were threaded from the fourth ventricle up the aqueduct to the caudal edge of the diencephalon yielded striking deficits in consciousness in cats and monkeys as operationalized by their failure to exhibit any apparent intentional behavior and their global lack of responsivity to emotional stimuli.[50] While forms of damage to many other higher areas of the brain can damage the "tools of consciousness," they typically do not impair the foundation of intentionality itself. PAG lesions do this with the smallest absolute destruction of brain tissue.[51] Moreover, lower intensities of electrical stimulation in this brain zone will arouse animals to a greater variety of coordinated emotional actions than stimulation at any other brain location. Accordingly, as a provisional hypothesis, I would suggest that the foundation of the most basic form of conscious activity, the generation of SELF-representation along with various basic affective states, arises from the intrinsic neurodynamics of the PAG, as well as the direct extensions of this tissue upward in the brain to intralaminar and midline thalamic areas, to widespread hypothalamic areas, and to various branches of the cerebral canopy.

Although it may seem unlikely that PAG tissue is sufficiently high along the neuroaxis to elaborate conscious awareness and intentionality, this doubt may be based more on our human pride in our extensive neocortical perceptual skills than on a critical evaluation of the empirical evidence and a consideration of what the foundation of consciousness must be like. Although high-level cognitive awareness is certainly not a local property of the PAG, such functions do emerge from the many higher brain areas that are especially closely linked to the PAG, including the frontal cortex.[52] As we have seen in so many of the preceding chapters, many affective processes seems to be intimately linked to networks that are interconnected with the PAG. To the best of our knowledge, this tissue is the most primal source of the anguished pain and suffering that suffuse consciousness during stressful circumstances. It is here that all forms of pain leave strong neuronal footprints, as indicated by *cfos* and Fos neuronal labeling. It is the PAG that allows creatures to first cry out in distress and pleasure.[53] It is largely here that pain arouses the unconditional state of fearfulness,[54] even though learning allows many other inputs, especially those from the amygdala and hippocampus, to also access the SELF.[55] All this is consistent with the postulate that our basic biological values, essential ingredients for a sense of self, are inextricably intertwined with the local properties of PAG tissue.

In sum, I doubt if we can explain secondary or higher contents of consciousness without first coming to terms with primitive SELF-representations and the ancient attentional work spaces with which they interact. Without the activities that transpire at the lower levels, the higher cerebral "observers" probably could not function efficiently, and if they could, they would probably suffer major deficits[56] as they stared into empty psychoaffective space. If all of the preceding is on the right track, we may eventually be able to measure the affective consciousness of animals in action by using modern electrophysiological and neurochemical techniques, especially when our probes are properly situated within the mesencephalic substrates of the SELF.[57] It is unfortunate that these brain areas are so inaccessible for analysis in humans, but neurochemical knowledge may eventually yield insights that can be evaluated using pharmacological probes.

The Neurochemistry of Consciousness

The primordial SELF is most probably organized around universally important, rapidly acting amino acid transmitter circuits such as glutamate. The closely related ARAS attentional networks, on the other hand, appear to have acetylcholine and norepinephrine at their core.[58] In addition, the SELF network may receive feedback concerning affective states via the many converging neuropeptide systems discussed throughout this book. Each separate emotional input may modify the reverberatory activity of the SELF in characteristic ways. Such changes in neural activity may ultimately be experienced as different emotional states of being. Obviously, the SELF mechanism also must have powerful outputs to control various higher brain activities as well as behaviors. The presence of nearby ascending serotonin, norepinephrine, and acetylcholine circuits provides such generalized neural substrates. Each of these systems has powerful and coherent effects on higher brain activities, yielding several ways in which all brain activity can be molded and controlled. For instance, cholinergic influences in the thalamus sustain processing in all sensory channels of the cortex and thereby control the flow of information that generates the perceptual contents of consciousness. Indeed, specific nuclei of the thalamus, the intralaminar nuclei and most especially the nucleus reticularis, may be critical for controlling the informational work space through which the specific contents of consciousness are created.[59] Although acetylcholine and GABA are key players in such thalamic functions, there are bound to be others. As we have seen in previous chapters, it is through specific neurochemical theories that most testable ideas concerning the nature of emotions, and thereby of primary-process affective consciousness, will be forged in the foreseeable future.

Although many neurochemical systems can modulate affective processes,[60] a key issue is whether disruptions of any single system will compromise all forms of affective consciousness without impairing general perceptual awareness. No such item is known at present, suggesting the two may be tightly linked. It seems certain that glutamate transmission is essential for both, for the simple reason that glutamate antagonists provoke such remarkable changes in the quality of consciousness. Drugs such as phencyclidine (PCP, street name "angel dust") dissociate sensory and motor processes to the point where cognitive coherence disintegrates.[61] Mild doses can cause panic attacks, while at high doses waking consciousness is so impaired that treated animals can undergo surgery without further anesthetic. Likewise, a study of the brain sites and mechanisms by which general anesthetics operate should provide key insights into the neurochemical nature of consciousness.[62]

Advances in clinical medicine have brought us many anesthetic agents that can completely compromise conscious activities. If we could identify the major brain circuits that such manipulations act upon, we would have the beginnings of a substantive neuroanatomy of consciousness. Unfortunately, critical sites in the brain remain to be identified, but judging by the evidence offered here concerning the nature of the SELF, I would predict that consciousness would be compromised most when such agents are placed into the PAG tissues of the midbrain and closely connected reticular areas of the diencephalon, perhaps all the way up to the front of the neural tube at the septal area.

Anesthetics have been used in novel ways to highlight the nature of consciousness in the human brain. In the study of epilepsy, neurologists have developed what is now called the *Wada test*, whereby short-acting barbiturate anesthetics are injected into one or the other carotid artery (see Figure 4.6), leading to a brief anesthetization of one whole cerebral mantle. Since much of the injection enters the anterior and lateral cerebral arteries, it is generally assumed that most of the effects are cortically as opposed to subcortically mediated. When one selectively "knocks out" the right cerebral hemisphere in this way, patients usually express little emotional concern about the matter, claiming everything is just fine; when the anesthetic wears off, they change their minds rapidly, making statements of their displeasure with the manipulation. This has led to the idea that each of the cerebral hemispheres can have distinct emotional feelings, which, if true, will tell us much about the higher nature of affective consciousness.[63]

In this vein, it is important to emphasize that scientists typically only respect theories that can be empirically evaluated, and those who are interested in the nature of consciousness should be willing to provide paradigmatic experiments that would highlight the workings of their theories. For me, the most telling experiments will be those that attempt to reveal the brain sites and neural mechanisms by which anesthetics operate and the study of the brain mechanisms that mediate affective experiences such as simple gustatory pleasures and aversion, as well as various forms of pain.[64] However, such primitive affective functions must link up with higher sensory-perceptual analyzers of the cortex.

Reflections of Emotions in the Higher Reaches of the Brain

Although the basic emotional "energies" arise from subcortical processes, the external details of emotional experiences are obviously encoded in the neural representations of time and space at higher cerebral levels. Usually, we do not just love, we love *someone*. We are not simply angry (a subcortical process), we are angry at something (a cortical process). We are not angry and in love for just a moment but for as long as our memories and relevant neurochemistries are aroused to sustain the neurodynamics of anger and love. Thus, affective and cognitive processes are inextricably intertwined in higher brain areas, such as the frontal and temporal cortices, which allows our brains to extend psychological events in time and space. Whether emotions in these higher brain systems also operate via the same neurochemical codes as in the lower reaches of the brain remains unknown. For instance, there are some corticotrophin releasing factor (CRF) cells in the cortex, as well as abundant CRF receptors, and it may well be that various stressful experiences are imbued with stressful affect in part by local cortical CRF dynamics.

Although emotions derive their rich cognitive resolution from interactions with higher brain functions, they can also be triggered at various levels of the neuroaxis by minimal stimuli as a function of conditioning—from the briefest glance to a nuance in someone's tone of voice. Once emotional systems are aroused, a variety of higher brain functions (from subtle appraisals to self-serving plans) are energized. Such cognition-emotion interactions constitute the details of people's lives, and we are more likely to recall specific events related to emotional episodes rather than reexperience the intensity of the aroused emotions themselves. The actual affective intensity that promoted the flow of action during emotional episodes seems to be easily forgotten. Only when the right "buttons" (i.e., the conditioned stimuli) are pushed again do the feelings return once more.

I will not dwell on cognitive details here, but it is important to consider how basic emotional systems might modify the higher cerebral processes that allow us to be the sophisticated, affectively cognitive creatures that we are. Indeed, it may well be that specific higher brain areas are specialized to help elaborate the cognitive contents of different types of affective processes (Figure 16.2). Thus, one general way to view many higher cortical functions is as providing ever more flexible ways for animals to deal with basic survival issues. One of the most important of these functions is the ability to utilize past experiences to inform future plans. The ability to extend action tendencies in time and space provides humans with remarkable advantages over animals that cannot gauge the passage of events as well.

It is generally accepted that the frontal lobes are capable of anticipating events and generating expectancies and foresights about the world. People with frontal lobe damage typically perseverate on old strategies and do not plan ahead effectively. They are susceptible to living within the present moment, in a more animal-like state of existence.[65] Because of rich cortical connections, the SEEKING system is especially strongly related to frontal cortical functions.[66] On the other hand, social-emotional sensitivities and feelings related to the PANIC system—namely, the affective dynamics of both positive and negative social interactions—appear to find a stronger focus of control within the cingulate cortex. For instance, the psychic tension that leads to panic disorders and agoraphobia is markedly diminished following cingulate cortex damage in humans, and changes in the arousability of this brain region have recently been implicated in the genesis of depression.[67] Neural computations that can activate FEAR, RAGE, and LUST appear to be especially well represented in the temporal lobes; indeed, the arousal of such emotions is based on perceptions that are processed in temporal cortical areas that have strong connections to specific regions of the amygdala.[68] People with damage to anterior temporal areas are often emotionally placid (the Klüver-Bucy syndrome); it is difficult to arouse such laid-back individuals to the point of irritability, anxiety, or lust. Indeed, it has recently been shown that people with amygdala lesions exhibit deficits in fearful memories, as has long been evident from animal brain research.[69]

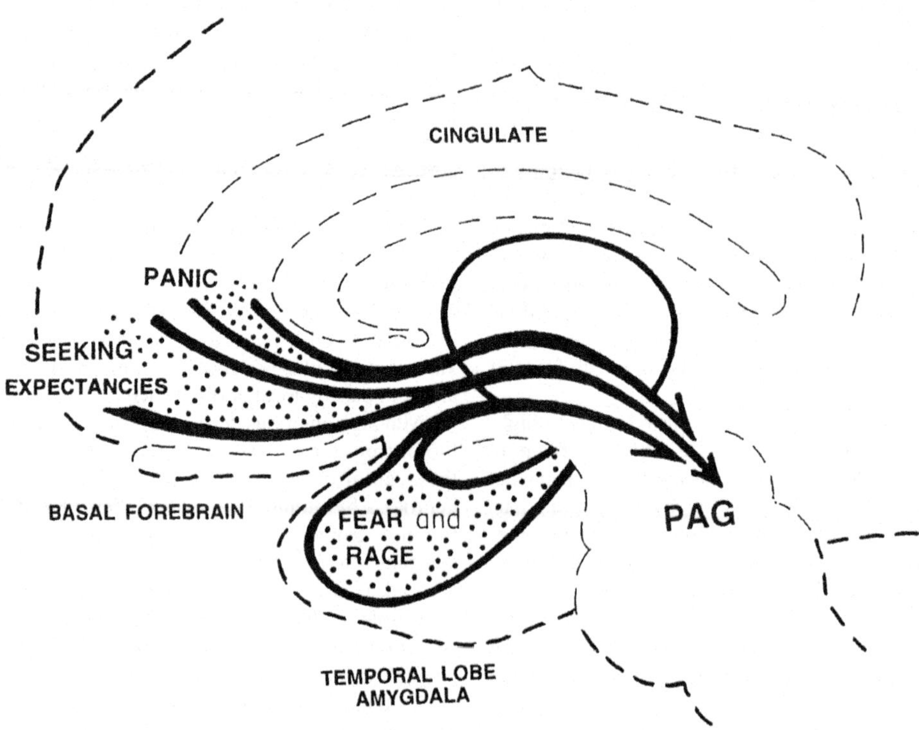

Figure 16.2. Overview of forebrain zones that are devoted to elaborating higher manifestations of basic emotional processes. Each of the emotional systems has higher spheres of influence, with FEAR and RAGE concentrated in the lateral and medial temporal lobes, SEEKING in the ventromedial frontal lobes, and various social emotional processes such as separation distress or PANIC in the anterior cingulate. All of these systems converge on the emotional and SELF representation zones of the midbrain. (Adapted from Panksepp, 1989; see n. 80.)

Although it is certain that the amygdala and nearby hippocampus are very important in processing cognitions and memories that can arouse various emotional responses, it is probably a mistake to believe that the affective entirety of such emotions as fear, anger, and sexuality is mediated locally just within medial temporal lobe structures. For instance, although it might be reasonable to expect that in males the sexually arousing effects of erotic images would be dramatically reduced by severing the pathways that transmit well-processed visual information from the occipital lobes into the temporal lobes, such brain damage should have much less of an effect on sexual arousal induced by touch, where the key connections are bound to be subcortical. Thus, even though it is likely that many conditional stimuli derive their emotional impact from local interactions within the amygdala, many other unconditional sensory inputs to the same functional systems may derive their affective impact by interacting with lower aspects of the emotional command systems (see Figures 10.1 and 16.1).

The main reason the amygdala may appear to be so important in generating affect may arise largely from the fact that most emotional episodes in adult animals are closely linked to learning and cognitive appraisals. These are the types of emotional stimuli that converge on the amygdala. Accordingly, the amygdala may gradually become a strong interface between higher information processing and emotional arousal as a function of development and various concrete life experiences,[70] but there is presently no clear evidence that the amygdala can generate emotional energy without the arousal of the lower functions situated in the hypothalamus, the PAG, and the rest of the periventricular gray. As we saw in Chapter 10, rage elicited from the amygdala is critically dependent on the integrity of the systems in the hypothalamus and the PAG (see Figure 10.4). Of course, it may well be that during ontogenetic development the higher functions assume such a prominent role in conscious life that the lower functions tend to become increasingly subconscious as organisms mature. Clearly, a great deal of work is needed before we will understand these processes with any assurance. Recent brain-imaging studies do suggest that only higher brain areas are aroused during emotional episodes, but, as indicated earlier, these techniques are quite likely to generate false-negatives as far as the lower brain stem areas are concerned. For simple anatomical reasons, such as the massive overlap of antagonistic circuits, the lower limbs and trunks of each emotional "tree" are less likely to "light up" than the more widely distributed branches.

One of the most intriguing findings is that positive emotional feelings are associated with EEG arousal of the frontal areas of the left hemisphere, while negative and depressive moods are associated with frontal arousal within the right hemisphere. These types of patterns also prevail in the resting EEGs of individuals with different temperaments—people who are depressed, or simply susceptible to depression, exhibit more right frontal arousal, while those who feel positive about life exhibit more left arousal.[71] These types of asymmetries are already evident in babies, with extroverted ones having more left arousal and inhibited ones having more right arousal.[72]

More recently, PET scanning studies have also provided glimmers of happiness and sadness in the brain; perhaps not surprisingly, sadness produces more arousal, while happiness produces neuronal relaxation.[73] This is not unexpected, since during sadness we have more cognitive problems to dwell on.[74] However, the laterality effects are not totally congruent with the electroencephalographic (EEG) data. Acute sadness leads to left frontal arousal, while depression has the opposite effect; only this latter effect is congruent with the EEG data, indicating left frontal underactivity in depression.

Considerable neuropsychological evidence indicates that characteristic emotional changes also result from damage to higher brain areas. In agreement with the aforementioned EEG data, the most robust finding is that damage to the left cerebral hemisphere (especially left frontal areas) appears to reduce positive affective tone, while similar damage to the right hemisphere does not.[75] Thus, following strokes to the right hemisphere, which is generally the sadder side of the brain, it is not uncommon for patients to deny that anything bad has happened; comparable damage to left cortical areas, the seemingly happier side, can promote feelings of catastrophic despair.[76]

Congruent effects during brain activation have been obtained with new techniques called rapid transcranial magnetic stimulation (rTMS). Preliminary results suggest that rTMS of the left frontal cortex can evoke feelings of sadness, while right stimulation enhances happiness. Of course, this is outwardly inconsistent with the aforementioned EEG data; however, the complexity of the underlying neural changes precludes definitive interpretation. It is certainly possible that the rTMS disrupts normal neural activity, causing a diminution of normal functions. In support of this possibility, the longer-term effect of right prefrontal stimulation was an increase in anxiety and worsening of mood in depressed individuals, while left stimulation provoked remarkable improvements in mood, even in medication-resistant individuals.[77]

It is generally believed that in addition to such positive and negative affective distinctions, the right hemisphere is more of a specialist for deep emotional communication as compared with the linguistically competent left hemisphere (see Appendix B), which is more focused on social niceties. While left hemisphere damage typically leads to deficits in understanding and expressing thoughts, right hemisphere damage disrupts one's ability to express and understand emotional inflections.[78] Although there are a great number of theories as to why the two hemispheres have different emotional specializations, as yet there is no clear evidence for any of them. One good idea is that the left hemisphere is more skillful in serial processing of information, as required for linear thinking such as math and language, while the right hemisphere provides more of an affective background for various experiences. Another intriguing possibility is that the left hemisphere specializes in the communication of socially constructed emotions, while the right hemisphere is more closely attuned to primal-process emotionality.[79]

Although a great deal of work has been devoted to differentiating how right and left hemispheres participate in various emotional functions, the idea that different cortical regions modulate specific emotions deserves greater attention in the future. It presently seems reasonable to suppose that in a mature organism the two hemispheres have different emotional strengths. However, it may be that these differences arise largely from learning, rather than from any deep and intrinsic differences in emotional competence.[80] For instance, the left hemisphere may appear more happy only as a secondary consequence of its linguistic functions, which are at least partly designed to reinforce the appearance of a positive "social front." This may leave the right hemisphere to dwell on the emotional realities that emerge from subcortical dynamics.

In addition, it also remains possible that various areas of the neocortex can be devoted to different emotions in relatively idiosyncratic ways, just as core memory space is devoted to software files in modern computers. Thus, there may be a great deal of variability in the higher representations of emotions among different individuals. In this context, it should again be emphasized that the new brain-scanning technologies are not as well suited for picking up distinct brain stem functions as they are for detecting differences in higher brain areas. In addition to concerns voiced earlier, most mood-induction procedures used for generating feelings in brain-imaging studies tend to employ mental imagery of one kind or another, which would automatically lead to better differentiation of higher rather than lower brain processes. To the best of our knowledge, the higher areas of the brain would remain emotionally cold without the psychological energies that emerge from the subcortical circuits described in this book. In other words, a distinction between higher cognitive/rational processes and the more primitive affective/passionate processes is essential if we are going to make sense of how the brain generates affective experiences and spontaneous emotional behaviors. Such a distinction is further affirmed by the ability of higher forms of brain damage in humans to impair voluntary facial expressions of emotions, while the more spontaneous emotionally driven expressions remain intact.[81]

How Does a Cognition Provoke Feelings?

Perhaps the most obvious experience of emotions that we humans have is that environmental events cause our feelings. As we have now seen, this is largely an illusion: Such events only activate intrinsic affective potentials of the nervous system. However, now that I have completed this provisional analysis of the deep nature of affective experience in the brain, we are in a better position to address the question: What does it mean, in brain terms, to experience the illusion that appraisals cause emotions?

I would suggest that this question boils down to how cognitive representations of the world get enmeshed within the extended neurodynamic process that we call affective states. If affective mood states are ultimately constituted of distinct reverberatory neural patterns within the extended SELF-representation networks of the brain, it is possible that each type of mood can be set in motion by a variety of inputs into the system. When the primitive emotional command circuits arouse the whole extended neural network, we have full-blown emotional states. On the other hand, when cognitive inputs, both conditioned and unconditioned attributions, initiate weaker types of reverberation in the system, we have mood states. Thus, because of our past experiences and history of conditioning, cognitions can come to reevoke strong feelings.

However, once a weak type of reverberation has been established, it can proceed along several paths. It has the potential to become a full-blown emotion if the reverberation recruits full arousal of the primitive emotional command systems. This is probably the path of least resistance in the brain, because of our many mood-congruent memory processes that can add fuel to each emotional fire. However, the reverberation also has the potential to fade rapidly, if one can divert cognitive resources to other points of view. This, I believe, is the main aim of various forms of self-discipline, including assisted ones such as cognitive behavior therapy. Thus, in adult humans, cognitive processes have the option of becoming enmeshed, ever further, within ongoing emotional dynamics, or they can extract themselves from any oncoming neural maelstrom. Emotional self-regulation is presumably made possible through our higher cerebral endowments. Our symbol systems are especially effective in allowing us to negotiate such rough terrain. Language allows us to regulate our emotions.

Conflicts between Cognitions and Emotions

If emotions and cognitions—or passion and reason, as they used to be called—are differentially, albeit interactively, organized in the brain, there are bound to be conflicts between the influences of the two systems. The dictates of emotional systems are bound to be more egocentric and unconditionally affective than those of cognitive systems, even though, as emphasized recently by proponents of evolutionary psychology, the goal of cognitive processes is to provide more subtle solutions to problems posed by states of emotional arousal.[82] Indeed, the evolution of certain higher symbolic abilities in hominids may have provided ways for organisms to solve conflicts that are simply too difficult from a simpleminded emotional perspective. For instance, explicit spoken or written contracts between humans help minimize disputes that would easily emerge if one merely followed the dictates of one's immediate wants and desires.

The ability for symbol systems to mediate conflict resolution has even been observed in chimpanzees. When confronted by a seemingly simple pointing task, where their desires are put in conflict with outcomes, chimps find it impossible to exhibit subtle self-serving cognitive strategies in the immediate presence of a desired reward. However, such tasks are mastered when an alternative symbol system is employed. Let me clarify: In one study, animals were confronted by a simple choice; two plates holding tasty food items were presented, each with a different number of treats. If the animal pointed to the plate having more treats, it would immediately be given to a fellow chimp in an adjacent cage, and the flustered subject would receive the smaller amount. After hundreds and hundreds of trials, these chimps could not learn to withhold pointing to the larger reward, even though it always resulted in the same undesired consequence of receiving the smaller of the desired alternatives. Although this outcome was commonly accompanied by howling and complaining, the task was simply too difficult for them to solve. However, these same chimps had already been taught the symbolic concept of simple numbers; when those numbers were placed on the plates as a substitute for the actual rewards, the chimps promptly learned to point to the smaller numbers first, thereby commandeering the larger rewards for themselves.[83]

In other words, in the immediate presence of a treat, chimps could not withhold their apparent self-referential desire for the bigger reward, but once a more affectively neutral numerical symbol system was introduced, they restrained themselves to achieve successfully selfish ends. The extent to which our various symbol systems, ranging from paper money to contracts, allow us to capitalize on our own selfish desires appears to be an unstudied dimension of human motivation. Obviously, money is equivalent to having the ability to make more choices in the world, and it is remarkable that even among chimpanzees a numerical symbol system was a more effective tool for acquisitiveness than the immediacy of their own wants when actually confronted by available rewards. Seemingly, the acquisition of numerical symbols expanded the options available for the chimp's higher levels of consciousness. Such work should make us suspect that human reason may still be inextricably intertwined with our self-centered animal needs.

If one is willing to dichotomize between cognitive functions and emotional functions—between reason and the passions (as many are no longer inclined to do in the present intellectual climate)[84]—then one can ask whether the downward cognitive controls or the upward emotional controls are stronger. If one looks at the question anatomically and neurochemically, the evidence seems overwhelming. The upward controls are more abundant and electrophysiologically more insistent; hence, one might expect that they would prevail if push came to shove. Of course, with the increasing influence of cortical functions as humans develop, along with the pressures for social conformity, the influences of the cognitive forces increase steadily during maturation. We can eventually experience emotions without sharing them with others. We can also easily put on false faces, which can make the facial analysis of emotions in real-life situations a remarkably troublesome business.[85]

Although we can employ our emotions with gradients of subtlety that other creatures simply cannot match, even using them for aesthetic or manipulative purposes, we would probably feel very little without the ancient subcortical source processes. And when those ancient sources become truly aroused, our cognitive apparatus shifts into fairly narrow grooves of obsessive ideation.[86]

In Sum

Although I have tried to clarify the neural foundations of affective experience in mammals, the actual manifestations of the neural circuits within living brains are so complex that many centuries of work will be needed to reveal how emotional systems really operate. In pursuing such matters empirically, we may find that there is a great deal more variability, plasticity, and flexibility in the underlying systems than I have suggested here. Many molecular underpinnings for neuronal plasticity have already been revealed (see Chapter 6), but no growth factor or gene has yet been identified that is specific to the growth and development of emotional systems. I suspect such molecules will be discovered, which may eventually open up a totally new area of psychiatric medicine.

Since we finally do have some precise knowledge concerning the neural substrates of a few emotional systems, we can begin to ask how these circuits change both structurally and functionally in response to various environmental events.[87] Ongoing work on electrical and psychostimulant sensitization (see "Afterthoughts," Chapters 5, 6, and 8) has already confirmed what William James surmised a long time ago when he wrote: "We are spinning our own fates, good or evil, and never to be undone. . . . The drunken Rip Van Winkle, in Jefferson's play, excuses himself for every fresh dereliction by saying, 'I won't count this time!' Well! he may not count it, and a kind Heaven may not count it; but it is being counted none the less. Down among his nerve cells and fibres the molecules are counting it, registering and storing it up to be used against him when the next temptation comes."[88]

We are spinning our own fates not only in our personal lives but also in our body politic. Until now, I have only alluded to the implications of this type of biological knowledge for cultural issues. A psychobiology text is not the most fitting place for such intellectual exercises, but I will take this final opportunity to share a few thoughts on the potential societal ramifications of emotional matters. I would emphasize, in closing, the obvious fact that our lives are outwardly swayed more by cultural issues than by biological ones. But even as we reside within the complexities of cultural structures and processes, our internal feelings will always be guided by powerful psychobiological tethers—our deep affective reactions to events in the world. Although such biological constraints on the human spirit have been denied by generations of scholars who prefer to think in terms of personal life histories rather than evolutionary terms, the evidence that such tethers exist is definitive. But the societal implications are not.

AFTERTHOUGHT: The Role of Brain Emotional Systems in the Construction of Social Systems

What consequences might a deeper understanding of emotions have on modes of thought in the humanities and social sciences? Can new information from psychobiology clarify issues in fields as distant as social, economic, and political thought? Hopefully they can. Although we remain remote from understanding the many interactions among brain circuits that govern the real-life flow of psychological responses in either animals or humans, our provisional knowledge allows us to explore some new lines of thought, hopefully without falling into the pit of *naturalistic fallacies*.[89] In this final "Afterthought," I will briefly probe the possible implications of the emerging psychobiological knowledge for the construction of social systems.[90]

To understand how affective processes are related to cultural institutions, we need to discuss how each emotional system of the brain might be related to existing social structures. This is a daunting task. Although we have many emotional systems in common with other mammals because of the long evolutionary journey we have shared, our cultural self-conceptions are not governed or constrained by our animal past. Nonetheless, they may be substantively clarified through the inclusion of affective dimensions in our discussions. For instance, the failure to fully recognize certain internal "forces" in human children may have already led to some very unusual societal practices in the United States.

Consider one troublesome example from our present educational practices—the widespread pathologization of rough-and-tumble play in the American school system. The widespread medical treatment of attention deficit, hyperactivity disorders, or hyperkinesis, as it used to be called, does not reflect an increased incidence of a neurological disorder in American children but an increased intolerance for childhood impulsivity. The use of drugs to control such symptoms in American schoolchildren has risen dramatically in the past few decades, to the point where many believe it has become a national scandal. The neuroscience data clearly indicate that psychostimulants such as methylphenidate and amphetamine can increase synaptic levels of catecholamines in the brain, and it is understandable why facilitation of noradrenergic tone in the cortex would increase attention spans in the classroom. The normal neurobiological function of this chemical system is to facilitate attentional processes, and the maturation of such systems during childhood is slow. This is one of the reasons young children are so impulsive and playful.

Obviously, these systems will mature more gradually in some children than in others, and psychostimulants certainly can increase attention span miraculously in children whose neurochemical development is slow. However, such drugs have many other effects on the brain. For instance, they markedly decrease playfulness—an effect that is well documented in animal studies (see Chapter 15). Are excessively playful children now being medicated to reduce their natural desire to play, on the pretext that they have some type of impulse-control disorder? This seems to be the case for at least some of the children who are being medicated. If so, it is unconscionable to give them antiplay drugs such as methylphenidate instead of providing substantial opportunities for rough-and-tumble play at the appropriate times of day, such as early in the morning when such urges are especially high. Even more frightening is the fact that the nervous system becomes sensitized to psychostimulants, and animal research indicates that such modifications of the nervous system can be permanent.[91] Are we now permanently altering the nervous systems of children with psychostimulant medications? Might we not actually be retarding the natural growth of the brain by reducing the normal influence of playful behaviors on central nervous system development?[92]

I believe that such effects are, in fact, occurring as a result of our present social policies, but the growing ethical debate on such matters is not yet being premised on our knowledge of the brain. The other basic emotional systems have equally important implications for our social practices, but they are also not being addressed because, as a society, we have yet to come to terms with the evolutionary epistemology of the nervous system.

As we have seen, the subcortical areas of the brain contain a large number of emotional systems that govern our moods and values. However, our cortical abilities have played a greater role in constructing social institutions than have our limbic circuits. The uniquely human neocortex, which allows our brains to elaborate complex ideas about the world, such as humanistic, scientific, and economic concepts, has evolved largely from sensory and attentional systems that harvest information from our external senses rather than from those that generate our internal feelings. Considering the likelihood that the evolution of human neocortical/cognitive processes was only partly constrained by the dictates of ancient limbic circuits, let me briefly explore the general impact on social institutions of our emerging understanding of subcortical emotional systems.

The human brain, like all other mammalian brains, has circuits that are designed to seek out positive rewards in the environment; this innate tendency can promote excessive materialism and greed (see Chapter 8). The brain also has systems that can induce anger toward perceived offenders to our liberties and freedom, which can lead to deep animosities among groups forced to compete for common resources (see Chapter 10). The brain mediates fear to detect those agents of change that threaten our safety and comfort; this can lead to xenophobia and the stigmatization of groups that do not appear to share our interests (see Chapter 11). We have brain systems that aspire for social pride and dominance, leading to the types of power politics that have been the hallmark of human history down through the ages.

Our mammalian brain also has systems that mediate social and sexual bonds, including parental nurturance (see Chapter 13) and the despair of being isolated from our fellows (see Chapter 14). As humans with sophisticated social sensitivities, we can also be overwhelmed with grief, shame, and embarrassment when we feel we have offended the strictures of our social contracts. Social systems that fail to recognize the importance and natural dynamics of these intrinsic urges are bound to make graver mistakes than those that do. The brain also elaborates hungers (see Chapter 9) and passions (see Chapter 12), and social systems that do not aspire to distribute necessary resources relatively evenly must tolerate increasing social chaos. The brain also contains circuits for social play and dominance (see Chapter 15), and no successful social system has stifled the dictates of those circuits. Emotional systems add immeasurably to the variety, chaos, meaning, and value of our lives. Without them, the cortex would have little to talk about and little to be excited about. Indeed, some deem it a moral imperative to live a passionate life. But our passions have no unambiguous power to dictate outcomes within complex social systems. Our feelings only encourage us to consider the options that are available to us.

There have already been too many political structures in human history that have promoted fear and aggression, but it should be possible to develop distinct social systems based on each of the emotions. If such social engineering is possible, the next question might be: At our present stage of cultural evolution, should a single system have priority in our deliberations about the future? Does one system have the intrinsic "right" or "worth" or "power" to predominate over the others? Many of us might agree that the social-emotional systems that allow us to be caring and giving, that promote deep sympathies for each other, have intrinsic worth, although they do not seem to have intrinsic power. Perhaps they could gradually recruit the necessary power by being more widely and realistically recognized within our cultural matrix, but there is no assurance that such values could prevail within the intrinsic emotional tendencies of the neurobiological mind. The urges for power and greed are probably as insistent in the brain circuits of the human species as the urges for nurturance.[93] But since we can now conceptualize the roles of the basic emotional systems more clearly, we are left with more choices.

It would be most interesting to imagine what form our society could eventually take if it chose to foster the feminine forces of nurturance and incentive-based altruism as opposed to materialism and male dominance. But how shall we construct stable and balanced economies that are not fueled by the self-serving forces of greed and materialism? Most prefer a bigger and bigger piece of the pie. How do we learn to divide the bounty of mother earth more equitably around the world so all her children can be reasonably satisfied? Perhaps a legislated cap on individual greed would be a move in the right direction, but to do so effectively, we may need to allow new and creative expressions for our dominance urges. As already exists in sports, we may have to widen compensatory doors for self-expression in the arts, humanities, and social services. These are psychobiological options that mammalian brain evolution offers for our consideration.

Although a full understanding of emotional systems may provide better alternatives for conceptualizing and creating new and better social institutions, our ancient emotional circuits cannot dictate the future. The neocortex, with its cognitive riches, shall remain the uneasy and pretentious master of the external realm, while emotions will remain the masters of our inner lives. Still, it is reasonable to suppose that new social systems will prosper only to the extent that they harmonize with the positive emotions of the greatest number, and will flounder to the extent that they do not. Social systems will flourish if they minimize the impact of negative emotions on the members of a society, and they will fail to the extent that they do not. However, within these constraints, there are all too many options to consider, including, as always, the dream of reason that creates monsters.[94]

This may be the most important overall message to take away from our consideration of the many emotional systems that exist within our human brain. These ancient neural systems, which constitute the foundations of our deeply felt personal values and standards of conduct, only give us options to consider in our social worlds. The relative importance we give to various emotional factors in each social equation will be determined as much by historical and ecological forces as by neurobiological ones. Environments where one must battle for resources will promote different social solutions than environments where circumstances are more generous and forgiving. This, of course, makes the study of cross-cultural differences in emotionality a remarkably difficult area of inquiry. Even though the different branches of the human family may have slightly different patterns of emotional responsivity, for both genetic and cultural reasons, it is now clear that we also share the same fundamental feelings. The same goes for the various genders.

What should scare us most is the 20th century recognition of the layers of deviousness that evolution may have bred within our intermediate cognitive systems (those areas of the higher limbic brain that intrinsically interface between primitive emotional systems and higher cognitive realms). Understanding human nature is surely not as simple as understanding the nature of the subcortical emotional systems we share with other mammals, even if they are the ancient centers of gravity for our affective value systems. On top of these systems we also have strong intrinsic potentials for Machiavellian deceit. The brain of "the lizard" still broadcasts its selfish messages widely throughout our brains. We have layers of human nature that sociobiologists and evolutionary psychologists are only beginning to decipher with the conceptual tools of inclusive fitness and game theories.

If we take their evolutionary stories to heart,[95] we can begin to grasp the nature of the psychopathic and sociopathic personalities that can sprout from the varieties of human SELVES. At some point in human evolution, it was probably adaptive for a certain number of individuals in each human society to have warrior temperaments—individuals who were highly pugnacious and relatively insensitive to the pain of others. If such adaptations thrived during human evolution, these traits probably remain with us, all too well prepared by our evolutionary heritage to wreak havoc and violence in social life, even during times of peace.[96] To some extent such urges may be rechanneled into sports and other forms of competition, or perhaps even modified by new social and pharmacological strategies.[97] However, if we see the cortex as a neuronal playground where multiple, evolutionarily adaptive strategies, some of them quite unseemly, can be played out, we have only modest reason for optimism and solace. It is sad to note that our sense of sympathy may be intrinsically weaker than our sense of retribution.

There are reasons to believe that cold reason, unfettered by the impulses of social emotions, can yield personalities that are egotistic, selfish, and willing to hurt others for their own gratification (as long as the perceived costs to themselves are not too high). There is no intrinsic reason that such personalities could not present themselves as highly extroverted and sensitive while seeking to skillfully take advantage of others in social and economic encounters. The existence of the social emotions within the human brain provides no shield against the existence and future evolution of cutthroat, self-serving individuals who have no desire to advance cooperative altruistic behavioral tendencies in human societies. It is troubling to contemplate that such individuals may be especially highly motivated to aspire to positions of political and economic power. The massive growth of the human neocortex now provides options such as these for the human spirit.

To grow fruitfully into the future, society must learn how to recognize and benignly discourage and shun those who have no wish or ability to practice and promote stable and honest cooperative strategies. It remains possible that some individuals pursue such avenues of life because of atypical responsivities of their basic emotional systems, while others pursue asocial life activities because of more personal choices. We may eventually be able to detect such personality traits at an early age, using sophisticated brain measurement procedures, a troublesome possibility that is almost at our doorstep.[98] It is hard to imagine how we might seek to measure and modify such emotional strengths and weaknesses of individuals without infringing on basic human rights and liberties.

It is a blessing that a modest sense of fair play has already been built into the value structures of our human brains. As game-theory analysis has affirmed, the most effective trading strategy is fairness: to punish your trading partners only if they have cheated, but then to forgive rapidly. This "tit-for-tat" strategy is also ingrained in our best social traditions such as "honesty is the best policy." Unfortunately, this strategy appears to be most effective in small groups where everyone knows each other and where shame can still motivate behaviors. In our anonymous megasocieties, the ancient stricture—*do unto others as you would have them do unto you*—may be gradually losing force. Wherever long-term social relationships are not stable, our commitments to traditional social contracts appear to weaken.[99] Since we are now so remote from the original evolutionarily adaptive environments where our brains were constructed, our best option may be to understand as honestly as possible the varieties of nature that can be nurtured within human minds.

Perhaps early emotional education could counter our potential for evil, but to do so, our school systems may need to cultivate new perspectives that explicitly recognize the nature and importance of *all* the basic emotions of our lives.[100] We should be willing to clearly and unambiguously teach future generations about the true nature of the affective forces that reside with-in the ancient structures of our brains. Public forums such as television, movies, and popular music can be increasingly coaxed and molded to uplift our spirits rather than to provide more and more shallow limbic and reptilian entertainment. We must learn to emotionally educate the whole brain. To do that well, we must come to terms with the biological sources of the human spirit.

Joy and woe are woven fine,
A clothing for the soul divine;
  Under every grief and pine
Runs a joy with silken twine.
  It is right it should be so;
Man was made for joy and woe;
And, when this we rightly know,
  Safely through the world we go.

William Blake,
"Auguries of Innocence" (1863)

Suggested Readings

Ardrey, R. (1974). *Social contract.* New York: Dell.
Barash, D. P. (1986). *The hare and the tortoise.* New York: Penguin.
Dennett, D. C. (1991). *Consciousness explained.* Boston: Little, Brown.
De Waal, F. (1982). *Chimpanzee politics: Power and sex among apes.* London: Jonathan Cape.
Edelman, G. M. (1992). *Bright air, brilliant fire.* New York: Basic Books.
Lumsden, D. J., & Wilson, E. O. (1983). *Promethean fire: Reflections on the origin of mind.* Cambridge, Mass.: Harvard Univ. Press.
Morris, R. (1983). *Evolution and human nature.* New York: Putnam.
Plato (1940). *The republic.* (B. Jowett, trans.). New York: Graystone.
Searle, J. (1984). *Minds, brains, and science.* Cambridge, Mass.: Harvard Univ. Press.
Walker, S. (1983). *Animal thought.* London: Routledge and Kegan Paul.
Wilson, P. J. (1983). *Man, the promising primate: The conditions of human evolution.* New Haven: Yale Univ. Press.

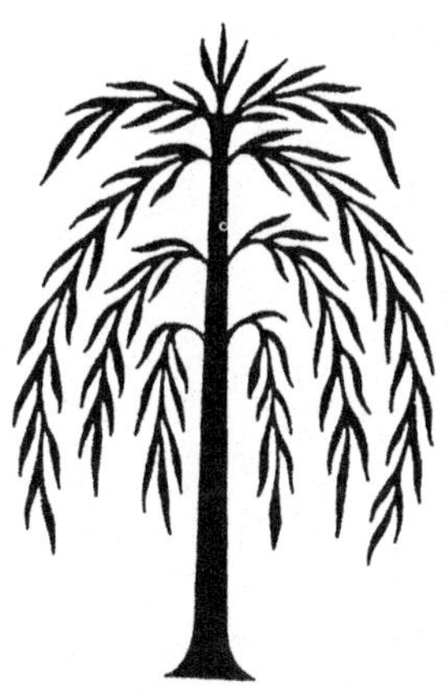

Appendix A
Bones, Brains, and Human Origins

In accepting the present view of the foundations of human nature, we need not deny the multifaceted possibilities of our human creativity and the complex intellectual perspectives that 20th century thought has impressed on our culture. Even as our postmodern imagination becomes increasingly engrossed by cultural relativism, we need to become conversant with evolutionary epistemology—the perspective that ancient emotional and motivational forces preceded the emergence of our cortical abilities in brain evolution. The aim of this appendix is to sketch the evolutionary passages that have created the human brain and mind. I will cover three questions: When did the human line diverge from prehuman ancestors? What factors promoted the divergence? And what is unique about the human psyche? Our most special ability, that of language—especially as it applies to our scientific pursuits—will be the focus of Appendix B.

Our Evolutionary Roots

Only a few decades ago, on the basis of fossil evidence, the accepted view was that the human line first diverged from that of the other great apes (chimpanzees and gorillas and, even more distantly, the orangutans and gibbons) some 20 to 30 million years ago on the now parched plains and rift valleys of East Africa.[1] As Robert Ardrey, that controversial and oft reviled popularizer of the evolutionary origins of humanity, intoned in moving hyperbole: "Not in innocence, and not in Asia, was mankind born. The home of our fathers was that African highland reaching north from the Cape to the Lakes of the Nile. Here we came about—slowly, ever so slowly—on a sky-swept Savannah glowing in menace."[2]

Analysis of molecular evidence from living species now suggests that we actually diverged from the other great apes more recently. The molecules suggest our divergence was finalized little more than 5 million years ago. This has not been a happy conclusion for those who believe in other creation stories. In any event, the fossil and molecular evidence of our past has enriched and complicated our view of ourselves. Our culture is still trying to come to terms with the lesson.[3]

Without the scientific discoveries of the 20th century to constrain them, storytellers of the past wove creation myths with relative abandon. Their tales often told of times and occurrences that were more closely related to the substance of our dreams and fantasies than our histories. Now, however, abundant fossil remains of our ancestors are available, and we have also learned to read the living book of evolution within the DNA-RNA-protein scripts that all living cells share. The degree of relatedness of different creatures can be estimated by comparing the base sequences of DNA, and the similarities in the resulting amino acid chains of proteins across living species is remarkable.[4]

The pace of divergence among species can now be estimated through the degree of molecular divergence. Since genetic mutations generally reflect random processes, such as the influence of cosmic rays, the accumulated changes in DNA, RNA, and proteins also compute the passage of time in an approximately linear fashion. Although the timing of the clock has to be anchored to geological evidence (e.g., radioisotope dating procedures), the molecular clock does affirm that we humans were not created as uniquely nor as recently as some had hoped.

The homologies in the molecular structures of our cells clearly reflect our shared heritage with all other vertebrates and even more "lowly" creatures. We humans are variants on a grand mammalian theme that started to blossom in earnest when the dynasties of large reptiles came to an end about 100 million years ago. That transition was probably precipitated by climatic and ecological changes resulting from volcanic activities and/or large asteroids striking the earth.[5]

The molecular data have now demonstrated that rather than taking separate paths 20 to 30 million years ago, as dating of the early bones had originally suggested, human, chimpanzee, and gorilla lines diverged less than 10 million years ago. While the protein data do not as clearly differentiate our divergence from our closest living relatives (chimps and gorillas), the DNA data are more discriminating.[6] They suggest that humans and chimpanzees diverged from a common ancestor about 7 million years ago and that both diverged from the line that led to gorillas about 9 million years ago. Our ancestral lines diverged from orangutans and gibbons perhaps 15 to 20 million years ago.

By such reckoning, we can conclude that hominid fossils younger than several million years may resemble our ancestors. There is little question that creatures such as *Homo habilis, Homo erectus*, and the other famous hominid remains are representatives of our line of ascent. Whether the existing fossil specimens are in a direct line to any existing humans remains unlikely, of course, but the evidence that *all living mammals* shared bloodlines within the last hundred million years or so is no longer controversial, at least among those who like to base their thinking on the evidence. As Vincent Sarich, one of the pioneers of molecular dating, so poignantly stated when he was still battling the "bone hunters" with regard to the approximate divergence dates, "I know my molecules had ancestors, the paleontologist can only hope that his fossils had descendants."[7]

At this distance of time, the bones can never reveal their precise lineage. Molecular analysis of living organisms can. For reasons such as these, we must now also estimate universal human abilities from a study of living humans rather than from any fossilized evidence, which can only give us a surface glimmer of the dimensions of ancestral brains and occasional samples of their artifacts. For similar reasons, the relevance of animal brain research for identifying certain mammalian universals should become an accepted fact.

The ancient bones speak reasonably clearly of the outward shapes of brains in our lineage. The best predivergence candidate for the ape and monkey lines, the ancient primate now called *Aegyptopithecus,* who roamed the banks of the Nile more than 30 million years ago, had brain surfaces that do not differ greatly from those of the monkeys that inhabit the world today. To the best of our knowledge, such brains could not generate symbolic representations more complex than those needed for immediate survival, and these creatures probably had only enough political savvy to establish simple social coalitions. In short, these creatures probably did not conduct any long-term community planning, even though modest social plans were no doubt routinely made and carried out. For instance, modern baboons, despite their immediate emotional ways, occasionally do exhibit a more subtle meeting of the minds. One striking example is the description of a coalition of older baboons in a colony that established a joint behavioral strategy to rid themselves of a marauding predator.[8] The level of social planning that can be achieved by chimpanzees has been strikingly detailed; there is even evidence that, like humans, they occasionally undertake warlike tribal skirmishes.[9]

Innumerable environmental pressures constrained and guided the trajectory of human brain evolution, as did our own emerging abilities. However, we will never unambiguously know the factors that led to the massive encephalization of our brains. Fossil records suggest this occurred in several steps, starting about 3 million years ago with the australopithecines, who had brains about a third the size of ours but had already achieved an upright stance. A critical stage in our cerebral progression began with the transitional phase of *Homo habilis* about 2 million years ago and culminated in *Homo erectus* about a million years ago. The final touches were completed about a hundred thousand years ago, when *Homo sapiens neanderthalensis* and Cro-Magnon walked the earth.

Homo habilis possessed a brain that was, in approximate terms, only about 60% of ours in size (about 700 cc on the average versus 1200+ cc for us), and that of *Homo erectus* (about 1000 cc) was only about 20% smaller than our cerebral crown. The various forms of early *Homo sapiens* (Neanderthal and Cro-Magnon) possessed cerebral endowments comparable to our own, at least as far as overall size was concerned. Most of this brain expansion had occurred in cortical areas, where we now display about a three-fold enlargement over the other modern apes. By contrast, the intermediate areas of our brain are only twice as enlarged in relative terms (i.e., corrected for body weight), while the lowest reaches, such as the medulla, retain ancestral proportions.[10]

In this context, it must be noted that the development of the human brain entailed more than simply an expansion in size. There is also evidence that new patterns of connectivities emerged in higher cortical areas, and hence the possibility of generating new ideas that can never be generated by the brains of other primates, not to mention the other mammals.[11] For this reason, it would be hard to fathom human cortical organization simply from studying rats and mice. All these creatures can provide is a clear sense of the internal organization of cortical *columns* (see Figure 4.9) and the ability of various columns to interrelate certain forms of information. By comparison, the more ancient functions in subcortical areas have apparently remained highly conserved, and hence a study of their function in animals should provide many reasonably accurate generalizations to human functions. Below the cortex, the brain of a mouse is not all that different in terms of overall organization from that of a man. If higher brain functions in humans have not imposed totally new organizational principles on lower functions, then our own subcortical processes can be understood from a study of those types of brain functions in other creatures.

The additional fact that allows us to have confidence in the generality of human brain functions across the world is the remarkable homogeneity of the human genome. Analysis of maternally transmitted mitochondrial DNA suggests that all humans on the earth shared essentially the same bloodline only some 200,000 years ago, even though some estimates go up to a million years.[12] This dating of a mythical "mitochondrial Eve" gives us special confidence that the study of one human group will highlight the general principles that govern the basic behavioral tendencies and mental lives of other human groups.

Factors Guiding Human Divergence and the Evolution of Unique Human Abilities

Although the ancestral remains of Neanderthals and Cro-Magnons suggest that the human brain evolved to its present state about a hundred thousand years ago, only within the past few centuries, through the accumulating riches of cultural evolution, has it yielded a technological world based on the power of our scientific imagination—ranging from the molecularly honed comforts of biological psychiatry to the anxieties of atomic despair. The potential of the human mind has finally outstripped what nature "intended"—which is, of course, an absurd thing to say. As Darwin taught us, nature intends nothing. It merely reels out unending and often seemingly arbitrary possibilities that either sink or swim on the basis of their adaptive merits. Only now, with the advent of genetic engineering, can we begin to modify biological traits with a precision that could only be approximated by traditional animal husbandry.

However, each new possibility is still tethered to the past. Thus, even as the potential of the human mind now reflects an intermixture of neural and cultural complexities not previously encountered on the earth, it continues to be constrained and guided by the brain structures and functions that preceded it. However, it is all too easy to make mistakes in such paleopsychological pursuits. For instance, on the basis of fragmentary evidence available to him and some faulty reasoning, Ardrey concluded: "Children of all animal kind, we inherited many a social nicety as well as the predator's way. But most significant of all our gifts, as things turned out, was the legacy bequeathed us by those killer apes, our immediate forebears. Even in the first long days of our beginnings we held in our hand the weapon, an instrument somewhat older than ourselves."[13]

Ardrey's attempt to trace the sources of human violence to a predatory heritage is belief rather than fact. First, brain evidence suggests that predatory urges emerge more from brain circuits that mediate SEEKING, rather than from the circuits of RAGE (as summarized in Chapter 8). It is vital to remember that these circuits mediate various forms of resource seeking rather than anger, and that human predation is more instrumental than it is instinctual. Indeed, the fossil evidence now suggests that our evolutionary roots are closer to those of herbivorous/omnivorous apes than to carnivorous ones, and there is no reason to believe that human SEEKING circuits are designed to mediate predatory intent in a manner resembling that found in carnivorous mammals. Human predation has probably been culturally molded from the higher dictates of the foraging systems that hunter-gatherers used to collect food efficiently. Ancient humans eventually developed the habit of stalking prey and eating meat (as do some present-day male chimpanzees in the wild), but this thread of character emerged independently of the intense and persistent carnivorous hunting urges of the cats and dogs of the ancient plains. The "killer apes" that Ardrey described were probably a figment of his imagination.

As the humanoid brain developed enough cortex to think and elaborate complex ideas, hunting became an acquired practice of the human lifestyle. In short, humans took their place at the pinnacle of the food chain not by the dictates of nature but by those of culture. This is not to deny that our SEEKING circuits are highly influential in potentiating our acquired hunting urges and practices.

Once ideas began to prevail over brute force, new avenues of development were opened, and the emerging behavioral opportunities surely contributed to the further evolution of our brains. In other words, our brain growth was guided not simply by natural selection but also by our own social selections, as well as by our ability to select and construct new environments in which to subsist. Still, the more ancient brain circuits continued to provide motivation for our newfound cognitive abilities. They still do, and some of the most striking universals of the human spirit will be found among the precognitive affective "energies" of those ancient circuits.

While Ardrey argued that the weapon in our hand ("an instrument somewhat older than ourselves") was a critical element in our cerebral evolution, other scholars have emphasized different factors. The fossil evidence clearly indicates that long before our divergence from the other apes, our ancestors had acquired flexible, fully rotatable shoulder joints along with our characteristic chest girdle, adaptations for hanging from branches and reaching for the ripest fruit. Monkeys do not possess such skills. Of course, our ancestral desire for ripe, richly colored fruits may have also promoted keen visual abilities, shared by all primates, long before our ancestors took to hanging from the branches. Such visual abilities, along with our remarkable shoulder flexibility, so beautifully refined in our distant cousins the gibbons, still serve us well. They allow us to swing hammers and mallets precisely, whether in the construction of homes or in our various destructive pursuits. These preadaptations gave us the option to hurl various projectiles at each other, but our choice to do so or not remains a cognitive issue that is deeply premised on our emotional concerns. Such exaptations now allow us to throw and hit various types of balls on the playing fields we have devised to exercise and refine the inborn urges of our ludic circuits. We can now choose to pursue competitive symbolic pursuits rather than dominance through the weapons of warfare.

Changes in weather patterns and the gradual shift to eating more seeds and tubers may have guided our ancestral descent from trees and the consequent assumption of upright postures and increasingly fine finger dexterity. For example, manual dexterity combined with an upright squatting position was a fine adaptation for large creatures to search the ground for small edible items such as seeds.

Ever so gradually, the survival advantages of group living may have guided the development of our prelinguistic ability to symbolize objects and events in gestures and vocal signs. But what was it that actually led to the final vast expansion of brain, the massive expansion of cortex, especially that devoted to speech—that most unique characteristic of our species? Although one could imagine the interplay of various social dynamics as being crucial, it is generally believed that one set of environmental events was decisive.

At about the time the earliest *Australopithecus* fossils were laid down, when our ancestors had brains only marginally superior to those of existing chimps and gorillas, a series of Ice Ages was set in motion. The accompanying hardships served as a powerful force for the emergence of deeper thoughts. Among those who had migrated north, survival at the edge of the advancing and receding ice sheets provided environments that required new solutions to the old problems of acquiring food and shelter, as well as many subtle problems related to the protection and distribution of resources. The fact that the human brain exhibited especially large growth spurts during the Ice Ages suggests that neural tissues that could weigh more subtle alternatives than brute force provided a substantial advantage for our survival. Archaeological evidence suggests that systematic hunting emerged as a key food-seeking strategy at about that time.

Prior to the Ice Ages, the human line probably subsisted like present-day apes and monkeys—surviving largely on plant foraging, occasionally supplemented by scavenged or caught meat. With the change in weather and the discovery of fire, the ability to capitalize on concentrated sources of protein energy would have been highly adaptive. However, a creature that had not been prepared for hunting through evolution needed to dwell on new ways to obtain the concentrated energy resource that meat provides.

As already mentioned, the truly "mighty hunters" of the time—the various cats, wolves, and bears—had achieved their prowess through the modification of primitive SEEKING circuits into ones that could energize predatory intent. By comparison, the new humanoid hunters of the Ice Ages were not instinctively equipped to hunt for meat. They eventually learned to achieve their hunting prowess through the application of thought and reason, often as coordinated social groups sharing joint long-term strategies, as opposed to simply using ingrained skills of physical speed, strength, and stealth. Although the idea that the potential rewards of a hunting lifestyle could have channeled human evolution has been criticized, the Paleolithic cave paintings of southern France and Spain,[14] as well as the collections of bones that have been unearthed from early dwelling sites,[15] attest to the emergence of new social orders related to the hunt. However, new ways of gathering were not neglected.

An important mental strategy that could have promoted survival in the harsher environments of the Ice Ages was the ability to bring food to central storage and provisioning areas. It is hard to imagine that an arboreal primate could ever have developed such practices, and indeed, there is little evidence for instinctual storage strategies in the human line, as there are in many rodents and birds.[16] Although early humans probably did not have the instinct to hoard, surely the human mind was already influenced by ancient circuits that promoted greediness—the desire to be first in line in access to resources. The instinct for greediness, without instinctual mechanisms for hoarding, could have led to new developments in economic thought and warlike competition, including new food storage strategies based on rational decision making. The distribution of stored resources would eventually become as important an issue for mental deliberation as was the organization of the hunt. Such matters could not be resolved without clear communication of some form. It was about at this time that language abilities evolved in the human cortex. However, the motivation for using the auditory as opposed to the gestural route of communication had been preconditioned by the evolution of various sociovocal signs. Obviously, sound is a better medium of communication than the other senses if one needs to compress a lot of information into a channel of information that can be used at some distance.

The ecological hardships of the Ice Ages, combined with the prior commitment of primates to living in extended social structures, probably added strongly to the confluence of forces that established the trajectory of cognitive evolution in the human brain. In the midst of hardships, social creatures must make ever more difficult and long-term decisions on how resources are to be distributed. Will the children get more food than the elderly? Will adolescents get less food than nursing mothers? Will the more effective hunters and gatherers get more than the less able? How much food should be saved? How can it be saved? Many of these questions can be seen to be "prisoner dilemma" scenarios—situations in which the economic goal of optimizing one's long-term needs cannot be achieved by the simple dictates of short-term wants. Because of social commitments that had already been established in the mammalian line, such as bonding and emotional dependencies between individuals, along with the unique commitment that humans had to show toward each other to survive in harsh environments, people could no longer just pursue their own personal "economic" advantage.

Still, when available resources are smaller than the desires of a highly social creature, the optimal evolutionary solution is not always simple greed but a judicious balance of tendencies where reciprocity ultimately rules the day. Without reciprocity, all participants in a social group may eventually be losers (at least on the evolutionary scale). Indeed, in formal mathematical analysis of various strategies that might be used in the competition for resources, the "tit-for-tat" approach typically prevails over all others.[17] This strategy affirms that one should consistently be honest, promptly punish any duplicitous offenses by competitors, and then forgive rapidly.[18]

With the further evolution of such mental abilities, it is not hard to envision how various cultural contrivances would have emerged from our ever-increasing abilities to symbolize, think, and make "rational" decisions. For instance, food gathering and storage would be enhanced by development of various means of conveyance, including baskets, slings, yolks, harnesses, and gradually more sophisticated modes of transport, such as could arise from the domestication of animals. The ability to pursue such activities required the emergence of a general-purpose, neuromental apparatus for thought, deliberation, decision, and action that now constitutes the cortical menagerie that can yield human rationality. Although these new abilities remained tethered to preexisting bodily needs and emotions, they continued to provide totally new social and intellectual environments for evolutionary selection to proceed. The newly emerging brain abilities provided many opportunities for brain evolution to progress via the refinement of cerebral potentials rather than the sharpening of bodily abilities. This passage to a new order of mind was marked by the emergence of modern human languages and cultures.

Still, considering the fact that an essentially modern human brain has probably existed for several hundred thousand years, our present level of cultural complexity is no mere consequence of encephalization; it is also a product of long-accumulated traditions. Our historical record of cultural evolution goes back a mere 10,000 years, and to the best of our knowledge, that passage has not promoted any dramatic advance in the complexity of the brain (although potential changes in internal organization issues cannot be empirically evaluated from the fossil evidence). For most of the ages that a fully human-type brain has viewed the world, it has had the intrinsic potential to be its "master," but it took a long time for the human species to create high culture. It took so long because even a human brain, without preexisting cultural supports, has to expend a considerable amount of time and effort simply to survive. A great deal of simple cultural growth had to accumulate before the time was ripe for the construction of our present world of science and technology.

Because of our ability to prevail in the natural world and to construct artificial worlds of creature comforts, we may now be at the threshold of a long period of cerebral stasis, comparable to that which the whales and dolphins have experienced. Their remarkable cerebral endowments have probably been their birthright for many more million years than ours, and there is little indication that their cognitive abilities have advanced much in that time. A constant environment, especially one full of creature comforts, may tend to put the brakes on the emergence of new faculties. Although it is not mandated, the comparatively stable environment we are presently constructing may eventually embalm our minds in a noncreative fog. Moreover, to increase our brain size much more seems impossible without a corresponding increase in the size of the birth canal. Of course, a doorway for new cerebral growth could be opened if babies can survive who are born more and more prematurely. Our only other option is to take the brain evolutionary path of cone-headedness.

Without such readjustments, it seems that human brain development has reached a plateau. Of course, reorganization of internal structures remains a possibility, and this could include new connections as well as new disconnections. The cerebral hemispheres may be increasing their influence a bit further at the expense of subcortical structures, so ancient brain areas of seemingly secondary importance are perhaps being disconnected from more recent cerebral developments.[19] Indeed, such a type of neurodevelopmental process seems evident in the anatomical patterns seen in the brains of autistic children.[20] Is it possible that autism and several other neurodevelopmental disorders reflect evolutionary shuffling of brain connections in ways that provide novel variants as fodder for the discriminating processes of natural selection? There is no way to tell yet.

On the Distinctiveness of the Human Psyche

What, then, is truly unique about the human mind and human nature? Our brains are obviously more encephalized than those of other creatures. This is especially prominent in areas designed for thought—the association cortices that blend information from the various sensory modalities. It is within the natural psychological "grooves" and depths of such new associative abilities that the defining uniqueness of human nature must be sought. Rational as well as irrational thoughts allow us to weigh alternative courses of action and to choose those that maximize the fulfillment of our desires and minimize our fears. It is also clear that we have much more of that subtle stuff called "free will" than do other creatures, which surely reflects the interactions of the SELF with higher cognitive structures.

In economic terms, rationality also allows humans to choose a course of action that will maximize returns from available resources and investments. Often the returns are largest if people work together, but they may also sometimes be greater when some people deceive and compete unfairly against others. Indeed, one of the functions of PLAY circuits in the human brain may be to hone such "winning" skills, as well as to learn how to lose gracefully. On the playing field, we learn to interact, to compete, to deceive, to test the perimeters of our knowledge and to learn about the skills and intentions of others.

Once thinking had become a major factor in the acquisition, distribution, and competition for resources, we might anticipate that there would also emerge evolutionary aberrations and excesses in these newfound skills. As with any natural process, the underlying mechanisms can go to extremes, and the price of certain evolutionary adaptations may be mental aberrations in a certain percentage of the population. For instance, the emergence of self-centered types of thought, where individuals persist in pursuing very limited and specialized lines of cognitive activity (should we call it "academic autism?"), beneficial up to a point, might also cascade into the excesses of obsessive-compulsive and full-blown autistic disorders. The former appear to arise from excessive frontal lobe activity,[21] while the latter are characterized by a disconnection of lower process (such as cerebellar and limbic emotional ones) from higher ones.[22]

Obviously, we humans are the most creative of all species, a trait that is a consequence of our cerebral evolution. We do not have to look to our opposable thumbs to recognize the abilities that now distinguish us from the other animals. We not only make tools but also make tools with tools. We not only build but also build models of buildings. We not only communicate but also communicate about communication. We not only think but also think about thinking. We also take special interest in the contents of other minds.

The constraints of traditional scientific languages pose enormous dilemmas for discussing and describing the intrinsic internal processes of the brain/mind. To pursue evolutionary epistemology to the fullest, we will need to rethink some of the constraints we have imposed on our scientific endeavors. We must try to study ancient brain processes that we cannot define. For such brain functions, the definitions will be achieved at the end of our scientific journey rather than at the outset. We may need to use metaphors more liberally, and we have to take seriously the types of brain processes that all the folks around us speak of so readily—our hungers and thirsts, our angers and fears, our ability to feel sadness and joy. We have to be able to conceptualize first-person issues, using third-person languages. Without some linguistic and conceptual flexibility, we cannot fathom the hidden realms of feelings that humans have discussed for millennia around the campfires of their lives.

Appendix B

The Brain, Language, and Affective Neuroscience

Next to being able to see and to think, our ability to speak is our most important scientific tool. The focus of much of this book has been on the prelinguistic processes that govern emotional organization in the brain. Animal behavior clearly tells us that basic emotions evolved long before human languages, which surely emerged to serve other functions than to talk about emotions. This may be one reason it is so difficult to speak about emotional matters in clear scientific terms. We cannot even generate a precise definition of emotions that everyone can agree with. Nonetheless, some scholars still hope that a substantive understanding of emotions can be generated through the mere use of language. This, of course, is not possible. Any credible scientific definition of basic emotions will have to include neural criteria (e.g., Figure 3.3). In this appendix, I will first elaborate on why human communication poses such difficulties in pursuing key issues in functional neuroscience, such as the study of basic emotions; I will then provide a brief overview of how the human brain generates language.

Linguistic Difficulties in the Psychological and Brain Sciences

The nature of human languages poses special dilemmas as it enters the arena of evolutionary epistemology—the genetically based knowledge that is embedded in the intrinsic patterns of brain organization. It is important to recall that our symbolic linguistic systems emerged only recently in human evolution, presumably for purposes other than the pursuit of science. Perhaps the earliest functions of vocal signs (which, of course, are different from language) were related to affective issues such as social communication, but human propositional speech that is the basis for science is only weakly linked to such signals. As we will see in the next section, propositional speech typically emerges from left hemisphere functions, while the affective intonations that still carry emotional messages arise from the opposite hemisphere. Thus, even though our spoken utterances are still colored by social and emotional intonations (allowing us even to socially "groom" each other at a distance), propositional speech emerged from our ability to symbolically interconnect the various events of the world that impress themselves on us through our various external senses.

With the evolution of connections between different sensory areas, vocal communication gradually emerged as an especially effective way for encoding the relationships among external events. In this role, it is ideal for discussing visually evident world events that constitute most of scientific inquiry; but as the ability to interrelate external events improved, it remained a deficient medium for discussing internal events that arise from deep evolutionary rather than environmental sources. These difficulties still haunt the application of language in scientific inquiries where we must speak of processes that cannot be seen. Emotions, of course, are such processes—for the only things we can "see" are the outward expressions, gestures, sounds, and other behavioral acts.

So what should scientists interested in such neuropsychological issues do? The traditional solution was "behaviorism," which denied the reality of issues that could not be directly seen. Most scientists still choose to work within excessively stringent linguistic constraints, limiting the range of their thinking, their expository style, and, all too often, what they are willing to pursue in the laboratory to the *visual* realm. The most common aspects of human experience were discarded from the list of problems psychologists needed to solve.

Unfortunately, it is often impossible to think about certain psychological issues unless one is willing to entertain the deep meaning of certain vernacular concepts. Thus a new view has been emerging in the study of scientific thought, one that I ascribe to in this text, which recognizes that many of our scientific concepts are initially metaphoric in form, as, for example, in the supposition that the brain behaves like a digital computer.[1] It follows that we should be willing to acknowledge and cultivate such sources of creativity in our scientific endeavors by entertaining more ideas along the lines of "*such* a psychological process, as indexed by *such* behaviors, is governed by *such* circuits and neurochemistries of the brain." Indeed, in psychology, carefully selected linguistic liberties along these lines, employing vernacular usages, may provide new insights more readily than the accepted strictures on scientific prose would lead us to believe. For this reason I decided to employ capitalized vernacular terms in this text.

It is sometimes easier to observe and think about new phenomena if we have first categorized them under an appropriate general conceptual label. When it comes to a study of integrative brain functions, especially those that were created by evolutionary processes, we must remain open to the existence of what at first seem to be fuzzy linguistic entities and to sustain a cautious flexibility in our lexical and linguistic tools. For instance, old emotional concepts need to be entertained in the field of behavioral neuroscience, not simply rejected out of hand. By entertaining novel interweaving of old concepts with new neuroscientific findings, we may gradually be able to overlay primal psychological functions onto brain functions in credible ways. A relaxation of the traditional lexical constraints (i.e., you can't talk about it unless you can define all your terms) may be justified simply on the basis of evolutionary considerations concerning the nature and sources of certain brain functions.

For instance, we obviously can never understand the deep nature of emotions without neuroscientific inquiry, and since we cannot study emotions without some type of linguistic guidance, we must learn to use emotional terms in ways that will further our experimental pursuits. This requires identifying coherent systems in the brain, labeling them with affective terms that will promote discussion and study, establishing operational behavioral definitions for the basic emotional processes so the underlying neural processes can be effectively investigated, and providing linkages for levels of discourse above (psychological) and below (physiological and biochemical) the neurobehavioral level of analysis. Obviously, a cross-species neural analysis can only hope to specify the necessary neural substrates of certain human emotions without making any claims about sufficiency.

Our failure to develop a more flexible attitude toward the study of the hidden evolutionary entities in the brain is partly due to the obvious linguistic difficulties, but it it goes deeper into the lopsided manner in which scientists are educated—namely, to be skeptical about absolutely everything that is difficult to measure, as opposed to being optimistically open to all of the complexities of the world. The proper focus of skepticism should be toward the end of inquiries, not at the beginning as it often tends to be in modern psychological and neural sciences. For instance, many still do not believe that a "social bond" or "brain mechanisms for social affiliation and affect" exist as objective brain functions, and, sadly, we originally experienced great difficulty publishing some of our work on rough-and-tumble play because we used the word *play*. We were advised to simply describe the behavior we saw. We have had similar experiences with distress vocalization (crying) and all the other emotional systems that are covered in this text. We decided not to cave in, for that would have compromised the future development of a scientifically credible affective neuroscience.

Skepticism is certainly a beneficial tool, to the extent that it yields a dialectic of ideas that can progress toward empirical resolution of difficult issues, but at present it is too commonly an attitude, a well-cultivated academic pretense, that leads to the neglect of important problems. Indeed, during the middle part of the 20th century, behavioral scientists asserted that we should ignore internal processes completely—a bias that is still common in behavioral neuroscience.

In light of the many unresolved problems that still exist, debate and disagreement are bound to continue to outweigh consensus within the psychobehavioral neurosciences. Although we all agree that evolution has created many intrinsic functions within the brain "computer," there is presently little agreement on how we should describe, discuss, and study those functions. We do know that internal neuropsychological functions can only be inferred from some combination of external signs, such as behavior and other bodily changes, along with basic psychological insights, but we still do not agree on how we can proceed in a coherent scientific fashion. Hopefully we will eventually reach a consensus on how we might begin to talk about these matters. One hope of this text has been to systematize this important area of knowledge so that a more open dialogue can be initiated between psychologists, neuroscientists, and all other disciplines interested in human nature. To this end, I used some plain emotional language in ways that have never been attempted before, at least in a basic science text.

The Brain Organization of Human Language and Comparable Functions in Animals

One of the greatest success stories of neuropsychology has been the identification of the brain areas that typically generate language, as well as their relatively clear division into areas for receptive and expressive skills, both of which are embedded in a broad field of neural tissue that generates thought. Propositional language is the highest achievement of the human brain, and probably the most recent major achievement in mammalian brain evolution, probably having emerged with early *Homo sapiens* perhaps a quarter of a million years ago. It is puzzling to consider that this is the one function, more than any other, with which we must conceptualize the many other functions of the brain. Thus, we are in the paradoxical position of trying to clarify everything that evolved before, using the most recent neural instrument in our toolbox of cognitive skills.

The locations of the language areas in the left cerebral hemisphere (Figure B.1), have now been affirmed

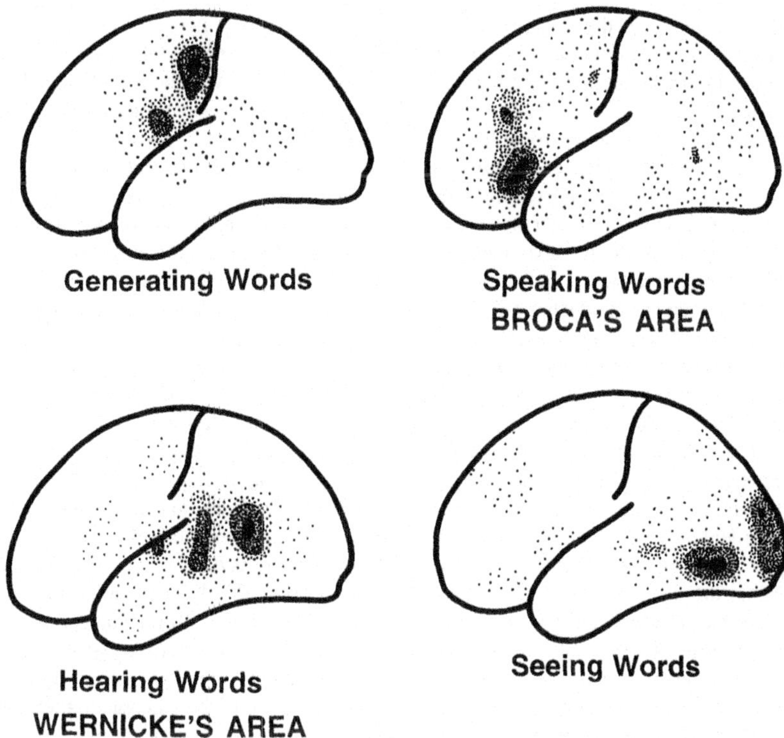

Figure B.1. Summary of language areas of the brain as determined by PET scans of individuals performing different aspects of language. Dark areas indicate highest levels of metabolic activity. When one is speaking words, Broca's area is most active. When one is hearing words, Wernicke's area is most active. When one is silently generating words or seeing words, other brain areas are active. (Adapted from a pet image by Marcus Reichle as depicted in Eccles, 1994, p. 175; see App. C, n. 9.)

by many techniques, but the actual processing of language is more complex than we could have imagined. One cortical zone, the so-called *Wernicke's area*, at the junction of the sensory cortices of parietal, occipital, and temporal lobes, is specialized for the reception of language. It is nestled between the areas of the brain that receive tactile, visual, and auditory information from those respective lobes. In other words, it is a higher-order sensory *association area*, ideally suited for synthesizing information from many modalities. From its central location, nestled among all the primary and secondary somatic-sensory processing areas of the cortex, Wernicke's area generates the essence of language—the symbolic representation of information from one sensory modality in another. This area sends information, via a pathway called the *arcuate fasciculus*, to the nearby premotor cortex, or *Broca's area*, which elaborates acts of speech. This area then transmits individual speech acts to nearby motor neurons that control the articulatory apparatus of mouth and throat (or gestures and other movements of the hands in the case of sign languages). The semantic information that is integrated in Wernicke's area, so readily translated into sounds, can also, after slow and arduous learning processes, be resymbolized in reading and writing. In other words, language is most naturally mediated by audiovocal processes, but it can also be instantiated in other sensory and motor realms. Thus, we must resist ascribing the *deep nature* of language systems of the human brain to specific zones of the brain such as Wernicke's and Broca's areas. Communication apparently can be elaborated by other brain areas, especially when we are young.[2]

When Wernicke's area is damaged in normal adults, people still hear language, but they make little sense of it. The ability to construct meaning has been lost. And even though their speech may sound fluent, it characteristically lacks coherent meaning. This suggests that the syntactic structures and basic urge to speak have remained intact. Because the natural flow of linguistic output appears to be an intrinsic function of Broca's area, when this area is lost, one has great difficulty articulating any coherent speech. However, the understanding of language is intact. When the large neural pathway between the two areas (i.e., the arcuate fasciculus) is damaged, patients show the expected mixture of symptoms: They understand what is said, but their fluent speech is incoherent.

So where does the urge to speak come from? It does not reside in Broca's area, since expressive aphasia is typically accompanied by a deep desire to communicate. It appears to be elaborated by yet another brain area, the *anterior cingulate cortex*, a zone that also mediates social motivation. This reinforces the conclusion that speech is fundamentally a social act, and it has only been tortuously bent for scientific ends. Parenthetically, dolphins and whales have rich neural expansions in this area of the brain,[3] and they do seem to be highly communicative. Following anterior cingulate damage, people exhibit *akinetic mutism,* which means that their apparent desire, but not competence, to talk has disappeared.

In this context, it is worth considering again that mysterious brain disorder known as Williams syndrome (described in Chapter 14). This childhood developmental problem highlights the distinction between brain mechanisms that generate fluid speech and those that generate meaning, revealing that it is not always the fastest and smoothest speakers who have the best ideas. Clearly, the motivational and neural carrier mechanisms for speech are distinct from those that infuse them with real significance. It is worth considering whether Williams syndrome might be accompanied by hypertrophy of the cingulate speech-motivation mechanisms that drive Broca's area, with a diminished influence on output by Wernicke's area. In contrast to this, most autistic children never pick up normal speech, and CAT and MRI brain scans indicate that many of them do not have enlarged left-hemisphere speech areas,[4] suggesting that the areas of the brain that elaborate linguistic meaning may not have matured properly in many of these children.[5] One hopes a neuronal growth factor will eventually be found that will allow that part of the brain to develop richer connections.

It is not clear why propositional language areas are better developed in the left cerebral hemisphere, but it may be related to right-handedness. The predominance of left hemispheric specialization for propositional language appears to be innate, for presently unknown reasons. Most newborn children have more cortical tissues in Wernicke's area on the left side of their brains than on the right. Because of this lateralization of function, mouth movements during speaking are asymmetrical in many people. Since descending motor systems cross in the brain stem, most people tend to speak a bit more out of the right side of their mouth, because the left cortex controls the right side of the face (however, in about 5% of individuals speech dominance is reversed). It would also be interesting to determine whether the motor dynamics change more on one side of the mouth than the other when people tell a lie. Such knowledge might suggest which hemisphere is the more truthful. I would anticipate that people are generally less truthful with the left hemisphere (since it is a specialist in social communication), and that at some deep and fundamental affective level, the right hemisphere is more in touch with true inner feelings and less liable to lie.

Of course, such an experiment would have to be conducted with considerable finesse, since the right hemisphere is reluctant to express itself. For instance, most analyses of hemispheric speech control, as can be done with split-brain individuals or those undergoing the Wada test (selective anesthetization of one hemisphere), find that language originating in the right hemisphere consists largely of simple labeling, with little ability to chain words together into semantic structures. However, this does not mean that the right hemisphere is intrinsically simpleminded or a slow learner. It has the ability to learn language quite well when we are young, and it understands more than it linguistically conveys.

Indeed, our ability to acquire language occurs most flexibly during the neural openness of our youth. If the left hemisphere is damaged early in life, the right side takes over remarkably well and permits normal acquisition of speech. This, unfortunately, is not the case for older folks. Following a stroke, speech impediments are often permanent, with only tortuous improvements over time, even with the best language therapies. Improvement is generally better in females after comparable damage, since they are more able than males to coordinate and use both hemispheres in unison.[6]

It is also noteworthy that different categories of words appear to come from different parts of the brain, from areas we might well have predicted simply from a knowledge of the general localization of sensory and motor processes. Nouns, those static descriptors of the world, appear to arise more from posterior sensory-analyzer parts of the brain close to Wernicke's area, while verbal action descriptors tend to emerge from frontal cortical areas that generate motor responses and plans for behavior—tissues that are closer to Broca's area.

The right hemisphere is not without sophisticated language functions. In addition to simple propositional skills, such as the generation of nouns, it is a specialist for conveying the emotional melody in language, or *prosody*. Even if one has lost left hemisphere speech, one can often still sing smoothly and expressively. Again, there are two general forms of this affective skill, receptive and expressive. Indeed, the expressive and receptive areas for prosody correspond anatomically to the areas of the brain designated as Broca's and Wernicke's areas in the left hemisphere. In other words, the cortical zone on the right side of the brain that corresponds to Wernicke's area allows us to interpret the emotional tone of speech, while the zone that corresponds to Broca's area mediates our ability to express emotional meaning and affective nuances in our utterances.

Without these right hemisphere functions, people exhibit specific deficits in communication. For instance, teachers who have had the misfortune to be inflicted with right cortical damage often find their ability to teach seriously compromised. They can still convey ideas, but the lyrical quality of their speech is impaired. Their lectures are monotonous, and learning in such classrooms becomes a tedious chore. Also, since they have difficulty conveying affective intonations to others (although they still feel them internally), they are not able to express conviction about their ideas, leaving students uninspired. It is easy to imagine why classroom control, especially in the lower grades, would be more difficult for teachers with such brain afflictions. In this context, it is also worth reemphasizing that the speech areas of the two hemispheres appear to function in a more coordinated fashion in women than in men, with men being much more dependent on their left hemisphere for the organization of speech. This may be one reason that the speech of women tends to be emotionally richer than that of men.

As with most other brain systems that have been studied, the vigorous use and disuse of the language-processing areas of the brain should yield measurable changes in the underlying neuronal architecture. A great deal of research on other brain systems has indicated that enriched environments facilitate the growth of cortical systems, especially in young animals.[7] Such effects have been especially well documented in the visual system. For instance, closing one eye in a young animal leads to permanent lifelong deficiencies in that eye's ability to process information, due to accumulating weaknesses in the underlying neural circuits.[8] Thus it has been of some interest to see how sign language is processed in deaf children, and preliminary brain mapping suggests that they process language in very different ways than depicted in the classic view (Figure B.1). For them, language is much more a function of information processing in somatosensory and somatomotor representations of the hand.[9] This remarkable finding suggests that in the young brain, many other areas than Broca's and Wernicke's are capable of elaborating the processing of linguistic material.

Do other species have cortex comparable to Wernicke's area, which brings together and intermixes many sensory impressions? In part, yes. In monkeys, the brain areas corresponding to Wernicke's area are also multimodal and thereby permit the animals to exhibit cross-modal learning. However, these areas do not appear to be important for the monkeys' rich repertoire of spontaneous communicative calls. Such vocal communication in "lower" mammals is typically organized by subcortical brain circuits that are closely linked to the generators of emotional states. A question that remains to be resolved is whether the cortical zones that control human language abilities are the same as those that allow other apes to pick up rudimentary forms of sign language.[10] Unfortunately, at present the rudimentary communications of other primates have not told us much about their minds, except that they can become quite adept at such social interactions. It remains possible that their willingness to participate in language games is motivated more by the joys of social interaction (and the treats they receive) than by any urge to convey their thoughts.

The poignant case of "Clever Hans," the calculating horse, is instructive here. Clever Hans became famous in the last century for his supposed ability to solve simple arithmetic problems. But alas, under close scientific scrutiny, it became all too evident that Clever Hans was merely responding to inadvertent cues from his master—a raised eyebrow or the quiver of a lip was enough to cue him to stop tapping his hoof and receive the desired reward. Hans had mastered no mathematics, only clever ways to obtain treats.

The ease with which we can be deceived has more recently surfaced in the practice of "facilitated communication," which is a nonverbal way to allow autistic and other linguistically impaired children to communicate on keyboards. As many careful scientific evaluations of the procedure have now indicated, most children were not communicating. The only linguistic production that was objectively evident emerged from the "Clever Hands" of the facilitators.[11]

Although language is the only way we can scientifically bridge the chasm between brain and mind, we should always remember that we humans are creatures that can be deceived as easily by logical rigor as by blind faith. Despite our scientific pride in using words precisely, the most important metrics for measuring our scientific insights are the predictions we can confirm and the useful products of our research. It is possible that some of the fuzzier concepts of folk-psychology may lead us to a more fruitful understanding of the integrative functions of the brain than the rigorous, but constrained, languages of visually observable behavioral acts. The dilemma that the "prison house of language" presently imposes on our modern scientific and cultural pursuits should not be underestimated.[12]

Appendix C
Dualism in the Neurosciences

What is the mind? Does it simply emerge from the biological functions of the brain? Most neuroscientists, who ascribe to *monistic* beliefs, now believe this is the case. Many others, who hold *dualistic* worldviews, do not agree. They believe mind and brain are fundamentally different, asserting in the most extreme cases that the two cannot be definitively joined through any neuroscientific or neuropsychological analysis. Some ascribe to a less radical form of dualism, believing that mental and neural activities interact at specific areas of the brain. The most famous champion of such views was the French philosopher René Descartes, who, perhaps as a matter of political-religious expediency,[1] suggested that the human mind and brain interact within the pineal gland. This left the province of the body to science and that of the human mind and soul to theology. The dilemma this debate embodies is as old as our ability to speak (see Appendix B), even though philosophers only started to worry about it in earnest after Descartes announced his unusual take on the matter.

Certainly dualism, or the mind-body problem, is tightly linked to the nature of language, historical records of which go back only about 20,000 years. Indeed, it is quite possible that the mind-body problem is merely a reflection of our brain's linguistic abilities—the ability to generate symbolic paradoxes and layers of *meaning* that do not exist in nature. Words can easily create semblances of meaning that are pure fantasies—but powerful ones that can change the world.

The remarkable idea that there is a mind that can operate independently of the complexities of the brain is not currently a popular one in modern neuroscience, but there are many cognitive scientists who are trying to simulate mental processes computationally.[2] Thus, the issue does need some attention by neuroscientists even in this modern era when the ready availability of computers has given us a powerful metaphor to make the mind-body dichotomy more understandable than it has traditionally been: Invisible, mindlike software functions, which consume very little energy, can easily control visible, body-type hardware functions, which consume much more.

We have come to recognize that information is an organized state of matter. Information flow is a distinct "semiphysical" process that can be conceptualized independently of specific forms of matter and energy by which it is instantiated.[3] The term *semiphysical* is used simply to focus our attention on the fact that the exact physical medium upon which information transfers occur is less important than the formal mathematical concepts that constitute the science of information processing. Thus, computer memories can be generated from a variety of physical substrates engineered to behave in similar ways. Of course, this does not mean that information can exist in our world without the physical instantiation provided by matter and energy. Information is a specific type of interaction between the two. Similarly, mind is an interaction of brain dynamics and environmental events.

Because it is now very clear how low-energy information processes within the brain can control high-energy body processes, most neuroscientists are not terribly interested in the old mind-body debates. Most thinkers are satisfied to believe that mind is simply the brain in action—namely, they ascribe to the *mind-brain identity* approach to the problem: For them, mind emerges as naturally from brain functions as digestion emerges from normal gastric processes. Although most brain scientists are happy to believe that mental events simply reflect the neurodynamic informational exchanges within many interacting networks of the brain, and nothing else, there is still substantial controversy among philosophically oriented investigators. Indeed, such issues are being most actively discussed in the ongoing debate about the nature of conscious experience.[4]

At one end of the opinion spectrum, some thinkers presently believe that consciousness emerges from quantum-level interactions within matter. To make sense of such ideas, one has to leap many gaps in knowledge—including neuroanatomical, neurophysiological, and neurochemical ones. Most neuroscientists are not willing to tolerate such large leaps of the imagination, and there are even greater leaps that take us well beyond the bounds of reason, firmly into the province of faith. Thus, on the weird side of the spectrum, some far-out thinkers are willing to entertain untestable ideas such as the notion that all blades of grass and even pebbles on the beach are imbued with some level of consciousness, but it is difficult to imagine the computational devices that might achieve those miracles. Of course, they would reply, consciousness is not computational. Most investigators hold more middle-of-the-road opinions and feel that mental events need to be understood as brain informational events that happen at circuit levels rather than any subatomic levels of organization.

In any case, scholars who try to explain how mind may emerge from material processes must contend with several distinct points of view in order to integrate all the available data. Like physicists who view electrons as either *particles* or *waves*, psychologists and brain scientists are coming to terms with the idea that the brain is a physical machine that transmits and processes information in highly complex ways—typically quite differently than digital computers. Although it seems unlikely that brain scientists will be able to specify *precisely* how mental events emerge from the dynamics of material events in the near future because of the sheer complexity of the task, most believe that mind is simply the brain participating in informational transaction that can already be envisioned in theory if not in practice.

Modern neuroscience has become relatively immune to the classic paradoxes of mentalism, but the issue of mind-brain dualism has not disappeared completely from neuroscience thinking. Indeed, it would be sad if it did, for then new generations of brain psychologists and philosophers would miss out on the fun of debating such perennial and "aweful" issues. We humans enjoy holding strange and often incredible beliefs. After all, above all else, we *are* storytelling creatures. We are bound to keep taking many diverse positions, and we will have to entertain many new ideas, especially those that may yield observable results, before we will have a practical description of the nature of human or animal consciousness. In any event, dualism is by no means dead in philosophical or neuroscientific discussions of brain functions.

Several prominent neuroscientists have continued to champion a variety of views along these lines, and they have provided several intellectual variants of this problem for our consideration. Here I will summarize the viewpoints of three prominent neuroscientists who have dwelled at length on issues of mind-brain dualism during the recent flowering of modern neuroscience. Even though they have not always spelled out their visions in ways that can be rigorously tested, their thoughts do allow us to view this ancient dilemma from a variety of intriguing perspectives.

During the past few decades, three esteemed senior neuroscientists have forcefully disagreed with the traditional and radically monistic *identity* view of the brain-mind debate, siding instead with the perspective that mind is in some essential way separable from the material entities of the brain. First I will summarize the views of Wilder Penfield, a pioneering neurosurgeon who first demonstrated that localized electrical stimulation of the temporal lobes could yield a remarkably faithful subjective reexperiencing of seemingly forgotten events. His findings suggested that vast unconscious stores of memories are locked away within our neural circuits. His work provided a major stimulus for the ongoing study of memory traces in temporal lobes, especially in tissues such as the hippocampus. Next, I will focus on the views of Roger Sperry, who won the Nobel Prize in 1981 for his work on the distinct and separate forms of awareness within each of the cerebral hemispheres (also see Chapter 16). Finally, I will summarize the more radical views of Sir John Eccles, a Nobel laureate in 1963, who worked out the details of how neurons synaptically generate electrical signals of excitation and inhibition (see Chapter 4).

After highly productive scientific careers, these scholars chose to dwell on the essential nature of the human spirit. Each found solace, understanding, and hope in the conviction that a distinction between mind and brain functions not only was real but also constituted a vital distinction for understanding the human brain and nature. Some of their views (especially Sperry's), with modest qualifications, might be usefully incorporated into the cognitive and affective neurosciences without a compromise of the types of monistic/materialistic principles upon which most modern brain and cognitive research is based. Some other ideas, especially the recent ones of Eccles, are distinctly more mystical.

Wilder Penfield made an especially dramatic contribution to our knowledge of human brain function. When certain areas of the temporal cortex (situated an inch inside the cranium from the top of the ear) are electrically stimulated in epileptic patients, these individuals experience past events almost as vividly as if they are reliving them. The experience unfolds psychologically like a videotape, with full experiential continuity, even while the patient remains aware of the reality of the surgical arena in which he or she is situated. To some extent these effects are dependent on neural tissue that has been primed by epilepsy. Such experiences were not easily reproduced in nonepileptic patients. Penfield summarized his findings and his philosophical views in 1975, a few years before his death, in a book entitled *The Mystery of the Mind*. Here he announced his decision, after many years of pondering the nature of human consciousness, to side with the idea that our mind is in fact not just the material reflection of brain functions, but that it is guided by some type of immaterial mind. As he phrased the issue: "One may ask this question: does the highest brain-mechanism provide the mind with its energy, and energy in such a changed form that it no longer needs to be conducted along neuroaxones? To ask such a question is, I fear, to run the risk of hollow laughter from the physicists. But, nonetheless, this is my question, and the suggestion I feel myself compelled to make." He proceeds to enunciate his dualistic view quite explicitly: "During brain action a neuro-physiologist can surmise where the conduction of potentials is being carried out and its pattern. It is not so in the case of what we have come to call mind-action. And yet the mind seems to act independently of the brain in the same sense that a programmer acts independently of his computer. . . . For my own part, after years of striving to explain the mind on the basis of brain-action alone, I have come to the conclusion that it is simpler (and far easier to be logical) if one adopts the hypothesis that our being does consist of two fundamental elements. . . . Because it seems to me certain that it will always be quite impossible to explain the mind on the basis of neuronal action within the brain." Penfield's straightforward conviction was that a dualist hypothesis is more reasonable than a monistic one. Hence he concludes that "the mind must be viewed as a basic *element* in itself. One might, then, call it a *medium*, an *essence*, a *soma*. That is to say, it has a *continuing existence*."[5]

Roger Sperry opened up the study of human consciousness with his startling findings concerning the distinct perceptual and cognitive abilities of the right and left hemispheres in folks whose *corpora callosa* had to be severed to control their epilepsies. From a rigorous behavioristic position, which ultimately proved incompatible with his personal worldview, Sperry formally presented his ideas concerning the dual functions of the brain in a series of theoretical papers in the preeminent journal for psychologically minded academicians, the *Psychological Review*. A synopsis of his view is captured in the following few sentences: "Current mind-brain theory no longer dispenses with conscious mind as just an 'inner aspect' of brain activity, or as some passive 'epiphenomenal,' metaphysical, or other impotent by-product, as has long been the custom; nor does it reject consciousness as merely an artifact of semantics or as being identical to the neural events. Consciousness, in these revised terms, becomes an integral, dynamic property of the brain process itself and a central constituent of brain action. Subjective experience is viewed . . . as a causal determinant in brain function and acquires emergent control influence in regulating the course of physico-chemical events in brain activity. No metaphysical interaction in the classical sense is implied; the causal relation primarily involves the power of the whole over its parts." In subsequent writings, it is quite clear that Sperry's monistic dualism is one of *emergent properties*, where the end result of simple processes is more complex than the sum of the whole—for instance, like the properties of water emerging from the molecular interaction of hydrogen and oxygen. He believes that a superordinate function of neural activity has ultimately formed a brain quality called consciousness, which then has the ability to directly modify brain activity. Sperry suggests that with the evolution of such superordinate functions, such as is present in our subjective experience, the flow of causal influences on behavior has become one where "top-down" regulation is the rule, and hence the science of mind has to come to terms with such emergent "mental" properties and how they influence the flow of information within the brain.[6]

There is a certain ambiguity in Sperry's ideas, since he really does not spell out how conscious awareness functions of the brain modify other neural activities. Yet he believes his viewpoint could be the foundation for a global ethic based on a science that promotes the overall welfare of our world rather than the one of personal greed that may have come close to destroying it.[7] Although Sperry's views often seem dualistic, they are actually a complex form of monism that accepts the complexities of neuromental representations. The evolution of such hierarchical controls must be taken seriously, asserts Sperry, before we can really understand the brain. He criticizes the traditional monistic reductionist approaches that only seek to "explain the whole in terms of 'nothing but' the parts" and thereby "leads to an infinite nihilistic regress in which eventually everything is held to be explainable in terms of essentially nothing."[8] The views espoused in the present text are compatible with Sperry's, in the sense that software functions can control hardware functions in computers, but the idea that affective consciousness is, in fact, an ancient brain process may be somewhat at odds with Sperry's view that subjective awareness is a recent phenomenon in brain evolution.

Sir John Eccles has provided the modern counterpart of a traditional religious view. In a series of books,[9] Eccles outlined a conception whereby a divinely created mind or soul could be infused into the developing human embryo. To give a flavor of his views, I will quote him from the final article in a 1982 Vatican symposium that he edited on mind-brain interrelations: "We have to be open to some deep dramatic significance in this earthly life of ours that may be revealed after the transformation of death. . . . We find ourselves here in this wonderfully rich and vivid conscious experience and it goes on through life; but is that the end? This self-conscious mind of ours has this mysterious relationship with the brain and as a consequence achieves experiences of human love and friendship, of the wonderful natural beauties, and of the intellectual excitement and joy given by appreciation and understanding of our cultural heritages. . . . In the context of Natural Theology I come to the belief that we are creatures with some supernatural meaning that is as yet ill defined."[10] In more recent works, he has attempted to refine his views to the point where they might be scientifically testable. Eccles does not equivocate about the fact that his viewpoint is deeply dualistic. The catchphrase in which he prefers to encapsulate his perspective is the "dualist-interactionist" view of mind.

His most recent statement on the matter is summarized recursively in the provocatively entitled *How the*

Self Controls Its Brain. After sharing an interesting history of his personal intellectual quest, the first third of the book dissects the many recent texts that have sought to explicate human consciousness from monistic neuroscientific points of view.[11] Eccles perform his surgery in both kindly and merciless fashion, and I could no more avoid the image of a quixotic knight-errant than I can avoid thinking about white elephants when told not to do so. The middle part of the book is a masterful analysis of cortical functions, ending with the crown jewel of his view—a chapter outlining a theory of how an insubstantial self might interact with brain matter without violating the energy conservation laws of physics.[12] In a nutshell, Eccles and his coauthor Friedrich Beck, a quantum physicist, suggest that "the self" may control activity in the cortex by altering the statistical probability of vesicular release of chemicals into synaptic endings, thus offering a putative explanation of how conscious thoughts may control brain activities. It is a clever maneuver, but the end result could be mediated by many other internal brain processes, including the epigenetic manifestations of the neural SELF described in Chapter 16. In any event, the bottom line is that no empirical evaluation of the idea was or has yet been provided. Thus, it remains an astonishing hypothesis or an untestable story, depending on your point of view. The end of the book is devoted to an enthusiastic summation of the battle he has waged on behalf of a neuroscientifically based dualism. Although Eccles does not profess to be religiously motivated in this book, in the final chapter he does again put his thinking in that context. Eccles concludes that "since materialists' solutions fail to account for our experienced uniqueness, I am constrained to attribute the uniqueness of the self or soul to a supernatural spiritual creation."[13]

In sum, Eccles's view is one of devout confrontation with the abiding mystery of existence, and he has chosen to accept an essentially religious view, with the complex embellishments of neuroscience. Like Descartes before him, Eccles has chosen to believe that the brain interacts with an immortal human soul, at specific neural locations like the "supplementary motor area" of the cortex, close to where a substantial amount of thought and voluntary behavior is, in fact, initiated. Because the two functions are interactive but separable, he leaves open the possibility of a spiritual afterlife. To put it perhaps a bit too simply: Eccles feels that our brains are touched by a benevolent life force of consciousness that may continue in some form after bodily death. Many individuals resonate with such beliefs, since they have difficulty accepting that the subtlety of their minds could have been constructed simply through the processes of biological evolution. It is hard for many to believe that one continues to live after death only in the thoughts and hearts of one's descendants. Many believe there must be a grander order that underlies our fundamental nature as living organisms. If so, it is presently outside the realm of science. However, many scientists, including myself, agree that there are mysteries in the universe that the human mind may never be able to understand. One hopes there will eventually be a world religion that will help us all, together, pay our respects to these abiding mysteries.

Although dualism remains a difficult view for most scientists to accept, many agree that mental and neural functions arise from the same grand complexity of brain organization. Brain scientists and psychologists are finally coming to terms with such complexities, without pretending that there must be any final answers to the old philosophical questions. We simply *experience* the things we do because of the types of brain functions we possess. Language can take these functions into realms of the imagination that are, hopefully, limitless. One of the biggest intellectual challenges of the 21st century will be to construct unified images of human nature that do not denigrate our animal past or our future potentials as members of the human family.

AFTERTHOUGHT: Neodualism and Other Alternative Views

Besides the garden varieties of dualism, which consider mind and brain to be constructed of fundamentally different stuff, there are various, more subtle and interesting versions that will no doubt remain with us for some time. Considering the complexity of the human mind and the likelihood that many higher mental processes are woven by pervasive neocortical transmitters such as glutamate, there is bound to remain some skepticism that a neural analysis can truly yield the level of scientific understanding concerning mental matters that we would like to achieve. If the nature of specific kinds of information processing cannot be solved by direct neurophysiological and neurochemical approaches, some argue that the computational approach is the only credible alternative. This type of "procedural dualism" suggests that a brain approach simply will not have the resolution needed to solve major issues in cognitive psychology, and hence, it is wiser to pursue other avenues of representational psychophysics—for instance, those that rely more on computerized simulation of mind functions than on the direct analysis of brain functions.

There is much to be said for such a view, but I will not attempt an analysis here, except to suggest that there is likely to be some significant chemical coding of cognitive dispositions in the higher reaches of the brain. As we have seen, the study of various neuropeptide systems is providing clear evidence for neurochemical specificity in the coding of a variety of emotional and motivational processes. Many of these systems interact with higher reaches of the mind (see corticotrophin releasing factor and cholecystokinin maps in Figure 6.7, as well as other transmitter systems in Figure 6.5), and we are barely beginning to fathom the nature of such interactions.[14] Although it is unlikely that these systems control the precise form of individual thoughts, it remains possible that many of these systems help guide cognitive processes in certain predictable paths. Thus, even if prevalent transmitters such as glutamate and GABA do control the construction of the specific form and shape of each thought, there may be various general neurochemical dispositions that guide the patterning of thoughts that no amount of computational work can clarify. Thus, I disagree with a prevailing cognitive psychological view that disregards the nature of the living brain in its deliberations about the nature of mental representations.

A very different functional form of neodualistic thought pervades behavioral neuroscience—the knee-jerk antagonism to considering the possibility that subjectively experienced representations of thoughts and emotions exist in the brains of other animals. I am tempted to call this "functional neodualism" since it is a well-cultivated intellectual stance implicitly based on a form of cross-species discrimination that creates a greater divide between the animal brain/mind and the human brain/mind than may truly exist—one that may be wider than the one originally posed by Descartes, since he at least accepted the reality of various animal passions. The emergence of unique representational abilities in humans, especially those instantiated by language, allows the great divide to be enforced with a great deal of assurance. Such convictions are based on a prevailing scientific bias—if you can't see it, you shouldn't talk about it. This has prevented the whole discipline of modern neuroscience from accepting the nature of emotions within the mammalian brain as a major topic of inquiry or even discussion.

This view, like the classic behaviorist one upon which it is based, is constrained by a special set of blinders that allow it to disregard the mass of converging evidence that suggests other creatures have strong emotional feelings akin to our own. It sees the world based on one overriding preconception—that reality can only be described through the assiduous applications of our senses, especially of the visual variety, and that theoretical inferences are not needed for us to truly comprehend the nature of the evolved brain. I disagree with this ultrapositivistic scientific view, and I believe that insightful observations always start with insightful preconceptions concerning the underlying nature of things. If we do not take initially unseen aspects of a phenomenon into consideration, the hidden underbelly of nature cannot be adequately revealed.

As should be evident by now, I have strong convictions about the importance of emotion research in the development of a scientific psychology as well as a credible integrative neuroscience, while the majority of my colleagues remain dubious of the reality of affective consciousness in the brains of other animals. The recent appearance of a fine book that shares both of the above beliefs, in a forthright and compelling manner, has convinced me to add this final "Afterthought," so as to contrast the raison d'être of the present work with the radical behaviorist perspective that still guides most work in this area.

After this book was submitted to the publisher, Joseph LeDoux's book, *The Emotional Brain* (1996), appeared in print. In addition to vigorously challenging the whole notion that emotional systems are concentrated in the limbic system, one of his central themes was that a consideration of emotional feelings or affective consciousness is more of a hindrance in the study of emotions than a key feature of the problem that needs to be solved. My own perspective on the matter is, of course, diametrically different. For me, the nature of affective feelings exists as a core problem for cross-species emotion research. Since so many of my colleagues still deny that a study of affective feelings is a key problem in emotion research, I have decided to use LeDoux's perspective as a foil for my final remarks. I do this with abundant admiration for LeDoux's empirical contributions.

At the end of his treatise, LeDoux struggles briefly with the nature of emotional feelings. He aspires to solve the dilemma by boiling affective experience down to the interaction of working memory mechanisms with some of the types of emotional systems described in this text. The "working memory" hypothesis surely contains more than a grain of truth, depending on precisely what we mean by that cognitive construct. At present, it remains a fairly empty category, at least in neural terms. LeDoux suggests that emotional consciousness is a mere byproduct, and a rather inconsequential one at that, of the higher memory mechanisms of the brain. According to LeDoux, affective feelings have little consequence in the regulation of emotional behaviors, and he proceeds, as did Descartes, to cast new versions of doubt on the existence of feeling states in most other mammalian species. He boldly asserts at the end: "The brain states and bodily responses are the fundamental facts of an emotion, and the conscious feelings are the frills that have added icing to the emotional cake."[15]

While I wholeheartedly agree that brain states and bodily responses are essential components of each integrated emotional response, I also accept emotional feelings as key attributes of emotional operating systems in action. Affective feelings are the here-and-now existential states created by these neuromechanisms as they interact with brain circuits that neurosymbolically represent the organism as a living creature. For instance, just as the unconditional, pleasant taste of sugar has little to do with working memory, I doubt if the feeling state of anger requires working memory, except as a modulatory influence to extend, shorten, or blend feelings in time. My point of view is that, rather than being created by memory systems, emotional systems are a major moving force within memory mechanisms. Thus, I would submit that the interaction of emotional feelings with working memory is, at best, only one of the many ways by which emotional states effectively control future behaviors.

Although my view affirms that the evolution of emotional feelings was linked, to a substantial degree, to the special needs of brain memory systems that must rapidly encode intrinsic biological values (see Chapters 1 and 2), I believe that the core of emotionality must be sought in more fundamental terms than as a mere subset of working memory, at least of the type that is typically conceptualized as a fairly high-level cortical function. In my research experience, animals with essentially no neocortex remain behaviorally, and probably internally, as emotional as ever, indeed more so.[16] I have argued, in agreement with investigators such as Paul MacLean, that the capacity to have affective feelings is an evolutionary birthright embedded within the intrinsic and ancient organizational dynamics of the mammalian brain, situated largely in subcortical realms known as the extended limbic system. I feel confident that this scheme remains a more defensible generalization than is suggested in LeDoux's severely critical analysis of the concept.

In sum, I doubt if emotional feelings need to be learned or extracted from dynamic memory stores. I think LeDoux is misguided, as was William James when he suggested that the cortex is the storehouse for our emotional feelings. Thus, while LeDoux asserts that we should confine our efforts largely to traditional behavioral and physiological realms in our study of emotions within the animal brain, I would advocate that we should, in addition, begin to study emotional feelings, indirectly, as essential foundation processes upon which many unique aspects of the human mind—from art to politics—have been created.

For those who would continue to deny the existence of emotional feelings in other animals (clearly a popular scientific stance), I would like to offer an allegorical devil's choice. Imagine that you have been cornered by the Evil One, and your options for life and freedom are constrained by his demanding sense of humor. Your hopes for a pleasant future hang on your ability to correctly answer one devilishly simple question: Do other mammals have internally experienced emotional feelings that control their behavioral tendencies or do they not? The devil knows the answer, and you must make the correct choice in order to enjoy the remaining days of your life. How would you reply? How many scientists would still be as bold as behaviorists and continue to deny that animals have feelings? My personal conviction is that we shall really not understand the brain or the nature of consciousness until we begin to take emotional feelings more seriously, as internally experienced neurosymbolic SELF-referenced representations of major evolutionary passages, in the animals that we study. Parenthetically, to do otherwise further widens the possibilities for many unethical behaviors in this troubled world of ours.

Fortunately, we do not need the correct answer to the devil's question in order to make scientific progress. We can collect many useful facts by subscribing to many points of view, and we should tolerate them *all*, as long as they do no harm and lead to new theoretical approaches and provocative findings that can be replicated, or negated, by others. Even though the view I have advanced in this text has been tolerated rather less than it should have been during the unusual intellectual history of 20th century psychology and modern neuroscience, we should remember that insightful observation of the systematic patterns in nature (whether easily visible or not) remains our second highest calling. In the final accounting, that is the most lovely aspect of science.

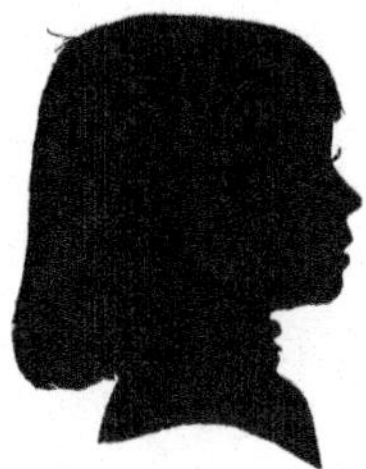

Notes

Chapter 1

1. Watson, J. B. (1924). *Psychology from the standpoint of a behaviorist*. Philadelphia: Lippincott.

2. Skinner, B. F. (1938). *The behavior of organisms*. New York: Appleton-Century-Crofts.

3. Gardner, H. (1985). *The mind's new science: A history of the cognitive revolution*. New York: Basic Books.

4. Barklow, J., Cosmides, L., & Tooby, J. (eds.) (1992). *The adapted mind: Evolutionary psychology and the generation of culture*. New York: Oxford Univ. Press.

5. A great number of writers have addressed this issue from different perspectives, and many key articles can be found in annual updates of *Advances in Animal Behavior*. Works that cover most of the critical issues are:

Hogan, J. A., & Roper, T. J. (1978). A comparison of the properties of different reinforcers. *Adv. Anim. Behav.* 8:155–255.

Marler, P., & Terrace, H. S. (eds.) (1984). *The biology of learning*. Berlin: Springer-Verlag.

Sherry, D. F., & Schacter, D. L. (1987). The evolution of multiple memory systems. *Psych. Rev.* 94:434–454.

6. Breland, K., & Breland, M. (1961). The misbehavior of organisms. *Am. Psychol.* 16:681–684.

7. Seligman, M. E. P., & Hager, J. L. (eds.) (1972). *Biological boundaries of learning*. New York: Appleton.

8. Panksepp, J. (1990). Psychology's search for identity: Can "mind" and behavior be understood without understanding the brain? *New Ideas Psychol.* 8:139–149.

9. Skinner, B. F. (1987). Whatever happened to psychology as the science of behavior? *Am. Psychol.* 42:780–786.

10. Plutchik, R. (1994). *The psychology and biology of emotions*. New York: HarperCollins College.

11. Lewis, M., & Haviland, J. M. (eds.) (1993). *Handbook of emotions*. New York: Guilford Press.

12. Wright, R. (1994). *The moral animal*. New York: Pantheon.

13. Two texts that cover most of the key issues are:

Posner, M. I., & Raichle, M. E. (1994). *Images of mind*. New York: Scientific American Library.

Roland, P. E. (1993). *Brain activation*. New York: Wiley-Liss.

14. Wright, R. (1995). The biology of violence. *New Yorker* (March 13).

Brain, P. F., & Haug, M. (1992). Hormonal and neurochemical correlates of various forms of animal "aggression." *Psychoneuroendocrinol.* 17:537–551.

15. One of the easiest ways to increase aggression is to precipitate withdrawal in opiate-addicted animals. See: Reiss, A., Miczek, K., & Roth, J. (eds.) (1994). *Understanding and preventing violence*. Vol. 2, *Biobehavioral influences*. Washington, D.C.: National Academy Press.

Brain opioids constitute a powerful antiaggressive system of the brain. See: Shaikh, M. B., Lu, C.-L., & Siegel, A. (1991). An enkephalinergic mechanism involved in amygdaloid suppression of affective defense behavior elicited from the midbrain periaqueductal gray in the cat. *Brain Res.* 559:109–117.

16. For current research and views on genetic dispositions in aggression, see: Special issue: The neurobehavioral genetics of aggression. *Behav. Genetics* 26:459–432.

For an overview of other biological controls, see: Marzuk, P. A. (1996). Violence, crime, and mental illness: How strong a link? *Arch. Gen. Psychiat.* 53:481–486.

17. Bouchard, T. J. (1994). Genes, environment, and personality. Science 264: 1700–1701.

Bouchard, T. J., Lykken, D. T., McGue, M., Segal, N. L., & Tellegen, A. (1990). Sources of human psychological differences: The Minnesota Study of Twins Reared Apart. *Science* 250:223–228.

18. Merzenich, M. M., & Sameshima, K. (1993). Cortical plasticity and memory. *Curr. Opin. Neurobiol.* 3:187–196.

Nudo, R. J., Milliken, G. W., Jenkins, W. M., & Merzenich, M. M. (1996). Use-dependent alterations of movement representations in primary motor cortex of adult squirrel monkeys. *J. Neurosci.* 16:785–807.

19. Elbert, T., Pantev, C., Wienbruch, C., Rockstroh, B., & Taub, E. (1995). Increased cortical representation of the fingers of the left hand in string players. *Science* 270:305–307.

20. Panksepp, J. (1985). Mood changes. In *Handbook of clinical neurology*. Vol. 1, *Clinical neuro-*

psychology (P. J. Vinken, G. W. Bruyn, & H. L. Klawans, eds.), pp. 272–285. Amsterdam: Elsevier.

21. Aronson, L. R., Tobach, E., Lehrman, D. S., & Rosenblatt, J. S. (eds.) (1970). *Development and evolution of behavior*. San Francisco: Freeman.

de Beer, G. G. (1958). *Embryos and ancestors* (3d ed.). London: Oxford Univ. Press.

22. A neologism that might be appropriate to denote genetic similarity on the level of function is *homogenic*, which could be taken to imply a common genetic source for an intrinsic function of the brain. In a similar vein, a term such as *logogenic* might be used to indicate innate perceptual sensitivities that are ingrained in certain brain systems because of direct genetic influences—for instance, the apparent unlearned fear of snakes that certain animals exhibit or the fear-evoking smell of predators discussed at the end of Chapter 1. Thus the existence of a similar neurodynamic basis for fear in the brains of all mammalian species may be considered *homogenic*, while the tendency of underlying circuits in different species to respond spontaneously to the perception of snakes or the odors of predators might be called *logogenic*.

Mineka, S., & Cook, M. (1988). Social learning and the acquisition of snake fear in monkeys. In *Social learning* (T. R. Zentall & B. G. Galef, eds.), pp. 51–73. Hillsdale, N.J.: Lawrence Erlbaum.

Morris, R., & Morris, D. (1965). *Men and snakes*. London: Hutchinson.

23. Gould, S. J. (1993). An earful of jaw and full of hot air. In *Eight little piggies: Reflection in natural history*, pp. 95–108, 109–120. New York: Norton.

24. Panksepp, J. (1996). Affective neuroscience: A paradigm to study the animate circuits for human emotions. In *Emotions: An interdisciplinary approach* (R. D. Kavanugh, B. Zimmerberg, & S. Fein, eds.), pp. 29–60. Hillsdale, N.J.: Lawrence Erlbaum.

25. Panksepp, J. (1991). Affective neuroscience: A conceptual framework of the neurobiological study of emotions. In *International review of studies on emotion*, vol. 1 (K. T. Strongman, ed.), pp. 59–99. Chichester, U.K.: Wiley.

26. Pagels, H. (1988). *The dreams of reason: The computer and the rise of the sciences of complexity*. New York: Simon and Schuster. Quotations on pp. 11–12.

27. Dudai, Y. (1989). *The neurobiology of memory*. New York: Oxford Univ. Press.

28. O'Keefe, J., & Nadel, L. (1978). *The hippocampus as a cognitive map*. Oxford: Clarendon Press.

29. Green, L., & Kagel, J. H. (eds.) (1996). *Advances in behavioral economics*. Vol 3, *Substance use and abuse*. Norwood, N.J.: Ablex.

30. "Discrete trial" behavioristic approaches to the treatment of autistic children have been remarkably successful. When such programs are conscientiously followed and well managed, the follow-up results have been outstanding. Initial findings were summarized in: Lovaas, O. I. (1987). Behavioral treatment and normal educational and intellectual functioning in young autistic children. *J. Consul. Clin. Psych.* 55:3–9.

More recent follow-up data are provided in: McEachin, J. J., Smith, T., & Lovaas, O. I. (1993). Long-term outcome for children with autism who received early intensive behavioral treatment. *Am. J. Ment. Retard.* 97:359–372.

31. See n. 29 and: Thompson, R. F. (1994). Behaviorism and neuroscience. *Psych. Rev.* 101:259–265.

Chapter 2

1. Truman, J. W. (1992). Hormonal regulation of behavior: Insights from invertebrate systems. In *Behavioral endocrinology* (J. B. Becker, S. M. Breedlove, D. Crews, eds.), pp. 423–450. Cambridge, Mass.: MIT Press. Quotation on pp. 434–435.

2. Although there is a tendency in brain sciences to focus on the diversity of details across species rather than the commonalities, the similarities at all levels—from genetic, to anatomical, to biochemical, to physiological, to behavioral, and perhaps even to certain basic psychological features—are so striking that when we have learned much about one mammalian species, we have typically learned a great deal about them all. Many examples are evident in the behavioral endocrinology text cited in the previous note, and this text is premised on the probable fruitfulness of such translations when we focus on the basic emotional circuits of the brain in mammalian species. The translations will be ever more difficult as one proceeds to ever more complex cognitive processes. Obviously, our complex intellectual abilities arise from higher cortical interconnections that most other species simply do not have. Indeed, the higher reaches of the human brain are unique. See: Willis, C. (1993). *The runaway brain: The evolution of human uniqueness*. New York: Basic Books.

For a modern view of the complexities of human brain development, see: Dawson, G., & Fischer, K. W. (1994). *Human behavior and the developing brain*. New York: Guilford Press.

3. The variety in the details of nature is endless, and here I intend to sustain a focus on principles that may have cross-species generality. Obviously, all emotional systems will be expressed somewhat differently in different species, but often the dissimilarities may be less modest than outward appearances would lead us to believe. For instance, as we will see in Chapter 8, apparently the SEEKING system can arouse exploration and appetitive approach behaviors in rodents and predatory stalking behaviors in cats. These behaviors have traditionally been studied as completely distinct behavioral systems, even though they both serve the function of obtaining food. In primates, this same system can increase visual scanning, which again is an important exploratory response that can serve the animal effectively in its search for resources. This exemplifies how a common underlying emotional/motivational system can mediate seemingly distinct behaviors in different species, but it would be an error to treat such species-typical behavioral manifestations as reflecting fundamentally distinct organizational principles in the nervous systems. A focus on what they have in common can often provide a more satisfactory understanding of behavioral control systems in the brain than a focus on the detailed differences. Even at the highest cerebral levels, some interesting commonalities are being found, such as in the affective specializations of the hemispheres. See:

Davidson, R. J., Kalin, N. H., & Shelton, S. E. (1993). Lateralized response to diazepam predicts temperamental style in rhesus monkeys. *Behav. Neurosci.* 107:1106–1110.

Hoptman, M. J., & Davidson, R. J. (1994). How and why do the two cerebral hemispheres interact? *Psych. Bull.* 116:195–219.

4. A discussion of the nature of affective consciousness will be an essential goal of this book. However, this troublesome topic will be left to the final chapter because the mechanism of consciousness, even though widely debated during the past decade, remains an unresolved dilemma. The overall position that undergirds the present coverage is that the nature of consciousness(es) is rapidly becoming an empirical question that is essential for understanding the nature of brain organization. For a recent overview of this topic, see: Gray, J. A. (1995). The contents of consciousness: A neuropsychological conjecture. *Behav. Brain Sci.* 18:659–722.

5. There have been several important debates concerning the degree to which emotions are precognitive functions of the brain. In one famous debate, Richard Lazarus supported the cognitive view and Robert Zajonc supported the precognitive perspective. See:

Lazarus, R. S. (1984). On the primacy of cognition. *Am. Psychol.* 39:124–129.

Zajonc, R. B. (1984). On the primacy of affect. *Am. Psychol.* 39:117–123.

In a second, less celebrated debate, two behavioral neuroscientists, J. A. Gray and J. Panksepp, took opposite points of view, with Gray supporting the view that emotions cannot be separated from cognitive processes and Panksepp arguing that they can. See:

Gray, J. A. (1990). Brain systems that mediate both emotion and cognition. *Cog. Emot.* 4:270–288.

Panksepp, J. (1990). Gray zones at the emotion/cognition interface: A commentary. *Cog. Emot.* 4:289–302.

6. Christianson, S.-A. (ed.) (1992). *The handbook of emotion and memory.* Hillsdale, N.J.: Lawrence Erlbaum.

7. Recent studies with EEG and other brain-imaging approaches (see chap. 1, n. 13) have indicated that various higher brain areas "light up" when humans experience emotions. For two important recent lines of research, see:

Davidson, R. A. (1992). Anterior cerebral asymmetry and the nature of emotion. *Brain Cog.* 20:125–151.

George, M. S., Ketter, T. A., Kimbrell, T. A., Steedman, J. M., & Post, R. M. (1996). What functional imaging has revealed about the brain basis of mood and emotion. In *Advances in biological psychiatry*, vol. 2 (J. Panksepp, ed.), pp. 63–114. Greenwich, Conn.: JAI Press.

However, it should be noted that such studies may not highlight the primary localization of emotional circuits in the brain, but rather the secondary reflections of emotional arousal in the higher regions of the brain. These brain-imaging techniques can highlight quite modest changes in brain activity in higher cortical regions, but they may often fail to highlight the arousal of fine subcortical emotional circuits because of the massive overlap with counteracting neural processes. The degree to which such techniques can highlight brain stem functions presently remains controversial.

8. Bell, I. R. (1996). Clinically relevant EEG studies and psychophysiological findings: Possible neural mechanisms for multiple chemical sensitivity. *Toxicology* 111:101–17.

Bell, I. R., Hardin, E. E., Baldwin, C. M., & Schwartz, G. E. (1995). Increased limbic system symptomatology and sensitizability of young adults with chemical and noise sensitivities. *Environ. Res.* 70:84–97.

Van der Kolk, B. A., McFarlane, A. C., & Weisaeth, L. (eds.) (1996). *Traumatic stress: The effects of overwhelming experience on mind, body, and society.* New York: Guilford.

9. There are now thousands of studies that have yielded such "stimulus-bound" emotional effects in animals and humans, but there has been a historical trend to interpret such effects either in terms of emotionally vacuous motor response effects or in terms of learning effects rather than in basic emotional terms. A fine overview of such issues is to be found in: Valenstein, E. (1973). *Brain control.* New York: Wiley.

10. Larimer, J. L. (1988). The command hypothesis: A new view using an old example. *Trends Neurosci.* 11:506–510.

11. Yeh, S. R., Fricke, R. A., & Edwards, D. H. (1996). The effect of social experience on serotonergic modulation of the escape circuit of crayfish, *Science* 271:366–369.

12. A thorough review of methodological issues is to be found in: Farthing, G. W. (1992). *The psychology of consciousness.* Englewood Cliffs, N.J.: Prentice Hall.

The classic citation highlighting how poorly humans identify the causes of their own behaviors is: Nisbett, R. E., & Wilson, T. D. (1977). Telling more than we can know: Verbal reports on mental processes. *Psych. Rev.* 84:231–259.

13. Weiner, J. (1995). *The beak of the finch: A story of evolution in our time.* New York: Vintage Books. Quotation on p. 161.

14. Coverage of such basic issues is available in practically any research methodology book. An especially clear summary of such logical issues can be found in: Ray, W. J. (1993). *Methods toward a science of behavior and experience.* Pacific Grove, Calif.: Brooks/Cole.

15. Cacioppo, J. T., & Tassinary, L. G. (eds.) (1990). *Principles of psychophysiology: Physiological, social and inferential elements.* New York: Cambridge Univ. Press.

Wagner, H., & Manstead, A. (eds.) (1989). *Handbook of social psychophysiology.* Chichester, U.K.: Wiley.

16. Gazzaniga, M. S. (ed.) (1995). *The cognitive neurosciences.* Cambridge, Mass.: MIT Press.

17. Gallistel, C. R. (ed.) (1992). *Animal cognition.* Cambridge, Mass.: MIT Press.

Gould, J. L., & Gould, C. G. (1994). *The animal mind.* New York: Scientific American Library.

Roitblat, T. G., Bever, H. S., & Terrace, H. (eds.) (1984). *Animal cognition.* Hillsdale, N.J.: Lawrence Erlbaum.

18. Rilling, M. E., & Neiworth, J. J. (1991). How animals use images. *Sci. Progress, Edinburgh* 75:439–452.

19. Chwalisz, K., Diener, E., & Gallagher, D. (1988). Autonomic arousal feedback and emotional experience: Evidence from the spinal cord injured. *J. Personal. Soc. Psychol.* 54:820–828.

20. Campos, J. J., Barret, K. C., Lamb, M., Goldsmith, H. H., & Stenberg, C. (1983). Socioemotional development. In *Handbook of child psychology.* Vol. 2, *Infancy and developmental psychobiology* (4th ed.) (M. Haith & J. J. Campos, eds.), pp. 783–916. New York: Wiley.

Campos, J. J., Mumme, D. L, Kermoian, R., & Campos, R. (1994). *A functionalist perspective on the nature of emotion.* Monographs of the Society for Research in Child Development 59 (Whole no. 240), pp. 284–303.

21. Lazarus, R. S. (1991). *Emotion and adaptation.* New York: Oxford Univ. Press.

22. See chap. 1, n. 4.

23. Davis, M., Gendelman, D. S., Tischler, M. D., & Gendelman, P. M. (1982). A primary acoustic startle circuit: Lesion and stimulation studies. *J. Neurosci.* 6:791–805.

24. A recent assertion that we do *not* need to consider subjective experience in studying emotional processes in animals is provided by: Rogan, M. T., & Le Doux, J. E. (1996). Emotion: Systems, cells, synaptic plasticity. *Cell* 85:469–475.

25. Although the initiation of the flexor reflex to pain, which has usually been studied in spinal animals, is typically less than 10 milliseconds, while pain responses such as screeching take about a second, it is important to note that no one, at least to my knowledge, has yet performed these two measures at the same time in the same animal. It is possible that in the normal animal, a fast flexor reflex is a conditioned response to the cues that predict pain. Thus, it would be important to analyze the preceding issues in very young animals that have not yet had much experience with pain.

In any event, if we consider a primal example of unconditioned human consciousness—the perception of pain in a baby—we find that only a second is required between the stimulus and the response, as demonstrated by the latency of normal 2-day-old infants to cry when their heels have been violated by the snap of a rubber band. See: Fisichelli, V. R., & Karelitz, S. (1963). The cry latencies of normal infants and those with brain damage. *J. Pediatrics* 62:724–734.

26. The history of this bias goes back to biblical perspectives concerning the mental chasm between animals and humans, and it was reified by Descartes in his suggestion that animals may be more akin to robots than to humans, who have a sentient soul. Modern versions of this bias are bolstered by the self-evident fact that we cannot directly see the internal feelings of other animals, and hence we should not talk about them in scientific circles. However, the present viewpoint is that if we do not talk about them and try to study them indirectly, we may be throwing away a major key to understanding the natural order of brain organization. As will be highlighted in Chapter 16, there are neuroscientific ways to conceptualize how internal feelings may emerge in animals. An essential prerequisite for such brain functions appears to be some type of neural representation of "the self."

27. James, W. (1884). What is an emotion? *Mind* 9:188–205. Quotation on pp. 189–190.

The most famous series of studies, which have proved quite difficult to replicate, were conducted by: Schacter, S., & Singer, J. E. (1962). Cognitive, social, and physiological determinants of emotional state. *Psych. Rev.* 69:379–399.

28. The idea that emotional and cognitive capacities of the nervous systems are so closely linked that they do not need to be distinguished remains a popular view in psychology, as well as in psychobiology (see n. 5). Here I advocate the classic position that affective feelings and cognitive deliberations about those feelings are distinctly organized in the brain.

29. Behavioral neuroscientists commonly claim that it is sufficient to study the neural correlates of behavior, without any regard for an animal's potential internal processes. The success of the behaviorist strategy has been great, filling the pages of many journals, and there has been little incentive for rigorous scientists to broaden their views to try to incorporate any types of affective processes in their conceptions of how animal behavior is controlled. Unfortunately, the failure to develop a systematic view of animal feelings has led to the insulation of the field of behavioral neuroscience from other disciplines working at higher levels (e.g., human psychology). Accordingly, there is little cross-fertilization between the disciplines, and contrary to the tradition in most other sciences, the higher levels now rarely seek explanatory linkages to the lower levels. Likewise, those working at the lower levels do not seek conceptual guidance from the higher levels. A goal of affective neuroscience is to provide a common language whereby individuals pursuing these different levels of analysis might begin to communicate and to benefit from each other's findings.

30. Carew, T. J. (1996). Molecular enhancement of memory formation. *Neuron* 16:5–8.

Frost, W. N., & Kandel, E. R. (1995). Structure of the network mediating siphon-elicited siphon withdrawal in *Aplysia. J. Neurophysiol.* 73:2413–2427.

Marcus, E. A., Emptage, N. J., Marois, R., & Carew, T. J. (1994). A comparison of the mechanistic relationships between development and learning in *Aplysia. Prog. Brain Res.* 100:179–188.

31. Wright, W. G., & Carew T. J. (1995). A single

identified interneuron gates tail-shock induced inhibition in the siphon withdrawal reflex of *Aplysia*. *J. Neurosci.* 15:790–797.

For a description of the natural repertoire of the *Aplysia*, see three papers in the series starting with: Kuenzi, F. M., & Carew, T. J. (1994). Head waving in *Aplysia californica*. I. Behavioural characterization of searching movements. *J. Exp. Biol.* 195:35–51.

32. Gallistel, C. R. (1980). *The organization of action: A new synthesis*. Hillsdale, N.J.: Lawrence Erlbaum.

33. For an overview of how the "strain gauge" like sensors from the joints of arthropods help them automatically control movements in a way that causes envy among engineers attempting to design mobile robots, see: Zill, S. N., & Seyfarth, E.-A. (1996). Exoskeletal sensors for walking. *Sci. Amer.* 275:86–90.

34. Schleidt, W. M. (1974). How "fixed" is the fixed action pattern? *Z. Tierpsychol.* 36:184–211.

Tinbergen, N. (1951). *The study of instinct*. Oxford: Oxford Univ. Press.

35. Ikemoto, S., & Panksepp, J. (1992). The effects of early social isolation on the motivation for social play in juvenile rats. *Devel. Psychobio.* 25:261–274.

36. Arnold, A. P., & Schlinger, B. A. (1993). Sexual differentiation of brain and behavior: The zebra finch is not just a flying rat. *Brain Behav. Evol.* 42:231–241.

Arnold, A. P. (1992). Developmental plasticity in neural circuits controlling birdsong: Sexual differentiation and the neural basis of learning. *J. Neurobiol.* 23:1506–1528.

Read, A. F., & Weary, D. M. (1992). The evolution of birdsong: Comparative analyses. *Philos. Trans. Royal Soc. Lond.* [*B*] 338:165–187.

37. Kuo, Z.-Y. (1967). *The dynamics of behavior development: An epigenetic view*. New York: Random House.

38. Rumbaugh, D. M. (1965). Maternal care in relation to infant behavior in the squirrel monkey. *Psych. Rep.* 16:171–176. Quotation on p. 174.

39. There has been remarkable progress in the neurobiological analysis of learning during the past few decades. Many important contributions are summarized in: McGaugh, J. L., Weinberger, N. M., & Lynch, G. (eds.) (1995). *Brain and memory: Modulation and mediation of neuroplasticity*. New York: Oxford Univ. Press.

40. Any of the fine psychobiology or neuroscience texts that have been written from a traditional perspective can serve this function well, including:

Carlson, N. R. (1994). *Physiology of behavior* (5th ed.). Boston: Allyn and Bacon.

Kalat, J. W. (1995). *Biological psychology* (5th ed.). Pacific Grove, Calif.: Brooks/Cole.

Kandel, E. R., & Schwartz, J. H. (1991). *Principles of neural science* (3d ed.). New York: Elsevier Science.

Pinel, J. P. J. (1997). *Biopsychology* (3d ed.). Boston: Allyn and Bacon.

41. See the Gray versus Panksepp debate (see n. 5) and: Panksepp, J. (1991). Affective neuroscience: A conceptual framework for the neurobiological study of emotions. In *International reviews of emotion research* (K. Strongman, ed.), pp. 59–99, Chichester, U.K.: Wiley.

42. For a discussion of the Kennard principle, see: Kolb, B. (1995). *Brain plasticity and behavior*. Mahwah, N.J.: Lawrence Erlbaum.

A striking example of the reverse principle for subcortical damage is evident in: Almli, C. R., & Golden, G. T. (1974). Infant rats: Effects of lateral hypothalamic destruction. *Physiol. Behav.* 13:81–90.

43. For a clear summary of Decartes's contributions and his other rules for pursuing the method of doubt, see: Williams, B. (1972). Descartes, René. In *The encyclopedia of philosophy* (P. Edwards, ed.), pp. 344–354. New York: Macmillan. Quotation on p. 344.

44. See chap. 1, n. 17, and: Tellegan, A., Lykken, D. T., Bouchard, T. J., Wilcox, K., Segal, N., & Rich, S. (1988). Personality similarity in twins reared apart and together. *J. Soc. Personal. Psych.* 54:1031–1039.

45. For evidence about the heritability of behavioral tendencies, see the many contributions in the journal that goes by this name—*Behavior Genetics*—as well as: Plomin, R. (1990). The role of inheritance in behavior. *Science* 248:183–188.

46. Maxson, S. C., Shrenker, P., & Vigue, L. C. (1983). Genetics, hormones, and aggression. In *Hormones and aggressive behavior* (B. B. Svare, ed.), pp. 179–196. New York: Plenum Press.

Also, see n. 48 and: Saudou, F., Amara, D. A., Dierich, A., LeMeur, M., Ramboz, S., Segu, L., Buhot, M. C., & Hen, R. (1994). Enhanced aggressive behavior in mice lacking 5–HT1B receptor. *Science* 265: 1875–1878.

47. Two of the first studies utilizing this strategy to clarify genetic systems that may control learning were:

Grant, S. G. N., O'Dell, T. J., Karl, K. A., Stein, P. L., Soriano, P., & Kandel, E. R. (1992). Impaired long-term potentiation, spatial learning, and hippocampal development in *fyn* mutant mice, *Science* 258: 1903–1910.

Silva, A. J., Paylor, R., Wehner, J. M., & Tonegawa, S. (1992). Impaired spatial learning in a alpha-calcium-calmodulin kinase II mutant mice. *Science* 257:206–211.

For a thorough analysis of such matters, see the special issue: Molecular genetic approaches to mammalian brain and behavior. *Behavior Genetics* 26 (May 1996), especially:

Wehner, J. M., Bowers, B. J., & Paylor, R. (1996). The use of null mutant mice to study complex learning and memory processes. *Behav. Gen.* 26:301–312.

Tonegawa, S., Li, Y., Erzurumlu, R. S., Jhaveri, S., Chen, C., Goda, Y., Paylor, R., Silva, A. J., Kim, J. J., & Wehner, J. M. (1995). The gene knockout technology for the analysis of learning and memory, and neural development. *Prog. Brain Res.* 105:3–14.

48. Nelson, R. J., Demas, G. E., Hunag, P. L., Fishman, M. C., Dawson, V. L., Dawson, T. M., & Snyder, S. H. (1995). Behavioural abnormalities in male mice lacking neuronal nitric oxide. *Nature* 378:383–386.

49. For a discussion of critical issues in the use of gene-deleted animals, see: Gerlai, R. (1996). Gene-targeting studies of mammalian behavior: Is it the mutation or the background genotype? *Trends Neurosci.* 19:177–181. Also see the accompanying three commentaries by J. W. Crawley, L. Lathe, and W. E. Crusio.

50. Simpleminded biological determinism has yielded many spin-offs into educational and social policy across the years—ranging from the use of IQ tests to evaluate certain human qualities to the restriction of educational opportunities for those whose intelligence is impaired. Many of these issues have been addressed in such books as: Gould, S. J. (1981). *The mismeasure of man.* New York: Norton.

One of the most recent and volatile volleys of the ongoing debate was: Herrnstein, R. J., & Murray, C. (1994). *The bell curve: Intelligence and class structure in American life.* New York: Free Press.

On the other side of the debate, the broadening of our conception of intelligence has been promoted by:

Gardner, H. (1993). *Multiple intelligences: The theory in practice.* New York: Basic Books.

Goleman, D. (1995). *Emotional intelligence.* New York: Bantam Books.

51. Scientists typically value rationality over emotionality. Perhaps as a consequence, there has been a long-standing bias in the academic community to minimize and downgrade emotional matters as a less than worthy area for scientific pursuit. This bias has been changing noticeably during the past few years, and many believe we are now on the verge of an "affective revolution" that will be as important as the preceding "cognitive revolution" in the development of a scientific psychology in the next few decades. At present, the neuroscience side of this new revolution is lagging noticeably behind the psychological side. However, a solid neuroscience base will be essential for the scientific maturation of the affective view. The bottom-line question—What is a feeling?—cannot be answered simply through psychologial or behavioral analysis.

52. Loehlin, J. C., Willerman, L., & Horn, J. M. (1988). Human behavior genetics. *Ann. Rev. Psych.* 39:101–133.

Plomin, R., De Fries, J. C., & McClearn, G. E. (1990). *Behavioral genetics.* New York: Freeman.

53. Such animals do exhibit different preferences for sweets, with the high self-stimulators consuming more. See: Ganchrow, J. R., Lieblich, I., & Cohen, E. (1981). Consummatory responses to taste stimuli in rats selected for high and low rates of self-stimulation. *Physiol. Behav.* 27:971–976.

54. Work at the neurochemical level is presently quite modest, but some animals such as high-acetylcholine animals may serve as models of depression. See: Overstreet, D. H. (1993). The Flinders Sensitive Line rats: A genetic animal model of depression. *Neurosci. Biobehav. Revs.* 17:51–68.

Also, it is noteworthy that temperaments in primates are being related to brain chemistries. See:

Higley, J. D., Thompson, W. W., Champoux, M., Goldman, D., Hasert, M. F., Kraemer, G. W., Scanalan, J. M., Suomi, S. J., & Linnoila, M. (1993). Paternal and maternal genetic and environmental contributions to cerebrospinal fluid monoamine metabolites in rhesus monkeys (*Macaca mulatta*). *Arch. Gen. Psychiat.* 50: 615–623.

Raleigh, M. J., McGuire, M. T., Brammer, G. L., Pollack, D. B., & Yuwiler, A. (1991). Serotonergic mechanisms promote dominance acquisition in adult male vervet monkeys. *Brain Res.* 559:181–190.

55. For a recent review of the role of genetics in psychiatric disorders, see: Le Boyer, M., & Gorwood, P. (1995). Genetics of affective disorders and schizophrenia. In *Advances in biological psychiatry*, vol. 1 (J. Panksepp, ed.), pp. 27–66. Greenwich, Conn.: JAI Press.

56. Young, A. B. (1995). Huntington's disease: Lessons from and for molecular neuroscience. *Neuroscientist* 1:51–58.

57. Gusella, J. F., & MacDonald, M. E. (1996). Trinucleotide instability: A repeating theme in human inherited disorders. *Ann. Rev. Med.* 47:201–209.

58. Lipton, S. A., & Rosenberg, P. A. (1995). Excitatory amino acids as a final common pathway for neurological disorders. *N. Eng. J. Med.* 330:613–622.

59. For a review of the extensive plasticity that has been documented in the visual system, see: Hirsch, H. V. B. (1986). The tunable seer: Activity-dependent development of vision. In *Handbook of behavioral neurobiology*. Vol. 8, *Developmental psychobiology and developmental neurobiology* (E. M. Blass, ed.), pp. 41–62. New York: Plenum Press.

For an overview of brain plasticity and behavior, see n. 42. For recent issues specifically related to learning and memory, see: McGaugh, J. L., Bermudez-Rattoni, F., & Prado-Alcala, R. A. (eds.) (1995). *Plasticity in the central nervous system.* Mahwah, N.J.: Lawrence Erlbaum.

Chapter 3

1. Taylor, G. J. (1987). Alexithymia: History and validation of the concept. *Transcult. Psychiat. Res. Rev.* 24:85–95.

Taylor, G. J., Bagby, R. M., & Parker, J. D. A. (1992). The revised Toronto Alexithymia Scale: Some reliability, validity, and normative data. *Psychother. Psychosom.* 57:34–41.

2. Although highly localized cortical stimulation cannot provoke emotions, widespread application of polarizing currents and intense, fluctuating magnetic feels can induce mood changes. See: Pascual-Leone, A., Catala, M. D., & Pascual-Leone, P. A. (1996). Lateralized effect of rapid-rate transcranial magnetic stimulation of the prefrontal cortex on mood. *Neurology* 46:499–502.

Certain drugs also provoke mood changes (both fear and euphoria with the same manipulation) because of widespread but distinct changes in the brain. See: Ketter, T. A., Andreason, P. J., George, M. S., Lee, C., Gill, D. S., Parekh, P. I., Willis, M. W., Herscovitch, P., & Post, R. M. (1996). Anterior paralimbic mediation of procaine-induced emotional and psychosensory experiences. *Arch. Gen. Psychiat.* 53:59–69.

Likewise, positive and negative moods generate different cortical patterns, with positive mood and happiness generally being characterized by left frontal cortical arousal, and depressive tendencies and sadness commonly accompanied by right frontal arousal. See: Davidson, R. J. (1993). The neuropsychology of emotion and affective style. In *Handbook of emotions* (M. Lewis and J. M. Haviland, eds.), pp. 143–154. New York: Guilford Press.

However, these effects appear to be mild compared with the effects that can be evoked by subcortical stimulation, and it remains possible that the effects obtained from higher brain areas are critically linked to descending modulation of subcortical emotional systems.

3. Recently it has been argued that the human brain has undergone major changes in its cortical connectivities, which yielded unique human cognitive abilities. See: Deacon, T. W. (1990). Rethinking mammalian brain evolution. *Am. Zool.* 30:629–705.

4. A comprehensive and readable discussion of emotional taxonomies has been provided by one of the pioneers of the field. See: Plutchik, R. (1980). *Emotion: A psychoevolutionary synthesis.* New York: Harper and Row.

Also, the issue of emotional primes within the brain has been championed by investigators who have done seminal work on the psychosocial aspects of emotions. See: Buck, R. (1985). Prime theory: An integrated view of motivation and emotion. *Psych. Rev.* 92:389–413.

5. The work of one of the main proponents of the social-constructivist view can be found in: Mandler, G. (1984). *Mind and body: The psychology of emotion and stress.* New York: Norton.

Since most investigators tend to view a phenomenon from their own parochial perspective, this view is most widely represented by social scientists whose work has not been concerned with brain issues. See: Harre, R. (1986). *The social construction of emotions.* Oxford: Basil Blackwell.

6. For a presentation of the componential approach, see: Ortony, A., & Turner, T. J. (1990). What's basic about basic emotions? *Psych. Rev.* 97:315–331.

7. The componential approach of Ortony and Turner was vigorously challenged by Paul Ekman, Caroll Izard, and Jaak Panksepp in separate commentaries published in volume 99 of *Psych. Rev.*, along with a response by Turner and Ortony:

Ekman, P. (1992). Are there basic emotions? *Psych. Rev.* 99:550–553.

Izard, C. E. (1992). Basic emotions, relations among emotions, and emotion-cognition relations. *Psych. Rev.* 99:561–565.

Panksepp, J. (1992). A critical role for "affective neuroscience" in resolving what is basic about basic emotions. *Psych. Rev.* 99:554–560. Quotation on p. 559.

Turner, T. J., & Ortny, A. (1992). Basic emotions: Can conflicting criteria converge? *Psych. Rev.* 99:566–571.

The most fully developed component-process theory of emotions is in: Scherer, K. R. (1984). Emotion as a multicomponent process: A model and some cross-cultural data. *Rev. Person. Soc. Psychol.*, no. 5:37–63.

8. Many of the controversies in the area of emotion are remarkably tedious because of the imprecision of concepts. Typically, there is no clear empirical way to resolve issues (see chap. 2, n. 5). As William James once commiserated, the descriptive literature on emotions "is one of the most tedious parts of psychology. And not only is it tedious, but you feel that its subdivisions are to a great extent either fictitious or unimportant, and that its pretences to accuracy are a sham," so that "reading of classic work on the subject" is as interesting as "verbal descriptions of the shapes of the rocks on a New Hampshire farm." (James, W. [1892]. *Psychology: The briefer course.* New York: Harper and Row. Quotation on p. 241.)

9. The simple arousal view was first presented by: Duffy, E. (1941). The conceptual categories of psychology: A suggestion for revision. *Psych. Rev.* 48:177–203.

The approach-avoidance perspective was first clearly enunciated by: Schneirla, T. C. (1949). Levels in the psychological capacities of animals. In *Philosophy for the future* (R. W. Sellars, V. J. McGill, & M. Farber, eds.), pp. 243–286. New York: Macmillan.

More recently, this simple view has been advanced in clinical neuropsychology by: Davidson, R. J., Ekman, P., Saron, C. D., Senulis, J. A., & Friesen, W. V. (1990). Approach-withdrawal and cerebral asymmetry: Emotional expression and brain physiology I. *J. Pers. Soc. Psychol.* 50:330–341.

10. For a recent paper using the positve and negative affect scales originally developed by A. Telegen, see: MacLeoad, A. K., Byrne, A., & Valentine, J. D. (1996). Affect, emotional disorder, and future-directed thinking. *Cog. Emot.* 10:69–86.

11. Without fully considering the neurological evidence, rational argumentation and semantic studies have little chance of shedding further light on the basic nature of emotions. Accordingly, much of what has been suggested of a theoretical nature in the existing psychological literature, especially when it is based merely on logical inference, will not be discussed here. Obviously, nature does not follow the dictates of semantic logic, even though our scientific *conclusions* always need to be cast in those terms. It is especially important to emphasize that without a full consideration of the brain data, all conclusions regarding the number and nature of the basic emotions must be deemed provisional.

12. Even though Ortony and Turner (see n. 6) strongly criticized the whole concept of "basic emotion," it is noteworthy that anger, fear, sorrow, and joy appear as fundamental constructs in practically all emotional taxonomies. My impression is that much of the confusion in the area arises from the nature and complexity of language rather than the complexity of the brain. The evidence for basic brain substrates for these emotions is massive, and those who choose to disagree with their existence have probably not read a sufficient amount of the available neurobehavioral literature. The main issue that should be controversial at present is the precise nature of the brain mechanisms that mediate such processes.

13. For a review of modern semantic analyses of the use of emotional words, see: Russell, J. A. (1991). Culture and the categorization of emotions. *Psych. Bull.* 110:426–450.

14. For an energetic debate concerning the facial analysis of emotions, see: Russell, J. A. (1994). Is there universal recognition of emotion from facial expression? A review of cross-cultural studies. *Psych. Bull.* 115:102–141.

For stinging rebuttals, see:

Ekman, P. (1994). Strong evidence for universals in facial expressions: A reply to Russell's mistaken critique. *Psych. Bull.* 115:263–287.

Izard, C. E. (1994). Innate and universal facial expressions: Evidence from developmental and cross-cultural research. *Psych. Bull.* 115:288–299.

15. Rinn, W. E. (1984). The neuropsychology of facial expression: A review of the neurological and psychological mechanisms for producing facial expressions. *Psych. Bull.* 95:52–77.

16. Andrews, R. J. (1963). The origin and evolution of the calls and facial expressions of the primates. *Behaviour* 20:1–109.

17. The classic distinction between feelings that arise from emotions and those that arise from motivations is based on the existence of distinct bodily referents for the latter (e.g., bodily energy, water, temperature), with no clearly regulated bodily states for the former (also see discussion in Chapter 9). As we come to recognize the neurochemical causes of emotions, especially the specificity provided by neuropeptide systems (see Chapter 5), this distinction has become less defensible.

18. Panksepp, J. (1992). A critical role for "affective neuroscience" in resolving what is basic about basic emotions. *Psych. Rev.* 99:554–560. Quotation on p. 554.

19. Kleinginna, P. R., & Kleinginna, A. M. (1981). A categorized list of emotion definitions, with suggestions for a consensual definition. *Motiv. Emot.* 5:345–379.

20. This neural defintion of emotion was first proposed in 1982 (see n. 26); to my knowledge, no one has yet generated an alternative brain-based definition of emotions.

21. James, W. (1905). The place of affectional facts in a world of pure experience. *J. of Phil. Psych and Sci. Methods* 2:281–282.

22. Obviously, there are many ways to carve up the natural world scientifically. The manner in which physicists came to accommodate the wave and particulate conceptions of subatomic particles is one of the most striking examples of the type of compromises that neuroscientists interested in the integrative functions of the brain will have to make in abundance. An intriguing assault on the claim that science can reveal absolute truth is to be found in: Johnson, G. (1995). *Fire in the mind: Science, faith, and the search for order*. New York: Knopf.

23. For many years, I have advocated the utility of introspection in guiding our thinking about emotional processes (for quotation see n. 26, p. 407). This view can easily be criticized on the basis of evidence showing how inaccurate introspection has been in generating substantive explanations of behavior in the past, as well as by those who have demonstrated how extensively our behavior is controlled by unconscious processes (see chap. 2, n. 12). Although such viewpoints are critically important, my support of the introspective view is premised not on an explanatory level but on the initial descriptive level: We need a method to identify fundamental psychobiological processes that can be clarified only through brain research. The evidence for certain types of emotional processes within the mammalian brain is overwhelming, but the mannner in which we should speak of them is by no means clear (see n. 12). The problem goes as deep as the very nature of language. In this context, we also need to remember that the speaking left hemisphere and the comparatively silent and more emotional right hemisphere have different agendas in the control of psychobehavioral processes (see Chapter 16 and Appendix B). Should we believe that all the semantic distinctions that can be created by the left hemisphere (see n. 13) reflect basic affective realities that exist in all mammals? Probably not, even though such socially constructed semantic realities are obviously real and important aspects of human social life. However, they may be instantiated in the epigenetically derived software functions of the brain rather than in the genetically coded hardware.

24. Changes in neural systems as a function of experience have become a powerful force in conceptualizing the epigenetic construction of the nervous system and mind. Some of the earlier work on this topic is succinctly summarized in: Rosenzweig, M. R., & Bennett, E. L. (1996). Psychobiology of plasticity: Effects of training and experience on brain and behavior. *Behav. Brain Sci.* 78:57–65.

More recent work that has probed the fine detail of such processes can be found in: Greenough, W. T., Black, J. E., & Wallace, C. S. (1987). Experience and brain development, *Child Devel.* 58:539–559.

Direct evidence for long-term functional changes in emotional systems is available in: Adamec, R. E. (1993). Lasting effect of FG-7142 on anxiety, aggression and limbic physiology in the rat. *J. Neurophysiol.* 7:232–248.

Obviously, the genetically provided operating systems of the brain do not mature normally unless they receive abundant input from the environment. Thus, if one keeps a young animal, such as a kitten, in a dark closet during the first months of life, it will never develop proper visual capacity (see chap. 2, n. 53).

25. I first utilized this type of chaining maneuver in: Panksepp, J. (1981). Hypothalamic integration of behavior: Rewards, punishments and related psychological processes. In *Handbook of the hypothalamus*. Vol. 3, part B, *Behavioral studies of the hypothalamus* (P. J. Morgane & J. Panksepp, eds.), pp 289–431. New York: Marcel Dekker.

The intent of the lexical chaining was to highlight the self-evident fact that all basic emotional system are bound to have many verbal referents.

26. The theory that is the basis for this text was first developed in the article cited in n. 25 and in: Panksepp, J. (1982). Toward a general psychobiological theory of emotions. *Behav. Brain Sci.* 5:407–467.

27. Some children are temperamentally prone to emotions that can promote depression. See: Kagan, J., & Snidman, N. (1991). Temperamental factors in human development. *Am. Psychol.* 46:856–862.

It is now evident that early childhood loss is one of the major risk factors for future depression, as well as the development of panic attacks, perhaps because of permanent developmental modification of the emotional substrates of separation distress. See: Faravelli, C., Webb, T., Ambonetti, A., Fonnsell, F., & Sessarego, A. (1985). Prevalance of traumatic early life events in 31 agoraphobic patients with panic attacks. *Am. J. Psychiat.* 142:1493–1494.

28. These effects are summarized in nn. 25 and 26. Although some investigators still believe such "stimulus-bound" behaviors are not accompanied by affective feelings, such a belief is not supported by the weight of existing data. When place preference and avoidance tasks have been conducted, animals indicate by their behavioral choices that they either like or dislike these kinds of brain stimulation (see Chapters 8 and 10).

29. It is presently generally accepted that schizophrenia is not a single disorder. According to one conceptual schema, two major forms have been characterized as Type I (more acute, with many positive, or florid, symptoms) and Type II (more chronic, with more negative symptoms). See: Mackay, A. V. P., & Crow, T. J. (1980). Positive and negative symptoms and the role of dopamine. *Br. J. Psychiat.* 137:379–386.

Ventricular enlargement in schizophrenia is more prominent in individuals with the more chronic, Type II form. See: Straube, E. R., & Oades, R. D. (1992). *Schizophrenia: Empirical research and findings.* San Diego: Academic Press.

30. Panksepp, J. (1994). Emotional development yields lots of "stuff" . . . especially mind "stuff" that emerges from brain "stuff." In *The nature of emotion: Fundamental questions* (P. Ekman & R. J. Davidson, eds.), pp. 367–372. New York: Oxford Univ. Press.

31. Panksepp, J., Knutson, B., & Pruitt, D. L. (1998). Toward a neuroscience of emotion: The epigenetic foundations of emotional development. In *What develops in emotional development?* (M. F. Mascolo & S. Griffin, eds.). New York: Plenum Press.

32. Panksepp, J., & Miller, A. (1996). Emotions and the aging brain. In *Handbook of emotion, adult development, and aging* (C. Magai & S. H. McFadden, eds.), pp. 3–26. San Diego: Academic Press.

33. See chap. 2, n. 27, and modern critique and update: Lang, P. J. (1994). The varieties of emotional experience: A meditation on James-Lange theory. *Psych. Rev.* 101:211–221.

34. See chap. 2, n. 27, and a critique of the Schacter and Singer approach in: Manstead, A. S. R., & Wagner, H. L. (1981). Arousal, cognition, and emotion: An appraisal of two-factor theory. *Curr. Psych. Revs.* 1:35–54.

35. Cannon, W. B. (1927). The James-Lange theory of emotions: A critical examination and an alternative theory. *Am. J. Psychol.* 39:106–124.

36. Gershon, M. D. (1981). The enteric nervous system. *Ann. Rev. Neurosci.* 4:227–272.

Panksepp, J. (1993). Neurochemical control of moods and emotions: Amino acids to neuropeptides. In *The handbook of emotions* (M. Lewis & J. Haviland, eds.), pp. 87–107. New York: Guilford Press.

37. Ekman, P., Levenson, R. W., & Friesen, W. V. (1983). Autonomic nervous system activity distinguishes between emotions. *Science* 221:1208–1210.

38. Harro, J., Vasar, E., Koszycki, D., & Bradwejn, J. (1995). Cholecystokinin in panic and anxiety disorders. In *Advances in biological psychiatry*, vol. 1 (J. Panksepp, ed.), pp. 235–262. Greenwich, Conn.: JAI Press.

39. Locke, S. E., & Hornig-Rohan, M. (eds.) (1983). *Mind and immunity: Behavioral immunology, annotated bibliography, 1976–1982.* New York: Institute for the Advancement of Health.

Rivier, C. (1993). Neuroendocrine effects of cytokines in the rat. *Revs. Neurosci.* 4:223–237.

40. Bluthe, R. M., Pawlowski, M., Suarez, S., Parnet, P., Pittman, Q., Kelley, K. W., & Dantzer, R. (1994). Synergy between tumor necrosis factor alpha and interleukin-1 in the induction of sickness behavior in mice. *Psychoneuroendocrinol.* 19:197–207.

Kent, S., Bluthe, R. M., Kelley, K. W., & Dantzer, R. (1992). Sickness behavior as a new target for drug development. *Trends Pharmacol. Sci.* 13:24–28.

41. Papez, J. W. (1937). A proposed mechanism of emotion. *Arch. Neurol. Psychiat.* 38:725–743.

42. Damasio, A. (1994). *Descartes' error.* New York: Putnam.

43. Vogt, B. A., & Gabriel, M. (eds.) (1993). *Neurobiology of cingulate cortex and limbic thalamus : A comprehensive handbook.* Boston: Birkhäuser.

44. Risold, P. Y., & Swanson, L. W. (1996). Structural evidence for functional domains in the rat hippocampus. *Science* 272:1484–1486.

45. Fanselow, M. S. (1991). Analgesia as a response to aversive Pavlovian conditional stimuli: Cognitive and emotional mediators. In *Fear, avoidance and phobias: A fundamental analysis* (M. R. Denny, ed.), pp. 61–86. Hillsdale, N.J.: Lawrence Erlbaum.

46. Papez's theory (see n. 41), initially ignored by most investigators, was given new life by: MacLean, P. (1949). Psychosomatic disease and the "visceral brain": Recent developments bearing on the Papez theory of emotion. *Psychosom. Med.* 11:338–353.

The concept of the limbic system was coined by: MacLean, P. (1952). Some psychiatric implications of physiological studies on frontotemporal portion of limbic system (visceral brain). *Electroenceph. Clin. Neurophysiol.* 4:407–418.

For comprehensive coverage of these issues, see: MacLean, P. (1990). *The triune brain in evolution.* New York: Plenum Press.

47. See chap. 2, n. 24, and contributions in: Aggleton, J. P. (ed.) (1992). *The amygdala: Neurobio-*

logical aspects of emotion, memory and mental dysfunction. New York: Wiley-Liss.

48. For instance, one of the main proponents of a facial analysis approach to understanding basic emotions, especially in children (i.e., Izard, C. E. [1971]. *The face of emotion*. Appleton-Century Crofts, New York), has shared an extensive neuroscience perspective in his recent theorizing. See: Izard, C. E. (1993). Four systems for emotion activation: Cognitive and noncognitive processes. *Psych. Rev.* 100:68–90.

It is noteworthy, however, that the main way the neuroscience of emotion is presently being assimilated into psychology is via a top-down approach, with a fairly selective focus on amygdaloid contributions to emotion (see n. 47). The goal of the present volume is to promote a more integrated view that includes the lower brain stem functions from which mammalian emotionality originally arose, and to which it is still strongly linked. This level will probably be more important for empirically untangling the neural nature of affective-feeling processes, while the higher levels will be essential for understanding how cognitions come to instigate and modulate feelings.

Chapter 4

1. Glezer, I. I., Jacobs, M. S., & Morgane, P. J. (1988). Implications of the "initial brain" concept for brain evolution in Cetacea. *Behav. Brain. Sci.* 11:75–116.

For an overview of the evolution of the brain, see: Sarnat, H. B., & Netsky, M. G. (1974). *Evolution of the nervous system*. New York: Oxford Univ. Press.

2. For full discussions of the frontal lobe functions, see:

Passingham, R. (1993). *The frontal lobes and voluntary action*. New York: Oxford Univ. Press.

Perecman, E. (ed.) (1987). *The frontal lobes revisited*. New York: IRBN Press.

3. Jacobs, M. S., McFarland, W. L., & Morgane, P. J. (1979). The anatomy of the brain of the bottlenose dolphin (*Tursiops truncatus*). Rhinic lobe (*rhinencephalon*): I. The archicortex. *Brain Res. Bull.* (suppl. 1):1–108.

4. Slotnick, B. M. (1967). Disturbances of maternal behavior in the rat following lesions of the cingulate cortex. *Behaviour* 24:204–236.

5. Araujo, D. M., Chabot, J.-G., & Quiron, R. (1990). Potential neurotrophic factors in the mammalian central nervous system: Functional significance in the developing and aging brain. *Int. Rev. Neurobiol.* 32:141–174.

Lindsay, R. M., Wiegand, S. J., Altar, C. A., & Di Stefano, P. S. (1994). Neurotrophic factors: From molecule to man. *Trends Neurosci.* 17:182–190.

Russell, D. S. (1995). Neurotrophins: New players, clinical uses? *The Neuroscientist* 3:119–122.

6. In a sense, the complexity of external representations is dependent on the complexity of the external world. To highlight this concept, Nobel laureate Herbert Simon wrote: "An ant, viewed as a behaving system, is quite simple. The apparent complexity of its behavior over time is largely a reflection of the complexity of the environment in which it finds itself" (Simon, H. [1969]. The sciences of the artificial [Cambridge, Mass.: MIT Press], quotation on p. 64). Recently, one of Simon's colleagues has detailed a theory of how complex cognitions might arise from the interactions of procedural and declarative knowledge. See: Anderson, J. (1996). ACT: A simple theory of complex cognition. *Amer. Psychol.* 51:355–365.

7. Besides differences in the types of information they collect (interoceptive versus exteroceptive), some of the key differences between the visceral and somatic nervous systems are anatomical location (visceral is more medially situated in the brain stem), electrophysiological (visceral-limbic neurons fire at a slower rate and hence consume less blood glucose), and neurochemical (many of the neuropeptide circuits that control the emotions I will discuss in this book are much more concentrated in the visceral-limbic nervous system). Finally, at an overall functional level, limbic and somatic seizures tend to have different symptoms and follow different channels of propagation within the nervous system. Also, we can obtain many emotional effects (both autonomic and behavioral) by electrically stimulating brain areas subsumed within the limbic system concept, but rarely from the higher reaches of the brain. Of course, somatic and visceral-limbic processes are highly interactive within the brain, but the distinction between limbic and somatic nervous systems is not an arbitrary conceptualization, as recently argued by some neuroanatomists, but one that is deeply ingrained within many organizational and functional patterns of the brain.

8. To my knowledge, such an experiment has never been published, even though I measured this phenomenon more than 20 years ago (Panksepp, 1974, unpublished data). Modulation of spinal reflexes by various stimuli is a well-established neurological finding. For instance, all one needs to do to intensify the patellar reflex is to tense the upper body by pressing the hands together in front of one's chest. For a recent demonstration of this type of an effect, see: Bonnet, M., Bradley, M. M., Lang, P. J., & Requin, J. (1995). Modulation of spinal reflexes: Arousal, pleasure, action. *Psychophysiol.* 32:367–372.

9. One way to conceptualize the evolution of higher brain functions is as providing ever-increasing "openness" to brain systems that control fairly stereotyped and relatively fixed behavior patterns. However, it must be remembered that all behaviors, even simple spinal reflexes, are modulated from above (see n. 8). This is one reason the classic study of reflexes has typically used decerebrate animals, especially ones whose brains are transected at the midcollicular level (i.e., the *cerveau isolé* preparation), so as to leave the tonic excitatory influences of the lower brain stem intact, which facilitates the study of reflexes, since a high spinal section leads gradually to a muscular flaccidity. For review see: Liddell, E. G. T. (1960). *Discovery of reflexes*. New York: Oxford Univ. Press.

10. Cajal's famous summary of brain anatomy, published in 1909 as a two-volume contribution in

French (*Histologie du system nerveux de l'homme et des vertebres*), is still widely considered the single most important work in neuroscience. The translated volumes have finally been republished in English as the sixth contribution in Oxford's History of Neuroscience series. See: Cajal, S. R. (1995). *Histology of the nervous systems of man and vertebrates*. New York: Oxford Univ. Press.

11. For a summary of the Nobel Prize–winning contributions in neuroscience, see: Jasper, H. H., & Sourkes, T. L. (1983). Nobel laureates in neuroscience: 1904–1981. *Ann. Rev. Neurosci.* 6:1–42. The quotations that accompany the citations of Nobel Prize--winning works in the next few chapters are the exact descriptors used by the Nobel Committee to recognize each of the cited neuroscientific breakthroughs.

12. The secondary source for this quotation is: Fischbach, G. D. (1992). Mind and brain. *Sci. Amer.* 267 (Sept.):48–57.

13. Levi-Montalcini, R. (1987). The nerve growth factor 35 years later. *Science* 237:1154–1162.

Levi-Montalcini, R., Skaper, S. D., Dal Toso, R., Petrelli, L., & Leon, A. (1996). Nerve growth factor: From neurotrophin to neurokine. *Trends Neurosci.* 19:514–520.

14. Duman, R. S., Vaidya, V. A., Nibuya, M., Morinobu, S., & Fitzgerald, L. R. (1995). Stress, antidepressant treatments, and neurotrophic factors: Molecular and cellular mechanisms. *The Neuroscientist* 1:351–360.

Finkbeiner, S. (1996). Neurotrophins and the synapse. *The Neuroscientist* 2:139–142.

15. Since much of what will be covered in this and the next two chapters is common knowledge in the field, literature citations will be used sparingly. Detailed coverage of these issues can be obtained from a multitude of neuroscience texts. One of the most popular and thorough is: Kandel, E. R., Schwartz, J. H., & Jessell, T. M. (eds.) (1991). *Principles of neural science* (3d ed.). New York: Elsevier. (Next edition due Oct. 1998.)

16. For a full summary of the triune brain concept, see: MacLean, P. (1990). *The triune brain in evolution*. New York: Plenum Press.

17. One of the most vigorous recent challenges against the limbic system concept has been mounted by Joe Le Doux, who has done some of the most impressive neuroscience work on emotions during the past decade. See: LeDoux, J. E. (1996). *The emotional brain: The mysterious underpinnings of emotional life*. New York: Simon and Schuster.

My view is that although the limbic system is certainly a vague entity anatomically, with the boundaries having been extended as we discover the interconnectivities of many of the higher limbic structures, it is an important functional-evolutionary conceptualization that can be supported by many lines of convergent evidence (see n. 7). If one wants to be totally rigorous about anatomical issues, one could argue that most brain anatomical designations are vague at the edges. For instance, where does the amygdala really begin and end? The amygdala has rich connections with the cortex and many brain stem areas. Obviously, all of the general neuroanatomical labels are terms of convenience, helping describe what our eyes behold, as opposed to concepts that are definitive by any accepted objective criterion. The limbic system is obviously more of a conceptual entity than many other anatomical terms, but it should be recognized and respected for the powerful heuristic conceptualization that it is.

Since much of this text focuses on hypothalamic functions, which contain the highest concentration of visceral functions in the brain, it is interesting to note how cleanly some hypothalamic proteins tend to highlight brain areas that traditionally constitute the limbic system. See: Gautvik, K. M., de Lecea, L., Gautvik, V. T., Danielson, P. E., Tranque, P., Dopazo, A., Bloom, F. E., & Sutcliffe, J. G. (1996). Overview of the most prevalent hypothalamus-specific mRNAs, as identified by directional tag PCR subtraction. *Proc. Natl. Acad. Sci.* 93:8733–8738.

Zhou, R., Copeland, T. D., Kromer, L. F., & Schulz, N. T. (1994). Isolation and characterization of Bsk, a growth factor receptor-like tyrosine kinase associated with the limbic system. *J. Neurosci. Res.* 37:129–143.

Also, the classic limbic system does appear to have some unique chemistries. See:

Levitt P. (1984). A monoclonal antibody to limbic system neurons. *Science* 223:299–301.

Zaccho, A., Cooper, V., Chantler, P. D., Fisher-Hyland, S., Horton, H. L., & Levitt, P. (1990). Isolation, biochemical characterization and structural analysis of the limbic system associated membrane protein (LAMP), a protein expressed by neurons comprising functional circuits. *J. Neurosci.* 10:73–90.

18. Traditionally, cortex has been divided into three types—neocortex, archicortex, and paleocortex—depending on its evolutionary age and cellular organization. The neocortex is most abundant in all higher mammals and has six cell layers, while archicortex and paleocortex have fewer cell layers and consist of ancient olfactory projection areas such as the piriform cortex and hippocampus.

19. In this regard we may consider the social abilities of dolphins. Recent work analyzing the play of dolphins has found that they appear to be as intrigued by certain forms of complex object play—for instance, the blowing of air-rings—as we are with some of our human games. See: Marten, K., Sharif, K., Psarakos, S., & White, D. J. (1996). Ring bubbles of dolphins. *Sci. Amer.* 275:2–7.

Although there will be vast differences in the details of behaviors exhibited by different species, the present assumption is that the basic urge to play arises from homologous brain systems in all mammals. It is sometimes assumed that play is a uniquely mammalian function, but it has been described in birds, and behavior resembling object play, perhaps the evolutionary progenitor of social play, has been described in turtles. See: Burghardt, G. M. (1988). Precocity, play, and the ectotherm-endotherm transition: Profound reorganization or superficial adapatation? In *Handbook of behavioral neurobiology*. Vol. 9, *Developmental psychobiology and behavioral ecology* (E. M. Blass, ed.), pp. 107–148. New York: Plenum Press.

20. Fletcher, P. C., Happe, F., Frith, U., Baker, S. C., Dolan, R. J., Frackowiak, R. S., & Frith, C. D. (1995). Other minds in the brain: A functional imaging study of "theory of mind" in story comprehension. *Cognition* 57:109–128.

21. Berntson, G. G., Boysen, S. T., & Cacioppo, J. T. (1993). Neurobehavioral organization and the cardinal principle of evaluative bivalence. *Ann. N.Y. Acad. Sci.* 702:75–102.

Boysen, S. T., Berntson, G. G., Hannan, M. B., & Cacioppo, J. T. (1996). Quantity-based interference and symbolic representations in chimpanzees. *J. Exp. Psych.: Anim. Behav. Proc.* 22:76–86.

22. Seyfarth, R. M., & Cheney, D. L. (1992). Meaning and mind in monkeys. *Sci. Amer.* 267 (Dec.):123–128.

23. Evans, C. S., Evans, L., & Marler, P. (1993). On the meaning of alarm calls: Functional reference in an avian vocal system. *Anim. Behav.* 46:23–38.

Evans, C. S., Macedonia, J. M., & Marler, P. (1993). Effects of apparent size and speed on the response of chickens, *Gallus gallus*, to computer-generated simulations of aerial predators. *Anim. Behav.* 46:1–11.

24. For a theory of emotions that focuses on higher appraisal issues, see: Roseman, I. J., Antoniou, A. A., & Jose, P. E. (1996). Appraisal determinants of emotions: Constructing a more accurate and comprehensive theory. *Cog. Emot.* 10:241–277.

25. Since there is practically no fossil evidence for internal brain structures, we must rely on the internal similarities in the brains of living species (see Appendix A).

26. It is noteworthy that cortical damage has much more severe effects in humans and other primates than in lower animals. Clearly, as organisms mature, their behavioral abilities become increasingly dependent on higher areas, all the more so with the degree of species-typical encephalization.

27. For an excellent discussion of cortex, see: Braitenberg, V., & Schulz, A. (1991). *Anatomy of the cortex*. New York: Springer-Verlag.

28. Folstein, S. E. (1989). *Huntington's disease: A disorder of families*. Baltimore: Johns Hopkins Univ. Press.

29. Harper, P. S. (ed.) (1991). *Huntington's disease*. London: Saunders.

30. Lavond, D. G., Kim, J. J., & Thompson, R. F. (1993). Mammalian brain substrates of aversive classical conditioning. *Ann. Rev. Psych.* 44:317–342.

31. Maren, S., De Cola, J. P., Swain, R. A., Fanselow, M. S., & Thompson, R. F. (1994). Parallel augmentation of hippocampal long-term potentiation, theta rhythm, and contextual fear conditioning in water-deprived rats. *Behav. Neurosci.* 108:44–56.

32. Thompson, R. F., & Krupa, D. J. (1994). Organization of memory traces in the mammalian brain. *Ann. Rev. Neurosci.* 17:519–549.

Swain, R. A., & Thompson, R. F. (1993). In search of engrams. *Ann. N.Y. Acad. Sci.* 702:27–39.

33. Freeman, W. J. (1994). Characterization of state transitions in spatially distributed, chaotic, nonlinear, dynamical systems in cerebral cortex. *Integrat. Physiol. and Behav. Sci.* 29:294–306.

34. Dusser de Barenne, J. G. (1920). Recherches experimentales sur les fonctions du système nerveux central, faites en particulier sur deux chat donc le neopallium a été enlevé. *Arch. Neurol. Physiol.* 4:31–123. This article provided an early description of the rage that followed decortication, noting how it could be elicited by "trivial and irrelevant" stimuli.

35. Decorticate rage is not obtained simply by eliminating the neocortex; one must selectively eliminate midline limbic cortex and certain other areas of the frontal and temporal lobes. See: Bard, P., & Mountcastle, V. B. (1948). Some forebrain mechanisms involved in expression of rage with special reference to suppression of angry behavior. *Res. Pub. Assoc. Nerv. Ment. Dis.* 27:362–404.

36. Klüver-Bucy syndrome was first observed in monkeys. See: Klüver, H., & Bucy, P. C. (1939). Preliminary analysis of functions of the temporal lobes in monkeys. *Arch. Neurol. Psychiat. (Chicago)* 42:979–1000.

This phenomenon was subsequently replicated in cats. See: Schreiner, L. H., & Kling, A. (1953). Behavioral changes following rhinencephalic injury in cats. *J. Neurophysiol.* 16:643–659.

Many of these phenomena have also been documented in humans. For a thorough review and analysis of such effects, see: Gloor, P. (1997). *The temporal lobe and limbic system*. New York: Oxford Univ. Press.

37. Brady, J. B., & Nauta, W. J. H. (1953). Subcortical mechanisms in emotional behavior: Affective changes following septal forebrain lesions in the albino rat. *J. Comp. Physiol. Psychol.* 46:339–346.

38. The initial hyperemotionality of a septal animal is gradually eliminated by handling, and the animals gradually become more social than normal. See: Yutzey, D. A., Meyer, P. M., & Meyer, D. R. (1964). Emotionality changes following septal and neocortical ablations in rats. *J. Comp. Physiol. Psychol.* 58:463–465.

The controversy surrounding the variability of some of these effects has been discussed by Meyer, D. R., Ruth, R. A., & Lavond, D. G. (1978). The septal social cohesiveness effect: Its robustness and main determinants. *Physiol. Behav.* 21:1027–1029.

39. Hess, W. R. (1954). *Diencephalon: Autonomic and extrapyramidal functions*. New York: Grune and Stratton.

40. Olds, M. E., & Olds, J. (1963). Approach-avoidance analysis of rat diencephalon. *J. Comp. Neurol.* 120:259–295.

Chapter 5

1. Caudill, M. (1992). *In our own image: Building an artificial person*. New York: Oxford Univ. Press.

Jubak, J. (1992). *In the image of the brain: Breaking the barrier between the human mind and intelligent machines*. Boston: Little, Brown.

2. The best examples of such relations come from biological psychiatry. Good sources for such issues can be found in journals such as *Archives of General Psychiatry*, *Biological Psychiatry*, and annual reviews such as *Advances in Biological Psychiatry* (Greenwich, Conn.: JAI Press). One of the most striking and well-replicated effects is the role of serotonin in controlling human mood, including relationships to aggression, depression, and suicidal tendencies in clinical populations (see Chapter 11). Of course, it is easier to do correlative rather than causal studies in humans, but the psychopharmacological literature for individuals with various clinical disorders is a compelling testament to the power of a vast number of neurochemical manipulations. Although there is no comparable database for normal individuals, there is now striking evidence of enhancement of positive moods in normal individuals given nutrients that facilitate serotonin and catecholamine activities in the brain. For an overview, see: Young, S. N. (1996). Behavioral effects of dietary neurotransmitter precursors: Basic and clinical aspects. *Neurosci. Biobehav. Revs.* 20:313–323.

3. The average bursting rate of neurons within thalamic and cortical sensory systems during information processing is probably about 40 Hz (which has also become a potential EEG signature for conscious information processing in the brain; see n. 28 and Chapter 16). It is probably the distribution of action potentials as much as the overall number that controls perceptual processes. Thus, when we perceive something, action potentials cluster in such a way as to highlight certain features of stimuli in the perceptual field. See: de Charms, R. C., & Merzenick, M. M. (1996). Primary cortical representation of sounds by the coordination of action-potential timing. *Nature* 381:610–613.

4. For more detailed coverage of synaptic transmission, see: Levitan, I. B., & Kaczmarek, L. K. (1991). *The neuron.* New York: Oxford Univ. Press.

5. The electroencephalograph (EEG) and magnetoencephalograph (MEG) monitor the electrical and magnetic field potential oscillations of large ensembles of neurons. In general the two measures tend to correlate highly, but the MEG allows more precise identification of the exact neuronal sources of fluctuating energy fields. See: Wikswo, J. P., Jr., Gevins, A., & Williamson, S. J. (1993). The future of the EEG and MEG. *Electroenceph. Clin. Neurophysiol.* 87:1–9.

6. I will not endeavor to detail or to provide citations for each of the historical discoveries, since they are covered in numerous physiological psychology and neuroscience texts. However, for a wonderfully illustrated text on the history of neuroscience, see: Corsi, P. (ed.) (1991). *The enchanted loom: Chapters in the history of neuroscience.* New York: Oxford Univ. Press.

7. Adrian, E. D. (1932). *The mechanism of nervous action: Electrical studies of the neurone.* Philadelphia: Univ. of Pennsylvania Press.

8. The simple fact that various areas of the "triune brain" have characteristically different firing patterns suggests that there are some broad neurophysiological differences between the limbic system and somatic sensory systems of the thalamic neocortical axis, as originally proposed by MacLean (see chap. 4, nn. 7 and 16). As we will see, there are also neurochemical distinctions between these general brain zones, which suggests that the "triune brain" concept is more than just an imaginary way to parcel the brain into evolutionary/functional components. It reflects a basic distinction that needs to be made between the somatic and visceral nervous systems (see chap. 4, n. 17).

9. Indeed, visualization of the flow of calcium into cells has been used to monitor neuronal activity in dramatic ways. See: O'Donovan, M. J., Ho, S., Sholomenko, G., & Yee, W. (1993). Real-time imaging of neurons retrogradely and anterogradely labeled with calcium-sensitive dyes. *J. Neurosci. Methods.* 46:91–106.

Yuste, R., & Katz, L. C. (1991). Control of postsynaptic Ca^{2+} influx in developing neocortex by excitatory and inhibitory neurotransmitters. *Neuron* 6:333–344.

10. Neher, E., & Sakmann, B. (1976). Single-channel currents recorded from membrane of denervated frog muscle fibres. *Nature* 260:799–802.

Catterall, W. A. (1988). Structure and function of voltage-sensitive ion channels. *Science* 242:50–61.

11. Le Vere, T. E. (1993). Recovery of function after brain damage: The effects of nimodipine on the chronic behavioral deficit. *Psychobiology* 21:125–129.

12. Although the initial finding of reduced potassium channels in the skin cells (fibroblasts) of Alzheimer's patients has not been well replicated (Gibson, G., Martins, R., Blass, J., & Gandy, S. [1996]. Altered oxidation and signal transduction systems in fibroblasts from Alzheimer patients. *Life Sci.* 59:477–489), another recent peripheral measure has been to monitor pupillary diameter as a function of stimulation with acetylcholine blocking agents, since both that visually evident reflex and the cognitive deficits of Alzheimer's are controlled by changes in acetylcholine neural systems. See: Scinto, L. F., Daffner, K. R., Dressler, D., Ransil, B., Rentz, D., Weintraub, S., Mesulam, M., & Potter, H. (1994). A potential noninvasive neurobiological test for Alzheimer's disease. *Science* 266:1051–1054.

13. The amounts and types of information that are available in the EEG remain controversial. The classic approaches have been to analyze the energy at specific frequencies (i.e., power spectrum analysis), which can be utilized in various ways such as ERS and ERD analyses (see nn. 36 and 37), which are being used in ever more sophisticated ways. See: Florian, G., & Pfurtscheller, G. (1995). Dynamic spectral analysis of event-related EEG data. *Electroencephal. Clin. Neurophysiol.* 95:393–396.

The amount of synchrony among waves in different brain areas (i.e., coherence analysis) is providing a measure of the degree to which different brain areas are working together. See: Rappelsberger, P., Pfurtscheller, G., & Filz, O. (1994). Calculation of event-related coherence: A new method to study short-lasting coupling between brain areas. *Brain Topography* 7:121–127.

It is remarkable that at present one can predict the behavior of animals by characterizing the population vectors of many firing neurons in such a way that we are beginning to get a true glimpse into the operation of their minds. See: Gothard, K. M., Skaggs, W. E., & McNaughton, B. L. (1996). Dynamics of mismatch correction in the hippocampal ensemble code for space: Interaction between path integration and environmental cues. *J. Neurosci.* 16:8027–8040.

Churchland, P. S., & Sejnowski, T. J. (1992). *The computational brain.* Cambridge, Mass.: MIT Press.

14. Milner, A. D., & Goodale, M. A. (1995). *The visual brain in action.* New York: Oxford Univ. Press.

15. Ullman, S. (1996). *High-level vision.* Cambridge, Mass.: MIT Press.

16. Houk, J. C., Davis, J. L., & Beiser, D. G. (eds.) (1995). *Models of information processing in the basal ganglia.* Cambridge, Mass.: MIT Press.

17. Brinkman, C., & Porter, R. (1983). Supplementary motor area and premotor area of the monkey cerebral cortex: Functional organization and activities of single neurons during performance of a learned movement. *Adv. Neurol.* 39:393–420.

Roland, P. E., Larsen, B., Lassen, N. A., & Skinhoj, E. (1989). Supplementary motor area and other cortical areas in organization of voluntary movements in man. *J. Neurophysiol.* 43:118–136.

18. Eccles, J. C. (1982). The initiation of voluntary movements by the supplementary motor area. *Arch. Psychiatr. Nervenkr.* 231:423–441.

Eccles, J. C. (1982). How the self acts on the brain. *Psychoneuroendocrinol.* 7:271–283.

19. The work of James Olds initiated the search for reward neurons (see Chapter 8); his seminal early work is summarized in: Olds, J. (1962). Hypothalamic substrates of reward. *Physiol. Rev.* 42:554–604.

20. Abbott, L. F., Rolls, E. T., & Tovee, M. J. (1996). Representational capacity of face coding in monkeys. *Cerebral Cortex* 6:498–505.

George, M. S., Ketter, T. A., Gill, D. S., Haxby, J. V., Ungerleider, L. G., Herscovitch, P., & Post, R. M. (1993). Brain regions involved in recognizing facial emotion or identity: An oxygen-15 PET study. *J. Neuropsychiat. Clin. Neurosci.* 5:384–394.

Rolls, E. T., Tovee, M. J., Purcell, D. G., Stewart, A. L., & Azzopardi, P. (1994). The responses of neurons in the temporal cortex of primates, and face identification and detection. *Exp. Brain Res.* 101:473–484.

21. Zivin, G. (ed.) (1985). *The development of expressive behavior: Biology-environment interactions.* Orlando, Fla.: Academic Press.

22. For a consideration of such issues and how they relate to basic vigilance states, see: Steriade, M., Contreras, D., & Amzica, F. (1994). Synchronized sleep oscillations and their paroxysmal developments. *Trends Neurosci.* 17:199–208.

23. The issue of whether the EEG actually contains meaningful psychological information has long been controversial and has only recently been resolved in the positive by some experts in the field. See: Petsche, H., & Rappelsberger, P. (1992). Is there any message hidden in the EEG? In *Induced rhythms of the brain* (E. Basar & T. Bullock, eds.), pp 65–87. Boston: Birkhäuser.

24. Although the 40-Hz gamma band has been the focus of many investigators interested in consciousness (see Chapter 16), it can also be used to analyze more mundane neuropsychological issues. See: Pfurtscheller, G., Flotzinger, D., & Neuper, C. (1994). Differentiation between finger, toe and tongue movement in man based on 40 Hz EEG. *Electroencephal. Clin. Neurophysiol.* 90:456–460.

25. Freeman, W. J., & Skarda, C. A. (1985). Spatial EEG patterns: Non-linear dynamics and perception: The neo-Sherrington view. *Brain Res. Rev.* 10:147–175.

26. No EEG frequency has a single function. For instance, there are several distinct theta waves in the brain (see n. 27). High levels of cortical theta have been related to frustrative responses and psychopathic tendencies in children. For overview, see: Panksepp, J., Knutson, B., & Bird, L. (1995). On the brain and personality substrates of psychopathy. *Behav. Brain Sci.* 18:568–600.

On the other hand, high theta also appears to be related to low anxiety and high extraversion. See: Mizuki, Y., Kajimura, N., Nishikori, S., Imaizumi, J., & Yamada, M. (1984). Appearance of frontal midline theta rhythm and personality traits. *Folia Psychiat. Neurol. Japonica.* 38:451–458.

27. For a thorough review of hippocampal theta generation, see: Vertes, R. P. (1982). Brain stem generation of the hippocampal EEG. *Prog. Neurobiol.* 19:159–186.

The role of theta in mediating information processing in the hippocampus is discussed by:

Klemm, W. R. (1976). Hippocampal EEG and information processing: A special role for theta rhythm. *Prog. Neurobiol.* 7:197–214.

Vanderwolf, C. H., & Robinson, T. E. (1981). Reticulo-cortical activity and behavior: A critique of the arousal theory and a new synthesis. *Behav. Brain. Sci.* 4:459–514.

Vinogradova, O. S. (1995). Expression, control, and probable functional significance of the neuronal theta-rhythm. *Prog. Neurobiol.* 45:523–583.

28. A feeling of psychological/perceptual coherence may arise from the ability of certain 40-Hz rhythms in the brain to bind the flow of sensory information in widespread areas of the brain. For example, see: Munk, M. H. J., Roelfsema, P. R., Konig, P., Engle, A. K., & Singer, W. (1996). Role of reticular activation in the modulation of intracortical synchronization. *Science* 272:271–274.

29. Early workers were fascinated by such possibilities. For a fine historical perspective, see: Walter, G. (1953). *The living brain.* New York: Norton.

30. For a detailed discussion of the idea that the P300 wave is an active information processing function (e.g., "context updating") of the brain, see: Donchin, E., & Coles, M. G. H. (1988). Is the P300 component a manifestation of context updating? *Behav. Brain Sci.* 11:357–374.

For a discussion of some other psychologically interesing event-related potentials that can be recorded from the cranial surface of humans, see: Naatanen, R. (1990). The role of attention in auditory information processing as revealed by event-related potentials and other brain measures of cognitive function. *Behav. Brain Sci.* 13:201–288.

31. The idea that the P300, instead of indicating ongoing cognitive processing, reflects the termination of such processing (i.e., a "context closure" hypothesis) has been advanced by: Verleger, R. (1988). Event-related potentials and cognition: A critique of the context updating hypothesis and an alternative interpretation of P3. *Behav. Brain Sci.* 11:343–427.

In discussing such issues, it might be important to remember that a positive-going wave in the cortical EEG typically corresponds to neuronal inhibition at the population level. For example, see Gloor, P., & Fariello, R. G. (1988). Generalized epilepsy: Some of its cellular mechanisms differ from those of focal epilepsy. *Trends Neurosci.* 11:63–67.

32. Pfurtscheller, G., Neuper, C., & Berger, J. (1994). Source localization using event-related desynchronization (ERD) within the alpha band. *Brain Topography* 6:269–275.

Gevins, A. (1995). High-resolution electroencephalographic studies of cognition. *Adv. Neurol.* 66:181–195.

33. Petsche, H., Lindner, K., Rappelsberger, P., & Gruber, G. (1988). The EEG: An adequate method to concretize brain processes elicited by music. *Music Percept.* 6:133–159.

For another type of imaging of the musical brain, see: Sergent, J. (1993). Mapping the musician brain. *Human Brain Mapping* 1:20–38.

Of course, during an epileptic fit, EEG activity is also very coherent, but brain information processing is compromised, indicating that there are limits to coherence analysis. However, it is noteworthy that the inherent ability of the brain to exhibit seizures may reflect the very nature of learning processes in the brain. For instance, it is widely recognized that epilepsy can be a learned phenomenon (as in "kindling"; see nn. 63–65, as well as the "Afterthought" of Chapter 5).

34. Gevins, A. (1996). High resolution evoked potentials of cognition. *Brain Topography* 8:189–199.

Gevins, A., Leong, H., Smith, M. E., Le, J., & Du, R. (1995). Mapping cognitive brain function with modern high-resolution electroencephalography. *Trends Neurosci.* 18:429–436.

Tucker, D. M. (1993). Spatial sampling of head electrical fields: The geodesic sensor net. *Electroencep. Clin. Neurophysiol.* 87:154–163.

35. Nunez, P. L. (ed.) (1995). *Neocortical dynamics and human EEG rhythms.* New York: Oxford Univ. Press.

Rugg, M. D., & Coles, M. G. H. (eds.) (1995). *Electrophysiology of mind.* New York: Oxford Univ. Press.

36. Pfurtscheller, G. (1991). EEG rhythm-event-related desynchronization and synchronization. In *Rhythms in physiological systems* (H. Haken & H. P. Koepchen, eds.), pp. 289–296. Berlin: Springer-Verlag.

37. Klimesch, W., Pfurtscheller, G., Mohl, W., & Schimke, H. (1990). Event-related desynchronization, ERD-mapping and hemispheric differences for words and numbers. *Intern. J. Psychophysiol.* 8:297–308.

38. Clynes, M. (1978). *Sentics: The touch of the emotions.* New York: Doubleday.

39. The pattern of brain changes for each of four seconds following each emotional expression is summarized elsewhere; chap. 1, n. 24.

40. Lensing, P., Schimke, H., Klimesch, W., Pap, V., Szemes, G., Klingler, D., & Panksepp, J. (1995). Clinical case report: Opiate antagonist and event-related desychronization in 2 autistic boys. *Neuropsychobiology* 31:16–23.

41. Some key lines of EEG research are summarized in nn. 33 and 71–73. A few other intriguing EEG studies on music are:

Breitling, D., Guenther, W., & Rondot, P. (1987). Auditory perception of music measured by brain electrical activity mapping. *Neuropsychologia* 25:765–774.

Hinrichs, H., & Machleidt, W. (1992). Basic emotions reflected in EEG-coherences. *Internat. J. Psychophysiol.* 13:225–232.

See n. 42 for the more modern approaches to visualizing emotions in the brain.

42. George, M. S., Ketter, T. A., Kimbrell, T. A., Speer, A. M., Steedman, J. M., & Post, R. M. (1996). What functional imaging has revealed about the brain basis of mood and emotion. In *Advances in biological psychiatry* (J. Panksepp, ed.), pp 63–113. Greenwich, Conn.: JAI Press.

Pardo, J. V., Pardo, P. J., & Raichle, M. E. (1993). Neural correlates of self-induced dysphoria. *Am. J. Psychiat.* 150:713–719.

It should be noted that these techniques generally have poor resolution for subcortical areas, not only because of the small size of the brain areas but also because of the density of overlapping neural systems in which opponent processes may be elaborated. Also, it is generally accepted that these techniques are better for monitoring functional changes occurring in synaptic fields than at cell bodies.

43. Success with this metabolic marker technique was achieved by treating animals with a form of sugar, 2-deoxy-D-glucose (2-DG), that could not be metabolized. 2-DG gains access to the inside of neurons just like ordinary glucose, but after the first metabolic step (a phosphorylation), it cannot be burned any further by the cellular furnace, nor can it be readily excreted from the cell. Thus, greater amounts of 2-DG linger within those neurons that extracted a lot of fuel from the bloodstream because of the increased generation of action potentials. In other words, 2-DG serves as a marker for the quantity of sugar a cell has consumed during a set period of time and hence of the amount of neuronal work that has transpired. For example, see: Everson, C. A., Smith, C. B., & Sokoloff, L. (1994). Effects of prolonged sleep deprivation on local rates of cerebral energy metabolism in freely moving rats. *J. Neurosci.* 14:6769–6778.

44. Schmidt, K. C., Lucignani, G., & Sokoloff L.

(1996). Fluorine-18-fluorodeoxyglucose PET to determine regional cerebral glucose utilization: A re-examination. *J. Nuclear Med.* 37:394–399.

Sokoloff, L. (1993). Sites and mechanisms of function-related changes in energy metabolism in the nervous system. *Devel. Neurosci.* 15:194–206.

45. Roberts, W. W. (1980). (^{14}C) Deoxyglucose mapping of first order projections activated by stimulation of lateral hypothalamic sites eliciting gnawing, eating and drinking in rats. *J. Comp. Neurol.* 194:617–638.

Also see: Gomita, Y., & Gallistel, C. R. (1982). Effects of reinforcement-blocking doses of pimozide on neural systems driven by rewarding stimulation of the MFB: A ^{14}C-2-deoxyglucose analysis. *Pharmac. Biochem. Behav.* 17:841–845.

46. McCabe, B. J., & Horn, G. (1994). Learning-related changes in Fos-like immunoreactivity in the chick forebrain after imprinting. *Proc. Nat. Acad. Sci.* 91:11417–11421.

McCabe, B. J., Davey, J. E., & Horn, G. (1992). Impairment of learning by localized injection of an N-methyl-D-aspartate receptor antagonist into the hyperstriatum ventrale of the domestic chick. *Behav. Neurosci.* 106:947–953.

47. Posner, M. I., & Raichle, M. E. (1994). *Images of the mind.* San Francisco: Freeman.

48. London, E. D. (ed.) (1993). Imaging drug action in the brain. Boca Raton, Fla.: CRC Press.

Phelps, M. E., & Mazziotta, J. C. (1985). Positron emission tomography: Human brain function and biochemistry. *Science* 228:799–809.

49. The D_2 receptor has been found to be elevated in schizophrenia (see n. 50), but it may participate in a wide variety of psychiatric disorders. See: Comings, D. E., et al., (1991). The dopamine D_2 receptor locus as a modifying gene in neuropsychiatric disorders. *J. Am. Med. Assoc.* 266:1793–1800.

Blum, K., Cull, J. G., Braverman, E. R., & Comings, D. E. (1996). Reward-deficiency syndrome. *Am. Sci.* 84:132–145.

50. Harris, G. J., & Hoehn-Saric, R. (1995). Functional neuroimaging in biological psychiatry. In *Advances in biological psychiatry*, vol. 1 (J. Panksepp, ed.), pp. 113–160. Greenwich, Conn.: JAI Press.

51. Morris, J. S., Frith, C. D., Perrett, D. I., Rowland, D., Young, A. W., Calder, A. J., & Dolan, R. J. (1996). A differential neural response in the human amygdala to fearful and happy facial expressions. *Nature* 383:812–815.

52. George, M. S., Wassermann, E. M., Williams, W., Steppel, J., Pascual-Leone, A., Basser, P., Hallett, M., & Post, R. M. (1996). Changes in mood and hormone levels after rapid-rate transcranial magnetic stimulation of the prefrontal cortex. *J. Neuropsychiatry Clin. Neurosci.* 8:172–180.

53. As will be seen repeatedly throughout this book, *cfos* is presently the most widely used tool for visualizing which areas of the brain participate in various behavioral functions. Since there has been a focus on kindling in this chapter, see: Clark, M., Post, R. M., Weiss, S. R., Cain, C. J., & Nakajima, T. (1991). Regional expression of c-fos mRNA in rat brain during the evolution of amygdala kindled seizures. *Mol. Brain Res.* 11:55–64.

For a recent example of how the *cfos* procedure picks up only new brain activity, see:

Watanabe, Y., Stone, E., & McEwen, B. S. (1994). Induction and habituation of c-fos and zif/268 by acute and repeated stressors. *Neuroreport.* 5:1321–1324.

Zhu, X. O., Brown, M. W., McCabe, B. J., & Aggleton, J. P. (1995). Effects of the novelty or familiarity of visual stimuli on the expression of the immediate early gene c-fos in rats. *Neuroscience* 69:821–829.

54. Obviously, there are many other techniques on the horizon that have not been covered here. For instance, another very promising technique has emerged from the discovery that the neuronal uptake of certain dyes changes as a function of voltage gradients that result from neuronal firing. Until recently, these dyes were used by neurophysiologists to study the electrical properties of isolated neurons, but they have now been found to be promising (albeit quite difficult and temperamental) tools for whole-animal studies. See: Dasheiff, R. M., & Sacks, D. S. (1992). Seizure circuit analysis with voltage-sensitive dye. *Seizure* 1:79–87.

After injecting animals with these dyes and exposing them to certain behaviorally interesting situations, one can visualize brain areas that had been most intensely activated. Of course, the technique also typically requires removing the brains from their crania and subjecting the tissue to microscopic analysis. See: Sacks, D. S., & Dasheiff, R. M. (1992). In vivo mapping of drug-induced seizures with voltage-sensitive dye. *Brain Res.* 595:79–86.

There are yet other promising techniques on the horizon. See: Bernroider, G. (1994). Processing biological images from very low light emissions. *J. Bioluminescence and Chemiluminescence* 9:127–133.

55. For a summary of Descartes's rules, see chap. 2, n. 43. Quotation on p. 344. Briefly, the first rule of his "method of doubt" was a commitment to *empiricism* (i.e., to accept nothing as true that could not be verified with one's own observations); the second was a commitment to *systematic analysis* (i.e., to divide up each difficulty into as many parts as possible); the third was a commitment to *simplification* (i.e., to begin with objects that were the most simple and easy to understand, and then to progress to complexities; and the fourth was a commitment to *thoroughness* (i.e., "to make enumerations so complete and reviews so general that I should be certain of having omitted nothing").

To all this Leibniz sneered that Descartes's celebrated rules added up to saying, "Take what you need, and do what you should, and you will get what you want" (as quoted in chap. 2, n. 43, p. 345).

56. Kleick, J. (1987). *Chaos: Making a new science.* New York: Penguin.

57. Elbert, T., Ray, W. J., Kowlaik, Z. J., Skinner, J. E., Fraf, K. E., & Birbaumer, N. (1994). Chaos and physiology: Deterministic chaos in excitable cell assemblies. *Physiol. Rev.* 74:1–47.

58. Freeman, W. J. (1991). The physiology of perception. *Sci. Am.* 264 (Feb.):78–85. Quotation on p. 83.

59. Freeman, W. J. (1995). *Societies of brain: A study in the neuroscience of love and hate.* Hillsdale, N.J.: Lawrence Erlbaum.

60. The traditional metaphoric image employed by chaos theorists is the potential effect of the fluttering of butterfly wings on distant weather patterns. In neurobiology, it is much easier to imagine how a small sensory-perceptual effect can have enormous consequences for the path that events take. World War I started with one man's relatively modest act of violence. World War II ended with a nuclear bomb, the idea for which arose from a modest idea—the possibility of a nuclear chain reaction—that occurred to a young physicist (von Neuman) one day while he paused for a red light in London. For a description, see: Bronowski, J. (1973). *The ascent of man.* Boston: Little, Brown.

61. For the variability of psychological effects produced by temporal lobe arousal, see: Fish, D. R., Gloor, P., Quesney, F. N., & Oliver, A. (1993). Clinical responses to electrical brain stimulation of the temporal and frontal lobes in patients with epilepsy: Pathophysiological implications. *Brain* 116:397–414.

For a full description of the types of emotional auras that precede temporal lobe fits, see: MacLean, P. (1990). *The triune brain in evolution.* New York: Plenum Press, pp. 412–516.

62. See MacLean's coverage in n. 61, and: Paradiso, S., Hermann, B. P., & Robinson, R. G. (1996). The heterogeneity of temporal lobe epilepsy. *J. Nerv. Ment. Dis.* 183:538–547.

63. For a variety of reviews of kindling, see: Teskey, G. C., & Cain, D. P. (1989). Recent developments in kindling. *Neurosci. Biobehav. Revs.* 13:251–322.

McNamara, J. O. (1988). Pursuit of the mechanisms of kindling. *Trends Neurosci.* 11:33–36.

Sato, M., Racine, R. J., & McIntyre, D. C. (1990). Kindling: Basic mechanisms and clinical validity. *Electrenceph. Clin. Neurophysiol.* 76:459–472.

64. Adamec, R. (1994). Modelling anxiety disorders following chemical exposures. *Toxicol. Indust. Health* 10:391–420.

Bell, I. R. (1994). Neuropsychiatric aspects of sensitivity to low-level chemicals: A neural sensitization model. *Toxicol. Indust. Health* 10:277–312.

Seyfried, T. N. (1979). Audiogenic seizures in mice. *Fed. Proc.* 38:2399–2404.

Probably these forms of sensitization, as well as those that lead to chronic emotional changes (see nn. 63 and 66), are mediated by chronic changes in excitatory amino acid systems of the brain. See: Faingold, C. L., Millan, M. H., Boersma, C. A., & Meldrum, B. S. (1988). Excitant amino acids and audiogenic seizures in the genetically epilepsy-prone rat: I. Afferent seizure initiation pathway. *Exp. Neurol.* 99:678–686.

65. Several different types of kindling reflect the interconnectivities of the brain. For instance, temporal lobe kindling tends to remain restricted to structures that typically fall under the rubric of the limbic system (see n. 63), while one can also evoke kindling, with many more trials, from the thalamic-neorcortical system. See: Cain, D. P. (1982). Kindling in sensory systems: Neocortex. *Exp. Neurol.* 76:276–283.

These distinct types of kindling respond differentially to antiepileptic drugs, with limbic kindling being inhibited more by benzodiazepines and neocortical kindling being inhibited better by hydantoins.

66. Adamec, R. E., & Morgan, H. D. (1994). The effect of kindling of different nuclei in the left and right amygdala on anxiety in the rat. *Physiol. Behav.* 55:1–12.

Adamec, R. E., & Stark-Adamec, C. (1989). Behavioral inhibition and anxiety: Dispositional, developmental, and neural aspects of the anxious personality of the domestic cat. In *Perspectives on behavioral inhibition* (J. Stevens, ed.), pp. 93–124. Chicago: Univ. of Chicago Press.

67. This finding has not been reported in the literature (Zolovick & Panksepp, 1980, unpublished data). However, sexually inactive male rats can be aroused with kindling. See: Paredes, R., Haller, A. E., Manero, M. C., Alvarado, R., & Ågmo, A. (1990). Medial preoptic area kindling induces sexual behavior in sexually inactive male rats. *Brain Res.* 515:20–26.

Also, it is noteworthy that the acute effects of a kindled seizure intensify the behavioral inhibition that normally follows sexual activity. See: Paredes, R. G., Manero, M. C., Haller, A. E., Alvarado, R., & Ågmo, A. (1992). Sexual behavior enhances postictal behavioral depression in kindled rats: Opioid involvement. *Behav. Brain Res.* 52:175–182.

68. For a discussion of LTP in learning, see:

Dudai, Y. (1989). *The neurobiology of memory.* Oxford: Oxford Univ. Press.

Martinez, J. L., Jr., & Derrick, B. E. (1996). Long-term potentiation and learning. *Ann. Rev. Psych.* 47: 173–203.

Nicoll, R. A., Kauer, J. A., & Malenka, R. C. (1988). The current excitement in long-term potentiation. *Neuron* 1:97–103.

69. The relationship between the LTP mechanisms and normal learning is still provisional. For one important study, see: Barnes, C. A. (1979). Memory deficits associated with senescence: A neurophysiological and behavioral study in the rat. *J. Comp. Physiol. Psychol.* 93:74–104.

For a thorough analysis of LTP issues, see: Baudry, M., & Davis, J. L. (eds.) (1991–1996). *Long-term potentiation.* 3 vols. Cambridge, Mass.: MIT Press.

70. Kalivas, P. W., Sorg, B. A., & Hooks, M. S. (1993). The pharmacology and neural circuitry of sensitization to psychostimulants. *Behav. Pharmacol.* 4: 315–334.

71. Ekman, P., Davidson, R. J., & Friesen, W. V. (1990). The Duchenne smile: Emotional expression and brain physiology II. *J. Person. Soc. Psych.* 58:342–353.

Ekman, P., & Davidson, R. J. (1993). Voluntary smiling changes regional brain activity. *Psych. Sci.* 4:342–345.

72. Davidson, R. J., Ekman, P., Sharon, C. D., Senulis, J. A., & Friesen, W. V. (1990). Approach-withdrawal and cerebral asymmetry: Emotional expression and brain physiology I. *J. Personal. Soc. Psych.* 58: 330–341.

Sobotka, S. S., Davidson, R. J., & Senulis, J. A. (1992). Anterior brain electrical asymmetries in response to reward and punishment. *Electroenceph. Clin. Neurophys.* 83:236–247.

73. Davidson, R. J. (1992). Anterior cerebral asymmetry and the nature of emotion. *Brain. Cog.* 20:125–151.

Henriques, J. B., & Davidson, R. J. (1991). Left frontal hypoactivation in depression. *J. Abnorm. Psych.* 100:535–545.

Wheeler, R. E., Davidson, R. J., & Tomarken, A. J. (1993). Frontal brain asymmetry and emotional reactivity: A biological substrate of affective style. *Psychophysiol.* 30:82–89.

74. Davidson, R. J., & Fox, N. A. (1989). Frontal brain asymmetry predicts infants' response to maternal separation. *J. Abnorm. Psych.* 98:127–131.

Dawson, G. (1994). Frontal electroencephalographic correlates of individual differences in emotion expression in infants: A brain systems perspective on emotion. *Monog. Soc. Res. Child Devel.* 59:135–151.

Dawson, G., Klinger, L. G., Panagiotides, H., Hill, D., & Spieker, S. (1992). Frontal lobe activity and affective behavior of infants of mothers with depressive symptoms. *Child Devel.* 63:725–737.

75. Robinson, R. G. (1996). Emotional and psychiatric disorders associated with brain damage. In *Advances in biological psychiatry,* vol. 2 (J. Panksepp, ed.), pp. 27–62. Greenwich, Conn.: JAI Press.

76. Posner, M. I., & Raichle, M. E. (1994). *Images of the mind.* San Francisco: Freeman.

77. Reiman, E. M., Raichle, M. E., Robins, E., Mintun, M. A., Fusselman, M. J., Fox, P. T., Price, J. L., & Hackman, K. A. (1989). Neuroanatomical correlates of a lactate-induced anxiety attack. *Arch. Gen. Psychiat.* 46:493–500.

78. George, M. S., Ketter, T. A., Parekh, P. I., Horwitz, B., Herscovitch, P., & Post, R. M. (1995). Brain activity during transient sadness and happiness in healthy women. *Am. J. Psychiat.* 152:341–351.

Chapter 6

1. For a thorough review of genetics and developmental biology, see: Lewin, B. (1993). *Genes V.* New York: Oxford Univ. Press.

Michel, G. F., & Moore, C. L. (1995). *Developmental Psychobiology.* Cambridge, Mass.: MIT Press.

2. For a more thorough review of neurochemistry, see: Cooper, J., Bloom, F., & Roth, R. (1996). *The biochemical basis of neuropharmacology (7th ed.).* New York: Oxford Univ. Press.

3. It is noteworthy that the third neucleotide of the "triplet code" is redundant and hence carries less information than the first two nucleotides, where a change always specifies a different amino acid. Accordingly, mutations of the third nucleotide are more neutral and hence are less likely to be "seen by" the selection processes of evolution. In a similar vein, genes are functional segments of DNA called *exons* that are interspersed with nonfunctional DNA sequences called *introns.* Mutations in exons are more likely to prove fatal than mutations in introns. Accordingly, mutations are more likely to be carried on to successive generations when they occur in the nonfunctional intron domains, and hence those mutations contribute more to tools such as "molecular clocks" that have been used to estimate the time of divergence of species from common ancestors. For a full discussion of such issues, see: Kimura, M. (1983). *The neutral theory of molecular evolution.* Cambridge: Cambridge Univ. Press.

4. Björklund, A., Hökfelt, T., & Kuhar, M. J. (eds.) (1984). *Handbook of chemical neuroanatomy.* Vol. 3, *Classical transmitters and transmitter receptors in the central nervous system, part 2.* New York: Elsevier.

Bonner, T. I. (1989). The molecular basis of muscarinic receptor diversity. *Trends Neurosci.* 12:148–151.

Zimmermann, H. (1994). *Synaptic transmission: Cellular and molecular basis.* New York: Oxford Univ. Press.

5. Levy, M. I., De Nigris, Y., & Davis, K. L. (1982). Rapid antidepressant activity of melanocyte inhibiting factor: A clinical trial. *Biol. Psychiat.* 17:259–263.

Van der Velde, C. D. (1983). Rapid clinical effectiveness of MIF-I in the treatment of major depressive illness. *Peptides* 4:297–300.

An important general concept is that complex peptides can be processed further into smaller peptides that often sustain or amplify only some of the effects of the parent peptide see: Kovacs, G. L., & De Wied, D. (1994). Peptidergic modulation of learning and memory processes. *Pharmacol. Revs.* 46:269–291.

6. Dawson, T. M., & Snyder, S. H. (1994). Gases as biological messengers: Nitric oxide and carbon monoxide in the brain. *J. Neurosci.* 14:5147–5159.

7. Olney, J. W. (1994). Excitotoxins in foods. *Neurotoxicology* 15:535–544.

Olney, J. W., & Farber, N. B. (1995). NMDA antagonists as neurotherapeutic drugs, psychotogens, neurotoxins, and research tools for studying schizophrenia. *Neuropsychopharmacology* 13:335–345.

8. Olney, J. W., & Farber, N. B. (1995). Glutamate receptor dysfunction and schizophrenia. *Arch. Gen. Psychiat.* 52:998–1007.

9. Only some peptides given peripherally do enter the brain in amounts large enough to modify behavior. See:

Banks, W. A., & Kastin, A. J. (1985). Permeability of the blood-brain barrier to neuropeptides: The case for penetration. *Psychoneuroendocrinol.* 4: 385–399.

Ermisch, A., Brust, P., Kretzschmar, R., & Ruhle, H.-J. (1993). Peptides and blood-brain barrier transport. *Physiol. Revs.* 73:489–527.

Many of the behavioral effects reported with peptides given peripherally are not due to direct brain effect. Especially well-documented indirect effects are the many memory-modulating actions of opioid peptides, which appear to be mediated indirectly through effects on the adrenal gland. See: Schulteis, G., & Martinez, J. L., Jr.

(1992). Peripheral modulation of learning and memory: enkephalins as a model system. *Psychopharmacol.* 109:347–1364.

Janak, P. H., Manly, J. J., & Martinez, J. L., Jr. (1994). [Leu]enkephalin enhances active avoidance conditioning in rats and mice. *Neuropsychopharmacol.* 10:53–60.

10. Opiate alkaloids found in plants have no established physiological role in the normal metabolism of plants. They may have evolved as functional adaptations to allow plants to interact with the nervous systems of other animals that might destroy them (hence serving a protective function) or facilitate their survival (hence serving their reproductive functions). For instance, if animals find the bitter taste of opiates aversive, they will avoid the plants. On the other hand, if certain animals find the internal effects of opiates pleasurable, they may serve poppies well by disbursing undigested seeds far afield in their feces. By mimicking the effects of endogenous brain molecules that animals find psychologically attractive, plant molecules may have evolved whose only function is to utilize animal behaviors in the service of their own survival. Also see n. 16.

11. The concept of "cosmetic psychopharmacology," whereby individuals might use psychopharmaceuticals to modify undesired personality traits, was introduced in: Kramer, P. D. (1993). *Listening to Prozac.* New York: Viking.

This type of application of new brain knowledge will be debated by society for a long time. In any event, there has been a great deal of promising research in the fields of neurochemistry and neuropharmacology, to the point that there is now an embarrassment of empirical riches in these areas. Detailed knowledge has accumulated far beyond our conceptualization of the meanings of the results—far beyond our current ability to draw meaningful functional inferences. Part of the problem lies in the reluctance of psychologists to grapple with the nature of the endogenous neuropsychic functions of the brain. Part of the problem may also lie in the fact that many neurochemical systems mediate rather broad and behaviorally nonspecific functions that are hard to conceptualize in precise terms (see Appendix B).

12. For a summary of the many serotonin-mediated effects, see n. 48 and: Bevans, P., Cools, A. R., & Archer, T. (eds.) (1989). *Behavioral pharmacology of 5-HT.* Hillsdale, N.J.: Lawrence Erlbaum.

13. For early optimism concerning chemical coding of behavior, see: Myers, R. D. (1974). *Handbook of drug and chemical stimulation of the brain.* New York: Van Nostrand Reinhold.

The great hope was dashed by the finding that many systems such as serotonin and norepinephrine participate in the modulation of every behavior. The discovery of neuropeptides is once again providing good reason to believe that psychobehavioral specificity exists in the brain. However, certain other transmitters, such as glutamate and GABA, are present everywhere in the brain and involved in everything the brain does. See: Conti, F., & Hicks, T. P. (eds.) (1996). *Excitatory amino acids and the cerebral cortex.* Cambridge, Mass.: MIT Press.

For these transmitters, it is more important to identify what they do in specific areas of the brain rather than seeking a unified psychobehavioral function. However, for neuropeptides, there is presently great hope that unifying functional themes will be found (as summarized throughout this book).

14. Panksepp, J. (1986). The neurochemistry of behavior. *Ann. Rev. of Psychol.* 37:77–107.

15. A continual distinction between *transmitter systems* (which actually propagate inhibitory and excitatory messages) and *modulatory systems* (which control the intensity of message generation without actually triggering excitatory and inhibitory postsynaptic potentials) can get semantically clumsy. Henceforth, I will conflate the two concepts and simply use the term *transmitter* in a generic way to cover both concepts when there is no special reason for distinctions to be made.

16. One intriguing fatty-acid transmitter is *anandamide*, which acts on the tetrahydrocannabinol receptor that helps mediate the types of psychological changes produced by marijuana. See: Adams, I. B., Ryan, W., Singer, M., Razdan, R. K., Compton, D. R., & Martin, B. R. (1995). Pharmacological and behavioral evaluation of alkylated anandamide analogs. *Life Sci.* 56: 2041–2048.

Musty, R. E., Reggio, P., & Consroe, P. (1995). A review of recent advances in cannabinoid research and the 1994 International Symposium on Cannabis and the Cannabinoids. *Life Sci.* 56:1933–1940.

The receptor distributions for these agents in areas such the cortex, temporal lobes, hippocampus, and basal ganglia readily help explain how certain drugs such as marijuana trigger their characteristic psychological, emotional, memory, and motor effects. New ways to pharmacologically modify this receptor will presumably yield new medicines for a variety of disorders: See Herkenham, M. (1992). Cannabinoid receptor localization in brain: relationship to motor and reward systems. *Ann. N.Y. Acad. Sci.* 654:19–32.

Howlett, A. C. (1995). Pharmacology of cannabinoid receptors. *Ann. Rev. Pharmacol. Toxicol.* 35:607–634.

Oviedo, A., Glowa, J., & Herkenham, M. (1993). Chronic cannabinoid administration alters cannabinoid receptor binding in rat brain: A quantitative autoradiographic study. *Brain Res.* 616:293–302.

17. For a review of the role of glutamate in memory and other cognitive processes, see: Collingridge, G. L., & Watkins, J. C. (1995). *The NMDA receptor.* New York: Oxford Univ. Press.

18. Two other excitatory and inhibitory amino acid transmitters are alanine and glycine, respectively. Parenthetically, glycine, which seems to control the atonia, or periodic loss of muscle tone, in REM sleep (see Chapter 7), is a devilishly sweet little amino acid, but surprisingly, it is not craved by lab animals such as rats, which usually exhibit an intense "sweet tooth" (Panksepp, 1975, unpublished data). Perhaps they avoid it because of its undesirable effects on neural functions. However, across the past 20 years it has repeatedly been found that megadoses of glycine can induce antipsychotic effects within the nervous system. For the most recent of several positive trials, see: Leiderman, E., Zylberman, I., Zukin, S. R., Cooper, T. B., & Javitt, D. C. (1996). Preliminary investigation of high-dose oral glycine on serum levels and negative symptoms in schizophrenia: An open-label trial. *Biol. Psychiat.* 39: 213–215.

Since glycine exhibits very weak penetrance into the brain, it is important to evaluate other glycine derivatives, such as dimethylglycine, in the treatment of schizophrenia. Also, there is a growing literature on the benefits of low doses of the glycine receptor agonist d-cycloserine in schizophrenia and Alzheimer's disease. See:

Goff, D. C., Tasai, G., Manoach, D. S., & Coyle, J. T. (1995). Dose-finding trial of d-cycloserine added to neuroleptics for negative symptoms in schizophrenia. *Am. J. Psychiat.* 152:1213–1215.

Schwartz, B. L, Hashtroudi, S., Herting, R. L., Schwartz, P., & Deutsch, S. I. (1996). d-Cycloserine enhances implicit memory in Alzheimer patients. *Neurology* 46:420–424.

19. A substantial part of the blood-brain barrier (BBB) is due to astrocytes. However, there are in fact many distinct barriers to the entry of molecules into the brain. Thorough discussions of such issues can be found in:

Davson, H., & Segal, M. B. (1996). *Physiology* of *the CSF and blood-brain barriers.* Boca Raton, Fla.: CRC Press.

Pardridge, W. M. (ed.) (1993). *The blood-brain barrier: Cellular and molecular biology,* New York: Raven Press.

20. A gradual decline in brain dopamine is a normal feature of brain aging; if this decline can be retarded, animals will presumably live longer. See: Knoll, J. (1988). The striatal dopamine dependency of lifespan in male rats: Longevity study with (-)deprenyl. *Mech. Aging and Devel.* 46:237–262.

21. The ability of tryptophan to control brain serotonin depends on a host of variables, including the levels of other neutral amino acids in the circulation. See: Fernstrom, J. D., & Wurtman, R. J. (1972). Brain serotonin content: Physiological dependence on plasma tryptophan levels. *Science* 173:149–152.

22. For a thorough discussion of these issues, see: Wurtman, R. J., & Wurtman, J. J. (eds.) (1986). *Nutrition and the brain.* Vol. 7, *Food constituents affecting normal and abnormal behaviors.* New York: Raven Press.

23. Young, S. N. (1996). Behavioral effects of dietary neurotransmitter precursors: Basic and clinical aspects. *Neurosci. Biobehav. Revs.* 20:313–323.

24. Williams, M. (1990). *Adenosine and adenosine receptors.* Clifton, N.J.: Humana Press.

25. De Kloet, E. R., & Sutanto, W. (1994). *Neurobiology of steroids.* San Diego: Academic Press.

26. Hamblin, A. S. (1993). *Cytokines and cytokine receptors.* Oxford: IRL.

Meager, A. (1991). *Cytokines.* Englewood Cliffs, N.J.: Prentice Hall.

27. The discovery of receptors was based on our ability to make the available drug ligands radioactive for tissue-binding studies. The basic technique for identifying opiate receptors—the first neurochemical receptor to be identified—was first developed by: Goldstein, A. (1971). Stereospecific and nonspecific interactions of the morphine congener levorphanol in subcellular fractions of mouse brain. *Proc. Nat. Acad. Sci.* 68:1742–1747.

This finding was rapidly refined in three separate labs: (1) L. Terenius in Sweden, (2) C. B. Pert and S. H. Snyder at Johns Hopkins, and (3) E. J. Simon, J. M. Hiller, and I. Edelman at New York University. Promptly, a race to identify the natural molecules that interact with these receptors was initiated and was won by J. Hughes and H. W. Kosterlitz at Aberdeen University. A full history of this intellectual journey can be found in: Levinthal, C. F. (1988). *Messengers of paradise: Opiates and the brain.* New York: Doubleday.

Similar approaches have been taken to many other receptors, and we now have maps for many transmitter and receptor systems in the brain. For a fine summary, see: Tohyama, M., & Takatsuji, K. (1997). *Atlas of neuroactive substances and their receptors in the rat.* New York: Oxford Univ. Press.

28. Giros, B., Jaber, M., Jones, S. R., Wightman, R. M., & Caron, M. G. (1996). Hyperlocomotion and indifference to cocaine and amphetamine in mice lacking the dopamine transporter. *Nature* 379:606–612.

29. Auta, J., Romeo, E., Kozikowski, A., Ma, D., Costa, E., & Guidotti. A. (1993). Participation of mitochondrial diazepam binding inhibitor receptors in the anticonflict, antineophobic and anticonvulsant action of 2–aryl-3–indoleacetamide and imidazopyridine derivatives. *J. Pharmacol. Exp. Therap.* 265:649–656.

Vidnyanszky, Z., Gorcs, T. J., & Hamori, J. (1994). Diazepam binding inhibitor fragment 33–50 (octadecaneuropeptide) immunoreactivity in the cerebellar cortex is restricted to glial cells. *Glia* 10:132–141.

30. To utilize *immunocytochemical* procedures, one needs a specific antibody for the molecule of interest. This is obtained by inoculating a donor animal with the neuropeptide or enzyme of interest and allowing the host animal to generate an antibody response to the "invading agent." Once the antibody is harvested and purified, it can be used to identify the precise locations of other molecules that resemble the "invading agent." All one needs to do is to histologically visualize the locations of the antibodies on the tissue sections; a variety of standard procedures are available. In general, one first exposes thin tissue sections to the primary antibody, which binds the antigen of interest, followed by a secondary antibody, which can recognize the primary antibody but has been linked to molecules (often heavy-metal or fluorescent ones) that permit visualization of the binding sites. Since neuropeptides are usually not taken back into neurons by reuptake mechanisms, and since synaptic replenishment of neuropeptides takes some time, immunocytochemical procedures also allow investigators to estimate peptide utilization during behavior. Less immunoreactivity after specific behaviors would suggest that the peptide was synaptically utilized during a behavioral episode.

31. Electrical transfer of information occurs via "gap junctions" between neurons. This rare mode of communication is most common in neural systems where rapid coordination of neurons is essential—for instance, the coordinated bursting of hypothalamic neurons that control milk secretion. See: Hatton, G. I., Modney, B. K., & Salm, A. K. (1992). Increases in dendritic bundling and dye coupling of supraoptic neurons after the induction of maternal behavior. *Ann. N.Y. Acad. Sci.* 652:142–155.

32. Mesulam, M. M. (1995). Cholinergic pathways and the ascending reticular activating system of the human brain. *Ann. N.Y. Acad. Sci.* 757:169–179.

33. For an overview of receptor mapping, see last book in note 27. As mentioned, a variety of ACh receptors have been isolated, purified, and partly characterized, but there may well be additional types of ACh receptors, besides the nicotinic and muscarinic varieties, that remain to be discovered. See: Patrick, J., Sequela, P., Vernino, S., Amador, M., Luetje, C., & Dani, J. A. (1993). Functional diversity of neuronal nicotinic acetylcholine receptors. *Prog. Brain Res.* 98:113–120.

For instance, placement of curare (a peripheral nicotinic receptor antagonist that causes paralysis when given peripherally) into the brains of experimental animals can yield what appears to be a state of extreme terror. Such animals repeatedly vocalize and exhibit spontaneous flight, but pharmacological studies suggest that the effect is not due to action on either nicotinic or muscarinic receptor types. Whether these effects are mediated by a third type of ACh receptor or some other receptor system remains unknown.

34. One of the first behavioral changes induced by increasing cholinergic activity in the rodent brain was voluminous drinking (e.g., Wolf, G., & Miller, N. E. [1964]. Lateral hypothalamic lesions: Effects on drinking elicited by carbachol in preoptic area and posterior hypothalamus. *Science* 143:585–587), leading to the idea that thirst was controlled by this system. For a discussion of other possibilities, see: Grossman, S. P. (1966). The VMH: A center for affective reactions, satiety, or both? *Physiol. Behav.* 1:1–10.

In any event, other species, such as cats, tended to exhibit only rage behavior from the same manipulations (see chap. 10, n. 91), suggesting different chemical coding of behavior across species. However, it remains possible that both behavioral effects simply reflected a nonspecific general arousal response and may highlight the fact that arousal is likely to funnel into different behavioral outputs in different species (see Chapter 8 for a discussion of just how such a process, evoked by "rewarding" brain stimulation, confused behavioral neuroscientists for a long time). If true, this example highlights the likelihood that a careful behavioral analysis without a concurrent conceptual analysis may readily yield faulty conclusions concerning the central functions of certain neurochemical systems.

35. For a review of cholinergic control of cognitive processes, see:

Deutsch, J. A. (1983). The cholinergic synapse and the site of memory. In *The physiological basis of memory* (J. A. Deutsch, ed.), pp. 367–386. New York: Academic Press.

Baldinger, B., Hasenfratz, M., & Battig, K. (1995). Comparison of the effects of nicotine on a fixed-rate and a subject-paced version of the rapid information processing task. *Psychopharmacology* 121:396–400.

Koelega, H. S. (1993). Stimulant drugs and vigilance performance: A review. *Psychopharmacology* 111:1–16.

Warburton, D. M. (1992). Nicotine as a cognitive enhancer. *Prog. Neuropsychopharmacol. Biol. Psychiat.* 16:181–191.

36. The cause of myasthenia gravis was first discovered when rabbits were injected with purified ACh receptors in order to have them produce antibodies for those molecules. As it turned out, the rabbits started to exhibit behavioral symptoms that characterize myasthenia gravis. See: Drachman, D. B. (ed.) (1987). *Myasthenia gravis: Biology and treatment.* Special issue of *Ann. N.Y. Acad. Sci.*, vol. 505. New York: New York Academy of Sciences.

37. Brandeis, R., Dachir, S., Sapir, M., Levy, A., Fisher, A. (1990). Reversal of age-related cognitive impairments by an M1 cholinergic agonist, AF102B. *Pharmacol. Biochem. Behav.* 36:89–95.

38. The identification of the precise mode of action for every psychoactive drug has been difficult, since each drug typically has many effects on the brain and body. For instance, in the early 1970s, it was thought that the potent and relatively specific antianxiety agents of the benzodiazepine class, such as diazepam (Valium) and chlordiazepoxide (Librium®), also achieved their effects by changing the turnover of biogenic amines, especially serotonin, but this view was soon overthrown by the discovery of specific benzodiazepine receptors that interacted with GABA receptors. The search for the endogenous molecule that acts on the benzodiazepine receptor has been intense. The role of one of the prime candidates for an anxiogenic ligand for this receptor, DBI (see n. 29), has become more controversial as it is being recognized that this peptide is synthesized primarily in glial cells and that one of its major effects appears to be the control of steroid synthesis in the body. See: Papadopoulos, V., & Brown, A. S. (1995). Role of the peripheral-type benzodiazepine receptor and the polypeptide diazepam binding inhibitor in steroidogenesis. *J. Steroid Biochem. Molec. Biol.* 53:103–110.

39. The endogenous activity of many brain systems is indicated by the fact that they continue to fire reasonably normally when small sections of tissue are studied following removal from the brain. The study of neuronal activity in brain slabs incubated in sustaining media has allowed investigators to work out the details of many systems. This technique has also indicated that the biogenic amine systems possess an intrinsic ability to generate action potentials. See: Andrade, R., & Aghajanian, G. K. (1984). Locus coeruleus activity in vitro: Intrinsic regulation by a calcium-dependent potassium conductance but not α_2 adrenoreceptors. *J. Neurosci.* 4:161–170.

40. Abercrombie, E. D., & Jacobs, B. L. (1987). Single-unit response of noradrenergic neurons in the locus coeruleus of freely moving cats: I. Acutely presented stressful and nonstressful stimuli. *J. Neurosci.* 7:2837–2843.

Aston-Jones, G., & Bloom, F. E. (1981). Norepinephrine-containing locus coeruleus neurons in behaving rats exhibit pronounced responses to non-noxious environmental stimuli. *J. Neurosci.* 1:887–900.

41. Considerable evidence indicates that norephinephrine is especially adept at increasing sensory processing in the brain by increasing signal-to-noise ratios within cortical projection areas, while dopamine is more effective in promoting motor arousal. See: Foote S. L., Bloom, F. E., & Aston-Jones, G. (1983). Nucleus locus coeruleus: New evidence of anatomical and physiological specificity. *Physiol. Revs.* 63:844–914.

42. Aston-Jones, G., Foote, S. L., & Bloom, F. E. (1984). Anatomy and physiology of locus coeruleus neurons: Functional implications. In *Norepinephrine: Clinical aspects* (M. G. Zeigler & C. R. Lake, eds.), pp. 92–116. Baltimore: Williams and Wilkins.

Goldman-Rakic, P. A. (1992). Dopamine-mediated mechanisms of the prefrontal cortex. *Seminar. Neurosci.* 4:149–159.

43. Yerkes, R. M., & Dodson, J. D. (1908). The relation of strength of stimulus to rapidity of habit-formation. *J. Comp. Neurol. Psychol.* 18:459–482.

44. Cook, E. H., Stein, M. A., Drajowski, M. D., Cox, W., Olkon, D. M., Keffer, J. E., & Leventhal, B. L. (1995). Association of attention-deficit disorder and the dopamine transporter gene. *Am. J. Human Genetics* 56:993–998.

Willerman, L. (1973). Activity level and hyperactivity in twins. *Child Devel.* 44:288–293.

45. Norepinephrine neurons in the locus coeruleus clearly mediate attentional processes, and the fine details of their special abilities are being well defined. See:

Aston-Jones G., Chiang C., & Alexinsky T. (1991). Discharge of noradrenergic locus coeruleus neurons in behaving rats and monkeys suggests a role in vigilance. *Prog. Brain Res.* 88:501–520.

Rajkowski J., Kubiak P., & Aston-Jones, G. (1994). Locus coeruleus activity in monkey: Phasic and tonic changes are associated with altered vigilance. *Brain Res. Bull.* 35:607–616.

46. Steriade, M., & Biesold, D. (1991). *Brain cholinergic systems.* New York: Oxford Univ. Press.

47. Although serotonergic raphe neurons show only a mild elevation of firing rate in response to emotionally provocative stimuli, as opposed to the massive elevations of firing in norpinephrine neurons (see. n. 40), they do powerfully change firing in response to behavioral state (i.e., waking versus sleep; see Chapter 7). Not only do these neurons have their own internal pacemakers, but they are powerfully controlled by inhibitory inputs such as GABA. See: Levine, E. S., & Jacobs, B. L. (1992). Neurochemical afferents controlling the activity of serotonergic neurons in the dorsal raphe nucleus: Microiontophoretic studies in the awake cat. *J. Neurosci.* 12:4037–4044.

When the activity of serotonin cells is diminished by facilitating GABA inhibition, animals exhibit a strong motor and motivational arousal. See: Klitenick, M. A., & Wirtshafter, D. (1989). Elicitation of feeding, drinking, and gnawing following microinjections of muscimol into the medial raphe nucleus of rats. *Behav. Neural Biol.* 51:436–441.

48. Coccaro, E. F., & Murphy, D. L. (eds.) (1990). *Serotonin in major psychiatric disorders.* Washington, D.C.: American Psychiatric Press.

Jacobs, B. L.,& Gelperin, A. (eds.) (1981). *Serotonin neurotransmission and behavior.* Cambridge, Mass.: MIT Press.

49. Although serotonin generally tends to produce a relaxed attitude in animals, some behaviorally oriented investigators still believe that it mediates anxiety (see chap. 11, n. 9). Their belief appears to be premised on the fact that serotonin can promote behavioral inhibition, and a variant of this response *is* common when animals are scared. Also, serotonin is released in the brain during stress, but this may be a counter regulatory antistress response. See: Shimizu, N., Take, S., Hori, T., & Oomura, Y. (1992). In vivo measurement of hypothalamic serotonin release by intracerebral microdialysis: Significant enhancement by immobilization stress in rats. *Brain Res. Bull.* 28:727–734.

Also, stimulation of one serotonin receptor can provoke intense fear in humans (see chap. 11, n. 72), but this receptor may be absent in humans!

50. Dalayeun, J. F., Nores, J. M., & Bergal, S. (1993). Physiology of β-endorphins: A close-up view and a review of the literature. *Biomed. Pharmacotherap.* 47:311–320.

Mansour, A., Khachaturian, H., Lewis, M. E., Akil, H., & Watson, J. (1988). Anatomy of CNS opioid receptors. *Trends Neurosci.* 11:308–314.

Reisine, T. (1995). Opiate receptors. *Neuropharmacol.* 34:463–472.

51. Dunn, A. J., & Berridge, C. (1990). Physiological and behavioral responses to corticotrophin-releasing factor administration: Is CRF a mediator of anxiety or stress responses? *Brain Res. Revs.* 15:71–100.

Souza, E. B. D., & Nemeroff, C. B. (eds.) (1995). *Corticotropin-releasing factor: Basic and clinical studies of a neuropeptide.* Boca Raton: Fla.: CRC Press.

52. Jard, S., & Jamison, R. (eds.) (1991). *Vasopressin.* London: John Libbery Eurotext.

Pedersen, C. A., Caldwell, J. D., Jirikowski, G. F., & Insel, T. R. (eds.) (1992). *Oxytocin in maternal, sexual, and social behaviors.* Special issue of *Ann. N.Y. Acad. Sci.*, vol. 652. New York: New York Academy of Sciences.

Van Wimersma Greidanus, T. B., & van Ree, J. M. (1990). Behavioral aspects of vasopressin. In *Current topics in neuroendocrinology*. Vol. 10, *Behavioral aspects of neuroendocrinology* (D. Ganten and D. Pfaff, eds.), pp. 61–80. Berlin: Springer-Verlag.

53. Bradwejn, J., & Koszycki, D. (1995). Cholecystokinin and panic disorder. In *Panic disorder: Clinical, biological, and treatment aspects* (G. M. Asnis & H. M. van Praag, eds.), pp. 99–109. New York: Wiley.

Harro, J., & Vasar, E. (1991). Cholecystokinin-induced anxiety: How is it reflected in studies of exploratory behavior? *Neurosci. Biobehav. Revs.* 15:473–477.

Lydiard, R. B. (1994). Neuropeptides and anxiety: Focus on cholecystokinin. *Clin. Chem.* 40:315–318.

54. See n. 18 and: Deutsch, S. I., Mastropaolo, J., Schwartz, B. L., Rosse, R. B., & Morihisa, J. M. (1989). A glutamatergic hypothesis of schizophrenia. *Clin. Neuropharmacol.* 12:1–13.

55. Strzelczuk, M., & Romaniuk, A. (1996). Fear induced by the blockade of $GABA_A$-ergic transmission in the hypothalamus of the cat. Behavioral and neurochemical study. *Behav. Brain Res.* 72:63–71.

56. Bauman, M. L., & Kemper, T. L. (1995). Neuroanatomical observations of the brain in autism. In *Advances in biological psychiatry,* vol. 1 (J. Panksepp, ed.), pp. 1–26. Greenwich, Conn.: JAI Press.

Bauman, M. L., & Kemper, T. L. (eds.) (1994). *The neurobiology of autism.* Baltimore: Johns Hopkins Univ. Press.

57. Ulrich, B., Shkaryov, Y. A., & Studhof, C. (1995). Cartography of neurexin: More than 1000 isolforms generated by alternative splicing and expressed in distinct subsets of neurons. *Neuron* 14:497–507.

58. Strittmatter, S. M., (1995). Neuronal guidance molecules: Inhibitory and soluble factors. *The Neuroscientist* 1:255–258.

59. Colamarino, S. A., & Tessier-Lavigne, M. (1995). The axonal chemoattractant netrin-1 is also a chemorepellant for trochlear motor axons. *Cell* 81:621–629.

60. Tatter, S. B., Galpern, W. R., & Isacson, O. (1995). Neurotrophic factor protection against excitotoxic neuronal death. *The Neuroscientist* 1:286–297.

61. Finkbeiner, S. (1996). Neurotrophins and the synapse. *The Neuroscientist* 2:139–142.

62. Ilag, L. L., et al., (1995). Pan-neurotrophin 1: A genetically engineered neurotrophic factor displaying multiple specificities in peripheral neurons in vitor and in vivo. *Proc. Natl. Acad. Sci.* 92:607–611.

63. Snider, W. D. (1994). Functions of the neurotrophins during nervous system development: What the knockouts are teaching us. *Cell* 77:627–638.

64. Martinez-Serrano, A., Lundberg, C., Hoellou, P., Fischer, W., Bentlage, C., Campbell, K., McKay, R. D., Mallet, J., & Björklund, A. (1995). CNS-derived neural progenitor cells for gene transfer of nerve growth factor to the adult rat brain: Complete rescue of axotomized cholinergic neurons after transplantation into the septum. *J. Neurosci.* 15:5668–5680.

65. Rosenzweig, M. R., & Bennett, E. L. (1996). Psychobiology of plasticity: Effects of training and experience on brain and behavior. *Behav. Brain Res.* 78:57–65.

66. This is an unproven therapy provided widely by occupational therapists, and is based on work and thinking such as: Ayers, A. J. (1964). Tactile functions: Their relations to hyperactive and perceptual motor behavior. *Amer. J. Occup. Therap.* 18:6–11.

67. Rimland, B., & Edelson, S. M. (1995). A pilot study of auditory integration training in autism. *J. Autism Devel. Dis.* 25:61–70.

68. Ghosh, A., Carnahan, J., & Greenberg, M. E. (1994). Requirement for BDNF in activity-dependent survival of cortical neurons. *Science* 263:1618–1623.

69. Lillrank, S. M., O'Connor, W. T., Oja, S. S., & Ungerstedt, U. (1994). Systemic phencyclidine administration is associated with increased dopamine, GABA, and 5-HIAA levels in the dorsolateral striatum of conscious rats: An in vivo microdialysis study. *J. Neural Trans.* 95:145–55.

Weiss, F., Hurd, Y. L., Ungerstedt, U., Markou, A., Plotsky, P. M., & Koob, G. F. (1992). Neurochemical correlates of cocaine and ethanol self-administration. *Ann. N.Y. Acad. Sci.* 654:220–241.

70. Boulton, A. A., Baker, G. B., & Adams, R. N. (eds.) (1995). *Voltammetric methods in brain systems.* Totowa, N.J.: Humana Press.

71. Panksepp, J., & Bishop, P. (1981). An autoradiographic map of (^{3}H)diprenorphine binding in rat brain: Effects of social interaction. *Brain Res. Bull.* 7:405–410.

For an overview of molecular imaging procedures, see: Sharif, N. A. (1994). *Molecular imaging in neuroscience.* New York: Oxford Univ. Press.

72. Eberwine, J. H., Valentino, K. L., & Barchas, J. D. (1994). *In situ hybridization in neurobiology: Advances in methodology.* New York: Oxford Univ. Press.

Wisden, W., & Morris, B. J. (eds.) (1994). *In situ hybridization protocols for the brain.* San Diego; Academic Press.

73. Schatzberg, A. F., & Nemeroff, C. B. (eds.) (1995). *The American Psychiatric Press textbook of psychopharmacology.* Washington, D.C.: American Psychiatric Press.

74. See chap. 9, n. 76.

75. Blum, K., Cull, J. G., Braverman, E. R., & Comings, D. E. (1996). Reward-deficiency syndrome. *Am. Sci.* 84:132–145.

Wise, R. A., & Bozarth, M. A. (1987). A psychomotor stimulant theory of addiction. *Psych. Rev.* 94: 469–492.

76. See n. 28.

77. Self, D. W., Barnhart, W. J., Lehman, D. A., & Nestler, E. J. (1996). Opposite modulation of cocaine-seeking behavior by D_1- and D_2–like dopamine receptor agonists. *Science* 271:1586–1589.

78. Carrera, M. R., Ashley, J. A., Parsons, L. H., Wirsching, P., Koob, G. F., & Janda, K. D. (1995). Suppression of psychoactive effects of cocaine by active immunization. *Nature* 378:727–730.

79. Suchecki, D., Nelson, D. Y., Van Oers, H., & Levine, S. (1995). Activation and inhibition of the hypothalamic-pituitary-adrenal axis of the neonatal rat: Effects of maternal deprivation. *Psychoneuroendocrinol.* 20:169–182.

Please note that many of the molecules of the pituitary-adrenal stress system, especially ACTH and its fragments, also serve many other functions in the brain. See: Strand, F. L., Rose, K. J., Zuccarelli, L. A., Kume, J., Alves, S. E., Antonawich, F. J., & Garrett, L. Y. (1991). Neuropeptide hormones as neurotrophic factors. *Physiol. Revs.* 72:1017–1046.

80. Sprott, R. L., Huber, R., Warner, T., & Williams, F. (eds.) (1993). *The biology of aging.* New York: Springer-Verlag.

81. It is noteworthy that granule cells can undergo mitosis, providing some type of continuing neural restoration in areas such as the hippocampus. Also, some hormone treatments reverse the natural age-related decline in hippocampal functions, as well as many other forms of neural damage. See:

Reul, J. M., Tonnaer, J. A., & De Kloet, E. R. (1988). Neurotrophic ACTH analogue promotes plasticity of type I corticosteroid receptor in brain of senescent male rats. *Neurobiol. Aging* 9:253–260.

82. Friedman, M. J., Charney, D. S., & Deutch, A. Y. (eds.) (1995). *Neurobiological and clinical consequences of stress: From normal adaptation to post-traumatic stress disorder.* Philadelphia: Lippincott-Raven Press.

McCubbin, J. A., Kaufmann, P. G., & Nemeroff, C. B. (1991). *Stress, neuropeptides, and systemic disease.* San Diego: Academic Press.

Stanford, S. C., & Salmon, P. (eds.) (1993). *Stress: From synapse to syndrome.* San Diego: Academic Press.

83. Gershon, M. D., & Tennyson, V. M. (1991). Microenvironmental factors in the normal and abnormal development of the enteric nervous system. *Prog. Clin. Biol. Res.* 373:257–276.

Gershon, M. D., Chalazonitis, A., & Rothman, T. P. (1993). From neural crest to bowel: Development of the enteric nervous system. *J. Neurobiol.* 24:199–214.

84. See n. 66 and:

Alexander, F. (1950). *Psychosomatic medicine: Its principles and applications.* New York: Norton.

Wolman, B. B. (1988). *Psychosomatic disorders.* New York: Plenum Medical.

Chapter 7

The decision to include the ambiguous concept of "mythmaking" in the title was based on the potential credibility of Jungian ideas regarding the archetypal images that emerge during dreaming. Also, an underlying premise of this chapter is that dreams, through poorly understood information-processing mechanisms, help create our beliefs and our sense of reality about the world. Such issues are eloquently explored in: Stevens, A. (1995). *Private myths.* Cambridge, Mass.: Harvard Univ. Press.

1. There are many levels of theorizing about dreaming and REM sleep. Most theories are limited to specific functions, while others take a more global view. As we will see, there is abundant evidence that memory consolidation is facilitated by REM sleep, but these important findings do not in themselves constitute a theory. A theory needs to be fairly comprehensive, explaining many diverse facts about REM. For instance, Francis Crick's theory (Crick, F., & Mitchinson, G. [1983]. The function of dream sleep. *Nature* 304:111–114) achieves that in suggesting that the function of REM is to dump unneeded information from memory. Unfortunately, the theory has practically no empirical evidence to support it.

In this same context, even though the categorization of sleep states is fairly well resolved, we should remember that there is still room for further refinements. See: Gottesmann, C. (1996). The transition from slow-wave sleep to paradoxical sleep: Evolving facts and concepts of neurophysiological processes underlying the intermediate stage of sleep. *Neurosci. Biobehav. Revs.* 20: 367–388.

2. The documentation of high levels of emotionality within dreams is not as impressive as one might think. Indeed, the dreams of young children seem to be fairly sparse in vivid emotional episodes (but this could also be a problem with dream reporting, as well as the safe environments in which these children have lived their lives). See: Foulkes, D. (1982). *Children's dreams: Longitudinal studies.* New York: Wiley.

However, the evidence that emotional processing occurs during REM is good. See: Greenberg, R. (1981). Dreams and REM sleep: An integrative approach. In *Sleep, dreams and memory: Advances in sleep research,* vol. 6 (W. Fishbein, ed.), pp. 125–133. New York: SP Medical.

3. Changes in neuropsychiatric disorders are summarized by:

Douglass, A. B. (1996). Sleep abnormalities in major psychiatric illnesses: Polysomnographic and clinical features. In *Advances in biological psychiatry,* vol. 2 (J. Panksepp, ed.), pp. 153–176. Greenwich, Conn.: JAI Press.

Ford, D., & Kamerow, D. (1989). Epidemiologic study of sleep disturbances in psychiatric disorders. *J. Am. Med. Assoc.* 262:1479–1484.

Gillin, J. C., & Wyatt, R. J. (1975). Schizophrenia: Perchance a dream? *Int. Rev. Neurobiol.* 17:297–342.

Zarcone, V., & Dement, W. (1969). Sleep disturbances in schizophrenia. In *Sleep: Physiology and pathology* (A. Kales, ed.), pp. 192–199. Philadelphia: Lippincott.

4. Heath, R. G., & Mickle, W. A. (1960). Evaluation of seven years' experience with depth electrode studies in human patients. In *Electrical studies on the unanesthetized brain* (E. R. Ramey & D. S. O'Doherty, eds.), pp. 214–247. New York: Paul B. Hoeber.

Heath, R. G. (1972). Marihuana: Effects on deep and surface electroencephalograms of man. *Arch. Gen. Psychiat.* 26:577–584.

5. Jouvet, M. (1967). Neurophysiology of the states of sleep. *Physiol. Rev.* 47:117–177.

Stern, W. C., Morgane, P. J., & Bronzino, J. D. (1972). LSD: Effects on sleep patterns and spiking activity in the lateral geniculate nucleus. *Brain. Res.* 41:199–204.

6. Initially there was an active attempt to blame the accident on the teenagers, probably because a policeman had been following the drunken driver for several miles without his siren or overhead lights. The case was eventually plea-bargained, since the hospital was withholding the blood-alcohol evidence (0.26%) from the legal system on the basis of doctor-patient confidentiality. The drunken driver's sentence was one year in jail.

7. Chase, M. H., & Morales, F. R. (1990). The atonia and myoclonia of active (REM) sleep. *Ann. Rev. Psychol.* 41:557–584.

8. Even minor stressors such as exposing organisms to new situations increases REM. See: Hartmann, E. (1981). The functions of sleep and memory processing. In *Sleep, dreams and memory: Advances in sleep research*, vol. 6 (W. Fishbein, ed.), pp. 111–124. New York: SP Medical.

9. Anch, A. M., Browman, C. P., Mitler, M. M., & Walsh, J. K. (1988). *Sleep: A scientific perspective.* Englewood Cliffs, N.J.: Prentice Hall.

10. Roffwarg, H. P., Muzio, J. N., & Dement, W. C. (1966). Ontogenetic development of the human sleep-dream cycle. *Science* 152:604–619.

11. Steriade, M. (1992). Basic mechanisms of sleep generation. *Neurology* 42(suppl.):9–18.

12. Sterman, M. B., & Wyrwicka, W. (1967). EEG correlates of sleep: Evidence for separate forebrain substrates. *Brain Res.* 6:143–163.

A specific SWS generator has provisionally been identified in the anterior hypothalamus. See: Sherin, J. E., Shiromani, P. J., McCarley, R. W., & Saper, C. B. (1996). Activation of ventrolateral preoptic neurons during sleep. *Science* 271:216–219.

13. Marquet, P., Peter, J.-M., Aerts, J., Delfiore, G., Degueldre, C., Luxzen, A., & Franck, G. (1996). Functional neuroanatomy of human rapid-eye-movement sleep and dreaming. *Nature* 383:163–166.

14. Vanderwolf, C. H., & Robinson, T. E. (1981). Reticulo-cortical activity and behavior: A critique of the arousal theory and a new synthesis. *Behav. Brain Sci.* 4:459–514.

Vertes, R. P. (1982). Brain stem generation of the hippocampal EEG. *Prog. Neurobiol.* 19:159–186.

15. Pavlides, C., & Winson, J. (1989). Influences of hippocampal place cell firing in the awake state on the activity of these cells during subsequent sleep episodes. *J. Neurosci.* 9:2907–2918.

Wilson, M. A., & McNaughton, B. L. (1994). Reactivation of hippocampal ensemble memories during sleep. *Science* 265:676–679.

Winson J. (1993). The biology and function of rapid eye movement sleep. *Cur. Opin. Neurobiol.* 3:243–248.

16. Chase, M. H., & Morales, F. R. (1989). The control of motorneuron during sleep. In *Principles and practice of sleep medicine* (M. H. Kryger, T. Roth, & W. C. Dement, eds.), pp. 74–85. Philadelphia: Saunders.

17. For a full description of the bodily changes during sleep, see n. 9 and: Kryger, M. H., Roth, T., & Dement W. C. (eds.) (1989). *Principles and practice of sleep medicine.* Philadelphia: Saunders.

18. Sniffing appears to be controlled by the same brain stem system that generates theta. See: Vertes, R. P. (1981). An analysis of ascending brain stem systems involved in hippocampal synchronization and desynchronization. *J. Neurophysiol.* 46:1140–1159.

19. Fischer, C., Gross, J., & Zuch, J. (1965). Cycle of penile erections synchronous with dreaming (REM) sleep. *Arch. Gen. Psychiat.* 12:29–45.

20. Schmidt, M. H.,Valatx, J. L., Schmidt, H. S., Wauquier, A., & Jouvet, M. (1994). Experimental evidence of penile erections during paradoxical sleep in the rat. *Neuroreport* 5:561–564.

21. Dement, W. C. (1974). *Some must watch while some must sleep.* San Francisco: Freeman.

22. Hartmann, E. (1984). *The nightmare: The psychology and biology of terrifying dreams.* New York: Basic Books.

23. Kleitman, N. (1963). *Sleep and wakefulness* (2d ed.). Chicago: Univ. of Chicago Press.

Sterman, M. B. (1973). The basic rest-activity cycle and sleep: Developmental consideration in man and cat. In *Sleep and the maturing nervous system* (C. Clemente, D. Purpura, & F. Mayer, eds.), pp. 175–197. New York: Academic Press.

24. Sterman, M. B., Lucas, E. A., & MacDonald, L. R. (1972). Periodicity within sleep and operant performance in the cat. *Brain Res.* 38:327–341.

25. Oswald, I., Merrington, J., & Lewis, H. (1970). Cyclical "on demand" oral intake by adults. *Nature* 225:959–960.

26. For an overview of SCN issues, see: Binkley, S. (1990). *The clockwork sparrow: Time, clocks and calenders in biological organisms.* Englewood Cliffs, N.J.: Prentice-Hall.

27. Mirmiran, M., Kok, J. H., Boer, K., & Wolf, H. (1992). Perinatal development of human circadian rhythms: Role of the foetal biological clock. *Neurosci. Biobehav. Revs.* 16:371–378.

Rusak, B., Abe, H., Mason, R., & Piggins, H. D. (1993). Neurophysiological analysis of circadian rhythm entrainment. Special issue: Neural mechanisms of the mammalian circadian system. *J. Biol. Rhythms* 8(suppl.): S39–S45.

Sollars, P. J., Kimble, D. P., & Pickard, G. E. (1995). Restoration of circadian behavior by anterior hypothalamic heterografts. *J. Neurosci.* 15:2109–2122.

28. Cassone, V. M., Roberts, M. H., & Moore, R. Y. (1988). Effects of melatonin on 2-deoxy-D-^{14}C glucose uptake within rat suprachiasmatic nucleus. *Am. J. Physiol.* 255:R332–R337.

Schwartz, W. J., & Gainer, H. (1977). Suprachiasmatic nucleus: Use of 14^{C}-labeled deoxyglucose uptake as a functional marker. *Science* 197:1089–1091.

Stehle, J., Vaneck, J., &Vollrath, L. (1989). Effects of melatonin on spontaneous electrical activity of neurons in rat suprachiasmatic nuclei: An in vitro iontophoretic study. *J. Neural Transm.* 78:167–177.

29. Klein, D., Moore, R. Y., & Reppert, S. M. (1991). *Suprachiasmatic nucleus: The mind's clock.* New York: Oxford Univ. Press.

30. Aschoff, J., Daan, S., & Gross, G. (eds.) (1982). *Vertebrate circadian systems*. Berlin: Springer.

Ibuka, N., & Kawamura, H. (1975). Loss of circadian rhythm in sleep-wakefulness cycle in the rat by suprachiasmatic nucleus lesions. *Brain Res.* 96:76–81.

Rusak, B., & Zucker, I. (1979). Neural regulation of circadian rhythms. *Physiol. Rev.* 59:449–526.

Stephan, F. K., & Zucker, I. (1972). Circadian rhythms in drinking behavior and locomotor activity of rats are eliminated by hypothalamic lesion. *Proc. Natl. Acad. Sci.* 69:1583–1586.

31. Miller, J. D., Morin, L. P., Schwartz, W. J., & Moore, R. Y. (1996). New insights into the mammalian circadian clock. *Sleep* 19:641–667.

Silver, R., Le Sauter, J., Tresco, P. A., & Lehman, M. N. (1996). A diffusible coupling signal from the transplanted suprachiasmatic nucleus controlling circadian locomotor rhythms. *Nature* 382:810–813.

32. Wetterberg, L. (ed.) (1993). *Light and biological rhythms in man*. Wenner-Gren International Series, vol. 63. Oxford: Pergamon.

Rusak, B., Robertson, H. A., Wisden, W., & Hunt, S. P. (1990). Light pulses that shift rhythms induce gene expression in the suprachiasmatic nucleus. *Science* 248:1237–1240.

33. Arendt, J. (1995). *Melatonin and the mammalian pineal gland*. London: Chapman and Hill.

34. Gauer, F., Masson-Pevet, J., Stehle, J., & Pevet, P. (1994). Daily variations in melatonin receptor density of rat pars tuberalis and suprachiasmatic nuclei are distinctly regulated. *Brain Res.* 641:92–98.

Shibata, S., Cassone, V. M., & Moore, R. Y. (1989). Effects of melatonin on neuronal activity in the rat suprachiasmatic nucleus in vitro. *Neurosci. Lett.* 97: 140–144.

35. Golombek, D. A., Pevet, P., & Cardinali, D. P. (1996). Melatonin effects on behavior: Possible mediation by the central GABAergic system. *Neurosci. Biobehav. Revs.* 20:403–412.

Nelson, E., Panksepp, J., & Ikemoto, S. (1994). The effects of melatonin on isolation distress in chickens. *Pharmac. Biochem. Behav.* 49:327–333.

Romijn, H. (1978). The pineal: A tranquilizing organ? *Life Sci.* 23:2257–2274.

36. Reiter, R. J., & Robinson, J. (1995). *Melatonin*. New York: Bantam Books.

37. Pierpaoli, W., & Regelson, W. (1995). *The melatonin miracle*. New York: Simon and Schuster.

However, it should be noted that so far longevity has been found only in mice that have an endogenous melatonin deficiency.

38. See nn. 33, 36, and 37, as well as good scientific documentation such as: Zhdanova, I. V., Wurtman, R. J., Morabito, C., Piotrovska, V. R., & Lynch, H. J. (1996). Effects of low oral doses of melatonin, given 2–4 hours before habitual bedtime, on sleep in normal young humans. *Sleep* 19:423–431.

39. Borbely, A. A., & Tobler, I. (1989). Endogenous sleep-promoting substance and sleep regulation. *Physiol. Rev.* 69:605–670.

Kapas, L., Obal, F., Jr., & Krueger, J. M. (1993). Humoral regulation of sleep. *Int. Rev. Neurobiol.* 35: 131–160.

40. Kruger, J. M., Opp, M. R., Toth, L. A., Johansen, L., & Kapas, L. (1990). Cytokines and sleep. In *Current topics in neuroendocrinology*. Vol. 10, *Behavioral aspects of neuroedocrinology* (D. Ganten & D. Pfaff, eds.), pp. 243–261. Berlin: Springer-Verlag.

41. Radulovacki, M., & Virus, R. M. (1985). Purine, 1–methylisoguanosine and pyrimidine compounds and sleep in rats. In *Sleep: Neurotransmitters and neuromodulators* (A. Wauquier, J. M. Monti, J. M. Gaillard, & M. Radulovacki, eds.), pp. 221–235. New York: Raven Press.

It is noteworthy that adenosine inhibits reticular cholinergic neurons, which mediate cortical arousal in both waking and REM. See: Rainnie, D. G., Grunze, H. C. R., McCarley, R. W., & Greene, R. W. (1994). Adenosine inhibition of mesoponine cholinergic neurons: Implications for EEG arousal. *Science* 263:689–692.

42. Radulovacki, M., Virus, R. M., & Djuricic-Nedelson, M. (1985). Adenosine and adenosine analogs: Effects on sleep in rats. In *Brain mechanisms of sleep* (D. J. McGinty, R. Drucker-Colin, A. R. Morrison, & P. L. Parmeggiani, eds.), pp. 221–240. New York: Raven Press.

43. Jus, A., Jus, K., Villeneuve, A., Pires, A., Lachance, R., Fortier, J., & Villeneuve, R. (1973). Studies on dream recall in chronic schizophrenic patients after prefrontal lobotomy. *Biol. Psychiat.* 6:275–293.

In this context it is also noteworthy that most areas of the normal brain appear to wake up (i.e., exhibit increased metabolic activity) during REM sleep, but the frontal lobes continue to exhibit reduced metabolic activity, just as they do during SWS. See: Maquet, P., Peters, J.-M., Aerts, J., Delfiore, G., Degueldre, C., Luxen, A., & Franck, G. (1996). Functional neuroanatomy of human rapid-eye-movement sleep and dreaming. *Nature* 383:163–166.

Neither cortical blindness nor retinal blindness impairs dream content (Oswald, I. [1962] *Sleeping and waking: Physiology and psychology*. Amsterdam: Elsevier). However, a lesion in middle-level processing—for instance, in the lateral geniculate nucleus—can cause empty spots in dream scenes, and the types of brain damage that lead to disconnection syndromes can markedly reduce dreaming. See: Doricchi, F., & Violani, C. (1992). Dream recall in brain-damaged patients: A contribution to the neuropsychology of dreaming through a review of the literature. In *The neuropsychology of sleep and dreaming* (J. S. Antrobus & M. Bertini, eds.), pp. 99–129. Hillsdale, N.J.: Lawrence Erlbaum.

44. Moruzzi, G. (1972). The sleep-waking cycle. *Ergeb. Physiol.* 64:1–165. Gottesmann, C. (1988). What the *cereveau isolé* preparation tells us nowadays about sleep-wake mechanisms. *Neurosci. Biobehav. Revs.* 12:39–48.

45. For a summary of transection brain stem work, see: Siegel, J. M. (1989). Brainstem mechanisms generating REM sleep. In *Principles and practice of sleep* *medicine* (M. H. Kryger, T. Roth, & W. C. Dement, eds.), pp. 104–120. Philadelphia: Saunders.

46. Siegel, J. M. (1985). Pontomedullary interactions in the generation of REM sleep. In *Brain mechanisms of sleep* (D. J. McGinty, R. Drucker-Colin, A. R. Morrison, & P. L. Parmeggiani, eds.), pp. 157–174. New York: Raven Press.

47. Batini, C., Moruzzi, G., Palestini, M., Rossi, G. F., & Zanchetti, A. (1958). Persistent patterns of wakefulness in the pretrigeminal midpontine preparation. *Science* 128:30–32.

For a striking PET image of the ARAS, see: Knomura, S., Larsson, J., Gluyas, B., & Roland, P. E. (1996). Activation by attention of the human reticular formation and thalamic intralaminar nuclei. *Science* 271:512–515.

For the most recent conception of how the ARAS sustains attention, see: Munk, M. H. J., Roelfsema, P. R., Konig, P., Engel., A. K., & Singer, W. (1996). Role of reticular activation in the modulation of intracortical synchronization. *Science* 272:271–274.

48. Siegel, J. M., Tomaszewski, K. S., & Nienhuis, R. (1986). Behavioral states in the chronic medullary and mid-pontine cat. *EEG Clin. Neurophysiol.* 63:274–288.

49. Shlaer, R., & Myers, M. L. (1972). Operant conditioning of the pretrigeminal cats. *Brain Res.* 38: 222–225.

50. Steriade, M., Gloor, P., Llinas, R. R., Lopes da Silva, F. H., & Mesulam, M.-M. (1990). Basic mechanisms of cerebral rhythmic activities. *EEG Clin. Neurophysiol.* 76:481–508.

51. Steriade, M. (1989). Brain electrical activity and sensory processing during waking and sleep states. In *Principles and practice of sleep medicine* (M. H. Kryger, T. Roth, & W. C. Dement, eds.), pp. 86–103. Philadelphia: Saunders.

52. Rossor, M. N., Garrett, N. J., Johnson, A. L. Mountjoy, C. Q., Roth, M., & Iversen, L. L. (1982). A post-mortem study of the cholinergic and GABA systems in senile dementia. *Brain* 105:313–330.

53. Panksepp, J., Jalowiec, J. E., Morgane, P. J., Zolovick, A. J., & Stern, W. C. (1973). Noradrenergic pathways and sleep-waking states in cats. *Exp. Neurol.* 41:233–245.

54. Jacobs, B. L. (1983). Single unit activity of brain monoaminergic neurons in freely moving animals: A brief review. In *Modulation of sensorimotor activity during alterations in behavioral states* (R. Bandler, ed.), pp. 99–120. New York: Liss.

Moore, R. Y., & Bloom, F. E. (1979). Central catecholamine neuron systems: Anatomy and physiology of the norepinephrine and epinephrine systems. *Ann. Rev. Neurosci.* 2:113–168.

It is also noteworthy that high locus coeruleus activity during waking sustains the ability of the brain to activate certain genetic programs in nerve cells. See: Cirelli, C., Pompeiano, M., & Tononi, G. (1996). Neuronal gene expression in the waking state: A role for the locus coeruleus. *Science* 274:1211–1215.

The whole topic of gene expression in the brain as a function of sleep states is summarized in *Sleep Research Society Bulletin* 2:(1996)1–28.

55. Aston-Jones, G., & Bloom, F. E. (1981). Norepinephrine-containing locus coeruleus neurons in behaving rats exhibit pronounced responses to non-noxious environmental stimuli. *J. Neurosci.* 8:887–900.

56. Abercrombie, E. D., & Jacobs, B. L. (1987). Single-unit response of noradrenergic neurons in the locus coeruleus of freely moving cats: II. Adaptation to chronically presented stressful stimuli. *J. Neurosci.* 7:2844–2848.

57. Redmond, D. E., Jr., & Hunag, Y. H. (1979). New evidence for a locus coeruleus–norepinephrine connection with anxiety. *Life Sci.* 25:2149–2162.

58. Jacobs, B. L., Heym, J., & Steinfels, G. F. (1984). Physiological and behavioral analysis of raphe unit activity. *Handb. Psychopharmacol.* 18:343–395.

McGinty, D., & Harper, R. M. (1976). Dorsal raphe neurons: Depression of firing during sleep in cats. *Brain Res.* 2101:569–575.

59. Wauquier, A., & Dugovic, C. (1990). Serotonin and sleep-wakefulness. *Ann. N.Y. Acad. Sci.* 600: 447–459.

60. Koella, W. P., Felstein, A., & Czicman, J. S. (1968). The effect of parachlorophenylalanine on the sleep of cats. *Electroencephal. Clin. Neurophysiol.* 37:161–166.

Dement, W. C., Miller, M. M., & Henrikson, S. J. (1972). Sleep changes during chronic administration of parachlorophenylalanine. *Rev. Can. Biol.* 31(suppl.): 239–246.

61. The early work finding powerful insomnia in cats following brain serotonin lesions is summarized in: Jouvet, M. (1972). The role of monoamines and acetylcholine-containing neurons in the regulation of the sleep-waking cycle. *Ergeb. Physiol.* 64:165–307.

More recent work indicating weaker effects with selective brain neurochemical manipulations are summarized in: Jones, B. E. (1989). Basic mechanism of sleep-wake states. In *Principles and practice of sleep medicine* (M. H. Kryger, T. Roth, & W. C. Dement, eds.), pp. 121–138. Philadelphia: Saunders.

Generally, the effects of serotonin depletion are substantial in cats (see nn. 59 and 60) but small or nonexistent in rats. See: Ross, C. A., Trulson, M. E., & Jacobs, B. L. (1976). Depletion of brain serotonin following intraventricular 5,7 dihydroxytryptamine fails to disrupt sleep in the rat. *Brain. Res.* 114:517–523.

62. Lammers, G. J., Arends, J., Declerck, A. C., Ferrari, M. D., Schouwink, G., & Troost, J. (1993). Gamma-hydroxybutyrate and narcolepsy: A double-blind placebo-controlled study. *Sleep* 16:216–220.

Scrima, L., Hartman, P. G., Johnson, F. H., Jr., Thomas, E. E., & Hiller, F. C. (1990). The effects of gamma-hydroxybutyrate on the sleep of narcolepsy patients: A double-blind study. *Sleep* 13:479–490.

In the preceding studies, gamma-hydroxybutyrate (GHB), a breakdown product of GABA metabolism, has been reported to be an effective medication for the treatment of REM-related sleep disorders such as narcolepsy. See: Mamelak, M. (1989). Gammahydroxybutyrate: An endogenous regulator of energy metabolism. *Neurosci. Biobehav. Revs.* 13:187–198.

By promoting normal SWS mechanisms, it is thought that GHB may stop the brain from making sudden early transitions from waking to REM, thus preventing narcoleptic individuals from collapsing in the middle of their waking activities. However, this mode of action may be problematic, since it has recently been demonstrated that GHB can strongly speed up the onset of REM sleep. See: Girodias, V., Godbout, R., Beaulieu, Schmitt, M., Bourguignon, J.-J., & Webster, H. H. (1996). Triggering of paradoxical sleep with gammahydroxybutyrate (GHB) in the rat is blocked by the GHB receptor antagonist NCS-382. *Sleep Res.* 25:9.

One of the most recent sleep-promoting factors found in the brain is a fatty acid. See: Cravatt, B. F., Prospero-Garcia, O., Siuzdak, G., Gilula, N. B., Herniksen, S. J., Boger, D. L., & Lernere, R. A. (1995). Chemical characterization of a family of brain lipids that induce sleep. *Science* 263:1506–1509.

63. See n. 45.

64. See n. 61.

65. Shiromani, P. J., Siegel, J. M., Tomaszewski, K. S., & McGinty, D. J. (1986). Alterations in blood pressure and REM sleep after pontine carbachol microinfusion. *Exp. Neurol.* 91:285–292.

Of course, there are multiple neurochemical controls over REM sleep. For instance, REM can be dramatically increased by promoting GABA activity in specific parts of the brain. See: Sastre, J. P., Buda, C., Kitahama, K., & Jouvet, M. (1996). Importance of the ventrolateral region of the periaqueductual gray and adjacent tegmentum in the control of paradoxical sleep as studied by muscimol microinjections in the cat. *Neuroscience* 74:415–426.

66. McCarley, R. W., & Hobson, J. A. (1971). Single neuron activity in cat gigantocellular tegmental field: Selectivity of discharge in desynchronized sleep. *Science* 174:1250–1252.

Siegel, J. M., & McGinty, D. J. (1977). Pontine reticular formation neurons: Relationship of discharge to motor activity. *Science* 196:678–680.

Also, it should be mentioned that some attempts to selectively destroy the FTG cells have not yielded striking changes in REM sleep. See: Sastre, J.-P., Sakai, K., & Jouvet, M. (1981). Are the gigantocellular tegmental field neurons responsible for paradoxical sleep? *Brain. Res.* 229:147–161.

67. See nn. 7 and 16.

68. Alyson, T., & Van Twiver, H. (1970). The evolution of sleep. *Nat. Hist.* 79:56–65.

69. Alyson, T., & Goof, W. R. (1968). Sleep in a primitive mammal, the spiny anteater. *Psychophysiol.* 5:200–201.

More recently, the apparent lack of REM in the echidna has become more controversial. Some have claimed to have measured the rudiments of a phylogenetically old sleep state in these creatures that may have combined aspects of slow wave and activated sleep. See: Siegel, J. M., Manger, P. R., Nienhuis, R., Fahringer, H. M., & Pettigrew, J. D. (1996). The echidna *Tachglossus aculeatus* combines REM and non-REM aspects in a single sleep state: Implications for the evolution of sleep. *J. Neurosci.* 16:3500–3506.

70. Rechtschaffen, A., Bergmann, B. M., Everson, C. A., Kushida, C. A., & Gillialand, M. A. (1989). Sleep deprivation in the rat: X. Integration and discussion of the findings. *Sleep* 12:68–87.

71. The bacterial blood infection hypothesis was put forward by: Everson, C. A. (1993). Sustained sleep deprivation impairs host defense. *Am. J. Physiol.* 265: R1148–R1158.

However, this conclusion has recently been challenged, since antibiotics do not reverse the sleep deprivation–induced demise. See: Begmann, B. M., Gilliland, M. A., Feng, P.-F., Russell, D. R., Shaw, P., Wright, M., Rechtschaffen, A., & Alverdy, J. C. (1996). Are physiological effects of sleep deprivation in the rat mediated by bacterial invasion? *Sleep* 19:554–562.

72. Horne, J. A. (1985). Sleep function, with particular reference to sleep deprivation. *Ann. Clin. Res.* 17:199–208.

Horne, J. (1988). *Why we sleep: The functions of sleep in humans and other mammals.* Oxford: Oxford Univ. Press.

73. VanderLaan, W. P., Parker, D. C., Rossman, L. G., & VanderLaan, E. F. (1970). Implications of growth hormone release in sleep. *Metabolism* 19:891–897.

74. Sassin, J. F., Parker, D. C., Mace, J. W., Gotlin, R. W., Johnson, L. C., & Rossman, L. G. (1969). Human growth hormone release: Relation to slow-wave sleep and sleep-waking cycles. *Science* 165:513–515.

75. Drucker-Colin, R. R., Spanis, C. W., Hunyadi, J., Sassin, J. F., & McGaugh, J. L. (1975). Growth hormone effects on sleep and wakefulness in the rat. *Neuroendocrinol.* 18:1–8.

Stern, W. C., Jalowiec, J. E., Shabshelowitz, H., & Morgane, P. J. (1975). Effects of growth hormone on sleep-waking patterns in cats. *Horm. Behav.* 6:189–196.

76. Growth hormone levels are much higher in youth. See:

Vigneri, R., & D'Agata, R. (1971). Growth hormone release during the first year of life in relation to sleep-wake periods. *J. Clin. Endocrinol. Metab.* 33: 561–563.

Brown, G. M (1976). Endocrine aspects of psychosocial dwarfism. In *Hormones, behavior and psychopathology* (E. J. Sachar, ed.), pp. 253–261. New York: Raven Press.

For a recent overview of psychosocial dwarfism related to GH deficiency, see: Skuse, D., Albanese, A., Stanhope, R., Gilmour, J., & Voss, L. (1996). A new stress-related syndrome of growth failure and hyperphagia in children, associated with reversibility of growth-hormone insufficiency. *Lancet* 348:353–358.

77. Sachar, E. J., Hellman, L., Roffward, H., Halpern, F., Fukushima, D., & Gallagher, T. F. (1973). Disrupted 24 hour patterns of cortisol secretion in psychotic depression. *Arch. Gen. Psychiat.* 23:289–298.

Weitzman, E. D., Fukushima, D., Nogeire, C., Roffward, H., Gallagher, T. F., & Hellman, L. (1971). Twenty-four hour pattern of the episodic secretion of cortisol in normal subjects. *J. Clin. Endocrinol.* 33:14–22.

78. Carroll, B. J. H., & Mendels, J. (1976). Neuroendocrine regulation in affective disorders. In *Hormones, behavior and psychopathology* (E. J. Sachar, ed.), pp. 193–224. New York: Raven Press.

79. See nn. 33, 36, and 37 and:

Arendt, J., Aldhous, M., English, J., Marks, V., & Arendt, J. H. (1987). Some effects of jet-lag and their alleviation by melatonin. *Ergonomics* 30:1379–1393.

Petrie, K., Dawson, A. G., Thompson, L., & Brook, R. (1993). A double-blind trial of melatonin as a treatment for jet-lag in international cabin crew. *Biol. Psychiat.* 33:526–530.

80. Sapolsky, R. (1992). Neuroendocrinology of the stress response. In *Behavioral endocrinology* (J. Becker, S. Breedlove, & D. Crews, eds.), pp. 287–322. Cambridge, Mass.: MIT Press.

81. McEwen, B., de Kloet, E., & Rostene, W. (1986). Adrenal steroid receptors and actions in the nervous system. *Physiol. Revs.* 66:1121–1163.

82. See n. 78 and: von Werder, K., & Muller, O. A. (1993). The role of corticotropin-releasing factor in the investigation of endocrine diseases. In *Corticotropin-releasing factor* (D. J. Chadwick, J. March, & K. Ackrill, eds.), pp. 317–336. Chichester, U.K.: Wiley.

83. See n. 77 and:

Branchey, L., Weinberg, U., Branchey, M., Linkowski, P., & Mendlewicz, J. (1982). Simultaneous study of 24-hour patterns of melatonin and cortisol secretion in depressed patients. *Neuropsychobiology* 8: 225–232.

Fullerton, D. T., Wenzel, F. J. Lohrenz, F. N., & Fahs, H. (1968). Circadian rhythm of adrenal cortical activity in depression. *Arch. Gen. Psychiat.* 19:674–681.

84. Interestingly, steroid therapy can evoke both mood elevation and depression. See:

Cleghorn, R. A. (1957). Steroid hormones in relation to neuropsychiatric disorders. In *Hormones, brain function and behavior* (H. Hoaland, ed.), pp. 3–25. New York: Academic Press.

Mendels, J. (ed.) (1973). *Biological psychiatry*. New York: Wiley.

85. Post, R. M., Kotin, J., & Goodwin, F. K. (1976). Effects of sleep deprivation on mood and central amine metabolism in depressed patients. *Arch. Gen. Psychiat.* 33:627–632.

The ability of antidepressants to reduce REM may predict their efficacy. See: Hochli, D., Riemann, D., Zulley, J., & Berger, M. (1986). Initial REM sleep suppression by clomipramine: A prognostic tool for treatment response in patients with a major depressive disorder. *Biol. Psychiat.* 21:1217–1220.

Bright light prolongs the antidepressant effect of sleep deprivation. See: Neumeister, A., Goessler, R., Lucht, M., Kapitony, T., Bamas, C., & Kasper, S. (1996). Bright light therapy stabilizes the antidepressant effect of partial sleep deprivation. *Biol. Psychiat.* 39:16–21.

86. Allison, T. (1972). Comparative and evolutionary aspects of sleep. In *The sleeping brain* (M. H., Chase, ed.), pp. 1–57. Los Angeles: UCLA Brain Research Institute.

Campbell, S. S., & Tobler, I. (1984). Animal sleep: A review of sleep duration across phylogeny. *Neurosci. Biobehav. Rev.* 8:269–300.

87. Crick, F., & Mitchinson, G. (1986). REM sleep and neural nets. Special issue: Cognition and dream research (R. E. Haskell, ed.). *J. Mind. Behav.* 7:229–250.

88. Jouvet, M. (1980). Paradoxical sleep and the nature-nurture controversy. In *Adaptive capabilities of the nervous system* (P. S. McConnell, ed.), pp. 331–346. Amsterdam: Elsevier.

89. Mirmiran, M., van de Poll, N. E., Corner, M. A., van Oyen, H. G., & Bour, H. L. (1981). Suppression of active sleep by chronic treatment with chlorimipramine during early postnatal development: Effects upon adult sleep and behavior in the rat. *Brain Res.* 204:129–146.

90. See n. 10 and: McGinty, D. J. (1971). Encephalization and the neural control of sleep. In *Brain development and behavior* (M. B. Sterman, D. J. McGinty, & A. M. Adinolfi, eds.), pp. 356–357. New York: Academic Press.

REM is also increased following various pharmacological challenges that may require brain repair. See: Oswald, I. (1969). Human brain protein, drugs and dreams. *Nature* 223:893–897.

Simply inhibiting protein synthesis pharmacologically can elevate REM, perhaps as a homeostatic attempt to restore compromised brain functions. See: Stern, W. C., Morgane, P. J., Panksepp, J., Zolovick, A. J., & Jalowiec, J. E. (1972). Elevation of REM sleep following inhibition of protein synthesis. *Brain Res.* 47:254–258.

91. Greenberg, R., & Pearlman, C. (1974). Cutting the REM nerve: An approach to the adaptive role of REM sleep. *Persp. Biol. Med.* 17:513–521.

For an update of such theories, see: Smith, C. (1996). Sleep states, memory processes and synaptic plasticity. *Behav. Brain Res.* 78:49–56.

92. See n. 93, and: Joy, R. M., & Prinz, P. N. (1969). The effect of sleep altering environment upon the acquisition and retention of a conditioned avoidance response. *Physiol. Behav.* 4:809–814.

Although simple learning tasks do not elevate REM, simply providing an enriched environment in which animals can exhibit many behaviors voluntarily does have that effect. See: Tagney, J. (1973). Sleep patterns related to rearing rats in enriched and impoverished environments. *Brain Res.* 53:353–361.

93. Pearlman, C., & Greenberg, R. (1973). Post-trial REM sleep: A critical period for consolidation of shuttlebox avoidance. *Anim. Learn. Behav.* 1:49–51.

Stern, W. C. (1971). Acquisition impairments following rapid eye movement sleep deprivation in rats. *Physiol. Behav.* 7:345–352.

A great deal of human data on memories and perceptual abilities are also available, with one of the more recent studies being: Karni, A., Tanne, D., Rubenstein, B. S., Askenasy, J. J. M., & Sagi, D. (1994). Dependence on REM sleep of overnight improvement of a perceptual skill. *Science* 265:679–682.

94. Sastre, P. J.-P., & Jouvet, M. (1979). Le Comportement onirique du chat. *Physiol. Behav.* 22:979–989.

Morrison, A. R. (1983). A window on the sleeping brain. *Sci. Am.* 248:94–102.

Morrison, A. R. (1988). Paradoxical sleep without atonia. *Arch. Ital. Biol.* 421:275–289.

95. Villablanca, J., & Marcus, R. J. (1972). Sleep-wakefulness, EEG and behavioral studies of chronic cats without neocortex and striatum: The "diencephalic" cat. *Arch. Ital. Biol.* 110:348–382.

96. See n. 95 and: Villablanca, J., & Marcus, R. J. (1972). Sleep-wakefulness, EEG and behavioral studies of chronic cats without the thalamus: The "athalamic" cat. *Arch. Ital. Biol.* 110:383–411.

97. Stern, W. C., & Morgane, P. J. (1974). Theoretical view of REM sleep function: Maintenance of catecholamine systems in the central nervous system. *Behav. Biol.* 11:1–32.

98. Siegel, J. M., & Rogawski, M. A. (1988). A function for REM sleep: Regulation of noradrenergic receptor sensitivity. *Brain Res. Revs.* 13:213–233.

At present, many researchers believe that various brain synaptic functions may be restored by sleep. For example, see: Kavanau, J. L. (1996). Memory, sleep, and dynamic stabilization of neural circuitry: Evolutionary perspectives. *Neurosci. Biobehav. Revs.* 20:289–311.

Some consider the function of REM sleep to be related more to processes that transpire during SWS than waking. See: Benington, J. H., & Heller, H. C. (1994). Does the function of REM sleep concern non-REM sleep or waking? *Prog. Neurobiol.* 44:433–448.

99. The serotonin restoration hypothesis has not been as well developed; it was originally suggested by: Panksepp, J. (1981). Hypothalamic integration of behavior: Rewards, punishments, and related psychological processes. In *Handbook of the hypothalamus*. Vol. 3, Part B, *Behavioral Studies of the Hypothalamus* (P. J. Morgane & J. Panksepp, eds.), pp.289–431. New York: Marcel Dekker. Probably the most extensive biochemical data relevant to this hypothesis suggested that REM-deprived animals use serotonin more rapidly than controls, suggesting that REM sleep helps conserve brain serotonin. See: Hery, F., Pujol, J.-F., Lopez, M., Macon, J., & Glowinski, J. (1970). Increased synthesis and utilization of serotonin in the central nervous system of the rat during paradoxical sleep deprivation. *Brain. Res.* 21:391–403.

At this point in time, few investigators believe that REM restores a single biochemical system in the brain. Many brain changes have already been found to be present in REM-deprived animals, and REM appears to restore many neurochemical functions within the brain, including functions related to general metabolism. See: Benington, J. H., & Heller, H. C. (1995). Restoration of brain energy metabolism as the function of sleep. *Prog. Neurobiol.* 45:347–60.

One intriguing function from the perspective that sleep may balance excitatory and inhibitory potentials of the brain is the ability of REM deprivation to increase glutamate, the most important excitatory transmitter of the brain. See: Bettendorff, L., Sallanon-Moulin, M., Touret, M., Wins, P., Margineanu, I., & Schoffeniels, E. (1996). Paradoxical sleep deprivation increases the content of glutamate and glutamine in rat cerebral cortex: *Sleep* 19:65–71.

One of the most recent brain findings following sleep deprivation has been a deficiency of certain proteins contained in postsynaptic membranes of the cortex and hippocampus. See: Neuner-Jehle, M., Denizot, J.-P., Borbely, A. A., & Mallet, J. (1996). Characterization and sleep deprivation–induced expression modulation of dendrin, a novel dendritic protein in rat brain neurons. *J. Neruosci. Res.* 46:138–151.

100. Myers, R. D. (1974). *Handbook of drug and chemical stimulation of the brain.* New York: Van Nostrand Reinhold.

101. Bishop, P. (1978). Serotonin replenishment: A possible function for activated sleep. Master's thesis, Bowling Green State University.

102. Milner, B., Corkin, S., & Teuber, H. L. (1968). Further analysis of the hippocampal amnesia syndrome: 14-year follow-up study of H. M. *Neuropsychologia* 6:215–234.

It is noteworthy that our inability to remember dreams well is reminiscent of the type of hippocampal amnesia exhibited by H. M. See: Badia, P. (1990). Memories in sleep: Old and new. In *Sleep and cognition* (R. R. Bootzin, J. F. Kihlstrom, & D. L. Schacter, eds.), pp. 67–76. Washington, D.C.: American Psychological Association.

103. Stern, W. C., (1981). REM sleep and behavioral plasticity: Evidence for involvement of brain catecholamines. In *Sleep, dreams and memory: Advances in sleep research*, vol. 6 (W. Fishbein, ed.), pp. 95–110. New York: SP Medical.

104. Aston-Jones, G., & Bloom, F. E. (1981). Activity of norepinephrine-containing locus coeruleus neurons in behaving rats anticipates fluctuations in the sleep-waking cycle. *J. Neurosci.* 8:876–886.

105. See n. 54 and: Steinfels, G. F., Heym, J., Strecker, R. E., & Jacobs, B. L. (1983). Behavioral correlates of dopaminergic unit activity in freely moving cats. *Brain Res.* 258:217–228.

Trulson, M. E., & Preussler, D. W. (1984). Dopamine-containing ventral tegmental area neurons in freely moving cats: Activity during the sleep-waking cycle and effects of stress. *Exp. Neurol.* 83:367–377.

106. See nn. 5 and 60, and: Brooks, D. C., & Gershon, M. D. (1971). Eye movement potentials in the oculomotor and visual systems of the cat: A comparsion of reserpine-induced waves with those present during wakefulness and rapid eye movment sleep. *Brain. Res.* 27:223–239.

107. Resnick, O., Krus, D. M., & Radkin, M. (1965). Accentuation of the psychological effects of

LSD-25 in normal subjects treated with reserpine. *Life Sci.* 4:1433–1437.

108. Resnick, O., Krus, D. M., & Raskin, M. (1964). LSD-25 action in normal subjects treated with a monoamine oxidase inhibitor. *Life Sci.* 3:1207–1214.

109. Halperin, J. M., Sharma, V., Siever, L. J., Schwartz, S. T., Matier, K., Worknell, G., & Newcorn, J. H. (1994). Serotonergic function in aggressive and nonaggressive boys with attention deficit hyperactivity disorder. *Am. J. Psychiat.* 151:243–248.

Linnoila, M., Virkkunen, M., Scheinin, M., Nuutilia, A., Rimon, R., & Goodwin, F. K. (1983). Low cerebrospinal fluid 5–HIAA concentration differentiates impulsive from nonimpulsive violent behavior. *Life Sci.* 33:2609–2614.

Roy, A., Adinoff, B., & Linnoila, M. (1988). Acting out hostility in normal volunteers: Negative correlation with levels of 5–HIAA in cerebrospinal fluid. *Psychiat. Res.* 24:187–194.

110. Asberg, M., Traksman, L., & Thoren, P. (1976). 5-HIAA in the cerebrospinal fluid: A biochemical suicide predictor? *Arch. Gen. Psychiat.* 33:1193–1197.

Brown, G. L., Ebert, M. H., Goyer, P. F., Jimerson, D. C., Klein, W. J., Bunney, W. E., & Goodwin, F. K. (1982). Aggression, suicide, and serotonin: Relationship to CSF amine metabolites. *Am. J. Psychiat.* 139: 741–746.

Coccaro, E. F. (1989). Central serotonin and impulsive aggression. *Br. J. Psychiatr.* 155:52–62.

In this context it is noteworthy that dominant individuals have high brain serotonin activity and tend to remain with their troops, while those with low activity tend to have less social competence and emigrate from their natal groups. See: Mehlamn, P. T., Higley, J. D., Faucher, I., Lilly, A. A., Taub, D. M., Vickers, J., Suomi, S. J., & Linnoila, M. (1995). Correlations of CSF 5–HIAA concentrations with sociality and the timing of emigration in free-ranging primates. *Am. J. Psychiat.* 152:907–913.

Chapter 8

1. See chap. 3, n. 25.

Also see: Panksepp, J. (1986). The anatomy of emotions. In *Emotions: Theory, research, and experience.* Vol. 3, *Biological foundations of emotions* (R. Plutchik & H. Kellerman, eds.), pp. 91–121. New York: Academic Press.

2. Jamison, K. R. (1993). *Touched with fire: Manic-depressive illness and the artistic temperament.* New York: Free Press.

3. The rationale for my terminology was first outlined in the work cited in chap. 3, n. 25. Gray continued to use the traditional term *reward system* and later elevated it to a more generalized status as the *Behavioral Activation System* (BAS). See: Gray, J. A. (1990). Brain systems that mediate both emotion and cognition. *Cog. Emot.* 4:269–288.

4. Depue, R. A., & Iacono, W. G. (1989). Neurobehavioral aspects of affective disorders. *Ann. Rev. Psychol.* 40:457–492.

5. Robinson, T. E., & Berridge, K. C. (1993). The neural basis of drug craving: An incentive-sensitization theory of addiction. *Brain Res. Revs.* 18:247–291.

6. The difficulty with the "EXPECTANCY" term was that it could also imply the anticipation of negative incentives, even though at the outset it was explicitly delimited to anticipatory eagerness from interacting with positive incentives.

The Behavioral Activation System terminology (see n. 3) is simply too broad, since there are many other forms of "behavioral activation," such as that accompanying RAGE and FEAR (see Chapters 10 and 11), which could easily promote semantic confusion.

The Behavioral Facilitation System terminology (see n. 4) attempts to provide the distinction that this system does not directly arouse behavior but indirectly promotes behavior, but it still contains the residual ambiguity of the BAS terminology.

The "wanting" terminology (see n. 5) is closer to the intent of the original "expectancy" terminology, but it may also imply a stronger psychological dimension than most behavioral neuroscientists would be willing to tolerate. Perhaps the SEEKING terminology has a sufficiently balanced blend of specific psychological and behavioral connotations, but it would be surprising if others in this contentious field would readily accept such a label.

7. Extensive discussion of anatomical issues will not be detailed here but can be found in a large number of sources, including:

Liebman, J. M., & Cooper, S. J. (eds.) (1989). *The neuropharmacological basis of reward.* Oxford: Clarendon Press.

Olds, J. (1977). *Drives and reinforcements: Behavioral studies of hypothalamic functions.* New York: Raven Press.

Rolls, E. T. (1975). *The brain and reward.* Oxford: Pergamon Press.

Stellar, J. R. (1985). *The neurobiology of motivation and reward.* New York: Springer-Verlag.

Routtenberg, A. (ed.) (1980). *Biology of reinforcement: Facets of brain stimulation reward.* New York: Academic Press.

Wauquier, A., & Rolls, E. T. (eds.) (1976). *Brain-stimulation reward.* Amsterdam: North-Holland.

8. Although we certainly understand that *procedures* of reinforcement, which follow the "law of effect" (i.e., positive rewards increase preceding responses and punishments reduce preceding responses), we are still far from understanding the process of reinforcement. See: Stein, L., Xue, B. G., & Belluzzi, J. D. (1994). In vitro reinforcement of hippocampal bursting: A search for Skinner's atoms of behavior. *J. Exp. Anal. Behav.* 61:155–168.

Some believe no such process exists, and animals develop cognitive knowledge about their world. We are beginning to understand how such cognitive abilities are created. See: McGaugh, J. L., Weinberger, N. M., & Lynch, G. (1995). *Brain and memory: Modulation and mediation of neuroplasticity.* New York: Oxford Univ. Press.

Whether there is also a "reinforcement" process within the brain, as traditionally understood, remains an open question. See:

Huston, J. P., Hasenohrl, R. U., Boix, F., Gerhardt, P., & Schwarting, R. F. (1993). Sequence-specific effects of neurokinin substance P on memory, reinforcement, and brain dopamine activity. *Psychopharmacol.* 112:147–162.

Montague, P. R., Dayan, P., & Sejnowski, T. J. (1996). A framework for mesencephalic dopamine systems based on predictive Hebbian learning. *J. Neurosci.* 16:1936–1947.

Rauschecker, J. P. (1991). Mechanisms of visual plasticity: Hebb synapses, NMDA receptors, and beyond. *Physiol. Rev.* 71:587–615.

9. There are descending glutamate synapses from the cortex to all of the basal ganglia, but so far there is little evidence that such synapses directly modulate self-stimulation "reward," even though it is generally accepted that they mediate cognitive abilities and behavioral arousal. See:

Taber, M. T., & Fibiger, H. C. (1995). Electrical stimulation of the prefrontal cortex increases dopamine release in the nucleus accumbens of the rat: Modulation by metabotropic glutamate receptors. *J. Neurosci.* 15:3896–3904.

Willick, M. L., & Kokkindis, L. (1995). The effects of ventral tegmental administration of $GABA_A$, $GABA_B$ and NMDA receptor agonists on medial forebrain bundle self-stimulation. *Behav. Brain Res.* 70:31–36.

10. At present, this proposal is largely a theoretical deduction from a conceptualization of the main function of SEEKING circuitry, and the assumption is that only reward-induced inhibition of SEEKING arousal will engage reinforcement. This idea, which remains to be formally tested, was first proposed in chap. 3, n. 25.

However, in this context, it should be noted that a reduction of lateral hypothalamic neuronal firing can also be rapidly induced by the onset of negative events. See: Kai, Y., Oomura, Y., & Shimizu, N. (1988). Responses of rat lateral hypothalamic neurons to periaqueductal gray stimulation and nociceptive stimuli. *Brain Res.* 461:107–117.

11. Hamburg, M. D. (1971). Hypothalamic unit activity and eating behavior. *Am. J. Physiol.* 220:980–985.

Aou, S., Takaki, A., Karadi, Z., Hori, T., Nishino, H., & Oomura, Y. (1991). Functional heterogeneity of the monkey lateral hypothalamus in the control of feeding. *Brain Res. Bull.* 27:451–455.

12. Rolls, E. T. (1986). Neural systems involved in emotion in primates. In *Emotion: Theory, research and experience.* Vol. 3, *Biological foundations of emotion* (R. Plutchik & H. Kellerman, eds.), pp.125–143. Orlando, Fla.: Academic Press.

13. Oomura, Y., Nishino, H., Karadi, Z., Aou, S., & Scott, T. R. (1991). Taste and olfactory modulation of feeding-related neurons in behaving monkeys. *Physiol. Behav.* 49:943–950.

14. Goldstein, M. D., & Keesey, R. E. (1969). Relationship of ICS onset and offset to centrally-elicited reinforcement. *Commun. Behav. Biol.* 3:73–80.

Poschel, B. P. H. (1963). Is centrally-elicited positive reinforcement associated with onset or termination of stimulation? *J. Comp. Physiol. Psychol.* 56:604–607.

15. Grastyan, E., Szabo, I., Molnar, P., & Kolta, P. (1968). Rebound, reinforcement, and self-stimulation. *Commun. Behav. Biol.* 2:235–266.

16. Typically, artificial activation of this system facilitates memory formation, but under other conditions, it can also promote amnesia. See:

Routtenberg, A. (1975). Self-stimulation pathways as substrate for memory consolidation. In *Nebraska symposium on motivation* (J. K. Cole & T. B. Sonderegger, eds.), pp. 161–182. Lincoln: Univ. of Nebraska Press.

Routtenberg, A., & Holzman, N. (1973). Electrical stimulation of substantia nigra, pars compacta disrupts memory. *Science* 181:83–85.

Aldavert-Vera, L., Segura-Torres, P., Costa-Miserachs, D., & Morgado-Bernal, I. (1996). Shuttle-box memory facilitation by posttraining intracranial self-stimulation: Differential effects in rats with high and low basic conditioning levels. *Behav. Neurosci.* 110:346–352.

17. It is noteworthy that animals will exhibit escape from the trains of self-stimulation that they initiated on previous occasions. See: Steiner, S. S., Beer, B., & Shaffer, M. M. (1969). Escape for self-produced rates of brain stimulation. *Science* 163:90–91

18. Ikemoto, S., & Panksepp, J. (1994). The relationship between self-stimulation and sniffing in rats: Does a common brain system mediate these behaviors? *Behav. Brain Res.* 61:143–162.

19. See n. 9 and many other studies analyzing converging influences on VTA dopamine neurons:

Bauco, P., Wang, Y., & Wise, R. A. (1993). Lack of sensitization or tolerance to the facilitating effect of ventral tegmental area morphine on lateral hypothalamic brain stimulation reward. *Brain Res.* 617:303–308.

Devine, D. P., & Wise, R. A. (1994). Self-administration of morphine, DAMGO, and DPDPE into the ventral tegmental area of rats. *J. Neurosci.* 14:1978–1984.

Heidbreder, C., Gewiss, M., De Mot, B., Mertens, I., & De Witte, P. (1992). Balance of glutamate and dopamine in the nucleus accumbens modulates self-stimulation behavior after injection of cholecystokinin and neurotensin in the rat brain. *Peptides* 13:441–449.

Yeomans, J. S., Mathur, A., & Tampakeras, M. (1993). Rewarding brain stimulation: Role of tegmental cholinergic neurons that activate dopamine neurons. *Behav. Neurosci.* 107:1077–1087.

20. For reviews of how these systems might participate in the genesis of schizophrenia, see chap. 3, n. 25, and: Ellison, G. (1994). Stimulant-induced psychosis, the dopamine theory of schizophrenia, and the habenula. *Brain Res. Revs.* 19:223–239

21. Heath, R. G. (ed.) (1964). *The role of pleasure in behavior.* New York: Harper and Row.

22. Izard, C. E., & Buechler, S. (1979). Emotion expressions and personality integration in infancy. In *Emotions in personality and psychopathology* (C. E. Izard, ed.), pp 447–472. New York: Plenum Press.

23. Positive Affect and Negative Affect scales are described by: Watson, L. A., Clark, L. A., & Tellegen, A. (1988). Development and validation of brief measures of positive and negative affect: The PANAS scales. *J. Person. Soc. Psych.* 54:1063–1070.

24. Zuckerman, M. (1984). Sensation-seeking: A comparative approach to a human trait. *Behav. Brain Sci.* 7:413–471.

25. Spielberger, C. D. (1975). The measurement of state and trait anxiety: Conceptual and methodological issues. In *Emotions: Their parameters and measurement* (L. Levi, ed.), pp. 713–725. New York, Raven Press.

Spielberger, C. D., Reheiser, E. C., & Sydeman, S. J. (1995). Measuring the experience, expression, and control of anger. *Iss. Comp. Ped. Nursing.* 18:207–232.

26. Heath, R. G. (1963). Electrical self-stimulation of the brain in man. *Am. J. Psychiat.* 120:571–577.

Quaade, F., Vaernet, K., & Larsson, S. (1974). Stereotaxic stimulation and electrocoagulation of the lateral hypothalamus in obese humans. *Acta Neurochir.* 30:111–117.

27. For a discussion of how pharmacological manipulation of these systems may modify affective responses, see commentaries in: Wise, R. A. (1982). Neuroleptics and operant behavior: The anhedonia hypothesis. *Behav. Brain Sci.* 5:39–88.

28. The following section is paraphrased from a previously published essay on the topic. Specific research citations supporting the assertions can be found in the original article: Panksepp, J. (1992). A critical role for "affective neuroscience" in resolving what is basic about basic emotions. *Psych. Rev.* 99:554–560.

29. Sacks, O. (1973). *Awakenings.* New York: Dutton.

30. See chap. 6, n. 28, and: Wise, R. A., & Rompre, P.-P. (1989). Brain dopamine reward. *Ann. Rev. Psychol.* 40:191–225.

31. An indication that psychology, 40-some years after its discovery, still does not quite know what to make of self-stimulation is highlighted by the fact that few introductory psychology texts give more than a passing mention to this phenomenon. Only gradually are psychologically oriented theoreticians beginning to recognize the importance of this brain system in the governance of many psychological processes (see nn. 3–5).

32. O'Keefe, J., & Nadel, L. (1978). The hippocampus as cognitive map. Oxford: Clarendon Press.

33. See chap. 5, nn. 26 and 27, and note that the theta within the hypothalamus is related to sniffing and exploratory locomotion. See: Slawinska, U., & Kasicki, S. (1995). Theta-like rhythm in depth EEG activity of hypothalamic areas during spontaneous or electrically induced locomotion in rats. *Brain Res.* 678:117–126.

Also note that high- and low-frequency thetas have opposite effects on hippocampal information processing. See: Barr, D. S., Lambert, N. A., Hoyt, K. L., Moore, S. D., & Wilson, W. A. (1995). Induction and reversal of long-term potentiation by low- and high-intensity theta pattern stimulation. *J. Neurosci.* 15: 5402–5410.

In this context, it is also important to remember that REM sleep is characterized by hippocampal theta, which is driven by lower, brain stem generators. See: Vertes, R. P., Colom, L. V., & Bland, B. H. (1993). Brainstem sites for the carbachol elicitation of the hippocampal theta rhythm in the rat. *Exp. Brain Res.* 96:419–429.

34. Vanderwolf C. H. (1992). Hippocampal activity, olfaction, and sniffing: An olfactory input to the dentate gyrus. *Brain Res.* 593:197–208.

35. See n. 7 and: Westerink, B. H. C., Kwint, H.-F., & deVries, J. B. (1996). The pharmacology of mesolimbic dopamine neurons: A dual-probe microdialysis study in the ventral tegmental area and the nucleus accumbens of the rat brain. *J. Neurosci.* 16:2605–2626.

36. Stellar, J. R., & Heard, K. (1976). Aftereffects of rewarding lateral hypothalamic brain stimulation and feeding behavior. *Physiol. Behav.* 17:865–867.

37. Deutsch, J. A. (1963). Learning and electrical self-stimulation of the brain. *J. Theor. Biol.* 4:193–214.

Gallistel, C. R., Shizgal, P., & Yeomans, J. S. (1981). A portrait of the substrate for self-stimulation. *Psych. Rev.* 88:228–273.

38. Trowill, J. A., Panksepp, J., & Gandelman, R. (1969). An incentive model of rewarding brain stimulation. *Psych. Rev.* 76:264–281.

39. Panksepp, J., & Trowill, J. A. (1967). Intraoral self-injection: II. The simulation of self-stimulation phenomenon with a conventional reward. *Psychon. Sci.* 9:407–408.

40. Damsma, G., Pfaus, J. G., Wenkstern, D., Phillips, A. G., & Fibiger, H. C. (1992). Sexual behavior increases dopamine transmission in the nucleus accumbens and striatum of male rats: Comparison with novelty and locomotion. *Behav. Neurosci.* 106:181–191.

Schultz, W., & Romo, R. (1990). Dopamine neurons of the monkey midbrain: Contingencies of responses to stimuli eliciting immediate behavioral reactions. *J. Neurophysiol.* 63:607–617.

Schultz, W. (1992). Activity of dopamine neurons in the behaving primate. *Semin. Neurosci.* 4:129–138.

However, it should be noted that hunger does increase the release of food intake–induced dopamine release, suggesting that dopamine release may also be related to palatability factors. See: Wilson, C., Nomikos, G. G., Collu, M., & Fibiger, H. C. (1995). Dopaminergic correlates of motivated behavior: Importance of drive. *J. Neurosci.* 15:5169–5178.

41. For summaries of anatomy, see n. 7. At present, investigators are focusing more on specific functional issues, usually on specific neurochemical questions, and many surprises are still being revealed. For example, see: Wagner, U., Segura-Torres, P., Weiler, T., & Huston, J. P. (1993). The tuberomammillary nucleus region as a reinforcement inhibiting substrate: Facilitation of ipsihypothalamic self-stimulation by unilateral ibotenic acid lesions. *Brain Res.* 613:269–278.

42. See n. 27, and: Hoebel, B. G. (1988). Neuroscience and motivation: Pathways and peptides that define motivational systems. In *Steven's handbook of experimental psychology.* Vol. 1, *Perception and motivation* (R. C. Atkinson, R. J. Herrenstein, G.

Lindzay, & R. D. Lance, eds.), pp. 547–597. New York: Wiley.

43. See commentaries in response to n. 27. Perhaps the biggest problem was that no investigator ever reported pleasure responses to stimulation of the human lateral hypothalamus, even though such effects were obtained from the septal area (see n. 21), which suggested that distinct functions were mediated by these brain areas (as affirmed by animal studies such as those in n. 44).

44. Stutz, R. M., Rossi, R. R., Hastings, L., & Brunner, R. L. (1974). Discriminability of intracranial stimuli: The role of anatomical connectedness. *Physiol. Behav.* 12:69–73.

45. Valenstein, E. S., Cox, V. C., & Kakolewski, V. C. (1970). Reexamination of the role of the hypothalamus in motivated behavior. *Psych. Rev.* 77:16–31.

Largely as a consequence of this paper, the amount of research activity on the psychobehavioral functions of self-stimulation circuitry diminished markedly. Only recently, a quarter century later, is there renewed interest in the underlying conceptual issues.

46. Berridge, K. C., & Valenstein, E. S. (1991). What psychological process mediates feeding evoked by electrical stimulation of the lateral hypothalamus? *Behav. Neurosci.* 105:3–14.

47. Smith, D. A. (1971). Lateral hypothalamic stimulation: Experience and deprivation as factors in rat's licking of empty drinking tubes. *Psychon. Sci.* 23:329–331.

48. Wise, R. A. (1971). Individual differences in effects of hypothalamic stimulation: The role of stimulation locus. *Physiol. Behav.* 6:569–572.

49. Valenstein, E. S. (1969). Behavior elicited by hypothalamic stimulation. *Brain Behav. Evol.* 2:295–316.

50. See chap. 10, n. 31.

51. The consequences of this failure are documented by the gradual demise of brain research in departments of psychology in the United States. See: Davis, H. P., Rosenzweig, M. R., Becker, L. A., & Sather, K. J. (1988). Biological psychology's relationship to psychology and neuroscience. *Am. Psychol.* 43:359–371.

This same trend is apparent in the steep decline in the number of students getting Ph.Ds in experimental psychology as opposed to other subareas during the past three decades. See Table 2 in Pion, G. M. et al. (1996). The shifting gender composition of psychology. *Amer. Psychol.* 31:509–528.

At the time these changes were beginning, I asserted that the utilization of some common psychological language (emotional terms) to discuss certain basic brain mechanisms might take us closer to the reality of brain organization than a sterile behavioral language. I still believe such conceptual bridges can help make functional neuroscience a foundation discipline for the rest of psychology, but that remains a minority opinion within the discipline.

52. Mendelson, J. (1972). Ecological modulation of brain stimulation effects. *Int. J. Psychobiol.* 1:285–304.

53. Rossi, J., III, & Panksepp, J. (1992). Analysis of the relationships between self-stimulation sniffing and brain-stimulation sniffing. *Physiol. Behav.* 51:805–813.

54. Rossi, J., III. (1983). An analysis of the relationship between electrically elicited sniffing behavior and self-stimulation in the rat. Ph.D. diss., Bowling Green State University.

55. It was a great surprise that dopamine blocking agents did not clearly reduce brain stimulation–induced sniffing at doses that totally eliminate exploratory sniffing (see n. 54). This indicates that brain stimulation can dissect subcomponents of the system that would not otherwise be evident. At present, we suspect that this dopamine-independent component of sniffing is directly controlled by descending glutamate transmission in the brain.

56. French, E. D., Mura, A., & Wang, T. (1993). MK-801, phencyclidine (PCP), and PCP-like drugs increase burst firing in rat A10 dopamine neurons: Comparison to competitive NMDA antagonists. *Synapse* 13:08–116.

57. Blackburn, J. R., Pfaus, J. G., & Phillips, A. G. (1992). Dopamine functions in appetitive and defensive behaviours. *Prog. Neurobiol.* 39:247–279.

58. Fibiger, H. C., & Phillips, A. G. (1986). Reward, motivation, cognition: Psychobiology of mesotelencephalic dopamine systems. In *Handbook of physiology*. Vol. 4, *The nervous system: Intrinsic regulatory systems of the brain*, pp. 647–675. Bethesda, Md.: American Physiological Society.

Mark, G. P., Smith, S. E., Rada, P. V., & Hoebel, B. G. (1994). An appetitively conditioned taste elicits a preferential increase in mesolimbic dopamine release. *Pharmacol. Biochem. Behav.* 48:651–660.

Phillips, A. G., Atkinson, L. J., Blackburn, J. R., & Blaha, C. D. (1993). Increased extracellular dopamine in the nucleus accumbens of the rat elicited by a conditional stimulus for food: An electrochemical study. *Can. J. Physiol. Pharmacol.* 71:387–393.

59. There is increasing evidence that aversive events can also increase mesolimbic DA release. See:

Salamone, J. D. (1994). The involvement of nucleus accumbens dopamine in appetitive and aversive motivation. *Behav. Brain Res.* 61:117–133.

Blackburn, J. R., Pfaus, J. G., & Phillips, A. G. (1992). Dopamine functions in appetitive and defensive behaviours. *Prog. Neurobiol.* 39:247–279.

However, it is still essential to fully evaluate whether release of dopamine by stressful events is linked more to the termination of aversive events (i.e., during the "relief" response) or to the onset of the bad events. When brain opioid release as a function of stress has been evaluated in this way, the evidence suggests that the release corresponds more to the offset of the stressful events than to their onset. See: Seeger, T. F., Sforzo, G. A., Pert, C. B., & Pert, A. (1984). In vivo autoradiography: Visualization of stress-induced changes in opiate receptor occupancy in the rat brain. *Brain Res.* 305:303–311.

60. This is not to deny that motivation-specific circuits exist in other parts of the brain, and that the SEEK-

ING system interacts with those systems. Some of the evident behavioral specificity that one occasionally sees in animals stimulated within the lateral hypothalamus (e.g., intense licking, gnawing, and copulatory urges) may also reflect the proximity of electrodes to neural interfaces between specific homeostatic detector systems, consummatory response systems, and the generalized SEEKING system (Figure 8.1). In other words, even though neural systems for motivational specificity do exist in the brain, they are not especially concentrated in the trajectory of the medial forebrain bundle, where the neural fibers that arouse animals to seek all possible worldly rewards reside. For a recent empirical consideration of this issue, see: Anderson, R., & Miliaressis, E. (1994). Does the MFB convey functionally different reward signals? *Behav. Brain Res.* 60:55–61.

For older views, see: Phillips, A. G. (1984). Brain reward circuitry: A case for separate systems. *Brain Res. Bull.* 12:195–201.

61. Bunney, B. S. (1979). The electrophysiological pharmacology of midbrain dopaminergic systems. In *The neurobiology of dopamine* (A. S. Horn, J. Korf, & B. H. Westerink, eds.), pp. 417–430. New York: Academic Press.

62. Chergui, K., Suaud-Chagny, M. F., & Gonon, F. (1994). Nonlinear relationship between impulse flow, dopamine release and dopamine elimination in the rat brain in vivo. *Neuroscience* 62:641–645.

63. Schultz, W., Apicella, P., & Ljungberg, T. (1993). Responses of monkey dopamine neurons to reward and conditioned stimuli during successive steps of learning a delayed response task. *J. Neurosci.* 13:900–913.

64. Nakano, Y., Lenard, L., Oomura, Y. , Nishino, H., Aou, S., & Yamamoto, T. (1987). Functional involvement of catecholamines in reward-related neuronal activity of the monkey amygdala. *J. Neurophysiol.* 57:72–91.

65. Rolls, E. T. (1990). A theory of emotion, and its application to understanding the neural basis of emotion. Special issue: Development of relationships between emotion, and cognition. *Cog. Emot.* 4:161–190.

66. Pfaus, J. G., & Phillips, A. G. (1991). Role of dopamine in anticipatory and consummatory aspects of sexual behavior in the male rat. *Behav. Neurosci.* 105: 727–743.

Fiorino, D. F., Coury, A., Fibiger, H. C., & Phillips, A. G. (1993). Electrical stimulation of reward sites in the ventral tegmental area increases dopamine transmission in the nucleus accumbens of the rat. *Behav. Brain Res.* 55:131–141.

67. Miliaressis, E. (1977). Serotonergic basis of reward in medial raphe of the rat. *Pharmacol. Biochem. Behav.* 7:177–180.

Self-stimulation from such sites is slow and methodical, as it is from many other brain areas such as the medial septum, as opposed to the highly excited self-stimulation one obtains from the trajectory of DA systems, suggesting that different underlying psychobiological functions are mediated by different systems that can sustain self-stimulation.

68. There is evidence that glutamate can both increase and decrease sniffing. See:

Kelland, M. D., Soltis, R. P., Boldry, R. C., & Walters, J. R. (1993). Behavioral and electrophysiological comparison of ketamine with dizocilpine in the rat. *Physiol. Behav.* 54:547–554.

Prinssen, E. P., Balestra, W., Bemelmans, F. F., & Cools, A. R. (1994). Evidence for a role of the shell of the nucleus accumbens in oral behavior of freely moving rats. *J. Neurosci.* 14:1555–1562.

It is noteworthy that certain glutamate antagonists appear to be rewarding within the trajectory of the main self-stimulation system. See: Carlezon, W. A., Jr., & Wise, R. A. (1996). Rewarding actions of phencyclidine and related drugs in nucleus accumbens. *J. Neurosci.* 16:3112–3122.

69. Kofman, O., & Yeomans, J. S. (1988). Cholinergic antagonists in ventral tegmentum elevate thresholds for lateral hypothalamic and brainstem self-stimulation. *Pharmacol. Biochem. Behav.* 31:547–559.

Nicotinic acetylcholine receptors are also important for self-stimulation. See: Bauco, P., & Wise, R. A. (1994). Potentiation of lateral hypothalamic and midline mesencephalic brain stimulation reinforcement by nicotine: Examination of repeated treatment. *J. Pharmacol. Exp. Therap.* 271:294–301.

70. For some neuropeptides in VTA see, n. 19; for others, see:

Glimcher, P. W., Giovino A. A., & Hoebel, B. G. (1987). Neurotensin self-injection in the ventral tegmental area. *Brain Res.* 403:147–150.

Huston, J. P., Hasenohrl, R. U., Boix, F., Gerhardt, P., & Schwarting, R. K. (1993). Sequence-specific effects of neurokinin substance P on memory, reinforcement, and brain dopamine activity. *Psychopharmacol.* 112:147–162.

Kalivas, P. W. (1993). Neurotransmitter regulation of dopamine neurons in the ventral tegmental. *Brain Res. Revs.* 18:75–113.

71. See n. 61, and:

Ikemoto, S., Glazier, B. S., Murphy, J. M., & McBride, W. J. (1995). Muscarinic receptors in the nucleus accumbens mediate a reinforcing effect. *Soc. Neurosci. Abst.* 21:1673.

Ikemoto, S., Murphy, J. M., & McBride, W. J. (1997). Self-infusion of $GABA_A$ antagonists directly into the ventral tegmental area and adjacent regions. *Behav. Neurosci.* 111:369–380.

72. Ikemoto, S., & Panksepp, J. (1996). Dissociations between appetitive and consummatory responses by pharmacological manipulations of reward-relevant brain regions. *Behav. Neurosci.* 110:331–345.

73. See n. 54 .

74. Olney, J. W., & Farber, N. B. (1995). NMDA antagonists as neurotherapeutic drugs, psychotogens, neurotoxins, and research tools for studying schizophrenia. *Neuropsychopharmacol.* 13:335–345.

75. For a synthesis of these studies, see n. 1 and: Olds, J., Disterhoft, J., Segal, M., Kornblith, C., & Hirsh, R. (1972). Learning centers of rat brain mapped by measuring latencies of conditioned unit responses. *J. Neurophysiol.* 35:202–219.

76. See nn. 40, 57, 58, 63, 64, and 66.

77. Bernardis, L. L., & Bellinger, L. L. (1993). The lateral hypothalamic area revisited: Neuroanatomy, body weight regulation, neuroendocrinology and metabolism. *Neurosci. Biobehav. Revs.* 17:141–193.

Campbell, B. A., & Baez, L. A. (1974). Dissociation of arousal and regulatory behaviors following lesions of the lateral hypothalamus. *J. Comp. Physiol. Psychol.* 87:142–149.

78. However, even in the middle of the behaviorist era, there were exceptions. The most famous renegade was Tolman, who believed that animals had internal representations of their world. See: Tolman, E. C. (1932). *Purposive behavior in animals and men.* New York: Appleton-Century.

Such views are now heralded by many, but in the updated jargon of cognitivism. See: Real, L. A. (1991). Animal choice behavior and the evolution of cognitive architecture. *Science* 253:980–986.

79. See n. 1 and: Clarke, S., Panksepp, J., & Trowill, J. A. (1970). A method of recording sniffing in the free-moving rat. *Physiol. Behav.* 5:125–126.

80. Delusional thinking is a core symptom of schizophrenia. Although delusional thinking may be adaptive, since it allows animals to anticipate rewards (see nn. 76 and 84–89), it remains to be fully considered whether a similar internally guided learning process does in fact help create the core delusions that characterize schizophrenic thinking.

81. Clark , S., & Trowill, J. A. (1971). Sniffing and motivated behavior in the rat. *Physiol. Behav.* 6:49–52.

82. At present, abundant evidence links both schizophrenic delusions and the urge to self-stimulate to excessive activity of dopamine synapses, especially the synapses of dopamine axons that project to the ventral striatum and frontal cortex—that is, the mesolimbic and mesocortical pathways, respectively. See: Le Moal, M., & Simon, H. (1991). Mesocorticolimbic dopaminergic network: Functional and regulatory roles. *Physiol. Revs.* 71:155–234.

83. For discussions of "confirmation bias," see: Tweney, R. D., Doherty, M. E., & Mynatt, C. R. (eds.) (1981). *On scientific thinking.* New York: Columbia Univ. Press.

84. Brown, P. L., & Jenkins, H. M. (1968). Autoshaping of the pigeon's key-peck. *J. Exp. Anal. Behav.* 11:1–8.

Williams, D. R., & Williams, H. (1969). Auto-maintenance in the pigeon: Sustained pecking despite contingent non-reinforcement. *J. Exp. Anal. Behav.* 12:511–520.

85. Phillips, A. G., McDonald, A. C., & Wilkie, D. M. (1981). Disruption of autoshaped responding to a signal of brain-stimulation reward by neuroleptic drugs. *Pharmacol. Biochem. Behav.* 14:543–548.

86. Falk, J. L. (1971). The nature and determinants of adjunctive behavior. *Physiol. Behav.* 6:577–588.

Falk, J. L., & Samson, H. H. (1975). Schedule-induced physical dependence on ethanol. *Pharmacol. Revs.* 27:449–464.

87. Skinner, B. F. (1948). "Superstition" in the pigeon. *J. Exp. Psychol.* 38:168–172.

88. Mittleman, G., & Valenstein, E. S. (1984). Ingestive behavior evoked by hypothalamic stimulation and schedule-induced polydipsia are related. *Science* 224:415–417.

Mittleman, G., Castaneda, E., Robinson, T. E., & Valenstein, E. S. (1986). The propensity for nonregulatory ingestive behavior is related to differences in dopamine systems: Behavioral and biochemical evidence. *Behav. Neurosci.* 100:213–220.

Piazza, P. V., Mittleman, G., Deminiere, J. M., Le Moal, M., & Simon, H. (1993). Relationship between schedule-induced polydipsia and amphetamine intravenous self-administration: Individual differences and role of experience. *Behav. Brain Res.* 55:185–193.

89. Wayner, M. J., Barone, F. C., & Loulis, C. C. (1991). The lateral hypothalamus and adjunctive behavior. In *Handbook of the hypothalamus.* Vol. 3, Part B, *Behavioral studies of the hypothalamus* (P. J. Morgane & J. Panksepp, eds.), pp.107–146. New York: Marcel Dekker.

90. Rapoport, J. L. (1989). *The boy who couldn't stop washing: The experience and treatment of obsessive-compulsive disorder.* New York: Dutton.

Woods, A., Smith, C., Szewczak, M., Dunn, R., Cornfeldt, M., & Corbett, R. (1993). Selective serotonin re-uptake inhibition decreases schedule-induced polydipsia in rats: A potential model for obsessive-compulsive disorder. *Psychopharmacol.* 112:195–198.

91. Antelman, S. M. (1991). Possible animal models of some of the schizophrenias and their response to drug treatment. In *Neuropsychology, psychophysiology, and information processing: Handbook of schizophrenia*, vol. 5 (S. R. Steinhauer, J. H. Gruzelier, & J. Zubin, eds.), pp. 161–183. Amsterdam: Elsevier Science.

92. One attractive idea is that mesolimbic dopamine bursting diminishes when a reward is found (see n. 11). This may be accompanied by a burst of glutamate transmission, which solidifies potential feedback connections from cortical analyzers back to the VTA system. Indeed, haloperidol mediates brain glutamate transmission at the level of the VTA and vice versa. See:

Fitzgerald, L. W., Ortiz, J., Hamedani, A. G., & Nestler, E. J. (1996). Drugs of abuse and stress increase the expression of GluR1 and NMDAR1 glutamate receptor subunits in the rat ventral tegmental area: Common adaptations among cross-sensitizing agents. *J. Neurosci.* 16:274–282.

Tung, C. S., Grenhoff, J., & Svensson, T. H. (1991). Kynurenate blocks the acute effects of haloperidol on midbrain dopamine neurons recorded in vivo. *J. Neural Transmis.* 84:53–64.

93. Andreassen, N. C., Swayze, V. W., Flaum, M., Yates, W. R., Arndt, S., & McChesney, C. (1990). Ventricular enlargement in schizophrenia evaluated with CT scanning. *Arch. Gen. Psychiat.* 47:1008–1015.

Crow, T. J. (1990). Abnormalities in the brain and schizophrenia. *N. Eng. J. Med.* 323:545–546.

Suddath, R. L., Christison, G. W., Torrey, E. F., Casanova, M. F., & Weinberger, D. R. (1990). Anatomical abnormalities in the brains of monozygotic twins discordant for schizophrenia. *N. Eng. J. Med.* 322:789–794.

94. Wong, D. F., et al. (1986). Positron emission tomography reveals elevated D_2 dopamine receptors in drug-naive schizophrenics. *Science* 234:1558–1563.

95. Reynolds, G. P. (1983). Increased concentrations and lateral asymmetry of amygdala dopamine in schizophrenia. *Nature* 305:527–529.

96. Borowsk, T. B., & Kokkinidis, L. (1992). Long-term influence of d-amphetamine on mesolimbic brain-stimulation reward: Comparison to chronic haloperidol and naloxone effects. *Pharmacol. Biochem. Behav.* 43:1–15.

97. See n. 21 and: Le Duc, P. A., & Mittleman, G. (1995). Schizophrenia and psychostimulant abuse: A review and re-analysis of clinical evidence. *Psychopharmacol.* 121:407–427.

98. Of course, stress has widespread neurochemical effects on the brain. See: Goldstein, L. E., Rasmusson, A. M., Bunney, B. S., & Roth, R. H. (1996). Role of the amygdala in the coordination of behavioral, neuroendocrine, and prefrontal cortical monoamine response to psychological stress in rats. *J. Neurosci.* 16:4787–4798.

99. See n. 5, and:

Kalivas, P., & Barnes, C. (eds.) (1988). *Sensitization in the nervous system.* Caldwell, N.J.: Telford Press.

Kalivas, P., & Stewart, J. (1991). Dopamine transmission in the initiation and expression of drug- and stress-induced sensitization of motor activity. *Brain Res. Revs.* 16:223–244.

100. Lang, A., Harro, J., Soosaar, A., Koks, S., Volke, V., Oreland, L., Bourin, M., Vasar, E., Bradwejn, J., & Mannisto, P. T. (1995). Role of N-methyl-D-aspartic acid and cholecystokinin receptors in apormorphine-induced aggressive behaviour in rats. *Naunyn-Schmiedebergs Arch. Pharmacol.* 351:363–370.

101. Steiner, S. S., & Ellman, S. J. (1972). Relation between REM sleep and intracranial self-stimulation. *Science* 177:1122–1124.

102. Zarcone, V., Azumi, K., Dement, W., Gulevich, G., Kraemer, H., & Pivik, T. (1975). REM phase deprivation and schizophrenia II. *Arch. Gen. Psychiat.* 32:1431–1436.

For a critical review of issues, see: Keshavan, M. S., Reynolds, C. F., & Kupfer, D. J. (1990). Electroencephalographic sleep in schizophrenia: A critical review. *Comp. Psychiatry.* 31:34–47.

103. Hunt, H. (1992). Dreams of Freud and Jung: Reciprocal relationships between social relations and archetypal/transpersonal imagination. *Psychiatry* 55: 28–47.

Weitz, L. J. (1976). Jung's and Freud's contributions to dream interpretation: A comparison. *Am. J. Psychother.* 30:289–293.

However, recent brain-mapping data do not support a strong relationship between schizophrenic arousal and that found in REM sleep. See: Weiler, M. A., Buchsbaum, M. S., Gillin, J. C., Tafalla, R., & Bunney, W. E., Jr. (1990–1991). Explorations in the relationship of dream sleep to schizophrenia using positron emission tomography. *Neuropsychobiology* 23:109–118.

104. Warnes, H. (1976–1977). An integrative model for the treatment of psychosomatic disorders: The place of sleep and dreams revisited. *Psychother. Psychosom.* 27:65–75.

Yeomans, J. S. (1995). Role of tegmental cholinergic neurons in dopaminergic activation, antimuscarinic psychosis and schizophrenia. *Neuropsychopharmacol.* 12:3–16.

Chapter 9

1. This quotation is from a letter in which Mr. Holwell, the officer in command for the Fort William garrison, describes the horrors of the imprisonment as it was printed in the British *Annual Register* for 1758. This excerpt is taken from Lewes, G. H. (1860). *The physiology of common life.* Leipzig: Bernhard Tauchnitz. Quotation on pp. 27–29.

2. Klein, D. F. (1993). False suffocation alarms, spontaneous panics, and related conditions: An integrative hypothesis. *Arch. Gen. Psychiat.* 50:306–317.

3. Vanter Wall, S. B. (1990). *Food hoarding in animals.* Chicago: Univ. of Chicago Press.

Early privation increases the sensitivity of the lateral hypothalamic seeking substrate that promotes hoarding behavior. See: Avery, D. D., Moss, D. E., & Hendricks, S. A. (1976). Food deprivation at weaning and adult behavior elicited by hypothalamic stimulation in the rat. *Behav. Biol.* 16:155–160.

4. Evidence for weight loss following social isolation can be found in:

Reite, M., & Capitanio, J. P. (1985). On the nature of social separation and social attachment. In *The psychobiology of attachment and separation* (M. Reite & T. Fields, eds.), pp. 223–255. Orlando, Fla.: Academic Press.

Hofer, M. A. (1973). The role of nutrition in the physiological and behavioral effects of early maternal separation on infant rats. *Psychosom. Med.* 35:350–359.

The social facilitation effects are reviewed in: Galef, B. G. (1988). Imitation in animals: History, definition and interpretation of data from the psychological laboratory. In *Social learning* (T. R. Zentall & B. G. Galef, eds.), pp. 3–28. Hillsdale, N.J.: Lawrence Erlbaum.

Also see: Zajonc, R. B. (1965). Social facilitation. *Science* 149:269–274.

Although a study of the brain substrates of social facilitation are poorly studied, there are some indications that it can be neurochemically modulated. For example, see: Henning, J. M., & Zentall, T. R. (1981). Imitation, social facilitation, and the effects of ACTH 4-10 on rats' bar-pressing behavior. *Am. J. Psychol.* 94:125–134.

5. For an overview, see: Panksepp, J. (1981). Hypothalamic integration of behavior. In *Handbook of the hypothalamus.* Vol. 3, part B, *Behavioral studies of the hypothalamus* (P. J. Morgane & J. Panksepp, eds.), pp. 289–431. New York: Marcel Dekker.

6. For anatomical details see: Morgane, P. J., & Panksepp, J. (eds.) (1979). *Handbook of the hypothalamus*. Vol. 1. *Anatomy of the hypothalamus*. New York: Marcel Dekker.

For Golgi stains, see: Millhouse, O. E. (1979). A Golgi anatomy of the rodent hypothalamus. In *Handbook of the hypothalamus*. Vol. 1, *Anatomy of the hypothalamus*. (P. J. Morgane & J. Panksepp, eds.), pp. 221–266. New York: Marcel Dekker.

7. See Oomura, Y. (1989). Sensitivity of endogenous chemical in control of feeding. In *Progress in sensory physiology*, vol. 9, pp. 171–191. Berlin: Springer-Verlag.

8. Blessing, W. W. (1997). *The lower brainstem and bodily homeostasis*. New York: Oxford Univ. Press.

Sawchenko, P. E., & Friedman, M. I. (1979). Sensory functions of the liver: A review. *Am. J. Physiol.* 236:R5–R20.

9. See Chapter 12 and: de Kloet, E. R., & Sutanto, W. (1994). *Neurobiology of steroids*. San Diego: Academic Press.

10. For a discussion of how such species-typical behavioral reflections of homologous brain systems (i.e., predatory aggression and the output of the SEEKING system) have led to confusion in the literature, see Chapters 8 and 10.

11. Indeed, the key anecdote here is that B. F. Skinner first built the Skinner box to save himself the tedium of having to observe the actual behavior of his animals. In any event, straightforward observation of animal behavior indicates that the agitation of a self-stimulating animal does not resemble the calm that overcomes a hungry animal that is allowed to indulge in the pleasure of eating. Of course, it could be pointed out that hungry animals that are given only very tiny treats do remain agitated. However, the interpretation of this arousal is that animals are sustained in the appetitive-SEEKING phase of behavior, since they are not given the opportunity to settle down into the consummatory phase for sustained periods. Indeed, as we will see, "rewarding" brain stimulation does not promote facial pleasure responses in rats (also see chap. 8, n. 46), which suggests that the desirability of this form of brain stimulation is not clearly related to a pleasure response.

12. Bolles, Robert C. (1975). *Theory of motivation*. New York: Harper and Row.

13. In unpublished work I have found overnight hunger to increase the human knee-jerk reflex, and it is well known that under hunger conditions animals have difficulty sleeping, while abundant food promotes sleep. See:

Borbely, A. A. (1977). Sleep in the rat during food deprivation and subsequent restitution of food. *Brain Res.* 124:457–471.

Danquir, J. (1987). Cafeteria diet promotes sleep in rats. *Appetite* 8:49–53.

Danquir, J., Gerard, H., & Nicolaidis, S. (1979). Relations between sleep and feeding patterns in the rat. *J. Comp. Physiol. Psychol.* 93:820–830.

At the same time, it should be noted that some manipulations that promote feeding, such as reducing glucose availability, can also markedly increase cortical slow-wave activity. See: Panksepp, J., Jalowiec, J. E., Zolovick, A. J., Stern, W. C., & Morgane, P. J. (1973). Inhibition of glycolytic metabolism and sleep-waking states in cats. *Pharmacol. Biochem. Behav.* 1:117–119.

14. For an analysis of the ecological variable that can modify feeding patterns, see: Galef, Jr., B. G. (1996). Food selection: Problems in understanding how we choose foods to eat. *Neurosci. Biobehav. Revs.* 20:67–74.

15. De Castro, J. M. (1996). How can eating behavior be regulated in the complex environments of free-living humans? *Neurosci. Biobehav. Revs.* 20:119–128.

16. Carpinelli, A. R., Machado, U. F., & Curi, R. (1996). Modulation of insulin secretion by feeding behavior and physical activity: Possible beneficial effects on obese and aged rats. *Neurosci. Biobehav. Revs.* 20:183–188.

17. Panksepp, J. (1975). Metabolic hormones and regulation of feeding: A reply to Woods, Decke, and Vasselli. *Psych. Rev.* 82:158–164.

Panksepp, J., Pollack, A., Krost, K., Meeker, R., & Ritter, M. (1975). Feeding in response to repeated protamine zinc insulin injections. *Physiol. Behav.* 14:487–493.

Panksepp, J., & Meeker, R. (1976). Suppression of food intake in diabetic rats by voluntary consumption and intrahypothalamic injection of glucose. *Physiol. Behav.* 16:763–770.

18. Schwartz, G. J., & Moran, T. H. (1996). Subdiaphragmatic vagal afferent integration of meal-related gastrointestinal signals. *Neurosci. Biobehav. Revs.* 20: 57–66.

19. Revusky, S. H., & Bedarf, E. W. (1967). Association of illness with prior ingestion of novel foods. *Science* 155:219–220.

Deutsch, G. A., & Hardy, W. T. (1977). Cholecystokinin produces bait shyness in rats. *Nature* 266:196.

20. See n. 19 and: Moore, B. O., & Deutsch, J. A. (1985). An antiemetic is antidotal to the satiety effects of cholecystokinin. *Nature* 315:321–322.

21. Harro, J., Vasar, E., Koszycki, D., & Bradwejn, J. (1995). Cholecystokinin in panic and anxiety disorders. In *Advances in biological psychiatry*, vol. 1 (J. Panksepp, ed.), pp. 235–262. Greenwich, Conn.: JAI Press.

22. Panksepp, J., Pollack, A., Meeker, R. B., & Sullivan, A. C. (1977). (-)-hydroxycitrate and conditioned aversions. *Pharmacol. Biochem. Behav.* 6:683–687.

23. Smith, G. P. (1996). The direct and indirect controls of meal size. *Neurosci. Biobehav. Revs.* 20:41–46.

24. I developed this test 30 years ago, but the work was never published. I share the results here for the first time. This test could be used as a measure of normal satiety, as can other tests, such as the one described in n. 25.

25. Siviy, S., & Panksepp, J. (1985). Energy balance and play in juvenile rats. *Physiol. Behav.* 35:435–441.

26. Turton, M. D., O'Shea, D., Gunn, I., Beak, S. A., Edwards, C. M. B., Meeran, K., Chol, S. J., Taylor, G. M., Heath, M. M., Lambert, P. D., Wilding, J. P. H., Smith, D. M., Ghatel, M. A., Herbert, J., & Bloom, S. R. (1996). A role for glucagon-like peptide-1 in the central regulation of feeding. *Nature* 379:69–72.

27. Panksepp, J., Bekkedal, M. Y. V., & Walter, M. (1996). Potent suppressive effects of the putative satiety agent GLP-1 on social-emotional behaviors. *Abst. Soc. Neurosci.* 22:16.

28. Panksepp, J. (1974). Hypothalamic regulation of energy balance and feeding behavior. *Fed. Proc.* 33:1150–1165.

For an update of a similar conception of energy regulation, see: Kaiyala, K. J., Woods, S. C., & Schwartz, W. W. (1995). New model for the regulation of energy balance and adiposity by the central nervous system. *Am. J. Clin. Nutr.* 62(suppl. 5):1123S-1134S.

29. For a study of the consequences of starvation in humans, see: Keys, A., Borzek, J., Henchel, A., Mickelsen, O., & Taylor, H. L. (1950). *The biology of human starvation.* Minneapolis: Univ. of Minnesota Press.

Excess feeding typically yields obesity in most animals. See: LeMagnen, J. (1983). Body energy balance and food intake: A neuroendocrine regulatory mechanism. *Physiol. Rev.* 63:314–386.

However, a substantial proportion of humans do not gain as much weight as might be expected from overfeeding, suggesting that their metabolism copes with the increased energy input. See: Sims, E. H. A., Danforth, E., Jr., Horton, E. S., Bray, G. A., Glennon, J. A., & Salans, L. B. (1973). Endocrine and metabolic effects of experimental obesity in man. *Recent Prog. Horm. Res.* 29:457–496.

30. Panksepp, J. (1976). On the nature of feeding patterns—primarily in rats. In *Hunger: Basic mechanisms and clinical implications* (D. Novin, W. Wyrwicka, & G. A. Bray, eds.), pp. 369–382. New York: Raven Press.

31. Collier, G., Hirsch, E., & Hamlin, P. (1972). The ecological determinants of reinforcement in the rat. *Physiol. Behav.* 9:705–716.

Collier, G., Johnson, D. F., & Morgan, C. (1992). The magnitude-of-reinforcement function in closed and open economies. *J. Exp. Anal. Behav.* 57:81–89.

Mathis, C. E., Johnson, D. F., & Collier, G. (1996). Food and water intake as functions of resource consumption costs in a closed economy. *J. Exp. Anal. Behav.* 65:527–547.

Morato, S., Johnson, D. F., & Collier, G. (1995). Feeding patterns of rats when food-access cost is alternately low and high. *Physiol. Behav.* 57:21–26.

32. Panksepp, J. (1973). A reanalysis of feeding patterns in the rat. *J. Comp. Physiol. Psychol.* 82:78–94.

Panksepp, J. (1978). Analysis of feeding patterns: Data reduction and theoretical implications. In *Hunger models* (D. A. Booth, ed.), pp. 143–166. London: Academic Press.

33. LeMagnen, J., Devos, M., Gaudilliere, J. P., Louis-Sylvestre, J., & Tallon, S. (1973). Role of a lipostatic mechanism in regulation by feeding of energy balance in rats. *J. Comp. Physiol. Psychol.* 84:1–23.

34. Schwartz, M. W., Fiuglewics, D. P., Baskin, D. G., Woods, S. C., & Porte, D., Jr. (1992). Insulin in the brain: A hormonal regulator of energy balance. *Endocrine Revs.* 13:387–414.

35. Powley, T. L. (1977). The ventromedial hypothalamic syndrome, satiety and a cephalic phase hypothesis. *Psychol. Rev.* 84:89–126.

36. LeMagnen, J. (1992). *Neurobiology of feeding and nutrition.* San Diego: Academic Press.

37. LeMagnen, J. (1981). The metabolic basis of dual periodicity of feeding in rat. *Behav. Brain Sci.* 4:561–607.

38. Removal of fat tissue has variable effects on obesity, largely because of the many factors from adipose tissue that can regulate feeding and body composition. See:

Harris, R. B., Martin, R. J., & Bruch, R. C. (1995). Dissociation between food intake, diet composition, and metabolism in parabiotic partners of obese rats. *Am. J. Physiol.* 268:R874–R883.

Hulsey, M. G., & Martin, R. J. (1992). An anorectic agent from adipose tissue of overfed rats: Effects on feeding behavior. *Physiol. Behav.* 52:1141–1149.

39. Anderson, G. H., & Kennedy, S. H. (eds.) (1992). *The biology of feast and famine: Relevance to eating disorders.* San Diego: Academic Press.

Bray, G. A., & York, D. A. (1979). Hypothalamic and genetic obesity in experimental animals: An autonomic and endocrine hypothesis. *Physiol. Rev.* 59:718–809.

Schneider, L. H., Cooper, S. J. H., & Halmi, K. A. (eds.) (1989). *The psychology of human eating disorders: Preclinical and clinical perspectives.* Special issue of *Annals of the New York Academy of Sciences*, vol. 574. New York: New York Academy of Sciences.

40. For a general review see n. 56 and:

Miller, R. J., & Bell, G. I. (1996). JAK/STAT eats the fat. *Trends Neurosci.* 19:159–161.

Halaas, J. L., Gajiwala, K. S., Maffei, M., Cohen, S. L., Chait, B. T., Rabinowitz D., Lallone, R. L. Burley, S. K., & Friedman, J. M.(1995). Weight-reducing effects of the plasma protein encoded by the obese gene. *Science* 269:543–546.

Pelleymounter, M. A., Cullen, M. J., & Baker, M. B. (1995). Effects of the *obese* gene product on body weight regulation in *ob/ob* mice. *Science* 269:540–543.

The weight-reducing effect of leptin may be mediated via inhibition of medial hypothalamic neuropeptide Y systems. See:

Stephens, T. W., Basinski, M., & Bristow, P. K. (1995). The role of neuropeptide Y in the antiobesity action of the *obese* gene product. *Nature* 377:530–532.

Schwartz, M. W., Baskin, D. G., Bukowski, T. R., Kuijper, J. L., Foster, D., Lasser, G., Prunkard, D. E., Porte, D., Jr., Woods, S. C., Seeley, R. J., & Weigle, D. S. (1996). Specificity of leptin action on elevated blood glucose levels and hypothalamic neuropeptide Y gene expression in *ob/ob* mice. *Diabetes* 45:531–535.

41. Considine, R. V., et al. (1996). Serum immunoreactive leptin concentration in normal-weight and obese humans. *New Engl. J. Med.* 334:292–295.

Levin, N., Nelson, C., Gurney, A., Vandlen, R., & De Sauvage, F. (1996). Decreased food intake does not completely account for adiposity reduction after ob protein infusion. *Proc. Natl. Acad. Sci.* 93:1726–1730.

42. Panksepp, J., Bishop, P., & Rossi, J. (1979). Neurohumoral and endocrine control of feeding. *Psychoneuroendocrinol.* 4:89–106.

The gender differences in gustatory responses and the regulation of feeding have been summarized by: Nance, D. M., Gorski, R. A., & Panksepp, J. (1976). Neural and hormonal determinants of sex differences in food intake and body weight. In *Hunger: Basic mechanisms and clinical implications* (D. Novin, W. Wyrwicka, & G. A. Bray, eds.), pp. 257–272. New York: Raven Press.

43. Booth, D. A. (1972). Postabsorptively induced suppression of appetite and the energostatic control of feeding. *Physiol. Behav.* 9:199–202.

Panksepp, J. (1971). Effects of fats, proteins and carbohydrates on food intake in rats. *Psychonomic Monograph Suppl.* 4, no. 5 (Whole no. 53):85–95.

Panksepp, J. (1975). Central metabolic and humoral factors involved in the neural regulation of feeding. *Pharmacol. Biochem. Behav.* 3(Suppl. 1):107–119.

44. For a summary of the classic parabiotic experiments, see: Panksepp, J. (1975). Hormonal control of feeding behavior and energy balance. In *Hormonal correlates of behavior*, vol. 2 (B. E. Eleftheriou & R. L. Sprott, eds.), pp. 657–695. New York: Plenum Press.

45. Panksepp, J. (1971). A re-examination of the role of the ventromedial hypothalamus in feeding behavior. *Physiol. Behav.* 7:385–394.

Panksepp, J., & Reilly, P. (1975). Medial and lateral hypothalamic oxygen consumption as a function of age, starvation and glucose administration in rats. *Brain Res.* 94:133–140.

46. Panksepp, J., & Rossi, J., III (1981). D-glucose infusion into the basal ventromedial hypothalamus and feeding. *Behav. Brain Res.* 3:381–392.

It is also noteworthy that chronic infusion of insulin or transplantation of insulin-secreting pancreatic beta cells into the hypothalamus can also reduce feeding. See:

Richardson, R. D., Ramsay, D. S., Lernmark, A., Scheurink, A. J., Baskin, D. G., & Woods, S. C. (1994). Weight loss in rats following intraventricular transplants of pancreatic islets. *Am. J. Physiol.* 266:R59–R64.

Woods, S. C., Porte, D., Jr., Bobbioni, E., Ionescu, E., Sauter, J. F., Rohnerje, F., & Jeanrena, B. (1985). Insulin: Its relationship to the central nervous system and to the control of food-intake and body weight. *Am J. Clin. Nutr.* 42:1063–1071.

47. See the 1967 *Handbook of physiology*. Sec. 6, *Alimentary canal*. Vol. 1, *Control of food and water intake*. Washington, D.C.: American Physiological Society.

48. Bernardis, L. L., & Bellinger, L. L. (1993). The lateral hypothalamic area revisted: Neuroanatomy, body weight regulation, neuroendocrinology and metabolism. *Neurosci. Biobehav. Revs.* 17:141–193.

49. Stricker, E. M., & Zigmond, M. K. (1976). Recovery of function after damage to central catecholamine-containing neurons: A neurochemical model for the lateral hypothalamic syndrome. *Prog. Psychobiol. Physiol. Psychol.* 6:121–188.

50. Powley, T. L., & Keesey, R. E. (1970). Relationship of body weight to the lateral hypothalamic syndrome. *J. Comp. Physiol. Psychol.* 70:25–36.

For a thorough recent review of lateral hypothalamic functions in feeding and other behavior, see n. 48 and: Bernardis, L. L., & Bellinger, L. L. (1996). The lateral hypothalamic area revisited: Ingestive behavior. *Neurosci. Biobehav. Revs.* 20:189–287.

51. It is clear that there are gustatory and olfactory inputs into the LH (see nn. 48 and 50), and that consummatory behaviors evoked there by ESB are exquisitely sensitive to palatability as well as starvation manipulations. See:

Burton, M. J., Rolls, E. T., & Mora, F. (1976). Effects of hunger on the response of neurons in the lateral hypothalamus to the sight and taste of food. *Exp. Neurol.* 51:668–677.

Karadi, Z., Oomura, Y., Nishino, H., & Aou, S. (1989). Olfactory coding in the monkey lateral hypothalamus: Behavioral and neurochemical properties of odor-responding neurons. *Physiol. Behav.* 45:1249–1257.

52. Novin, D., Sanderson, J., & Gonzalez, M. (1979). Feeding after nutrient infusions: Effects of hypothalamic lesions and vagotomy. *Physiol. Behav.* 22:107–113.

Young, J. K. (1981). Current evidence for a role of glucose as a regulator of hypothalamic function and caloric homeostasis. *Psychoneuroendocrinol.* 6:281–299.

For a discussion of the complexities in conceptualizing short-term glucostatic controls of normal feeding behavior, see: Grossman, S. P. (1986). The role of glucose, insulin and glucagon in the regulation of food intake and body weight. *Neurosci. Biobehav. Revs.* 10:295–315.

53. Panksepp, J. (1971). Is satiety mediated by the ventromedial hypothalamus? *Physiol. Behav.* 7:381–384.

Panksepp, J., & Nance, D. M. (1972). Insulin, glucose and hypothalamic regulation of feeding. *Physiol. Behav.* 9:447–451.

54. Insulin is high in VMH animals, and one can rapidly induce obesity with such a manipulation. As soon as insulin injections are terminated, animals begin to undereat and return to normal body weights (see n. 17).

55. For a while, it was believed that most of the appetite and weight effects following medial hypothalamic damage were due to damage of fibers from the paraventricular nucleus (PVN). See: Gold, R. M., Jones, A. P., Sawchenko, P. E., & Kapatos, G. (1977). Paraventricular area: Critical focus of a longitudinal neurocircuitry mediating food intake. *Physiol. Behav.* 18: 1111–1119.

However, that hypothesis has proved to be only a small part of the story. See:

Kirchgessner, A. L., & Sclafaini, A. (1988). PVN-hindbrain pathway involved in the hypothalamic hyperphagia-obesity syndrome. *Physiol. Behav.* 42:517–528.

Leibowitz, S. F., Hammer, N. J., & Chang, K. (1981). Hypothalamic paraventricular nucleus lesions produce overeating and obesity in the rat. *Physiol. Behav.* 27:1031–1040.

56. For a general review of the leptin story, see:

Barinagea, M. (1995). "Obese" protein slims mice. *Science* 269:475–476.

Bray, G. A. (1996). Leptin and leptinomania. *Lancet* 348:140–141.

57. Zhang, Y., Proenca, R., Maffei, M., Barone, M., Leopold, L., & Friedman, J. M. (1994). Positional cloning of the mouse obese gene and its human homologue. *Nature* 372:425–432.

58. For a summary of the parabiotic experiments that eventually led to the discovery of leptin, see n. 44 and: Hamilton, B. S., et al. (1995). *Nature Med.* 1:953–956.

Usually obese humans produce sufficient leptin, suggesting that their problem is related more to leptin insensitivity, or its failure to reach the receptors in the brain. See:

Caro, J. F., Kolaczynski, J. W., Nyce, M. R., Ohannesian, P., Opentanova, I., Goldman, W. H., Lynn, R. B., Zhang, P.-L., Sinha, M. K., & Considine, R. V. (1996). Decreased cerebrospinal-fluid/serum leptin ratio in obesity: A possible mechanism for leptin resistance. *Lancet* 348:159–161.

Lonnqvist, F., Arner, P., Nordfors, L., & Schalling, M. (1995). Overexpression of the obese (*ob*) gene in adipose tissue of human subjects. *Nature Med.* 1:950–953.

59. Mantzoros, C. S., Qu, D., Frederich, R. C., Susulic, V. S., Lowell, B. B., Maratos-Flier, E., & Flier, J. S. (1996). Activation of beta(3) adrenergic receptors suppresses leptin expression and mediates a leptin-independent inhibition of food intake in mice. *Diabetes* 45:909–914.

60. Frederich, R. C., Hamann, A., Anderson, S., Lollmann, B., Lowell, B. B., & Flier, J. S. (1995). Leptin levels reflect body lipid content in mice: Evidence for diet-induced resistance to leptin action. *Nature Med.* 1:1311–1314.

61. In addition to those summarized in nn. 27 and 56, for other recently proposed satiety factors see:

Oomura, Y. (1989). Sensing of endogenous chemical in control of feeding. *Progress in sensory physiology*, vol 9, pp. 171–191. Berlin: Springer-Verlag.

Sasaki, K., Li, A.-J., Oomura, Y., Muto, T., Hanai, K., Tooyama, I., Kimura, H., Yanaihara, N., Yagi, H., & Hori, T. (1994). Effect of fibroblast growth factors and related peptides on food intake by rats. *Physiol. Behav.* 56:211–218.

It has also been proposed that urocortin may mediate suppression of feeding without producing other symptoms of stress. See: Spina, M., Merlo-Pich, E., Chan, R. K. W., Basso, A. M., Rivier, J., Vale, W., & Koob, G. F. (1996). Appetite-suppressing effects of urocortin, a CRF-related neuropeptide. *Science* 273: 1561–1564. However, in unpublished work, we have observed that urocortin potentiates separation distress in chicks as much as CRF.

62. Cummings, D. E., Brandon, E. P., Planas, J. V., Motamed, K., Idzerda, R. L., & McKnieght, G. S. (1996). Genetically lean mice result from targeted disruption of the RIIß subunit of protein kinase A. *Nature* 382:622–626.

63. See nn. 28 and 46.

64. Kasser, T. R., Harris, B. S., & Martin, R. J. (1985). Level of satiety: Fatty acid and glucose metabolism in three brain sites associated with feeding. *Am. J. Physiol.* 243:R447–R452.

Kasser, T. R., Harris, B. S., & Martin, R. J. (1985). Level of satiety: GABA and penose shunt activities in three brain sites associated with feeding. *Am. J. Physiol.* 243:R453–R458.

There are also brain areas where feeding may be related to other metabolic processes such as lipid metabolism. See: Beverly, J. L., & Martin, R. J. (1991). Influence of fatty acid oxidation in lateral hypothalamus on food intake and body composition. *Am. J. Physiol.* 261:R339–R343.

65. McGowan, M. K., Andrews, K. M., & Grossman, S. P. (1992). Chronic intrahypothalamic infusions of insulin or insulin antibodies alter body weight and food intake in the rat. *Physiol. Behav.* 51:753–766.

Woods, S. C., Chavez, M., Park, C. R., Riedy, C., Kaiyala, K., Richardson, R. D., Figlewicz, D. P., Schwartz, M. W., Porte, D., Jr., & Seeley, R. J. (1996). The evaluation of insulin as a metabolic signal influencing behavior via the brain. *Neurosci. Biobehav. Revs.* 20:139–144.

66. Debons, A. F., Krimsky, I., From, A., & Pattinian, H. (1974). Phlorizin inhibition of hypothalamic necrosis induced by gold thioglucose. *Am. J. Physiol.* 226:574–578.

67. Panksepp, J., & Meeker, R. B. (1980). The role of GABA in the ventromedial hypothalamic regulation of food intake. *Brain Res. Bull.* 5(suppl.):453–460.

However, GABA has effects in all parts of the brain, and there are many sites in the hypothalamus where GABA can promote feeding, perhaps by reducing hunger-induced agitation or perhaps even negative emotionality, in the same way that antianxiety agents can increase feeding. See: Kelly, J., Alheid, G. F., Newberg, A., & Grossman, S. P. (1977). GABA stimulation and blockade in the hypothalamus and midbrain: Effects on feeding and locomotor activity. *Pharmac. Biochem. Behav.* 7:537–541.

Our assumption here is that increased GABA can increase feeding in the short term, but that the long-term consequences are an inhibition of feeding, based on the fact that blockade of GABA-transaminase has a powerful effect on depressing appetite in the long term.

68. Cooper, B. R., Howard, J. L., While, H. L., Soroko, F., Ingold, K., & Maxwell, R. A. (1980). Anorexic effects of ethanolamine-O-sulfate and muscimol in the rat: Evidence that GABA inhibits ingestive behavior. *Life Sci.* 26:1997–2002.

Nobrega, J. N., & Coscina, D. V. (1982). Inhibition of acute feeding response to systemic 2-deoxyglucose or insulin in rats pretreated with the GABA-transaminase blocker ethanolamine-O-sulfate (EOS). *Pharmac. Biochem. Behav.* 17:1145–1148.

For the effects of nutrition on GABA shunt activity in the VMH, see a series of papers by Beverly and Martin, ending with: Beverly, J. L., & Martin, R. J. (1991). Effect of glucoprivation on glutamate decarboxylase activity in the ventromedial hypothalamus. *Physiol. Behav.* 49:295–299.

It should be noted that an alternative line of data suggests that overeating and obesity are characterized by high levels of GABA within the VMH. See: Beverly, J. L., & Martin, R. J. (1989). Increased GABA shunt activity in VMN of three hyperphagic rat models. *Am. J. Physiol.* 25:R1225–R1231.

But also see: Coscina, D. V., & Lloyd, K. G. (1980). Medial hypothalamic obesity: Association with impaired hypothalamic GABA synthesis. *Brain Res. Bull.* 5:793–796.

69. See third citation in n. 43 and: Snead, O. C. (1977). Minireview: Gamma hydroxybutyrate. *Life Sci.* 20:1935–1944.

70. Leibowitz S. F. (1995). Brain peptides and obesity: Pharmacologic treatment. *Obesity Res.* 3 (suppl. 4):573S–589S.

Morley, J. E. (1995). The role of peptides in appetite regulation across species. *Amer. Zool.* 35:437–445.

Morley, J. E., & Blundell, J. E. (1988). The neurobiological basis of eating disorders: Some formulations. *Biol. Psychiat.* 23:53–78.

71. Gray, R. W., & Cooper, S. J. (1995). Benzodiazepines and platability: Taste reactivity in normal ingestion. *Physiol. Behav.* 58:853–859.

72. For an overview and key references for NPY, see: Colmers, W. F., & Wahlestedt, C. (eds.) (1993). *The biology of neuropeptide Y.* New York: Humana Press. Other key articles are:

Kalra, S. P., & Kalra, P. S. (1990). Neuropeptide Y: A novel peptidergic signal for the control of feeding behavior. In *Current topics in neuroendocrinology,* vol. 10 (D. Ganten & D. Pfaff, eds.), pp. 191–221. Berlin: Springer-Verlag.

Liewbowitz, S. F. (1991). Brain neuropeptide Y: An integrator of endocrine metabolic, and behavioral processes. *Brain Res. Bull.* 21:905–912.

Wahlestedt, C., & Reis, D. J. (1993). Neuropeptide Y–related peptides and their receptors: Are the receptors potential therapeutic drug targets? *Ann. Rev. Pharmacol. Toxicol.* 33:309–352.

Myers, R. D., Wooten, M. H., Ames, C. D., & Nyce, J. W. (1995). Anorexic action of a new potential neuropeptide Y antagonist infused into the hypothalamus of the rat. *Brain Res. Bull.* 37:237–245.

73. Helig, M., & Widerlov, E. (1990). Neuropeptide Y: An overview of central distribution, functional aspects, and possible involvement in neuropsychiatric illnesses. *Acta Psychiat. Scand.* 82:95–114.

NPY is changed not only in the brains of those with appetite problems but also in the brains of persons with many other psychiatric disorders. See: Boulenger, J., Jerabek, I., Jolicoeur, F. B., & Lavallee, Y. J. (1996). Elevated plasma levels of neuropeptide Y in patients with panic disorder. *Am. J. Psychiat.* 153:114–116.

74. Beck, B., Burlet, A., Bazin, R., Nicolas, J. P., & Burlet, C. (1993). Elevated neuropeptide Y in the arcuate nucleus of young obese Zucker rats may contribute to the development of their overeating. *J. Nutr.* 123:1168–1172.

Nearby dynorphin and galanin systems can also increase feeding. See:

Kyrkouli, S. E., Stanley, B. G., Hutchinson, R., Seirafi, R. I., & Leibowitz, S. F. (1990). Peptide-amine interactions in the hypothalamic paraventricular nucleus: Analysis of galanin and neuropeptide Y in relation to feeding. *Brain Res.* 521:185–191.

Lambert, P. D., Wilding, J. P. H., Al-Dokhayel, A., & Gilbey, S. G. (1993). The central effect of central blockade of kappa-opioid receptors on neuropeptide Y–induced feeding in the rat. *Brain Res.* 629:146–148.

Morley, J. E., Levine, A. S., Grace, M., & Kneip, J. (1982). Dynorphin-(1-13), dopamine and feeding in rats. *Pharmacol. Biochem. Behav.* 16:701–705.

75. Tempel, D. L., Leibowitz, K. J., & Leibowitz, S. F. (1988). Effects of PVN galanin on macronutrient selection. *Peptides* 9:309–314.

76. Animals missing NPY seemingly exhibit normal food intake regulation. See: Erickson, J. C., Clegg, K. E., & Palmiter, R. D. (1996). Sensitivity to leptin and susceptibility to seizures of mice lacking neuropeptide Y. *Nature* 381:415–421.

However, reducing brain NPY with "antisense" RNA techniques, which block the expression of the NPY gene, can reduce feeding and body weight in the long term. See: Hulsey, M. G., Pless, C. M., White, B. D., & Martin, J. (1995). ICV administration of anti-NPY antisense oligonucleotide: Effects on feeding behavior, body weight, peptide content and peptide release. *Reg. Peptides* 59:207–214.

In this context it is worth noting that in the short term, NPY blockade can increase food intake, perhaps by making animals more anxious. See: Sipols, A. J., Brief, D. J., Ginter, K. L., Saghafi, S., & Woods, S. C. (1992). Neuropeptide Y paradoxically increases food intake yet causes conditioned flavor aversions. *Physiol. Behav.* 51:1257–1260.

77. Rozin, P., & Kalat, J. W. (1972). Specific hungers and poison avoidance as adaptive specializations of learning. *Psychol. Rev.* 78:459–486.

78. Berridge, K. C. (1996). Food reward: Brain substrates of wanting and liking. *Neurosci. Biobehav. Rev.* 20:1–26.

79. Cabanac, M. (1971). Physiological role of pleasure. *Science* 173:1103–1107.

Cabanac, M. (1992). Pleasure: The common currency. *J. Theor. Biol.* 155:173–200.

80. Booth, D. A., Lovett, D., & McShery, G. M. (1972). Postingestive modulation of the sweetness preference gradient in the rat. *J. Comp. Physiol. Psychol.* 78:485–512.

81. Panksepp, J., & Meeker, R. (1977). Effects of insulin and hypothalamic lesions on glucose preference in rats. In *Food intake and the chemical senses* (T. Katsui, M. Satao, S. Takagi, & Y. Oomura, eds.), pp. 343–356. Tokyo: Tokyo Univ. Press.

82. Chiva, M. (1983). Taste and non-verbal communication of infants. [French: Gout et communication non verbale chez le jeune enfant.] *Enfance* 1–2:53–64.

Steiner, J. E. (1979). Human facial expressions in response to taste and smell stimulation. *Adv. Child Devel. Behav.* 13:257–295.

83. Grill, H. J., & Berridge, K. C. (1985). Taste reactivity as a measure of the neural control of palatability. In *Progress in psychobiology and physiological psychology* (J. M Sprague & A. N. Epstein, eds.), pp. 1–61. Orlando, Fla.: Academic Press.

84. Berridge, K. C., & Pecina, S. (1995). Benzodiazepines, appetite, and taste palatability. *Neurosc. Biobehav. Revs.* 19:121–131.

Pecina, S., & Berridge, K. C. (1995). Central enhancement of taste pleasure by intraventricular morphine. *Neurobiology* 3:269–280.

85. See chap. 8, n. 46.

86. Spyraki, C., Fibiger, H., & Phillips, A. (1982). Attenuation by haloperidol of place preference conditioning using food reinforcement. *Psychopharmacol.* 77:379–382.

87. Deems, D. A., & Garcia, J. (1986). Involvement of dorsomedial hypothalamus in taste aversion learning: Possible alterations in general sensitivity to illness. *Nutr. Behav.* 3:91–100.

Galverna, O., Seeley, R. J., Berridge, K. C., Grill, H. J., Schulkin, J., & Epstein, A. N. (1993). Lesions of the central nucleus of the amygdala: 1. Effects on taste reactivity, taste aversion learning and sodium appetite. *Behav. Brain. Res.* 59:11–17.

Gold, R. M., & Proulx, D. M. (1972). Baitshyness is impaired by VMH lesions that produce obesity. *J. Comp. Physiol. Psychol.* 79:201–209.

Roth, S. R., Schwartz, M., & Teitelbaum, P. (1973). Failure of recovered lateral hypothalamic rats to learn specific food aversions. *J. Comp. Physiol. Psychol.* 83:184–197.

Simbayi, L. C., Boakes, R. A., & Burton, M. J. (1986). Effects of basolateral amygdala lesions on taste aversions produced by lactose and lithium chloride in the rat. *Behav. Neurosci.* 100:455–465.

There are also forms of brain damage that increase conditioned taste aversions. See: Cromwell, H. C., & Berridge, K. C. (1993). Where does damage lead to enhanced food aversion: The ventral pallidum/substantia innominata or lateral hypothalamus? *Brain Res.* 624:1–10.

88. Humans and animals readily develop cravings for drugs that facilitate brain dopamine activity (amphetamines, cocaine, etc.); more precisely, this psychological dependence is, to a substantial extent, due to arousal of the A10 mesolimbic dopamine system (see Chapter 8). Although psychostimulant seeking and self-administration are diminished by destruction of mesolimbic dopamine systems, it remains unclear what type of neuropsychic reinforcing event is mediated by dopamine. Does the induced psychological process resemble consummatory pleasure or some other form of desirable psychic arousal? The present position is that the psychological state is akin to a generalized desire or reward-seeking urge rather than any type of pleasure that typically accompanies consummatory acts. Generally, this is in accord with the most common subjective reports from human subjects, which indicate that what is being experienced are feelings of positive energization, arousal, power, effectiveness, and being on top of things. These are not the types of psychic characteristics that people typically attribute to consummatory pleasures. From this perspective, it would seem unlikely that the pleasurable aspects of taste are directly controlled by brain dopamine, but in addition to the substantial data for opioids, there is quite a bit of data suggesting that taste responsivity may be modulated by brain dopamine. For a discussion of such issues, see n. 78 and: Wise, R. A. (1982). Neuroleptics and operant behavior: The anhedonia hypothesis. *Behav. Brain Sci.* 5:39–87.

89. Chapter 8 focused on the fact that ascending brain dopamine systems are essential for arousing the appetitive phase of behavior, which leads animals to seek out needed resources, and pleasure is probably linked to the consummatory activities that reduce the impulse to forage. However, there is some evidence that certain hypothalamic dopamine systems are activated not only prior to but also during feeding behavior. See: Hoebel, B. G. (1988). Neuroscience and motivation: Pathways and peptides that define motivational systems. In *Stevens' handbook of experimental psychology* (R. C. Atkinson, R. J. Herrenstein, G. Lindzey, & R. D. Luce, eds.), pp. 547–626. New York: Wiley.

It remains possible that these systems may be distinct from the long-axoned, ventral tegmental and substantia nigra systems discussed in the previous chapter. For instance, some of the relatively sparse dopamine cell groups higher up in the hypothalamus (A11 to A15) may help elaborate the rewarding value of food intake, while the more caudally located systems elaborate foraging activities. In any event, it is clear that blockade of dopamine systems can markedly reduce the intake of palatable substances, especially sweets, without having strong effects on regulatory eating, that is, intake of calories needed to maintain body weight. However, in humans, such dopamine blocking agents as antipsychotic drugs typically produce dysphoric feelings that are generally deemed to be unpleasant. Still, this may not be related to any specific regulatory behavior, but merely may be due to the psychological lassitude that one feels when arousal of the SEEKING system has been pharmacologically diminished. For a discussion of such issues, see: Phillips, A. G. (1996). Neural basis of food reward. *Neurosci. Biobehav. Revs.* 20.

Of course, many neurochemical systems contribute to taste reactivity. Among the better-studied ones are the benzodiazepine-responsive systems of the brain. See n. 84 and: Cooper, S. J., & Estall, L. B. (1985). Behavioural pharmacology of food, water and salt intake in relation to drug actions at benzodiazepine receptors. Neurosci. *Biobehav. Revs.* 9:5–19.

90. Fantino, M., Hosottle, J., & Apfelbaum, M. (1986). An opioid antagonist, naltrexone, reduces preference for sucrose in humans. *Am. J. Physiol.* 251: R91–R96.

But see:

Hetherington, M. M., Vervaet, N., Blass, E., & Rolls, B. J. (1991). Failure of naltrexone to affect the pleasantness or intake of food. *Pharmacol. Biochem. Behav.* 40:185–190.

Lynch, W. C. (1986). Opiate blockade inhibits saccharin intake and blocks normal preference acquisition. *Pharmacol. Biochem. Behav.* 24:833–836.

Parker, L. A., Maier, S., Rennie, M., & Crebolder, J. (1992). Morphine- and naltrexone-induced modification of palatability analysis by the taste reactivity test. *Behav. Neurosci.* 106:999–1010.

Siviy, S. M., Calcagnetti, D. J., & Reid, L. D. (1982). Opioids and palatability. In *The neural basis of feeding and reward* (B. G. Hoebel & D. Novin, eds.), pp. 517–524. Brunswick, Maine: Haer Institute.

For a series of overviews of how opiate antagonists modify various gustatory urges, see: Reid, L. D. (ed.) (1990). *Opioids, bulimia, and alcohol abuse and alcoholism.* New York: Springer-Verlag.

91. Blass, E. M., & Shah, A. (1995). Pain-reducing properties of sucrose in human newborns. *Chemical Senses* 20:29–35.

Blass, E. M., & Shide, D. J. (1994). Some comparisons among the calming and pain-relieving effects of sucrose, glucose, fructose and lactose in infant rats. *Chemical Senses* 19:239–249.

92. Dum, J., Gramsch, C. H., & Herz, A. (1983). Activation of hypothalamic ß-endorphin pools by reward induced by highly palatable food. *Pharmacol. Biochem. Behav.* 18:443–447.

93. In this context it is noteworthy that individuals undergoing opiate withdrawal exhibit a heightened appetite for sweets; this, in turn, may help activate endogenous brain opioid systems, which may help alleviate withdrawal symptoms (see n. 91).

94. It is possible that knowledge of this kind will eventually clarify such ancient principles as *chi* in traditional Chinese medicine, which seems to encapsulate the broad concept of homeostasis as the search for a balanced life. The general pleasure produced by brain opioid systems may be related to an interesting effect that can be produced by high doses of externally administered opioids—a quieting of the body that at its most extreme takes the form of catalepsy: When animals are given high doses of opiates, their bodies become rigidly "waxy," so that one can mold them into almost any shape. Perhaps a mild form of this type of immobility characterizes animals that have no regulatory imbalances—ones that are completely satisfied.

95. Bakshi, V. P., & Kelley, A. E. (1993). Feeding induced by opioid stimulation of the ventral striatum: Role of opiate receptor subtypes. *J. Pharmacol. Exp. Ther.* 265:1253–1260.

Gosnell, B. A. (1987). Central structures involved in opioid-induced feeding. *Fed. Proc.* 46:163–167.

Stanley, B. G., Lanthier, D., & Leibowitz, S. F. (1988). Multiple brain sites sensitive to feeding stimulation by opioid agonists: A cannula-mapping study. *Pharmacol. Biochem. Behav.* 31:825–832.

96. Davies, R. F. , Rossi, J., Panksepp, J., Bean, N. J., & Zolovick, A. J. (1983). Fenfluramine anorexia: A peripheral locus of action. *Physiol. Behav.* 30:723–730.

97. Johnson, A. K., & Edwards, G. L. (1990). The neuroendocrinology of thirst: Afferent signalling and mechanisms of central integration. In *Behavioural aspects of neuroedocrinology.* Vol. 10, *Current topics in neuroendocrinology* (D. Ganten & D. Pfaff, eds.), pp.149–190. Berlin: Springer-Verlag.

98. Stricker, E. M. (ed.) (1990). *Handbook of behavioral neurobiology.* Vol. 10, *Neurobiology of food and fluid intake.* New York: Plenum Press.

99. Schulkin, J. (1991). *Sodium hunger: The search for a salty taste.* Cambridge: Cambridge Univ. Press.

100. Krieckhouse, E. E. (1970). "Innate recognition" aids rats in sodium regulation. *J. Comp. Physiol. Psychol.* 73:117–122.

101. Braverman, N. S., & Bronstein, P. (eds.) (1985). *Experimental assessments and clinical applications of conditioned food aversions.* Special issue of *Ann. N.Y. Acad. Sci.*, vol. 443. New York: New York Academy of Sciences.

102. Galef, B. G., Jr. (1988). Communication of information concerning distant diets in a social, central-place foraging species: *Rattus norvegicus.* In *Social learning: Psychological and biological perspectives* (T. R. Zentall & B. G. Galef, Jr., eds.), pp. 119–140. Hillsdale, N.J.: Lawrence Erlbaum.

Rozin, P. (1988). Social learning about food by humans. In *Social learning: Psychological and biological perspectives* (T. R. Zentall & B. G. Galef, Jr., eds.), pp. 165–188. Hillsdale, N.J.: Lawrence Erlbaum.

103. Booth, D. A. (1977). Satiety and appetite are conditioned reactions. *Psychosom. Med.* 39:76–81.

Booth, D. A. (1980). Acquired behavior controlling energy intake and output. In *Obesity* (A. J. Stunkard, ed.), pp 101–143. Philadelphia: Saunders.

Booth, D. A. (1985). Food-conditioned eating preferences and aversions with interoreceptive elements, conditioned appetites, and satieties. *Ann. N.Y. Acad. Sci.* 443:22–41.

In the context of everything that has been discussed in this chapter, it should be remembered that foodstuffs can have many direct effects on brain transmitters and hence on behavioral and psychological dispositions (see chap. 6, nn. 22 and 23).

Chapter 10

1. See Lorenz, K. (1966). *On aggression.* New York: Harcourt, Brace, and World.

For an interesting recent survey of aggression in primates, see: Mason, W. A., & Mendoza, S. P. (eds.) (1993). *Primate social conflict*. Albany: State Univ. of New York Press.

2. Dominance is a complex phenomenon, and it appears likely that animals can exhibit different dominance hierarchies for different resources. For a thorough review of issues, see: Berenstein, I. S. (1981). Dominance: The baby and the bathwater. *Behav. Brain Sci.* 4:419–458.

3. Goodall, J. (1986). *The chimpanzees of Gombe*. Cambridge, Mass.: Harvard Univ. Press.

4. For a fine essay on such events in modern urban societies, see: Wright, R. (1995). The biology of violence. *New Yorker*, March 13.

5. Benus, R. F., Bohus, B., Koolhaas, J. M., & Van Oortmerssen, G. A. (1991). Heritable variation of aggression as a reflection of individual coping strategies. *Experientia* 47:1008–1019.

Hyde, J. S., & Sawyer, T. F. (1980). Selection for agonistic behavior in wild female mice. *Behav. Genetics* 10:349–359.

In interpreting genetic effects on aggression, or any other behavior for that matter, one must also consider the differential consequences of rearing environments such as selective maternal effects. When the appropriate cross-fostering experiments have been conducted, some supposed genetic effects have turned out to be environmental ones. See: Carlier, M., Roubertoux, P. L., & Pastoret, C. (1991). The Y chromosome effect on intermale aggression in mice depends on the maternal environment. *Genetics* 129:231–236.

Many relevant issues concerning the genetics of aggression have been summarized in 10 contributions to the special issue: The Neurobehavioral Genetics of Aggression. *Behavior Genetics* 26:459–532.

6. Mealey, L. (1995). The sociobiology of sociopathy: An integrated evolutionary model. *Behav. Brain Sci.* 18:529–599.

7. Brunner, H. G., Nelen, M., Breakfield, X. O., Ropers, H. H., & van Oost, B. A. (1993). Abnormal behavior associated with a point mutation in the structural gene for monoamine oxidase A. *Science* 262: 578–580.

Also, mice with a deletion of this gene exhibit heightened aggression. See: Cases, O., Seif, I., Grimsby, J., Gaspar, P., Chen, K., Pournin, S., Uller, U., Aquet, M., Babinet, C., Shih, J. C., & De Maeyer, E. (1995). Aggressive behavior and altered amounts of brain serotonin and norepinephrine in mice lacking MAO-A. *Science* 268:1763–1766.

8. For a summary of serotonin control of aggression in animals and humans, see: Coccaro, E. F. (1996). Neurotransmitter correlates of impulsive aggression in humans. *Ann. N.Y. Acad. Sci.* 794:82–89.

But note that some of these effects interact with rearing environments. See: Kraemer, G. W., & Clark, S. (1996). Social attachment, brain function, and aggression. *Ann. N.Y. Acad. Sci.* 794:121–135.

9. For a discussion of "organizational and activational" issues, see Chapter 12. A thorough discussion of hormones and aggression can be found in: Svare, B. B. (ed.) (1983). *Hormones and aggressive behavior*. New York: Plenum Press.

Many fine recent summaries of such issues are to be found in: Ferris, C. F., & Grisso, T. (eds.) (1996). *Understanding aggressive behavior in children*. Special issue of *Ann. N.Y. Acad. Sci.*, vol. 794. New York: New York Academy of Sciences.

10. Monaghan, E. P., & Glickman, S. E. (1992). Hormones and aggressive behavior. In *Behavioral endocrinology* (J. B. Becker, S. M. Breedlove, & D. Crews, eds.), pp. 261–285. Boston, Mass.: MIT Press.

11. Campos, J., Mumme, D. L., Kermoian, R., & Campos, R. (1994). A functionalist perspective on the nature of emotion. *Monog. Soc. Res. Child Devel.* 59: 284–303.

12. The importance of dealing fully with the emotional dynamics that underlie psychiatric disorders is receiving increasing attention in psychotherapy. See: Korman, L. M., & Greenberg, L. S. (1996). Emotion and therapeutic change. In *Advances in biological psychiatry*, vol. 2 (J. Panksepp, ed.), pp. 1–25. Greenwich, Conn.: JAI Press.

13. The issue of "free will" is obviously a difficult one to biologize, but it is presumably a central nervous system reflection of our conscious abilities to reflect upon the consequences of different courses of action (see Chapter 16). Our ability to utilize such reflective abilities depends critically on our past experiences, as well as on the intensity of arousal within our basic motivational and emotional systems. The stronger the arousal of these primal circuits, the more difficult it will presumably be for individuals to select a course of action based on deliberation rather than emotional impulse.

14. Gallup, G. G., Jr. (1974). Animal hypnosis: Factual status of a fictional concept. *Psych. Bull.* 81: 836–853.

15. The study of learning within aggression systems of the brain is remarkably meager. Certainly, animals and humans can become temperamental following temporal lobe kindling (see MacLean, P. [1993]. Cerebral evolution of emotion. In *Handbook of emotions* [M. Lewis & J. M. Haviland, eds.], pp. 67–83. New York: Guilford Press), but there is no data base comparable to the learning of fears that will be covered in Chapter 11. However, some investigators have taken the position that all aggression is learned, on the basis of the fact that animals can be trained to be vigorous fighters (Scott, J. P. [1966]. Agonistic behavior in mice and rats. *Amer. Zool.* 6:683–701). This type of important data should not, however, be taken as support of a conclusion that all aggression is learned. Certainly, the types that are promoted by anger emerge from the natural potential of the nervous system to generate that feeling.

16. Averill, J. R. (1982). *Anger and aggression: An essay on emotion*. New York: Springer-Verlag.

Frijda, N. H. (1986). *The emotions*. Cambridge: Cambridge Univ. Press.

17. Miczek, K. A. (1987). The psychopharmacology of aggression. In *Handbook of psychopharmacology*. Vol. 19, *New directions in behavioral pharma-*

cology (L. L. Iversen, S. D. Iversen, & S. H. Snyder, eds.), pp. 183–328. New York: Plenum Press.

Miczek, K., Haney, M., Tidey, J., Vivian, J., & Weerts, E. (1994). Neurochemistry and pharmacotherapeutic management of aggression and violence. In *Understanding and preventing violence*. Vol. 2, *Biobehavioral influences* (A. Reiss, K. Miczek, & J. Roth., eds.), pp 245–514. Washington, D.C.: National Academy Press.

18. Zivin, G. (ed.) (1985). *The development of expressive behavior: Biology-environment interactions*. Orlando, Fla.: Academic Press.

19. Christianson, S.-A. (ed.) (1992). *The handbook of emotion and memory: Research and theory*. Hillsdale, N.J.: Lawrence Erlbaum.

Stein, N. L., Leventhal, B., & Trabasso, T. (eds.) (1990). *Psychological and biological approaches to emotion*. Hillsdale, N.J.: Lawrence Erlbaum.

20. For a summary of frontal lobe functions, see: Krasnegor, N. A., Lyon, G., & Goldman-Rakic, S. (eds.) (1997). Development of the prefrontal cortex. Baltimore: Paul H. Bookes.

21. Hutchinson, R. R., & Renfrew, J. W. (1978). Functional parallels between the neural and environmental antecedents of aggression. *Neurosci. Biobehav. Revs*. 2:33–58.

22. Dodge, K. A. (1986). Social information-processing variables in the development of aggression and altruism in children. In *Altruism and aggression: Biological and social origins* (C. Zahn-Waxler, E. M. Cummings, & R. Iannotti, eds.), pp., 280–302. Cambridge: Cambridge Univ. Press.

23. For a discussion of these issues, see: Gray, J. A. (1982). *The neuropsychology of anxiety: An enquiry into the functions of the septo-hippocampal system*. Oxford: Oxford Univ. Press.

24. For a discussion of emotional changes following frontal lobe damage: see, Damasio, A. R. (1994). *Descartes' error*. New York: Putnam.

25. Moyer, K. E. (1976). *The psychobiology of aggression*. New York: Harper and Row.

26. Valzelli, L. (1981). *Psychobiology of aggression and violence*. New York: Raven Press.

27. One reason for this very dramatic display was that I had inadvertently left the current switch on the times 10 setting and hence had administered more current than I had intended. Clearly, the intensity of all the stimulus-bound behaviors discussed in this book is directly related to how strongly the underlying circuits are stimulated. In a comparable way, the intensities of our naturally evoked emotions are probably due to the degree to which the underlying circuits are aroused. The variability in emotional temperaments reflects, in part, the degree to which our emotional circuits can be aroused. Excessive and sustained arousal is probably a hallmark of psychiatric disturbances.

28. Flynn, J. P. (1967). The neural basis of aggression in cats. In *Neurophysiology and emotion* (D. C. Glass, ed.), pp. 40–60. New York: Rockefeller Univ. Press.

29. Masserman, J. H. (1941). Is the hypothalamus a center of emotion? *Psychosom. Med*. 3:3–25.

30. There are many striking descriptions of rage in humans during brain stimulation, especially of medial amygdaloid sites. See:

Hitchcock, E., & Cairns, V. (1973). Amygdalotomy. *Postgrad. Med*. 49:894–904.

King, H. E. (1961). Psychological effects of excitation in the limbic system. In *Electrical stimulation of the brain* (D. E. Sheer, ed.), pp. 477–486. Austin: Univ. of Texas Press.

Mark, V. H., Ervin, F. R., & Sweet, W. H. (1972). Deep temporal lobe stimulation in man. In *The neurobiology of the amygdala* (B. E. Eleftheriou, ed.), pp. 485–507. New York: Plenum Press.

31. Panksepp, J. (1971). Aggression elicited by electrical stimulation of the hypothalamus in albino rats. *Physiol. Behav*. 6:321–329.

32. Flynn, J. P. (1976). Neural basis of threat and attack. In *Biological foundations of psychiatry* (R. G. Grenell & S. G. Abau, eds.), pp. 275–295. New York: Raven Press.

33. See n. 31.

34. Kruk, M. R., Van der Poel, A. M., & De Vos-Frerichs, T. P. (1979). The induction of aggressive behaviour by electrical stimulation in the hypothalamus of male rats. *Behaviour* 70:292–322.

35. See n. 31.

36. Panksepp, J., Gandelman, R., & Trowill, J.A. (1970). Modulation of hypothalamic self-stimulation and escape behavior by chlordiazepoxide in the rat. *Physiol. Behav*. 5:965–969.

37. Panksepp, J. (1971). Drugs and "stimulus-bound" attack. *Physiol. Behav*. 6:317–320.

38. Panksepp, J. (1975, unpublished data). Also see: Kruk, M. R., Van der Poel, A. M., Lammers, J. H. C. M., Hagg, T., De Hey, A. M. D. M., & Oostwegel, S. (1987). Ethopharmacology of hypothalamic aggression in the rat. In *Ethopharmacology of agonistic behaviour in animals and humans* (B. Olivier, J. Mos, & P. F. Brain, eds.), pp. 33–45. Dordrecht: Martinus Nijhoff.

39. Siegel, A., & Brutus, M. (1990). Neural substrates of aggression and rage in the cat. In *Progress in psychobiology and physiological psychology*, vol. 14 (A. N. Epstein & A. R. Morrison, eds.), pp. 135–233. San Diego: Academic Press.

40. See n. 31.

41. Bandler, R. (1988). Brain mechanisms of aggression as revealed by electrical and chemical stimulation: Suggestion of a central role for the midbrain periaqueductal gray region. In *Progress in psychobiology and physiological psychology*, vol. 13 (A. N. Epstein & A. R. Morrison, eds.), pp 67–154. San Diego: Academic Press.

42. See n. 39.

43. See n. 31 and:

Alexander, M., & Perachio, A. A. (1973). The influence of target sex and dominance on evoked attack in rhesus monkeys. *Amer. J. Phys. Anthrop*. 38:543–547.

Delgado, J. M. R. (1969). *Physical control of the mind: Toward a psychocivilized society*. New York: Harper and Row.

44. See n. 37.

45. De Molina, A. F., & Hunsperger, R. W. (1962). Organization of the subcortical system governing defense and flight reactions in the cat. *J. Physiol. (London)* 160:200–213.

46. Thorpe, S. J., Rolls, E. T., & Maddison, S. (1983). Neuronal activity in the orbitofrontal cortex of the behaving monkey. *Exp. Brain Res.* 49:93–115.

47. Rolls, E. T. (1990). A theory of emotion, and its application to understanding the neural basis of emotion. *Cogn. Emot.* 4:161–190.

48. See n. 41.

49. Mancia, G., & Zanchetti, A. (1971). Hypothalamic control of autonomic functions. In *Handbook of the hypothalamus*. Vol. 3, part B, *Behavioral studies of the hypothalamus* (P. J. Morgane & J. Panksepp, eds.), pp. 147–202. New York: Marcel Dekker.

50. Animals for such studies typically are preselected to not exhibit spontaneous attack toward a prey object. In rats, quiet-biting attack could be obtained only from animals that were temperamentally very close to exhibiting the behavior spontaneously, as indicated by their intense interest in the prey object.

51. See n. 31.

52. Hutchinson, R. R., & Renfrew, J. W. (1966). Stalking attack and eating behaviors elicited from the same sites in the hypothalamus. *J. Comp. Physiol. Psychol.* 61:360–367.

The idea that aggression, and the expression of other seemingly negative emotional behaviors, may have positive affective consequences for an animal was first developed by: Glickman, S. E., & Schiff, B. B. (1967). A biological theory of reinforcement. *Psychol. Rev.* 74:81–109.

53. MacDonnell, M. F., & Flynn, J. P. (1966). Control of sensory fields by stimulation of hypothalamus. *Science* 152:1406–1408.

54. Smith, D. A. (1972). Increased perioral responsiveness: A possible explanation of the switching of behavior observed during lateral hypothalamic stimulation. *Physiol. Behav.* 8:617–621.

55. Bandler, R., & Flynn, J. P. (1972). Control of somatosensory fields for striking during hypothalamically elicited attack. *Brain Res.* 38:197–201.

56. Bandler, R., & Flynn, J. P. (1971). Visually patterned reflex during hypothalamically elicited attack. *Science* 171:817–818.

57. In this context, it is worth noting that in agonistic encounters, primates prefer to keep sight of their opponents in their left visual fields, which sends input into the right hemisphere, which is specialized for emotional processing of information. See: Casperd, J. M., & Dunbar, R. I. M. (1996). Asymmetries in the visual processing of emotional cues during agonistic interactions by gelada baboons. *Behavioural Processes* 37: 57–65.

58. Beagley, W. K., & Holley, T. L. (1977). Hypothalamic stimulation facilitates contralateral visual control of a learned response. *Science* 196:321–322.

59. The "female selection hypothesis" for male aggression, put forward by several sociobiologists, is another interesting "evolutionary story" that cannot be empirically evaluated. The essence of this idea was first proposed by: Fisher, R. A. (1930). *The genetical theory of natural selection*. Oxford: Clarendon Press.

For several recent discussions of such issues, and how they relate to human behavior, see:

Cronin, H. (1991). *The ant and the peacock: Altruism and sexual selection from Darwin to today*. New York: Cambridge Univ. Press.

Ridley, M. (1994). *The Red Queen: Sex and the evolution of human nature*. New York: Macmillan.

Taylor, T. (1966). *The prehistory of sex: Four million years of human sexual culture*. New York: Bantam Books.

60. Albert, D. J., Walsh, M. L., & Jonik, R. H. (1993). Aggression in humans: What is its biological foundation? *Neurosci. Biobehav. Revs.* 17:405–426.

61. Although sex and aggression produced substantially different *cfos* labeling in the medial area, there were areas of overlap, suggesting a shared feature to male sex and aggression. See: Kollack-Walker, S., & Newman, S. W. (1995). Mating and agonistic behavior produce different patterns of FOS immunolabelling in the male Syrian hamster brain. *Neuroscience* 66: 721–736.

62. DeVries, G. J., Buijs, R. M., Van Leeuwen, F. W., Caffe, A. R., & Swaab, D. F. (1985). The vasopressinergic innervation of the brain in normal and castrated rats. *J. Comp. Neurol.* 233:236–254.

63. DeVries, G. J., Crenshaw, B. J., & Ali Al-Shamma, H. (1992). Gonadal steroid modulation of vasopressin pathways. *Ann. N.Y. Acad. Sci.* 652:387–396.

64. Sokol, H. W., & Valtin, H. (eds.) (1982). *The Brattleboro rat*. Special issue of *Ann. N.Y. Acad. Sci.*, vol. 394. New York: New York Academy of Sciences.

65. Koolhaas, J. M., van den Brink, T. H. C., Roozendaal, B., & Boorsma, F. (1990). Medial amygdala and aggressive behavior: Interaction between testosterone and vasopressin. *Aggres. Behav.* 16:223–229.

It is noteworthy that part of testosterone-induced aggression may be mediated by conversion to estrogen. See: Compaan, J. C., Wozniak, A., De Ruiter, A. J., Koolhaas, J. M., & Hutchison, J. B. (1994). Aromatase activity in the preoptic area differs between aggressive and nonaggressive male house mice. *Brain Res. Bull.* 35:1–7.

66. Ferris, C. F. (1992). Role of vasopressin in aggressive and dominant/subordinate behaviors. *Ann. N.Y. Acad. Sci.* 652:212–226.

Ferris, C. F., & Delville, Y. (1994). Vasopressin and serotonin interaction in the control of agonistic behavior. *Psychoneuroendocrinol.* 19:593–601.

67. See n. 66 and: Potegal, M., & Ferris, C. F. (1989). Intraspecific aggression in male hamsters is inhibited by intrahypothalamic vasopressin-receptor antagonists. *Aggres. Behav.* 15:311–320.

68. Gandelman, R. (1980). Gonadal hormones and the induction of intraspecific fighting in mice. *Neurosci. Biobehav. Rev.* 4:130–140.

Kruk, M. R. (1991). Ethology and pharmacology of

hypothalamic aggression. *Neurosci. Biobehav. Rev.* 15:527–538.

69. Testosterone levels have been correlated to intensity of aggression in humans, especially in adolescents (e.g., Dabbs, J. M., Jurkovic, G. J., & Frady, R. L. [1991]. Salivary testosterone and cortisol among late adolescent male offenders. *J. Abnorm. Child. Psychiat.* 19:469–478). However, it has been difficult to demonstrate elevated levels of aggression and subjective anger in normal males given supplementary testosterone (e.g., Bjorkqvist, K., Nygren, T., Björklund, A.-C., & Bjorkqvist, S.-E. [1994]. Testosterone intake and aggressiveness: Real or anticipation? *Aggres. Behav.* 20:17–26). Of course, considering that normal adult males have learned to regulate their aggressive impulses, it would seem far-fetched that they would be prone to report elevated anger or exhibit aggression, unless truly provoked. To my knowledge, such provocation studies remain to be done.

70. The idea that aggression is largely learned has been advocated by:

Scott, J. P. (1958). *Aggression.* Chicago: Univ. of Chicago Press.

Scott, J. P. (1966). Agonistic behavior in mice and rats. *Am. Zool.* 6:683–701.

However, others have had difficulty training animals to fight, and further analysis has indicated that such behavioral traits may be acquired only by animals that have been housed in isolation for a long period. See: Cairns, R. B. (1972). Ontogenetic contributions to aggressive behavior. In *Determinants of behavioral development* (F. J. Monks, W. W. Hartup, & J. de Wit, eds.), pp. 395–400. New York: Academic Press.

71. Booth, A., Shelley, G., Mazure, A., Tharp, G. & Kittok, R. (1989). Testosterone and winning and losing in human competition. *Horm. Behav.* 23:556–571.

Rose, R. M. (1980). Endocrine responses to stressful psychological events. In *Advances in psychoneuroendocrinology* (E. J. Sachar, ed.), pp. 251–276. Philadelphia: Saunders.

72. Mazur, A., & Lamb, T. A. (1980). Testosterone, status, and mood in human males. *Horm. Behav.* 14: 236–246.

73. The effects of estrogen and progesterone are complex, depending on the type of aggression being studied, as well as the developmental stage at which they are administered. For instance, neonatal estrogen masculinizes the brain and increases aggression, while in adulthood estrogen typically reduces aggression. For an overview of the complexities, see: Brain, P. F. (1983). Pituitary-gonadal influences on social aggression. In *Hormones and aggressive behavior* (B. B. Svare, ed.), pp. 3–25. New York: Plenum Press. Also see other chapters in that book.

Also see: Simon, N. G., McKenna, S. E., Lu, S.-F., & Cologer-Clifford, A. (1996). Development and expression of hormonal systems regulating aggression. *Ann. N.Y. Acad. Sci.* 794:8–17.

74. Prescott, J. W. (1971). Early somatosensory deprivation as an ontogenetic process in the abnormal development of brain and behavior. *Proceedings of the Second Conference on Experimental Medicine and Surgery in Primates* (E. I. Goldsmith & J. Mody-Janokowski, eds.), pp. 356–375. Basel: Karger.

In this context, it is worth emphasizing that one of the main ways investigators induce high aggressive tendencies in animals is through long-term social isolation (see n. 26). Without additional research, it cannot be concluded that this is simply due to lack of touch, but it is a possibility worth considering.

75. Hrdy, S. B. (1977). Infanticide as a primate reproductive strategy. *Amer. Sci.* 65:40–49.

Hrdy, S. B. (1979). Infanticide among animals: A review, classification and examination of the implications for the reproductive strategies of females. *Ethol. Sociobiol.* 1:13–40.

76. Mennella, J., & Moltz, H. (1988). Infanticide in rats: Male strategy and female counter-strategy. *Physiol. Behav.* 42:19–28.

77. McCarthy, M. M., Low, L.-M., & Pfaff, D. W. (1992). Speculations concerning the physiological significance of central oxytocin in maternal behavior. *Ann. N.Y. Acad. Sci.* 652:70–82.

78. Goodall, J. (1977). Infant-killing and cannibalism in free-living chimpanzees. *Folia Primatol.* 28: 259–282.

79. Hutchinson, R. R., & Renfrew, J. W. (1978). Functional parallels between the neural and environmental antecedents of aggression. *Neurosci. Biobehav. Revs.* 2:33–58.

80. For a comprehensive summary of drugs, including ß-blockers, that can be used to reduce aggression in children, see: Connor, D. F., & Steingard, R. J. (1996). A clinical approach to the pharmacotherapy of aggression in children and adolescents. *Ann. N.Y. Acad. Sci.* 794:290–307.

81. See n. 17.

Recent work on the neurochemistry of aggression systems is summarized in: Siegel, A., & Schubert, K. (1995). Neurotransmitters regulating feline aggressive behavior. *Revs. Neurosci.* 6:47–61.

Recent brain work has affirmed the ability of alcohol and glutamate systems to potentiate aggression. See:

Schubert, K., Shaikh, M. B., Han, Y., Poherecky, L., & Siegel, A. (1996). Differential effects of ethanol on feline rage and predatory attack behavior: An underlying neural mechanism. *Alcoholism: Clin. Exp. Res.* 20:882–889.

Schubert, K., Shaikh, M. B., & Siegel, A. (1996). NMDA receptors in the midbrain periaqueductal gray mediate hypothalamically evoked hissing behavior in the cat. *Brain Res.* 762:80–90.

The ability of GABA to modulate predatory aggression is summarized in: Han, Y., Shaikh, M. B., & Siegel, A. (1996). Medial amygdaloid suppression of predatory attack behavior in the cat: II. Role of a GABAergic pathway from the medial to the lateral hypothalamus. *Brain Res.* 716:72–83.

82. Shaikh, M. B., Steinberg, A., & Siegel, A. (1993). Evidence that substance P is utilized in medial amygdaloid facilitation of defensive rage behavior in the cat. *Brain Res.* 625:283–294.

It should be noted that this pathway also suppresses quiet-biting attack, further affirming the distinction between the two forms of aggression. See: Han, Y., Shaikh, M. B., & Siegel, A. (1996). Medial amygdaloid suppression of predatory attack behavior in the cat: Role of a substance P pathway from the medial amygdala to the medial hypothalamus. *Brain Res.* 716:59–71.

83. Olivier, B., Mos, J. R., & Rasmussen, D. L. (1991). Behavioral pharmacology of the serenic, eltoprazine. *Drug Metab. Drug Interact.* 8:31–83.

84. Sijbesma, H., Schipper, J., de Kloet, E. R., Most, J., van Aken, H., & Olivier, B. (1991). Postsynaptic 5-HT1 receptors and offensive aggression in rats: A combined behavioural and autoradiographic study with eltoprazine. *Pharmac. Biochem. Behav.* 38:447–458.

85. Valzelli, L., & Bernasconi, S. (1979). Aggressiveness by isolation and brain serotonin turnover changes in different strains of mice. *Neuropsychobiol.* 5:129–135.

86. Bevan, P., Cools, A. R., & Archer, T. (eds.) (1989). *Behavioral pharmacology of 5-HT.* Hillsdale, N.J.: Lawrence Erlbaum.

Fuller, R. W. (1996). Fluoxetine effects on serotonin function and aggressive behavior. *Ann. N.Y. Acad. Sci.* 794:90–97.

Olivier, B., Mos, J., & Rasmussen, D. L. (1990). Offensive aggressive paradigms. *Rev. Drug Metab. Drug Interact.* 8:34–55.

87. It is a well-established finding that as a group, people who commit suicide have low brain serotonin levels. See: Linnoila, V. M., & Virkkunen, M. (1992). Aggression, suicidality and serotonin. *J. Clin. Psychiatry.* 53(suppl.):46–51.

In this context, it is also noteworthy that low plasma cholesterol levels promote suicide in humans and increase aggression in animals, apparently because of reduced brain serotonin production. See: Fontenot, M. B., Kaplan, J. R., Shively, C. A., Manuck, S. B., & Mann, J. J. (1996). Cholesterol, serotonin, and behavior in young monkeys. *Ann. N.Y. Acad. Sci.* 794:352–354.

88. Coccaro, E. F. (1989). Central serotonin and impulsive aggression. *Br. J. Psychiatr.* 155:52–62.

Kruesi, M., Rapoport, J., Hanberger, S., Hibbs, E., Potter, W., Levane, M., & Brown, G. (1990). Cerebrospinal fluid monoamine metabolites, aggression and impulsivity in disruptive behavior disorders of children and adolescents. *Arch. Gen. Psychiat.* 47:419–426.

89. Raleigh, M. J., & McGuire, M. T. (1994). Serotonin, aggression, and violence in vervet monkeys. In *The neurotransmitter revolution* (R. Masters & M. T. McGuire, eds.), pp. 129–145. Carbondale: Southern Illinois Univ. Press.

90. Brown, G. L., Goodwin, F. K., Ballenger, J. C., Goyer, P. F., & Major, L. F. (1979). Aggression in humans correlates with cerebrospinal fluid amine metabolites. *Psychiat. Res.* 1:131–139.

91. Brudzynski, S. M., Eckersdorf, B., & Golebiewski, H. (1993). Emotional-aversive nature of the behavioral response induced by carbachol in cats. *J. Psychiat. Neurosci.* 18:38–45.

MacPhail, E. M., & Miller, N. E. (1968). Cholinergic stimulation in cats: Failure to obtain sleep. *J. Comp. Physiol. Psychol.* 65:499–503.

92. Sometimes such threat displays are not a prelude to aggression. For instance, young opossums exhibit such a response to approach, but one can typically pick them up with impunity. Such brain circuits have been mapped in opossums with ESB. See: Roberts, W. W., Steinberg, M. L., & Means, L. W. (1967). Hypothalamic mechanisms of sexual, aggressive, and other motivational behaviors in the opossum, *Didelphis Virginiana. J. Comp. Physiol. Psychol.* 64:1–15.

93. Bandler, R., Carrive, P., & Zhang, S. P. (1991). Integration of somatic and autonomic reactions within the midbrain periaqueductal grey: Viscerotopic, somatotopic and functional organization. *Prog. Brain Res.* 87:67–154.

Depaulis, A., Keay, K. A., & Bandler, R. (1992). Quiescence and hyporeactivity evoked by activation of cell bodies in the ventrolateral midbrain periaqueductal gray of the rat. *Exp. Brain Res.* 90:75–83.

94. Glutamate appears to be a final common pathway for all emotional behaviors. The powerful ability of glutamate blockade to reduce rage in the PAG has been demonstrated by: Shaikh, M. B., Schubert, K., & Siegel, A. (1994). Basal amygdaloid facilitation of midbrain periaqueductal gray elicited defensive rage behavior in the cat is mediated through NMDA receptors. *Brain Res.* 635:187–195.

95. "Defense motivation" systems have been proposed to exist in the brain, but presently we are still in a semantic quagmire, with different people using such terms in different ways. I believe that defensive behavior is a mixture of activities in FEAR and RAGE systems and do not believe that credible data exist to distinguish those integrative systems from a defense system. Of course, this may be largely a semantic issue (a carryover from the behaviorist era), and some discussion of these points can be found elsewhere. See: Masterson, F. A., & Crawford, M. (1982). The defense motivation system: A theory of avoidance behavior. *Behav. Brain Sci.* 5:661–696.

96. Nelson, R. J., Demas, G. E., Hunag, P. L., Fishman, M. C., Dawson, V. L., Dawson, T. M., & Snyder, S. H. (1995). Behavioral abnormalities in male mice lacking neuronal nitric oxide synthetase. *Nature* 378:383–386.

97. Heath, R. G., Llewellyn, R. C., & Rouchell, A. M. (1980). The cerebellar pacemaker for intractable behavioral disorders and epilepsy: Follow-up report. *Biol. Psychiat.* 15:254–256.

98. Bernston, G. G., & Micco, D. J. (1976). Organization of brainstem behavioral systems. *Brain Res. Bull.* 1:471–483.

99. See n. 98.

100. Pascual-Leone, A., Grafman, J., & Cohen, L. G. (1995). Transcranial magnetic stimulation: A new tool for the study of higher cognitive functions in humans. In *Handbook of neuropsychology* (J. Grafman & F. Boller, eds.). Amsterdam: Elsevier.

101. George, M. S., Wassermann, E. M., Williams,

W. A., Callahan, A., Ketter, T. A., Basser, P., Hallett, M., & Post, R. M. (1995). Daily repetitive transcranial magnetic stimulation (rTMS) improves mood in depression. *Neuroreports* 6:1853–1856.

Pascual-Leone, A., Rubio, B., Pallardo, F., & Catala, M. D. (1996). Rapid-rate transcranial magnetic stimulation of left dorsolateral prefrontal cortex in drug-resistant depression. *Lancet* 348:233–237.

Chapter 11

1. American Psychiatric Association (1994). *Diagnostic and statistical manual of mental disorders, DSM IV*. Washington, D.C.: American Psychiatric Association.

2. The nature of this response is fully described in: Panksepp, J. (1990). The psychoneurology of fear: Evolutionary perspectives and the role of animal models in understanding anxiety. In *Handbook of anxiety*. Vol. 3, *The neurobiology of anxiety* (G. D. Burrows, M. Roth, & R. Noyes, Jr., eds.), pp. 3–58. Amsterdam: Elsevier.

3. For many additional excellent reviews of anxiety from the biological point of view, see other chapters in the book cited in n. 2, as well as the following:

Davis, M., Campeau, S., Kim, M., & Falls, W. A. (1995). Neural systems of emotion: The amygdala's role in fear and anxiety. In *Brain and memory: Modulation and mediation of neuroplasticity* (J. L. McGaugh, N. M. Weinberger, & G. Lynch, eds.), pp. 3–40. New York: Oxford Univ. Press.

Fanselow, M. S. (1994). Neural organization of the defensive behavior system responsible for fear. *Psychon. Bull. Rev.* 1:429–438.

Graeff, F. G., Silveira, M. C. L., Nogueira, R. L., Audi, E. A., & Olivera, R. M. W. (1993). Role of the amygdala and periaqueductal gray in anxiety and panic. *Behav. Brain Res.* 18:123–131.

Johnson, M. R., & Lydiard, R. B. (1995). The neurobiology of anxiety disorders. *Psychiatric Clin. N. Amer.* 18:681–725.

Le Doux, J. E. (1995). Emotion: Clues from the brain. *Ann. Rev. Psychol.* 46:209–235.

Pratt, J. (1992). The neuroanatomical basis of anxiety. *Pharmac. Ther.* 55:149–181.

4. At the present time, most investigators (e.g., see n. 3), conceptualize the FEAR system as simply an output pathway for an integrative system for fear in the amygdala. On the other hand, I have advocated the view that this system is also essential for integrating the entire genetically based fear response, including the affective experiential or subjective experiences of fear.

5. This issue has been discussed extensively by: Panksepp (see n. 2).

6. For a summary of CER procedures, see: Church, R. M. (1972). Aversive behavior. In *Woodworth and Schlosberg's experimental psychology* (J. W. Kling & L. A. Riggs, eds.), pp. 703–742. New York: Holt, Rhinehart and Winston.

7. Davis, M. (1996). Fear-potentiated startle in the study of animal and human emotion. In *Emotion: An interdisciplinary approach* (R. Kavanaugh, B. Zimmerberg, & S. Fine, eds), pp. 61–89. Hillsdale, N.J.: Lawrence Erlbaum.

8. Lang, P. J., Bradley, M. M., & Cuthbert, B. N. (1990). Emotion, attention, and the startle reflex. *Psych. Rev.* 97:377–395.

Lang, P. J. (1995). The emotion probe. *Am. Psychol.* 50:372–385.

9. Graeff, F. G., Guimares, F. S., De Andrade, T. G., & Deakin, J. F. (1996). Role of 5-HT in stress, anxiety, and depression. *Pharmacol. Biochem. Behav.* 54:129–141.

Soubrie, P. (1986). Reconciling the role of central serotonin neurons in human and animal behavior. *Behav. Brain Sci.* 92:319–364.

10. For reviews, see: Bevan, P., Cools, A. R., & Archer, T. (1989). *Behavioural pharmacology of 5-HT*. Hillsdale, N.J.: Lawrence Erlbaum.

11. Gray, J. A. (1982). *The neuropsychology of anxiety: An enquiry into the functions of the septo-hippocampal system*. Oxford: Oxford University Press.

12. These steroid measures are relatively nonspecific for all forms of stress and hence cannot be taken to be specific measures of fear. See: Sapolsky, R. M. (1992). *Stress, the aging brain, and the mechanisms of neuron death*. Cambridge, Mass.: MIT Press.

13. Costall, B., Hendrie, C. A., Kelly, M. E., & Naylor, R. J. (1987). Actions of sulpiride and tiapride in a simple model of anxiety in mice. *Neuropharmacology* 26:195–200.

14. File, S. E. (1987). The contribution of behavioural studies to the neuropharmacology of anxiety. *Neuropharmacology* 26:877–886.

15. Pellow, S., Chopin, P., File, S. E., & Briley, M. (1985). Validation of open:closed arm entries in an elevated plus-maze as a measure of anxiety in the rat. *J. Neurosci. Meth.* 14:149–167.

16. See n. 15 for original BZ plus-maze data. The evaluation of BZs on play suppressed by cat smell remains unpublished but was presented by: Crepeau, L., & Panksepp, J. (1987). Effects of chlordiazepoxide and morphine on CER attenuated juvenile rat play. *Soc. Neurosci. Abst.* 13:1323.

For the long-term effects of cat smell, see Figure 1.1 and: Adamec, R. E., & Shallow, T. (1993). Lasting effects on rodent anxiety of a single exposure to a cat. *Physiol. Behav.* 54:101–109.

17. See n. 16. The fact that the BZ antianxiety agents and opiates have very different profiles on various tests of anxiety strongly suggests the existence of several anxiety-mediating systems in the brain. For a comprehensive review, see n. 2, and for the ability of morphine to actually facilitate avoidance, see: Davis, W. M., & Smith, T. P. (1975). Morphine enhancement of shuttle avoidance prevented by alpha-methyltyrosine. *Psychopharmacologia* 44:95–97.

However, also see: Rodriguez R. (1992). Effect of various psychotropic drugs on the performance of avoidance and escape behaviors in rats. *Pharmacol. Biochem. Behav.* 43:1155–1159.

18. Fanselow, M. S. (1991). Analgesia as a response

to aversive Pavlovian conditional stimuli: Cognitive and emotional mediators. In *Fear, avoidance and phobias: A fundamental analysis* (M. R. Denny, ed.), pp. 61–86. Hillsdale, N.J.: Lawrence Erlbaum.

19. Pinel, J. P. J., & Treit, D. (1978). Burying as a defensive response in rats. *J. Comp. Physiol. Psychol.* 92:708–712.

20. For review, see n. 2. These effects were originally described in: Hess, W. R. (1957). *The functional organization of the diencephalon.* New York: Grune and Stratton.

21. Panksepp, J., Sacks, D. S., Crepeau, L. J., & Abbott, B. B. (1991). The psycho- and neuro-biology of fear systems in the brain. In *Aversive events and behavior* (M. R. Denny, ed.), pp. 7–59. Hillsdale, N.J.: Lawrence Erlbaum.

22. Panksepp, J., Normansell, L., Herman, B., Bishop, P., & Crepeau, L. (1988). Neural and neurochemical control of the separation distress call. In *The physiological control of mammalian vocalizations* (J. D. Newman, ed.), pp. 263–300). New York: Plenum Press.

23. Klein, D. F. (1981). Anxiety reconceptualized. In *Anxiety: New research and changing concepts* (D. F. Klein & J. Rabkin, eds.), pp. 235–264. New York: Raven Press.

24. Although the subjective emotional effects are not well described in DSM-IV (see n. 1), such patterns have been documented using diary reports. See: Oatley, K. (1992). *Best-laid schemes: The psychology of emotions.* New York: Cambridge Univ. Press.

25. Klein, D. F. (1993). False suffocation alarms, spontaneous panics, and related conditions. *Arch. Gen. Psychiat.* 50:306–317.

Gorman, J. M., Liebowitz, M. R., Fyer, A. J., & Stein, J. (1989). A neuroanatomical hypothesis for panic disorder. *Am. J. Psychiatry* 146:148–161.

26. Schweizer, E., Rickels, K., Weiss, S., & Zavodnick, S. (1993). Maintenance drug treatment of panic disorder: I. Results of a prospective, placebo-controlled comparison of alprazolam and imipramine. *Arch. Gen. Psychiat.* 50:51–60.

27. Charney, D. S., Deutch, A. Y., Krystal, J. H., Southwick, S. M., & Davis, M. (1993). Psychobiologic mechanisms of posttraumatic stress disorders. *Arch. Gen. Psychiat.* 50:294–300.

28. Adamec, R. E., & Stark-Adamec, C. (1989). Behavioral inhibition and anxiety: Dispositional, developmental, and neural aspects of the anxious personality of the domestic cat. In *Perspective on behavioral inhibition* (J. Stevens, ed.), pp. 93–124. Chicago: Univ. of Chicago Press.

29. Rosen, J. B., Hamerman, E., Sitcostke, M., Glowa, J. R., & Schulkin, J. (1996). Hyperexcitability: Exaggerated fear-potentiated startle produced by partial amygdala kindling. *Behav. Neurosci.* 110:43–50.

30. Altemus, M. (1995). Neuroendocrinology of obsessive-compulsive disorder. In *Advances in biological psychiatry*, vol. 1 (J. Panksepp, ed.), pp. 215–233. Greenwich, Conn.: JAI Press.

31. Kunovac, J. L., & Stahl, S. M. (1995). Future directions in anxiolytic pharmacotherapy. *Psychiatric Clin. N. Amer.* 18:895–909.

32. For review, see: Puglisi-Allegra, S., & Oliverio, A. (eds.) (1990). *Psychobiology of stress.* Dordrecht: Kluwer Academic.

33. Gorman, J. M., Liebowitz, M. R., Fyer, A. J., & Stein, J. (1989). A neuroanatomical hypothesis for panic disorders. *Am. J. Psychiat.* 146:148–161.

34. Redmond, D. E., & Huang, Y. H. (1979). New evidence for a locus coeruleus norepinephrine connection with anxiety. *Life Sci.* 25:2149–2162.

35. Graeff, F. G., Quintero, S., & Gray, J. A. (1980). Median raphe stimulation, hippocampal theta rhythm and threat-induced behavioural inhibition. *Physiol. Behav.* 25:253–261.

36. See n. 11.

37. Davis, M., Rainnie, D., & Cassell, M. (1994). Neurotransmission in the rat amygdala related to fear and anxiety. *Trends Neurosci.* 17:208–214.

38. Panksepp, J., Gandelman, R., & Trowill, J. (1970). Modulation of hypothalamic self-stimulation and escape behavior by chlordiazepoxide. *Physiol. Behav.* 5:965–969.

39. The idea that such brain stimulation evoked pseudoemotions was first proposed by: Masserman, J. H. (1941). Is the hypothalamus a center of emotion? *Psychosom. Med.* 5:3–25. A thorough review and critique of studies indicating that fear would not condition readily can be found in n. 2.

40. Panksepp, J. (1996). Modern approaches to understanding fear: From laboratory to clinical practice. In *Advances in biological psychiatry*, vol. 2 (J. Panksepp, ed.), pp. 207–228. Greenwich, Conn.: JAI Press.

41. A summary of such affective responses to brain stimulation in humans can be found in: Panksepp, J. (1985). Mood changes. In *Handbook of clinical neurology.* Revised series, vol. 1 (45), *Clinical neuropsychology* (P. J. Vinken, G. W. Buyn, & H. L. Klawans, eds.), pp. 271–285. Amsterdam: Elsevier Science.

42. Le Doux, J. E. (1993). Emotional memory systems in the brain. *Behav. Brain Res.* 58:69–79.

43. Bandler, R., & Shipley, M. T. (1994). Columnar organization in the midbrain periaqueductal gray: Modules for emotional expression. *Trends Neurosci.* 17:379–389.

44. For coverage of these issues, see references cited in nn. 2, 3, and 41.

45. Bolles, R. C., & Fanselow, M. S. (1980). A perceptual-defensive-recuperative model of fear and pain. *Behav. Brain Sci.* 3:291–301.

46. Basbaum, A. I., & Fields, H. L. (1984). Endogenous pain control systems: Brainstem spinal pathways and endorphin circuitry. *Ann. Rev. Neurosci.* 7:309–338.

47. Ohman, A. (1993). Fear and anxiety as emotional phenomena: Clinical phenomenology, evolutionary perspectives, and information-processing mechanisms. In *Handbook of emotions.* (M. Lewis & J. M. Haviland, eds.), pp. 511–536. New York: Guilford Press.

48. Ono T., McNaughton, B. L., Molotchnikoff, S., Rolls, E. T., & Nishijo, H. (eds.) (1996). *Perception, memory and emotion: Frontiers in neuroscience*. Amsterdam: Elsevier.

49. Gray, J. A. (1987). *The psychology of fear and stress*. New York: Cambridge Univ. Press.

50. Aggleton, J. P. (ed.) (1992). *The amygdala: Neurobiological aspects of emotion, memory, and mental dysfunction*. New York: Wiley-Liss.

51. Kapp, B. S., Whalen, P. J., Supple, W. F., & Pascoe, J. P. (1992). Amygdaloid contributions to conditioned arousal and sensory information processing. In *The amygdala: Neurobiological aspects of emotion, memory, and mental dysfunction* (J. P. Aggleton, ed.), pp. 229–245. New York: Wiley-Liss.

52. Hitchcock, J. M., & Davis, M. (1991). Efferent pathway of the amygdala involved in conditioned fear as measured with the fear-potentiated startle paradigm. *Behav. Neurosci.* 104:826–842.

53. Le Doux, J. (1993). Emotional networks in the brain. In *Handbook of emotions* (M. Lewis & J. M. Haviland, eds.), pp. 109–118. New York: Guilford Press.

54. Le Doux, J. E., Cicchetti, P., Xagoraris, A., & Romanski, L. M. (1990). The lateral amygdaloid nucleus: Sensory interface of the amygdala in fear conditioning. *J. Neurosci.* 10:1062–1069.

55. Davis, M. (1992). The role of the amygdala in fear and anxiety. *Ann. Rev. Psychol.* 43:353–375.

56. Le Doux, J. E. (1995). Emotion: Clues from the brain. *Ann. Rev. Psychol.* 46:209–235.

57. Davis, M., Campeau, S., Kim M., & Falls, W. A. (1995). Neural systems of emotion: The amygdala's role in fear and anxiety. In *Brain and memory: Modulation and mediation of neuroplasticity* (J. L. McGaugh, N. M. Weinberger, & G. Lynch, eds.), pp. 3–40. New York: Oxford Univ. Press.

58. Campeau, S., Miserendino, M. J. D., & Davis, M. (1992). Intra-amygdala infusion of the N-methyl-D-aspartate receptor antagonist APV blocks acquisition but not expression of fear-potentiated startle to an auditory conditioned stimulus. *Behav. Neurosci.* 106:569–574.

Fanselow, M. S., & Kim, J. J. (1994). Acquisition of contextual Pavlovian fear conditioning is blocked by application of an NMDA receptor antagonist D,L-2-amino-5-phosphonovaleric acid to the basolateral amygdala. *Behav. Neurosci.* 108:210–212.

59. Chaill, L., Prins, B., Weber, M., & McGaugh, J. L. (1994). ß-Adrenergic activation and memory for emotional events. *Nature* 371:702–704.

60. Fanselow, M. S., Kim, J. J., Yipp, J., & De Oca, P. (1994). Differential effects of the N-methyl-D-aspartate antagonist D,L-2-amino-5-phosphonovalerate on acquisition of fear of auditory and contextual cues. *Behav. Neurosci.* 108:235–240.

Phillips, R. G., & Le Doux, J. E. (1992). Differential contribution of amygdala and hippocampus to cued and contextual fear conditioning. *Behav. Neurosci.* 106:274–285.

61. Falls, W. A., Miserendino, M. J. D., & Davis, M. (1992). Extinction of fear-potentiated startle: Blockade by infusion of an excitatory amino acid antagonist into the amygdala. *J. Neurosci.* 12:854–863.

Le Doux, J. E., Romanski, L. M., & Xagoraris, A. E. (1989). Indelibility of subcortical emotional memories. *J. Cog. Neurosci.*, 1:238–243.

62. Gray, T. S. (1989). Autonomic neuropeptide connections of the amygdala. In *Hans Selye symposia on neuroendocrinology and stress*. Vol. 1, *Neuropeptides and stress* (Y. Tache, J. E. Morley, & M. R. Brown, eds.), pp. 92–106. Berlin: Springer-Verlag.

Smith, G. S. T., Savery, D., Marden, C., Costa, J. J. L., Averill, S., Priestly, J. V., & Rattray, M. (1994). Distribution of messenger RNAs encoding enkephalin, substance P, somatostatin, galanin, vasoactive intestinal polypeptide, neuropeptide Y, and calcitonin gene-related peptide in the midbrain periaqueductal gray in the rat. *J. Comp. Neurol.* 350:23–40.

63. Tallman, J. F., & Gallagher, D. W. (1985). The GABA-ergic system: A locus of benzodiazepine action. *Ann. Rev. Neurosci.* 8:21–44.

64. Young, W. S., & Kuhar, M. J. (1980). Radiohistochemical localization of benzodiazepine receptors in the rat brain. *J. Pharmcol. Exp. Ther.* 212:337–346.

65. Miczek, K. A., Weerts, E. M., Vivian, J. A., & Barros, H. M. (1995). Aggression, anxiety and vocalizations in animals: $GABA_A$ and 5-HT anxiolytics. *Psychopharmacologia* 121:38–56.

66. Olsen, R. W., & Wenter, J. C. (eds.) (1986). *Benzodiazepine/GABA receptors and chloride channels: Structural and functional properties*. New York: Alan R. Liss.

67. Indeed, BZs can selectively reduce arousal of left frontal cortical areas in primates, an electrical pattern that is known to accompany negative affective states in humans. See: Davidson, R. J., Kalin, N. H., & Shelton, S. E. (1992). Lateralized effects of diazepam on frontal brain electrical asymmetries in rhesus monkeys. *Biol. Psychiat.* 32:438–451.

68. Adamec, R. E. (1993). Lasting effect of FG-7142 on anxiety, aggression and limbic physiology in the rat. *J. Neurophysiol.* 7:232–248.

69. Haefely, W. E. (1990). The GABA-benzodiazepine receptor: Biology and pharmacology. In *Handbook of anxiety*. Vol. 3, *The neurobiology of anxiety* (G. D. Burrows, M. Roth, & R. Noyes, Jr., eds.), Amsterdam: Elsevier.

70. Whether DBI is an endogenous inverse agonist anxiety-inducing agent acting at the benzodiazepine receptor remains highly controversial, with little definitive work on the topic. However, the binding of this agent in the brain overlaps extensively with the FEAR system. See: Alho, H., Costa, E., Ferrero, P., Fujimoto, M., Cogenza-Murphy, D., & Guidotti, A. (1985). A neuropeptide located in selected neuronal populations of rat brain. *Science* 229:179–182.

For some of the complexities that have emerged with this putative fear transmitter, see:

Ferrarese, C., Appollonio, I., Bianchi, G., Frigo, M., Marzorati, C., Pecora, N., Perego, M., Pierpaoli, C., & Frattola, L. (1993). Benzodiazepine receptors and diazepam binding inhibitor: A possible link between stress, anxiety and the immune system. *Psychoneuroendocrinol.* 18:3–22.

Weizman, R., & Gavish, M. (1993). Molecular cellular and behavioral aspects of peripheral-type benzodiazepine receptors. *Clin. Neuropharmacol.* 16:401–417.

There are other benzodiazepine inverse agonist candidates on the horizon. See: Rigo, J. M., Belachew, S., Lefebvre, P. P., Leprince, P., Malgrange, B., Rogister, B., Kettenmann, H., & Moonen, G. (1994). Astroglia-released factor shows similar effects as benzodiazepine inverse agonists. *J. Neurosci. Res.* 39:364–376.

71. Panksepp, J. (1986). The neurochemistry of behavior. *Ann. Rev. Psychol.* 37:77–107

72. Charney, D. S., Woods, S. W., Goodman, W. K., & Heninger, G. R. (1987). Serotonin function in anxiety: II. Effects of the serotonin agonist MCPP in panic disorder patients and healthy subjects. *Psychopharmacology* 92:14–24.

73. Eckersdorf, B., Gol biewski, H., & Konopacki, J. (1996). Kainic acid versus carbachol induced emotional-defensive response in the cat. *Behav. Brain Res.* 77:201–210.

74. Bandler, R., & Keay, K. A. (1996). Columnar organization in the midbrain periaqueductal gray and the integration of emotional expression. In *Progress in brain research*, vol. 107 (G. Holstege, R. Bandler, & C. B. Saper, eds.), pp. 285–300. Amsterdam: Elsevier.

75. Panksepp, J. (1993). Neurochemical control of moods and emotions: Amino acids to neuropeptides. In *The handbook of emotions* (M. Lewis & J. Haviland, eds.), pp. 87–107. New York: Guilford Press.

76. Candor, M., Ahmed, S. H., Koob, G. F., Le Moal, M., & Stinus, L. (1992). Corticotropin-releasing factor induces a place aversion independent of its neuroendocrine role. *Brain Res.* 597:304–309.

Dunn, A. J., & Berridge, C. (1990). Physiological and behavioral responses to corticotrophin-releasing factor administration: Is CRF a mediator of anxiety or stress responses? *Brain Res. Revs.* 15:71–100.

Kalin, N. H., & Takahashi, L. K. (1990). Fear-motivated behavior induced by prior shock experience is mediated by corticotropin-releasing hormone systems. *Brain Res.* 509:80–81.

77. Chalmers, D. T., Lovenberg, T. W., Grigoriadis, D. E., Behan, D. P., & De Souza, E. B. (1996). Corticotrophin-releasing factor receptors: From molecular biology to drug design. *Trends Neurosci.* 17: 166–172.

78. Panksepp, J., & Abbott, B. B. (1990). Modulation of separation distress by α-MSH. *Peptides* 11:647–653.

Panksepp, J., & Normansell, L. (1990). Effects of ACTH (1-24) and ACTH/MSH (4-10) on isolation-induced distress vocalization in domestic chicks. *Peptides* 11:915–919.

79. Harro, J., Vasar, E., Koszycki, D., & Bradwejn, J. (1995). Cholecystokinin in panic and anxiety disorders. In *Advances in biological psychiatry,* vol. 1 (J. Panksepp, ed.), pp. 235–262. Greewich, Conn.: JAI Press.

80. Heilig, M., Koob, G. F., Ekman, R., & Britton, K. T. (1994). Corticotropin-releasing factor and neuropeptide Y: Role in emotional integration. *Trends Neursoci.* 17:80–85.

Pedersen, C. A., Caldwell, J. D., Jirikowski, G., & Insel, T. R. (eds.) (1992). *Oxytocin in maternal, sexual, and social behavior.* Special issue of *Ann. N.Y. Acad. Sci.*, vol. 652. New York: New York Academy of Sciences.

81. Kalra, S. P., & Kalra, P. S. (1990). Neuropeptide Y: A novel peptidergic signal for the control of feeding behavior. In *Current topics in neuroendocrinology.* Vol. 10, *Behavioral aspects of neuroendocrinology* (D. Ganten & D. Pfaff, eds.), pp. 191–222. Berlin: Springer-Verlag.

82. Majewska, M. D. (1995). Neuronal actions of dehydroepiandrosterone. *Ann. N.Y. Acad. Sci.* 774:111–120.

Paul, S. M., & Purdy, R. H. (1992). Neuroactive steroids. *FASEB J.* 6:2311–2322.

83. For a history of these pre-benzodiazepine agents, see n. 11. It is noteworthy that most of these older agents are now known to also interact with the BZ-GABA receptor complex.

84. Randall, L. O., Schallek, W., Heise, G. A., Keith, E. F., & Bagdon, R. E. (1960). The psychosedative properties of methaminodiazepoxide. *J. Pharmacol. Exp. Ther.* 129:163–171.

85. Petursson, H., & Lader, M. (1984). *Dependence on tranquilizers.* Oxford: Oxford Univ. Press.

86. Greenblatt, D. J., & Schader, R. I. (1974). *Benzodiazepines in clinical practice.* New York: Raven Press.

87. Costa, E. (ed.) (1983). *The benzodiazepines: From molecular biology to clinical practice.* New York: Raven Press.

88. Muller, W. E. (1987). *The benzodiazepine receptor.* New York: Cambridge Univ. Press.

89. Hindmarch, I., Ott, H., & Roth, D. (eds.) (1984). *Sleep, benzodiazepines and performance.* Berlin: Springer-Verlag.

90. Roy-Byrne, P. P., & Cowley, D. S. (1991). *Benzodiazepines in clinical practice: Risks and benefits.* Washington, D.C.: American Psychiatric Press.

91. Eison, A. S., & Temple, D. L. (1986). Buspirone: Review of its pharmacology and current perspective on its mechanism of action. *Am. J. Med.* 80 (suppl. 3B):1–9.

92. Schweizer, E., Rickels, K., & Lucki, I. (1986). Resistance to the anti-anxiety effect of buspirone in patients with a history of benzodiazepine use. *New Engl. J. Med.* 314:719–720.

93. Stahl, S. M., Gastpar, M., & Keppel Hesselink, J. M. (eds.) (1992). *Serotonin 1_A receptors in depression and anxiety.* New York: Raven Press.

94. Nutt, D. J. (1990). The pharmacology of human anxiety. *Pharmac. Ther.* 47:233–266.

95. Liebowitz, M. R. (1988). Pharmacotherapy of personality disorders. In *Emotions and psychopathology* (M. Clynes & J. Panksepp, eds.), pp. 77–94. New York: Plenum Press.

96. The issue of affective consciousness is considered in Chapter 16. The idea will be developed that the various emotional feelings arise from the influences of emotional command circuits on the basic midbrain representation of an animal as an active creature in the world. Fear is envisioned to reflect a specific type of neurodynamic effect on this system, which promotes a change in bodily motor tone leading to behavior patterns such as those depicted in Figure 11.2.

97. Beck, C. H. M., & Fibiger, H. (1995). Conditioned fear-induced changes in behavior and the expression of the immediate early gene *c-fos*: With and without diazepam pretreatment. *J. Neurosci.* 15:709–720.

Silveira, M. C., Graeff, F. G., & Sandner, G. (1994). Regional distribution of Fos-like immunoreactivity in the rat brain after exposure to fear-inducing stimuli. *Braz. J. Med. Biol. Res.* 27:1077–1081.

Rauch, S. L., Savage, C. R., Alpert, N. M., Miguel, E. C., Baer, L., Breiter, H. C., Fischman, A. J., Manzo, P. A., Moretti, C., & Jenike, M. A. (1995). A positron emission tomographic study of simple phobic symptom provocation. *Arch. Gen. Psychiat.* 52:20–28.

98. Drevets, W. C., Videen, T. O., MacLeod, A. K., Haller, J. W., & Raichle, M. E. (1992). PET images of blood flow changes during anxiety: Correction. *Science* 256:1696.

99. Irwin, W., Davidson, R. J., Lowe, M. J., Mock, F. J., Sorenson, J. A., & Turski, P. A. (1996). Human amygdala activation detected with echo-planar functional magnetic resonance imaging. *NeuroReports* 7:1765–1769.

Ketter, T. A., Adreason, P. J., George, M. S., Lee, C., Gill, D. S., Parekh, P. J., Wills, M. W., Herscovitch, P., & Post, R. M. (1996). Anterior paralimbic mediation of procaine-induced emotional and psychosensory experiences. *Arch. Gen. Psychiat.* 53:59–69.

100. Adolphs, R., Tranel, D., Damasio, H., & Damasio, A. (1994). Impaired recognition of emotion in facial expressions following bilateral damage to the human amygdala. *Nature* 372:669–672.

Bechara, A., Tranel, D., Damasio, H., Adolphs, R., Rockland, C., & Damasio, A. R. (1995). Double dissociation of conditioning and declarative knowledge relative to the amygdala and hippocampus in humans. *Science* 269:1115–1118.

Young, A. W., Hellawell, D. H. J., van de Wal, C., & Johnson, M. (1996). Facial expression processing after amygdalotomy. *Neuropsychologia* 34:31–40.

101. Tranel, D., & Damasio, A. R. (1990). Covert learning of emotional valence in patient Boswell. *J. Clin. Exp. Neuropsych.* 12:27.

Tranel, D., & Damasio, A. R. (1990). The covert learning of affective valence does not require structures in hippocampal system or amygdala. *J. Cog. Neurosci.* 5:79–88.

102. For instance, in association with one of our studies of decorticate animals, we analyzed the contextual freezing response of such animals; even though they exhibited wariness of the environment, they would not stay still in one place like normal animals. See: Deyo, R. A., Panksepp, J., & Abbott, B. (1990). Perinatal decortication impairs performance on an 8-arm radial maze task. *Physiol. Behav.* 11:647–653.

103. The lowest area of the brain where the FEAR response is integrated is the PAG. For a comprehensive source for the many functions of this brain area, see: Depaulis, A., & Bandler, R. (eds.) (1991). *The midbrain periaqueductal gray matter: Functional anatomical and neurochemical organization.* New York: Plenum Press.

104. Schechter, M. D., & Calcagnetti, D. J. (1993). Trends in place preference conditioning with a cross-indexed bibliography, 1957–1991. *Neurosci. Biobehav. Revs.* 17:21–41.

105. London, J. (1963). *White Fang and other stories.* New York: Dodd, Mead.

106. Blanchard, R. J., Yudko, E. B., Rodgers, R. J., & Blanchard, D. C. (1993). Defense system psychopharmacology: An ethological approach to the pharmacology of fear and anxiety. *Behav. Brain Res.* 58:155–156.

107. Panksepp, J., Knutson, B., & Pruitt, D. L. (1998). Toward a neuroscience of emotion: The epigenetic foundations of emotional development. In *What develops in emotional development?* (M. F. Mascolo & S. Griffin, eds.), pp. 53–84. New York: Plenum Press.

Valentine, C. W. (1930). The innate bases of fear. *J. Genet. Psychol.* 37:394–419.

108. Winans, S. S., Lehman, M. N., & Powers, J. B. (1982). Vomeronasal and olfactory CNS pathways that control male hamster mating behavior. In *Olfaction and endocrine regulation* (W. Breipohl, ed.). Oxford: IRL Press.

109. Crepeau, L., & Panksepp, J. (1988). Selective lesions of the dual olfactory system and cat smell attenuate play behavior among juvenile rats. *Neurosci. Abst.* 14:1104.

110. Monti-Bloch, L., Jennings-White, C., Dolberg, D. S., & Berliner, D. L. (1994). The human vomeronasal system. *Psychoneuroendocrinol.* 19:673–686.

Silver, R. (1992). Environmental factors influencing hormone secretion. In *Behavioral endocrinology* (J. B. Becker, S. M. Breedlove, & D. Crews, eds.), pp. 401–422. Cambridge, MA: MIT Press.

Chapter 12

All quotations from Tolstoy's *Kreutzer Sonata* in this chapter are from L. Tolstoy, *The Kreutzer Sonata and Other Tales*, translated by Aylmer Maude (London: Oxford University Press, 1889/1924). Page numbers of quotations are given in the text.

1. Even in species where reproduction occurs by nonsexual parthogenesis, sexual activity continues, apparently as a way to keep the reproductive apparatus healthy. See: Crews, D. (1992). Diversity of hormone-behavior relations in reproductive behavior. In *Behavioral endocrinology* (J. B. Becker, S. M. Breedlove, & D. Crews, eds.), pp. 143–186. Cambridge, Mass.: MIT Press.

2. Buss, D. M. (1994). The strategies of human mating. *Amer. Sci.* 82:238–249.

Buss, D. M. (1994). *The evolution of desire: Strategies of human mating*. New York: Basic Books.

3. Heath, R. G. (1972). Pleasure and brain activity in man. *J. Nerv. Ment. Dis.* 154:3–18.

4. MacLean, P. D., & Ploog, D. W. (1962). Cerebral representation of penile erection. *J. Neurophysiol.* 25:29–55.

The idea that the brain contains an "organ of orgasm" was first introduced by: Davidson, J. M. (1980). The psychobiology of sexual experience. In *The psychobiology of consciousness* (J. M. Davidson & R. J. Davidson, eds.), pp. 271–332. New York: Plenum Press.

5. Carter, S. C., DeVries, A. C., & Getz, L. L. (1995). Physiological substrates of mammalian monogamy: The prairie vole model. *Neurosci. Biobehav. Revs.* 19:303–314.

6. Short, R. V., & Balaban, E. (eds.). *The difference between the sexes*. Cambridge: Cambridge Univ. Press.

One of the few exceptions to the general mammalian pattern of stronger nurturant behavior in mothers is found in titi monkeys. See: Mendoza, S. P., & Mason, W. A. (1997). Attachment relationships in new world primates. *Ann N.Y. Acad. Sci.* 807:203–218.

7. Children without fathers are obviously more common than children without mothers. The fact that nurturance is biologically weaker in fathers than mothers in most mammals is a self-evident aspect of life. See: Barash, D. P. (1976). Some evolutionary aspects of parental behavior in animals and man. *Amer. J. Psychol.* 89:195–217.

This does not mean that decreased nurturance in males cannot be changed through education. See: Gubernick, D. J., & Klopfer, P. H. (eds.) (1981). *Parental care in mammals*. New York: Plenum Press.

8. Just consider the variability in bonding and sexuality patterns among the great apes: Gibbons tend to mate in pairs for life; gorillas tend to be a harem species, with a single silverback having long-term relationships with several females; orangutans come together for sexual activity but then go their separate ways; chimpanzees tend to be rather promiscuous, with dynamic dominance hierarchies and temporary coalitions and pairings guiding the flow of social events. Humans seem to be capable of all these patterns. Still, human males appear to exhibit more devotion to their offspring than do any of the great apes, although gibbon fathers are also remarkably nurturant. See: Yogman, M. W. (1990). Male parental behavior in humans and nonhuman primates. In *Mammalian parenting* (N. A. Krasnegor & R. S. Bridges, eds.), pp. 461–488. New York: Oxford Univ. Press.

9. Muscarella, F., & Cunningham, M. R. (1996). The evolutionary significance and social perception of male pattern baldness and facial hair. *Ethol. Sociobiol.* 17:99–117.

10. Alexander, R. D. (1979). *Darwinism and human affairs*. Seattle: Univ. of Washington Press.

Barlow, G. W., & Silverberg, J. (eds.) (1980). *Sociobiology: Beyond nature/nurture?* Boulder, Colo.: Westview Press.

Trivers, R. (1985). *Social evolution*. Menlo Park, Calif.: Benjamin/Cummings.

11. Berthold, A. A. (1849). Transplantation der Hoden. *Arch. Anat. Physiol. Wissensch. Med.* 42–46.

12. Knobil, E., & Neill, J. D. (eds.) (1988). *The physiology of reproduction*. New York: Raven Press.

13. Baker, R. R., & Bellis, M. A. (1994). *Human sperm competition: Copulation, masturbation and infidelity*. New York: Chapman and Hall.

Batten, M. (1992). *Sexual strategies: How females choose their mates*. New York: Putnam.

14. There are many examples of psychologists' attempts to propose that sexual matters largely reflect issues of environmental stimulation and personal choice rather than neurobiological destiny. Obviously, all these factors are involved, but the desire to deny biological issues is often clever and deceptive. For a recent example of this genera of thought, see: Bem, D. J. (1966). Exotic becomes erotic: A developmental theory of sexual orientation. *Psych. Rev.* 103:320–335.

15. Goodall, J. (1986). *The chimpanzees of Gombe*. Cambridge, Mass.: Harvard Univ. Press.

16. Gur, R. C., Mozley, L. H., Mozley, P. D., Resnick, S. M., Karp, J. S., Alavi, A., Arnold, S. E., & Gur, R. E. (1995). Sex differences in regional cerebral glucose metabolism during a resting state. *Science* 267:528–531.

17. Moore, F. L., & Miller, L. J. (1983). Arginine vasotocin induces sexual behavior of newts by acting on cells in the brain. *Peptides* 4:97–102.

18. De Vries, G. J., Buijs, R. M., Van Leeuwen, F. W., Caffe, A. R., & Swaab, D. F. (1985). The vasopressinergic innervation of the brain in normal and castrated rats. *J. Comp. Neurol.* 233:236–254.

Pedersen, C. A., Caldwell, J. D., Jirikowski, G. F., & Insel, T. R. (eds.) (1992). *Oxytocin in maternal, sexual, and social behaviors*. Special issue of *Ann. N.Y. Acad. Sci.*, vol. 652. New York: New York Academy of Sciences.

19. Caldwell, J. D., Johns, J. M., Faggin, B. M., Senger, M. A., & Pedersen, C. A. (1994). Infusion of an oxytocin antagonist into the medial preoptic area prior to progesterone inhibits sexual receptivity and increases rejection in female rats. *Horm. Behav.* 28: 288–302.

20. Argiolas, A. M., Melis, M. R., Gessa, G. L., & Serra, G. (1988). The oxytocin antagonist d(CH_2)5Tyr (Me)-Orn^8–vasotocin inhibits male copulatory behavior in rats. *Eur. J. Pharmacol.* 149:389–392.

21. Argiolas, A., & Gessa, G. L. (1991). Central functions of oxytocin. *Neurosci. Biobehav. Revs.* 15: 217–231.

22. Of course, such subtle feelings are impossible to measure in animals, but the postejaculatory pause is lengthened by lesioning major oxytocin-containing nuclear groups of the paraventricular nucleus of the hypothalamus. However, this type of damage includes much more than oxytocin neurons, and the fact that the postejaculatory refractory period is decreased by oxytocin treatment in rats (see n. 81) would suggest that oxytocin actually arouses sexuality, which is also suggested by the induction of erections by central injections of oxytocin (see n. 21). However, as is evident (see

n. 23), many peptides exhibit opposite effects at high doses than they do at low doses, which leaves open the possibility that higher doses may provoke postejaculatory behavioral inhibition.

23. Inverted U-shaped functions for peptides are common. For instance, for a long time it has been found that oxytocin is an amnesic peptide, but high doses of peptide were usually employed. When low doses were finally used (see n. 24), oxytocin was found to facilitate social memories. Many other examples exist in the literature. For example, see: Hara, C., & Kastin, A. J. (1986). Biphasic effects of MIF-1 and Tyr-MIF-1 on apomorphine-induced stereotypy in rats. *Pharmacol. Biochem. Behav.* 25:757–761.

24. Popik, P., & van Ree, J. M. (1991). Oxytocin, but not vasopressin, facilitates social recognition following injection into the medial preoptic area of the rat brain. *Eur. J. Neuropsychopharmacol.* 1:555–560.

25. Panksepp, J., Nelson, E., & Bekkedall, M. (1997). Brain systems for the mediation of social separation-distress and social-reward. *Ann. N.Y. Acad. Sci.* 807:78–100.

26. Crews, D. (ed.) (1987). *Psychobiology of reproductive behavior.* Englewood Cliffs, N.J.: Prentice-Hall.

Everitt, B. J., & Bancroft, J. (1991). Of rats and men: The comparative approach to male sexuality. *Ann. Rev. Sex Res.* 2:77–117.

Melis, M. R., & Argiolas, A. (1995). Dopamine and sexual behavior. *Neurosci. Biobehav. Revs.* 19:19–38.

Van Furth, W. R., Wolterink, G., & van Ree, J. M. (1995). Regulation of masculine sexual behavior: Involvement of brain opioids and dopamine. *Brain Res. Revs.* 21:162–184.

27. Hamer, D., & Copeland P. (1994). *The science of desire: The search for the gay gene and the biology of behavior.* New York: Simon and Schuster.

Hamer, D., Hu, S., Magnuson, V. L., Hu, N., & Pattatucci, A. A. (1993). A linkage between DNA markers on the X chromosome and male sexual orientation. *Science* 261:321–327.

LeVay, S., & Hamer, D. H. (1994). Evidence for a biological influence in male homosexuality. *Sci. Amer.* 270:44–49.

28. Swaab, D. F., & Hofman, M. A. (1995). Sexual differentiation of the human hypothalamus in relation to gender and sexual orientation. *Trends Neurosci.* 18:264–270.

Although the biological control of sexual feelings is no doubt profound, the degree of biological control in human sexual practices will remain as debatable as ever until direct evidence is obtained: See n. 14 and:

Byne, W., & Parsons, B. (1993). Human sexual orientation: The biological theories reappraised. *Arch. Gen. Psychiat.* 50:228–239.

Bailey, J. M., & Benishay, D. S. (1993). Familial aggregration of female sexual orientation. *Amer. J. Psychiat.* 150:272–277.

Bailey, J. M., & Pillard, R. C. (1991). A genetic study of male sexual orientation. *Arch. Gen. Psychiat.* 48:1089–1096.

29. Berta, P., Hawkins, J. R., Sinclair, A. H., Taylor, A., Griffiths, B. L., & Goodfellow, P. N. (1990). Genetic evidence equating SRY and the testis-determining factor. *Nature* 348:448–450.

30. Toran-Allerand, C. D. (1984). On the genesis of sexual differentiation of the central nervous system: Morphogenetic consequences of steroidal exposure and possible role of α-fetoprotein. In *Sex differences in the brain.* Special issue of *Prog. Brain Res.* (G. J. De Vries, J. P. C. De Bruin, H. B. M. Uylings, & M. A. Corner, eds.) 61:63–98.

31. Breedlove, S. M. (1992). Sexual differentiation of the brain and behavior. In *Behavioral endocrinology* (J. B. Becker, S. M. Breedlove, & D. Crews, eds.), pp. 39–70. Cambridge, Mass.: MIT Press.

Le Vay, S. (1993). *The sexual brain.* Cambridge, Mass.: MIT Press.

32. Gorski, R. A. (1988). Sexual differentiation of the brain: Mechanisms and implications for neuroscience. In *From message to mind: Direction in developmental neurobiology* (S. S. Easter, Jr., K. F. Barald, & B. M. Carlson, eds.), pp. 256–271. Sunderland, Mass.: Sinauer.

33. Ehrhardt, A. A., Meyer-Bahlburg, H. F. L., Rosen, L. R., Feldman, J. F., Veridiano, N. P., Zimmerman, I., & McEwen, B. S. (1985). Sexual orientation after prenatal exposure to exogenous estrogen. *Arch. Sex. Behav.* 14:57–78.

34. Imperato-McGinley, J., Peterson, R. E., Gautier, T., & Sturla, E. (1979). Androgens and the evolution of male-gender identity among male pseudohermaphrodites with 5-alpha-reductase deficiency. *N. Eng. J. Med.* 300:1233–1237.

35. Kincl, F. A. (1990). *Hormone toxicity in the newborn.* Berlin: Springer-Verlag.

36. See nn. 14 and 28 for discussion of key issues. But note that some believe that morally reprehensible behaviors such as child abuse and rape may have evolutionary adaptive value. See: Palmer, C. T. (1991). Human rape: Adaptation or by-product? *J. Sex Res.* 28:365–386.

37. Zhou, J.-N., Hofman, M. A., Gooren, L. J. G., & Swaab, D. F. (1995). A sex difference in the human brain and its relation to transsexuality. *Nature* 378: 68–70.

38. Shaywitz, B. A., Shaywitz, S. E., Pugh, K. R., Constable, R. T., Skudlarski, P., Fulbright, R. K., Bronen, R. A., Fletcher, J. M., Shankweller, D. P., Katz, L., & Gore, J. C. (1995). Sex differences in the functional organization of the brain for language. *Nature* 373: 607–609.

Witelson, S. F. (1991). Neural sexual mosaicism: Sexual differentiation of the human temporo-parietal region for functional asymmetry. *Psychoneuroendocrinol.* 16:131–153.

39. See n. 32. The original paper demonstrating this difference in rats was: Gorski, R. A., Bordon, J. H., Shyrne, J. E., & Southam, A. M. (1978). Evidence for a morphological sex difference within the medial preoptic area of the rat brain. *Brain Res.* 143:333–346.

40. Allen, L. S., Hines, M., Shryne, J. E., & Gorski, R. A. (1989). Two sexually dimorphic cell groups in the human brain. *J. Neurosci.* 9:497–506.

Le Vay, S. (1991). A difference in hypothalamic structure between heterosexual and homosexual men. *Science* 253:1034–1037.

41. Heimer, L., & Larsson, K. (1966–1967). Impairment of mating behavior in male rats following lesions in the preoptic-anterior hypothalamic continuum. *Brain. Res.* 3:248–263.

42. Twiggs, D. G., Popolow, H. B., & Gerall, A. A. (1978). Medial preoptic lesions and male sexual behavior: Age and environmental interactions. *Science* 200: 1414–1415.

Leedy, M. G., Vela, E. A., Popolow, H. B., & Gerall, A. A. (1980). Effect of prepubertal medial preoptic area lesions on male rat sexual behavior. *Physiol. Behav.* 24:341–346.

43. Leedy, M. G., & Hart, B. L. (1986). Medial preoptic-anterior hypothalamic lesions in prepubertal male cats: Effects on juvenile and adult sociosexual behaviors. *Physiol. Behav.* 36:501–506.

44. Baum, M. J. (1992). Neuroendocrinology of sexual behavior in the male. In *Behavioral endocrinology* (J. B. Becker, S. M. Breedlove, & D. Crews, eds.), pp. 97–130. Cambridge, Mass.: MIT Press.

45. Oomura, Y., Yoshimatsu, H., & Aou, S. (1983). Medial preoptic and hypothalamic neuronal activity during sexual behavior. *Brain Res.* 266:340–343.

Aou, S., Oomura, Y., & Yoshimatsu, H. (1988). Neuron activity of the ventromedial hypothalamus and the medial preoptic area of the female monkey during sexual behavior. *Brain Res.* 455:65–71.

46. Blaustein, J. D., & Olster, D. H. (1989). Gonadal steroid hormone receptors and social behaviors. In *Advances in comparative and environmental physiology*. Vol. 3, *Molecular and cellular basis of social behavior in vertebrates* (J. Balthazart, ed.), pp. 31–104. Berlin: Springer-Verlag.

It should also be noted that a reversal of male- and female-typical cognitive skills in humans has recently been achieved by cross-sex administration of hormones, presumably because of the existence of the appropriate receptors at maturity. See: Van Goozen, S. H., Cohen-Kettenis, P. T., Gooren, L. J., Frijda, N. H., & Van de Poll, N. E. (1995). Gender differences in behaviour: activating effects of cross-sex hormones. *Psychoneuroendocrinol.* 20:343–363.

47. Clark, A. S., Davis, L. A., & Roy, E. J. (1985). A possible physiological basis for the dud-stud phenomenon. *Horm. Behav.* 19:227–230.

48. Newman, S. W., Parfitt, D. B., & Kollack-Walker, S. (1997). Mating-induced *c-fos* expression patterns complement and supplement observations after lesions in the male Syrian hamster brain. *Ann. N.Y. Acad. Sci.* 807:239–259.

49. Breedlove, S. M., & Arnold, A. A. (1980). Hormone accumulation in a sexually dimorphic motor nucleus of the rat spinal cord. *Science* 210:564–566.

Breedlove, S. M. (1992). Sexual dimorphism in the vertebrate nervous system. *J. Neurosci.* 12:4133–4142.

Gerall, A. A., Moltz, H., & Ward, I. L. (eds.) (1992). *Sexual differentiation*. Vol. 11, *Handbook of behavioral neurobiology*. New York: Plenum Press.

50. Archer, J. (1975). Rodent sex differences in emotional and related behavior. *Behav. Biol.* 14:451–479.

Beatty, W. W. (1979). Gonadal hormones and sex differences in nonreproductive behaviors in rodents: Organizational and activational influences. *Horm. Behav.* 12:112–163.

For a discussion of gender differences in feeding and energy balance regulation, see: Nance D. M. (1983). The developmental and neural determinants of the effects of estrogen on feeding behavior in the rat: a theoretical perspective. *Neurosci. Biobehav. Revs.* 7:189–211.

51. Of course, evolutionary speculations concerning the adapative functions of behavioral traits can never be proved, but the increased incidence of homosexual and bisexual male offspring from stressed mothers is well documented, at least in laboratory rats. See: Ward, I. L. (1984). The prenatal stress syndrome: Current status. *Psychoneuroendocrinol.* 9:3–11.

52. Kinsley, C. H., & Bridges, R. S. (1988). Prenatal stress and maternal behavior in intact virgin rats: Response latencies are decreased in males and increased in females. *Horm. Behav.* 22:76–89.

53. Ward, I. L., & Ward, O. B. (1985). Sexual behavior differentiation: Effects of prenatal manipulations in rats. In *Handbook of behavioral neurobiology*, vol. 7 (N. Adler, D. Pfaff, & R. W. Goy, eds.), pp. 77–98. New York: Plenum Press.

Ward, I. L. (1992). Sexual behavior: The product of perinatal hormonal and prepubertal social factors. In *Sexual differentiation*. Vol. 11, *Handbook of behavioral neurobiology* (A. A. Gerall, H. Moltz, & I. L. Ward, eds.), pp. 157–178. New York: Plenum Press.

54. Jacobson, C. D., & Gorski, R. A. (1981). Neurogenesis of the sexually dimorphic nucleus of the preoptic area in the rat. *J. Comp. Neurol.* 196:519–529.

55. Ward, O. B., Monaghan, E. P., & Ward, I. L. (1986). Naltrexone blocks the effects of prenatal stress on sexual behavior differentiation in male rats. *Pharmacol. Biochem. Behav.* 25:573–576.

56. Neonatal opiate exposure has been found to enhance feminine sexual behavior in male hamsters. See: Johnston, H. M., Payne, A. P., & Gilmore, D. P. (1992). Perinatal exposure to morphine affects adult sexual behavior of the male golden hamster. *Pharmac. Biochem. Behav.* 42:41–44.

However, male rats have not been affected this way by prenatal morphine exposure, even though sexual behavior of females was diminished. See: Vathy, I. U., Etgen, A. M., & Barfield, R. J. (1985). Effects of prenatal exposure to morphine on the development of sexual behavior in rats. *Pharmac. Biochem. Behav.* 22:227–232.

57. Kinsley, C. H. (1990). Prenatal and postnatal influences on parental behavior in rodents. In *Mammalian parenting: Biochemical, neurobiological and behavioral determinants* (N. S. Krasnegor & R. S. Bridges, eds.), pp. 347–371. New York: Oxford Univ. Press.

However, it is noteworthy that sex differences in nurturant tendencies among juvenile rats tend to disappear with repeated testing experience. See: Pellegrini, V., & Dessi-Fulgheri, F. (1994). Sex differences in maternal behaviors of immature rats: The role of emotionality. *Aggress. Behav.* 20:257–265.

58. Rosenblatt, J. S. (1967). Nonhormonal basis of maternal behavior in the rat. *Science* 156:1512–1514.

59. Dorner, G., Geier, T., Ahrens, L., Krell, L., Munx, G., Sieler, H., Kittner, E., & Muller, H. (1980). Prenatal stress as possible aetiogenetic factor of homosexuality in human males. *Endokronologie* 75:365–368.

60. Herrenkohl, L. R. (1986). Prenatal stress disrupts reproductive behavior and physiology in offspring. *Ann. N.Y. Acad. Sci.* 474:120–128.

61. Quotation by I. L. Ward, n. 51, p. 9.

62. Money, J. (1987). Human sexology and psychoneuroendocrinology. In *Psychobiology of reproductive behavior* (D. Crews, ed.), pp 323–343. Englewood Cliffs, N.J.: Prentice-Hall.

63. See n. 48.

64. Baker, R. (1996). *Sperm wars: Infidelity, sexual conflict and other bedroom battles*. London: Fourth Estate.

65. For descriptions of male and female sexual behaviors, see nn. 44 and 67.

66. McClintock, M. K. (1987). A functional approach to the behavioral endocrinology of rodents. In *Psychobiology of reproductive behavior* (D. Crews, ed.), pp. 176–203. Englewood Cliffs, N.J.: Prentice-Hall.

67. Pfaff, D. W. (1980). *Estrogens and brain function: Neural analysis of a hormone-controlled mammalian reproductive behavior*. New York: Springer-Verlag.

68. Steinach, E. (1940). *Sex and life: Forty years of biological and medical experiments*. New York: Viking.

For a full description of the sexual motivation of the female rat, see n. 67 and: Meyerson, B. J., & Lindstrom, L. H. (1973). Sexual motivation in the female rat. *Acta Physiol. Scand.* (suppl. 389):1–80.

69. Pfaff, D. W., & Schwartz-Giblin, S. (1988). Cellular mechanisms of female reproductive behaviors. In *The physiology of reproduction* (E. Knobil & J. Neill, eds.), pp. 1487–1568. New York: Raven Press.

70. Recently it has been found that when the excess body weight of genetically obese *ob/ob* mice is reduced with injections of leptin (see Chapter 9), fertility is markedly increased. See: Chehab, F. F., Lim, M. E., & Ronghua, L. (1996). Correction of the sterility defect in homozygous obese female mice by treatment with the recombinant human ob protein. *Nature Genet.* 12: 318–320.

71. Adler, N. T. (ed.) (1981). *Neuroendocrinology of reproduction: Physiology and behavior*. New York: Plenum Press.

72. Morris, N., Udry, J., Khan-Dawood, F., & Dawood, M. (1987). Marital sex frequency and midcycle female testoterone. *Arch. Sex. Behav.* 16:27–37.

73. See n. 18. The testosterone controls of such neuropeptide expression are evident in more ancient animals, such as lizards and birds, that possess only the vasopressin precursor, vasotocin. See: Stoll, C. J., & Voorn, P. (1985). The distribution of hypothalamic and extrahypothalamic vasotocinergic cells and fibers in the brain of a lizard, *Gekko gecko*: Presence of a sex difference. *J. Comp. Neurol.* 239:193–204.

74. It is currently believed that the reduction in sexual activity following POA lesions is due largely to deficiencies in physical rather than psychological arousal. Rhesus monkeys with such lesions lose their copulatory activity, but they are apparently aroused by females and have been observed to continue masturbation. See: Slimp, J. C., Hart, B. L., & Goy, R. W. (1975). Heterosexual, autosexual and social behavior of adult male rhesus monkeys with medial preoptic-anterior hypothalamic lesions. *Brain Res.* 142:105–122.

Also, rats with such lesions continue to work for access to receptive females even though they are no longer able to copulate. See: Everitt, B. J. (1990). Sexual motivation: A neural and behavioral analysis of the mechanisms underlying appetitive and copulatory responses of male rats. *Neurosci. Biobehav. Rev.* 14: 217–232.

75. Davidson, J. M. (1966). Activation of male rat's sexual behavior by intracerebral implantation of androgen. *Endocrinol.* 79:783–794.

Kierniesky, N. C., & Gerall, A. A. (1973). Effects of testosterone propionate implants in the brain on the sexual behavior and peripheral tissue of the male rat. *Physiol. Behav.* 11:633–640.

76. Sachser, N., Lick, C., & Stanzel, K. (1994). The environment, hormones, and aggressive behaviour: A 5-year-study in guinea pigs. *Psychoneuroendocrinology* 19:697–707.

Schurman, T. (1980). Hormonal correlates of agonistic behavior in adult male rats. In *Adaptive capabilities of the nervous system* (P. S. McConnell, G. J. Boer, H. J. Romijin, N. E. van de Poll, & M. A. Corner, eds.). Amsterdam: Elsevier/North Holland.

77. Sokol, H. W., & Valtin, H. (eds.) (1982). *The Brattleboro rat*. Special issue of *Ann. N.Y. Acad. Sci.*, vol. 394. New York: New York Academy of Sciences.

78. Sodersten, P., Henning, M., Melin, P., & Ludin, S. (1983). Vasopressin alters female sexual behaviour by acting on the brain independently of alterations in blood pressure. *Nature* 301:608–610.

79. Landgraf, R., Neumann, I., Russell, J. A., & Pittman, Q. J. (1992). Push-pull perfusion and microdialysis studies of central oxytocin and vasopressin release in freely moving rats during pregnancy, parturition, and lactation. *Ann. N.Y. Acad. Sci.* 652:326–339.

80. Jirikowski, G. F., Caldwell, J. D., Pilgrim, C., Stumpf, W. E., & Pedersen, C. A. (1989). Changes in immunostaining of oxytocin in the forebrain of the female rat during late pregnancy, parturition and early lactation. *Cell Tissue Res.* 256:411–417.

81. The suggestion that oxytocin may promote sexual satisfaction may seem contradictory with some of the available behavioral data. Most data indicate that oxytocin promotes both male and female sexual arousal: Male sexuality is dramatically reduced by blocking the brain oxytocin system (see n. 20), and so is the receptivity of female rats (see n. 19). Furthermore, precopulatory oxytocin tends to facilitate sexuality, especially in sluggish animals. See: Arletti, R., Benelli, A., & Bertolini, A. (1992). Oxytocin involvement in male and female sexual behavior. *Ann. N.Y. Acad. Sci.* 652:180–193.

The supposition made here is that the increase of oxytocin after orgasm promotes emotional-erotic satisfaction, but this state also has the intrinsic potential to promote additional sexual activity. In any event, it is well known that oxytocin is also released at orgasm in humans. See: Richard, P., Moos, F., & Freund-Mercier, M.-J. (1991). Central effects of oxytocin. *Physiol. Rev.* 71:331–370.

82. Carter, C. S. (1992). Oxytocin and sexual behavior. *Neurosci. Biobehav. Revs.* 16:131–144.

83. Johnson, A. E. (1992). The regulation of oxytocin receptor binding in the ventromedial hypothalamic nucleus by gonadal steroids. *Ann. N.Y. Acad. Sci.* 652:357–373.

Schumacher, M., Coirini, H., Flanagan, L. M., Frankfurt, M., Pfaff, D. W., & McEwen, B. S. (1992). Ovarian steroid modulation of oxytocin receptor binding in the ventromedial hypothalamus. *Ann. N.Y. Acad. Sci.* 652:374–386.

84. Caldwell, J. D., Barakat, A. S., Smith, D. D., Hruby, V. J., & Pedersen, C. A. (1990). A uterotonic antagonist blocks the oxytocin-induced facilitation of female sexual receptivity. *Brain Res.* 103:655–662.

85. See n. 19.

86. See n. 20.

87. Carmichael, M. S., Humbert, R., Dixen, J., Palmiana, G., Greenleaf, W., & Davidson, J. M. (1987). Plasma oxytocin increase in the human sexual response. *J. Clin. Endocrinol. Metab.* 64:27–31.

Murphy, M. R., Seckl, J. R., Burton, S., Checkley, S. A., & Lightman, S. L. (1990). Changes in oxytocin and vasopressin secretion during sexual activity in men. *J. Clin. Endocrinol. Metab.* 65:738–741.

More recently, it has been found that in multiorgasmic women, there is a positive relationship between the subjective intensity of orgasm and the amount of oxytocin secretion: Carmichael, M. S., Warburton, V. L., Dixen, J., & Davidson, J. M. (1994). Relationships among cardiovascular, muscular, and oxytocin responses during human sexual activity. *Arch. Sex. Behav.* 23:59–79.

However, it should also be noted that blocking opioid secretion inhibits the orgasm-related oxytocin secretion and significantly diminishes the subjective arousal and pleasure that is experienced: Murphy, M. R., Checkley, S. A., Seckl, J. R., & Lightman, S. L. (1990). Naloxone inhibits oxytocin release at orgasm in man. *J. Clin. Endocrinol. Metab.* 71:1056–1058.

88. Winslow, J. T., Hastings, N., Carter, C. S., Harbaugh, C. R., & Insel, T. R. (1993). A role for central vasopressin in pair bonding in mongamous prairie voles. *Nature* 365:544–548.

89. Moss, R. L., & Dudley, C. A. (1984). The challenge of studying the behavioral effects of neuropeptides. In *Handbook of psychopharmacology*, vol. 18 (L. L. Iversen, S. D. Iversen, & S. H. Snyder, eds.), pp. 397–454. New York: Plenum Press.

90. Ågmo, A., & Berenfeld, R. (1990). Reinforcing properties of ejaculation in the male rat: Role of opioids and dopamine. *Behav. Neurosci.* 104:177–182.

It is noteworthy that copulation-induced place preference is also evident in female rats, but this requires sexual priming. See: Oldenburger, W. P., Everitt, B. J., & de Jonge, F. H. (1992). Conditioned place preference induced by sexual interaction in female rats. *Horm. Behav.* 26:214–228.

Other evidence also suggests that female rats do regard sexual activity as a positive incentive. See: Johnson, W. A., (1977). Female rats' self-paced responding for artificial sexual stimulation. *Behav. Biol.* 21:405–411.

91. Ågmo, A., & Gomez, M. (1993). Sexual reinforcement is blocked by infusion of naloxone into the medial preoptic area. *Behav. Neurosci.* 107:812–818.

92. Burger, H., Hailes, J., Nelson, J., & Menelaus, M. (1987). Effect of combined implants of estradiol and testosterone on libido in postmenopausal women. *Br. Med. J.* 294:936–939.

Sherwin, B. B., & Gelfand, M. (1987). Differential symptom response to parenteral estrogen and/or androgen administration in the surgical menopause. *Amer. J. Obst. Gynecol.* 151:153–162.

In this context, it is also worth noting that male sexuality may be critically dependent on estrogen receptors in the brain (Roselli, C. E., Thornton, J. E., & Chambers, K. C. [1993]. Age-related deficits in brain estrogen receptors and sexual behavior of male rats. *Behav. Neurosci.* 107:202–209), and the sensitivity of vasopressin within the POA is dependent on levels of circulating estrogen (Huhman, K. L., & Albers, H. E. [1993]. Estradiol increases the behavioral response to arginine vasopressin [AVP] in the medial preoptic-anterior hypothalamus. *Peptides* 14:1049). These complex interdependencies, along with the aforementioned effects of oxytocin (see n. 81), highlight how intertwined are the biological underpinnings of male and female sexuality.

93. Nottebohm, F. (1984). Birdsong as a model in which to study brain processes related to learning. *The Condor* 86:227–236.

94. Alvarez-Buylla, A., Theelen, M., & Nottebohm, F. (1988). Birth of projection neurons in the higher vocal center of the canary forebrain before, during, and after song learning. *Proc. Natl. Acad. Sci.* 85:8722–8726.

Nordeen, K., & Nordeen E. J. (1988). Projection neurons within a vocal motor pathway are born during song learning in zebra finches. *Nature* 334:149–151.

95. Volman, S. F., & Khanna, H. (1995). Convergence of untutored song in group-reared zebra finches. *J. Comp. Psych.* 109:211–221.

96. Unfortunately, all such claims have been made in anectodal reports at scientific meetings, and there appears to be no systematic study of this effect. However, a great number of intranasal oxytocin studies have been done, where no such effect has been reported (albeit questions concerning genital arousal had not beer asked). For example, see: Fehm-Wolfsdorf, G., & Born, J. (1991). Behavioral effects of neurohypophyseal peptides in healthy volunteers: 10 years of research. *Peptides* 12:1399–1406.

97. For a review of the many agents that can modify human sexuality, see:

Crenshaw, T., & Goldberg, J. P. (1996). *Sexual pharmacology: Drugs that affect sexual functioning.* New York: Norton.

Riley, A. J., & Wilson, C. (eds.) (1993). *Sexual pharmacology.* New York: Oxford Univ. Press.

98. Knoll, J. (1992). (-)Deprenyl-medication: A strategy to modulate the age-related decline of the striatal dopaminergic system. *J. Amer. Geriat. Soc.* 40:839–847.

99. Kreutz, L. E., Rose, R. M., & Jennings, J. R. (1972). Suppression of plasma testosterone levels and psychological stress. *Arch. Gen. Psychiat.* 26:479–483.

Mazur, A., & Lamb, T. A. (1980). Testosterone, status, and mood in human males. *Horm. Behav.* 14:236–246.

100. McClintock, M. K. (1983). Synchronizing ovarian and birth cycles by female phermones. In *Chemical signals in vertebrates*, vol. 3 (D. Muller-Schwarze & R. M. Siverstein, eds.), pp. 159–178. New York: Plenum Press.

101. McClintock, M. K. (1983). Phermonal regulation of the ovarian cycle: Enhancement, suppression and synchrony. In *Pheromones and reproduction in mammals* (J. G. Vandenbergh, ed.), pp. 113–149. New York: Academic Press.

102. For a review of the many lines of evidence for olfactory control of human reproduction, as well as that of other primate species, see Chapter 13 and: Surbey, M. K. (1990). Family composition, stress, and the timing of human menarche. In *Socioendocrinology of primate reproduction* (T. E. Ziegler & F. B. Bercovitch, eds.), pp. 11–32. New York: Wiley-Liss.

Chapter 13

1. Burton, R. (1621/1927). *The anatomy of melancholy.* New York: Tudor Pub. Co. Quotation on p. 284.

2. Balikci, A. (1970). *The Netsilik eskimo.* New York: Natural History Press.

3. For a description of the Digo way of child rearing, see: De Vries, M. W., & Sameroff, A. J. (1984). Culture and temperament: Influences on infant temperament in 3 East African societies. *Am. J. Orthopsychiat.* 54:83–96.

Certainly, communities that do not allow risk factors to accumulate—poverty, domestic violence, drug and sexual abuse, the absence of male nurturance—are more likely to have successful children than those in which individuals are less accountable for their actions. The opportunities provided by society open doors to healthy growth in children, but at the foundation of all such endeavors there must exist an abundance of individual feelings of nurturance. A discussion of such issues for raising children in America has been put forth by: Clinton, H. R. (1996). *It takes a village: And other lessons children teach us.* New York: Simon and Schuster.

4. Bartholomew, K. (1993). From childhood to adult relationships: Attachment theory and research. In *Learning about relationship* (S. Duck, ed.), pp. 30–62. Newbury Park, Calif.: Sage.

Bowlby, J. (1988). *A secure base: Parent-child attachment and healthy human development.* New York: Basic Books.

5. For popular summaries of the discovery of brain opioids, see:

Davis, J. (1984). *Endorphins: New waves in brain chemistry.* Garden City, N.Y.: Dial Press.

Goldberg, J. (1988). *Anatomy of a scientific discovery: The race to discover the secret of human pain and pleasure.* New York: Bantam Books.

Levinthal, C. F. (1988). *Messengers of paradise: Opiates and the brain.* New York: Doubleday.

6. Rosenblatt, J. S. (1990). Landmarks in the physiological study of maternal behavior with special reference to the rat. In *Mammalian parenting* (N. A. Krasnegor & R. S. Bridges, eds.), pp. 40–60. New York: Oxford Univ. Press.

Rosenblatt, J. S., Siegel, H. I., & Mayer, A. D. (1979). Progress in the study of maternal behavior in the rat: Hormonal, nonhormonal, sensory, and developmental aspects. In *Advances in the study of behavior*, vol. 10 (J. S. Rosenblatt, R. A. Hinde, C. G. Beer, & M.-C. Busnel, eds.), pp. 225–311. New York: Academic Press.

7. There is an abundance of data indicating that the smell of home is a potent alleviator of separation distress in rodents. Indeed, animals will rapidly learn to navigate a maze to be close to their homes, even though their mothers are not there. See: Panksepp, J., & DeEskinazi, F. G. (1980). Opiates and homing. *J. Comp. Physiol. Psychol.* 94:650–663.

8. Although there are bound to be other key brain chemistries that we do not yet know about, molecules such as opioids, oxytocin and prolactin are the most reasonable candidates as key mediators of social bonding. See: Panksepp, J., Nelson, E., & Bekkedal, M. (1997). Brain systems for the mediation of social separation-distress and social-reward: Evolutionary antecedents and neuropeptide intermediaries. *Ann. N. Y. Acad. Sci.* 807:78–100.

9. Nyberg, F., Linstrom, L. H., & Terenius, L. (1988). Reduced ß-casein levels in milk samples from patients with postpartum psychosis. *Biol. Psychiat.* 23: 115–122.

10. An endogenous opioid theory of autism was first suggested by: Panksepp, J. (1979). A neurochemical theory of autism. *Trends Neurosci.* 2:174–177.

The most recent support for such a theory at the present time, at least for the treatment of children, is to be found in: Bouvard, M. P., Leboyer, M., Launay, J. M., Recasens, C., Plumet, M.-H., Waller-Perotte, D., Tabuteau, F., Bondoux, D., Dugas, M., Lensing, P., & Panksepp, J. (1995). Low-dose naltrexone effects on plasma chemistries and clinical symptoms in autism: A double-blind, placebo-controlled study. *Psychiat. Res.* 58:191–201

Kolmena, B. K., Feldman, H. M., Handsen, B. L., &

Janosky, J. E. (1995). Naltrexone in young autistic children: A double-blind, placebo-controlled crossover study. *J. Am. Acad. Child Adolesc. Psychiat.* 34:223–231.

However, some have not found increases in social behavior, but the doses used were quite high. See: Willemsen-Swinkels, S. H., Buitelaar, J. K. , Weijnen, F. G., & van Engeland, H. (1995). Placebo-controlled acute dosage naltrexone study in young autistic children. *Psychiat. Res.* 58:203–215.

Evidence that casomorphins may be one factor in the disorder has been provided by: Reichelt, K.-L., Scott, H., Knivsberg, A.-M., Wiig, K., Lind, G., & Nødland, M. (1990). Childhood autism: A group of hyperpeptidergic disorders. Possible etiology and tentative treatment. In *B-casomorphins and related peptides* (F. Nyberg & V. Brantl, eds.), pp. 163–173. Uppsala: Fyris-Tryck.

11. There are now many studies indicating that the separation calls of young animals arouse parents, especially mothers, into action. One of the first studies was by: Pettijohn, T. F. (1977). Reaction of parents to recorded infant guinea pig distress vocalizations. *Behav. Biol.* 21:438–442.

12. Jacob, F. (1977). Evolution and tinkering. *Science* 196:1161–1166. Quotation on pp. 1163–1164.

13. The secure-base concept was first developed by: Ainsworth, M. D. S., Blehar, M., Waters, E., & Wall, S. (1978). *Patterns of attachment: Strange situation behavior of one year olds.* Hillsdale, N.J.: Lawrence Erlbaum.

The fact that early abuse can have permanent effects on the brain has been highlighted recently by long-term deficits in short-term memory abilities. See: Bremner, J. D., Randall, P., Scott, T. M., Capelli, S., Delaney, R., McCarthy, G., & Charney, D. S. (1995). Deficits in short-term memory in adult survivors of childhood abuse. *Psychiat. Res.* 59:97–107.

Specific brain changes have also been documented in combat veterans with PTSD. See: Bremner, J. D., Randall, P., Scott, T. M., Bronen, R. A., Seibyl, J. P., Southwick, S. M., Delaney, R. C., McCarthy, G. Charney, D. S., & Innis, R. B. (1995). MRI-based measurement of hippocampal volume in patients with combat-related posttraumatic stress disorder. *Am. J. Psychiat.* 152:973–981.

14. Figler, R. A., MacKenzie, D. S., Owens, D. W., Licht, P., & Amoss, M. S. (1989). Increased levels of arginine vasotocin and neurophysin during nesting in sea turtles. *Gen. Comp. Endocrinol.* 73:223–232.

The fact that similar neurochemical events transpire in mammals is indicated by work by: Kendrick, K. M., & Keverne, E. (1992). Control of synthesis and release of oxytocin in the sheep brain. *Ann. N.Y. Acad. Sci.* 652:102–121.

15. Practically all of the data cited in this chapter can be found in the excellent review papers contained in n. 6. Another key general reference is: *Oxytocin in maternal, sexual, and social behavior* (C. A. Pedersen, J. D. Caldwell, G. F. Jirikowski, & T. R. Insel, eds.). Special issue of *Annals of the New York Academy of Sciences*, vol. 652. New York: New York Academy of Sciences.

More recent reviews on this topic are to be found in: Winberg, J., & Kjellmer, I. (eds.) (1994). The neurobiology of infant-parent interaction in the newborn period. *ACTA Paediatrica* 83(suppl. 397).

16. Rosenblatt, J. (1992). Hormone-behavior relations in the regulation of parental behavior. In *Behavioral endocrinology* (J. B. Becker, S. M. Breedlove, & D. Crews, eds.), pp. 219–259. Cambridge, Mass.: MIT Press.

Berman, P. W. (1980). Are women more responsive than men to the young? A review of developmental and situational variables. *Psych. Rev.* 88:668–695.

17. Bridges, R. S., & Mann, P. E. (1994). Prolactin-brain interactions in the induction of maternal behavior in rats. *Psychoneuroendocrinol.* 19:611–622.

18. Bridges, R. S. (1990). Endocrine regulation of parental behavior in rodents. In *Mammalian parenting* (N. A. Krasnegor & R. S. Bridges, eds.), pp. 93–117. New York: Oxford Univ. Press.

19. Insel, T. R., & Shapiro, L. E. (1992). Oxytocin receptors and maternal behavior. *Ann. N.Y. Acad. Sci.* 652:122–141.

Jirikowski, G. F. (1992). Oxytocinergic neuronal systems during mating, pregnancy, parturition, and lactation. *Ann. N.Y. Acad. Sci.* 652:253–270.

Rosenblatt, J. S., Wagner, C. K., & Morrell, J. I. (1994). Hormonal priming and triggering of maternal behavior in the rat with special reference to the relations between estrogen receptor binding and ER mRNA in specific brain regions. *Psychoneuroendocrinol.* 19: 543–552.

20. Modney, B. K., & Hatton, G. I. (1990). Motherhood modifies magnocellular neuronal interrelationships in functionally meaningful ways. In *Mammalian parenting* (N. A. Krasnegor & R. S. Bridges, eds.), pp. 305–323. New York: Oxford Univ. Press.

21. Landgraf, R., Neumann, I., Russell, J. A., & Pittman, Q. J. (1992). Push-pull perfusion and microdialysis studies of central oxytocin and vasopressin release in freely moving rats during pregnancy, parturition and lactation. *Ann. N.Y. Acad. Sci.* 652:326–339.

22. For a review of the early studies, see: Slotnick, B. M. (1975). Neural and hormonal basis of maternal behavior in the rat. In *Hormonal correlates of behavior*, vol. 2 (B. E. Eletheriou & R. L. Sprott, eds.), pp. 585–656. New York: Plenum Press.

23. Pedersen, C. A., Ascher, J. A., Monroe, Y. L., & Prange, A. J. (1982). Oxytocin induces maternal behavior in virgin female rats. *Science* 216:648–649.

24. Keverne, E. B., & Kendrick, K. M. (1992). Oxytocin facilitation of maternal behavior in sheep. *Ann. N.Y. Acad. Sci.* 652:83–101.

25. Bolwerk, E. L. M., & Swanson, H. H. (1984). Does oxytocin play a role in the onset of maternal behaviour in the rat? *J. Endocrinol.* 101:353–357.

It is now clear that even though oxytocin promotes the onset of maternal behavior in many species, it is not an absolutely essential ingredient, for "knockout" mice missing the gene for the manufacture of oxytocin exhibit seemingly normal maternal behavior, even though their pups do not survive unless milk letdown is facilitated by external oxytocin supplementation. See: Nishimori, K., Young, L. J., Guo, Q., Wang, Z., Insel, T. R., & Matzuk, M. M. (1996). Oxytocin is required for nursing but is not essential for parturition or reproductive behavior. *Proc. Natl. Acad. Sci., USA* 92:11699–11704.

In this context, it is also noteworthy that mice lacking the gene for the *fosB* protein are severely lacking in maternal behavior, apparently because the cascade of genetic activation within nurturant circuits emanating from the preoptic area is deficient. See: Brown, J. R., Ye, H., Bronson, R. T., Dikkes, P., & Greenberg, M. E. (1996). A defect in nurturing in mice lacking the immediate early gene *fosB*. *Cell* 86:297–309.

26. Fleming, A. S., & Rosenblatt, J. S. (1974). Olfactory regulation of maternal behavior in rats: I. Effects of olfactory bulb removal in experienced and inexperienced lactating and cycling females. *J. Comp. Physiol. Psychol.* 86:221–232.

Kendrick, K. M., Levy, F., & Keverne, E. B. (1992). Changes in the sensory processing of olfactory signals induced by birth in sheep. *Science* 256:833–836.

Cellular evidence for plasticity in maternal circuits has recently been provided. See: Fleming, A. S., & Korsmit, M. (1996). Plasticity in the maternal circuit: Effects of maternal experience on Fos-Lir in hypothalamic, limbic, and cortical structures in the postpartum rat. *Behav. Neurosci.* 110:567–582.

27. The olfactory memory appears to be mediated by norepinephrine within the olfactory bulbs. See: Pissoinier, D., Thiery, J. C., Fabre-Nys, C., Poindron, P., & Keverne, E. B. (1985). The importance of olfactory bulbs and noradrenaline for maternal recognition in sheep. *Physiol. Behav.* 35:361–363.

In animals like sheep, the social attraction becomes highly discriminating very rapidly, and mothers tend to reject other sheep soon after the bond has formed. On the other hand, mother rats develop their olfactory bond more to the nest than to the pups, which makes cross-fostering of animals an easy manipulation.

28. For a summary of the confusion that accompanied the initial observation of oxytocin-induced maternal behavior, see page 59 in Pedersen, C. A., Caldwell, J. D., Peterson, G., Walker, C. H., & Mason, G. A. (1992). Oxytocin activation of maternal behavior in the rat. *Ann. N.Y. Acad. Sci.* 652:58–69.

In brief: The original groups of animals in which oxytocin precipitated maternal behavior had chronic respiratory ailments that reduced their olfactory acuity. Now we know that in animals whose ability to smell is impaired by the removal of the olfactory bulbs, oxytocin is quite effective in triggering maternal behavior. See: Wamboldt, M. Z., & Insel, T. R. (1987). The ability of oxytocin to induce short-latency maternal behaviour is dependent on peripheral anosmia. *Behav. Neurosci.* 101:439–441.

29. Fahrbach, S. E., Morrell, J. I., & Pfaff, D. W. (1986). Effect of varying the duration of pretest cage habituation on oxytocin induction of short-latency maternal behavior. *Physiol. Behav.* 37:135–139.

30. Van Leengoed, E., Kerker, E., & Swanson, H. H. (1987). Inhibition of post-partum maternal behavior in the rat by infusion of an oxytocin antagonist into the cerebral ventricles. *J. Endocrinol.* 112:275–282.

31. Insel, T. R. (1990). Oxytocin and maternal behavior. In *Mammalian parenting* (N. A. Krasnegor & R. S. Bridges, eds.), pp. 260–280. New York: Oxford Univ. Press.

32. Walsh, R. J., Slaby, F. J., & Posner, B. I. (1987). A receptor-mediated mechanism for the transport of prolactin from blood to cerebrospinal fluid. *Endocrinol.* 120:1846–1850.

33. The more prevalent report is of opiates suppressing maternal behavior, but there are good reasons to believe such studies were simply detecting the sedative effects of modest opiate doses. Low doses can increase various social behaviors. The controversy is discussed fully in: Panksepp, J., Nelson, E., & Siviy, S. M. (1994). Brain opioids and mother-infant social motivation. *Acta Paediatrica* 397(suppl.):40–46.

34. Insel, T. R., & Harbaugh, C. R. (1989). Lesions of the hypothalamic paraventricular nucleus disrupt the initiation of maternal behavior. *Physiol. Behav.* 45: 1033–1041.

35. For a review see n. 6. This experience-dependent development of maternal behavior was originally called "concaveation" by: Wiesner, B. P., & Sheard, N. M. (1933). *Maternal behavior in the rat.* London: Oliver and Boyd.

When rediscovered, it was call "sensitization." See: Rosenblatt, J. S. (1967). Nonhormonal basis of maternal behavior in the rat. *Science* 156:1512–1514.

36. Soloff, M. S., Alexandrova, M., & Fernstrom, M. J. (1979). Oxytocin receptors: Triggers for parturition and lactation? *Science* 204:1313–1314.

37. Insel, T. R. (1986). Postpartum increases in brain oxytocin binding. *Neuroendocrinol.* 44:515–518.

Insel, T. R. (1992). Oxytocin: A neuropeptide for affiliation—evidence from behavioral, autoradiographic and comparative studies. *Psychoneuroendocrinol.* 17: 3–35.

38. Numan, M. (1988). Maternal behavior. In *The physiology of reproduction* (E. Knobil & J. Neill, eds.), pp. 1569–1645. New York: Raven Press.

39. Hansen, S., & Kohler, C. (1984). The importance of the peripeduncular nucleus in the neuroendocrine control of sexual behavior and milk ejection in the rat. *Neuroendocrinol.* 39:563–572.

40. Jirikowski, G. F., Caldwell, J. D., Stumpf, W. E., & Pedersen, C. A. (1988). Estradiol influences oxytocin immunoreactive brain systems. *Neuroscience* 25:237–248.

41. Numan, M. (1990). Neural control of maternal behavior. In *Mammalian parenting* (N. A. Krasnegor & R. S. Bridges, eds.), pp. 231–259. New York: Oxford Univ. Press.

42. Numan, M. (1994). A neural circuitry analysis of maternal behavior in the rat. *Acta Paediatrica* 397 (suppl.):19–28.

An intriguing way to study nurturance circuits in males has been through their tendency to exhibit "maternal" aggression following hormonal pretreatment. See: Rosenblatt, J. S., Hazelwood, S., & Poole, J.

(1996). Maternal behavior in male rats: Effects of medial preoptic area lesions and presence of maternal aggression. *Horm. Behav.* 30:201–215.

43. Pedersen, C. A., Caldwell, J. D., Walker, C., Ayers, G., & Mason, G. A. (1994). Oxytocin activates the postpartum onset of rat maternal behavior in the ventral tegmental area and medial preoptic areas. *Behav. Neurosci.* 108:1163–1171.

44. Hansen, S., Harton, C., Wallin, E., Lofberg, L., & Svensson, K. (1991). Mesotelencephalic dopamine system and reproductive behavior in the female rat: Effects of ventral tegmental 6-hydroxydopamine lesions on maternal and sexual responsiveness. *Behav. Neurosci.* 105:588–598.

Numan, M., & Numan, M. J. (1991). Preoptic-brainstem connections and maternal behavior in rats. *Behav. Neurosci.* 105:1013–1029.

45. Hansen, S., & Ferreira, A. (1986). Food intake, aggression, and fear behavior in the mother rat: Control by neural systems concerned with milk ejection and maternal behavior. *Behav. Neurosci.* 100:64–70.

46. The medial amygdala, in its role of mediating aggressive and sexual behavior, inhibits maternal behavior by actions on the preoptic area. See:

Fleming, A. S., Miceli, M., & Morretto, D. (1983). Lesions of the medial preoptic area prevent the facilitation of maternal behavior produced by amygdaloid lesions. *Physiol. Behav.* 31:502–510.

Calamandrei, G., & Keverne, E. B. (1994). Differential expression of Fos protein in the brain of female mice dependent on pup sensory cues and maternal experience. *Behav. Neurosci.* 108:113–120.

Fleming, A. S., Such, E. J., Korsmit, M., & Rusak, B. (1994). Activation of Fos-like immunoreactivity in the medial preoptic area and limbic structures by maternal and social interactions in rats. *Behav. Neurosci.* 108:724–734.

47. Fleischer, S., & Slotnick, B. M. (1978). Disruption of maternal behavior in rats with lesions of the septal area. *Physiol. Behav.* 21:189–200.

48. Slotnick, B. M. (1975). Neural and hormonal basis of maternal behavior in the rat. In *Hormonal correlates of behavior*, vol. 2 (B. E. Eleftheriou & R. L. Sprott, eds.), pp. 585–656. New York: Plenum Press.

49. Bowlby, J. (1980). *Attachment and loss.* Vol. 1, *Attachment.* New York: Basic Books.

Bowlby, J. (1988). *A secure base: Parent-child attachment and healthy human development.* New York: Basic Books.

50. Panksepp, J. (1981). Brain opioids: A neurochemical substrate for narcotic and social dependence. In *Progress in theory in psychopharmacology* (S. Cooper, ed.), pp. 149–175. London: Academic Press.

51. See n. 15.

52. See nn. 8, 33, 50, 52 and: Carter, S., Kirkpatrick, B., & Lederhendler, I. I. (eds.) (1997). *Neurobiology of affiliation.* Special issue of *Annals N.Y. Acad. Sci.*, vol. 807. New York: New York Academy of Sciences.

53. Panksepp, J., Herman, B. H., Vilberg, T., Bishop, P., & De Eskinazi, F. G. (1980). Endogenous opioids and social behavior. *Neurosci. Biobehav. Revs.* 4:473–487.

54. Ågmo, A., & Berenfeld, R. (1990). Reinforcing properties of ejaculation in the male rat: Role of opioids and dopamine. *Behav. Neurosci.* 107:812–818.

55. Cocteau, J. (1957). *Opium: The diary of a cure.* New York: Grove Press.

56. Alexander, B. K., Coambs, R. B., & Hadaway, P. F. (1978). The effect of housing and gender on morphine self-administration in rats. *Psychopharmacol.* 58:175–179.

Panksepp, J., Herman, B. H., Vilberg, T., Bishop, P., & DeEskinazi, F. G. (1980). Endogenous opioids and social behavior. *Neurosci. Biobehav. Revs.* 4:473–487.

57. For a thorough review of imprinting, see: Hess, E. H. (1973). *Imprinting; Early experience and the developmental psychobiology of attachment.* New York: Van Nostrand Reinhold.

58. Nelson, E., & Panksepp, J. (1996). Oxytocin mediates acquisition of maternally associated odor preferences in preweanling rat pups. *Behav. Neurosci.* 110:583–592.

Hansen, S., Harton, C., Wallin, E., Lofberg, L., & Svensson, K. (1991). Mesotelencephalic dopamine system and reproductive behavior in the female rat: Effects of ventral tegmental 6–hydroxydopamine lesions on maternal and sexual responsiveness. *Behav. Neurosci.* 105:588–598.

59. Lorenz, K. (1935). Der Kumpan in der Umwelt des Vogels. *J. Ornithologie* 83:137–213.

Lorenz, K. (1965). *Evolution and modification of behavior.* Chicago: Univ. of Chicago Press.

60. Kovacs, G. L., & Van Ree, M. V. (1985). Behaviorally active oxytocin fragments simultaneously attenuate heroin self-administration and tolerance in rats. *Life Sci.* 37:1895–1900.

Krivan, M., Szabo, G., Sarnyai, Z., Kovacs, G. L., & Telegdy, G. (1995). Oxytocin blocks the development of heroin-fentanyl cross-tolerance in mice. *Pharmacol. Biochem. Behav.* 52:591–594.

61. Winslow, J. T., Hastings, N., Carter, C. S., Harbaugh, C. R., & Insel, T. R. (1993). A role for central vasopressin in pair bonding in monogamous prairie voles. *Nature* 365:544–548.

62. See nn. 8 and 54.

63. Thor, D. H., & Holloway, W. R. (1982). Social memory of the male laboratory rat. *J. Comp. Physiol. Psychol.* 98:908–913.

64. Dantzer, R., Bluthe, R. M., Koob, G. F., & Le Moal, M. (1988). Modulation of social memory in male rats by neurohypophyseal peptides. *Psychopharmacol.* 91:363–368.

Dantzer, R., Koob, G. F., Bluthe, R. M., & Le Moal, M. (1988). Septal vasopressin modulates social memory in male rats. *Brain Res.* 457:143–147.

65. Popik, P., Vetulani, J., & Van Ree, J.M. (1992). Low doses of oxytocin facilitate social recognition in rats. *Psychopharmacol.* 106:71–74.

66. Although the most sensitive site for induction of erection is in the paraventricular nucleus of the hypothalamus, the hippocampus is a surprisingly sensitive site. See: Melis, M. R., Argioolas, A., & Gessa, G. L. (1986). Oxytocin-induced penile erection and yawning: Site of action in the brain. *Brain Res.* 398:259–265.

67. Prescott, J. W. (1971). Early somatosensory deprivation as an ontogenetic process in the abnormal development of brain and behavior. In *Proceedings of the Second Conference on Experimental Medicine and Surgery in Primates* (E. I. Goldsmith & J. Mody-Janokowski, eds.), pp. 356–375. Basel: Karger.

68. See Chapter 12 and: McCarthy, M. M. (1990). Oxytocin inhibits infanticide in wild female house mice (*Mus domesticus*). *Horm. Behav.* 24:365–375.

69. Hausfater, G., & Hrdy, S. B. (eds.) (1984). *Infanticide: Comparative and evolutionary perspectives.* New York: Aldine.

Malkin, C. M., & Lamb, M. E. (1994). Child maltreatment: A test of sociobiological theory. *J. Comp. Family Stud.* 25:121–133.

70. McCarthy, M. M., Low, L.-M., & Pfaff, D. W. (1992). Speculations concerning the physiological significance of central oxytocin in maternal behavior. *Ann. N.Y. Acad. Sci.* 652:70–82.

71. Mennella J. A., & Moltz, H. (1988). Infanticide in rats: Male strategy and female counter-strategy. *Physiol. Behav.* 42:19–28.

72. Stern, J. M. (1997). Offspring-induced nurturance: Animal-human parallels. *Devel. Psychobiol.* 31: 19–37. See: Jirikowski, G. F. (1992). Oxytocinergic neuronal systems during mating, pregnancy, parturition, and lactation. *Ann. N.Y. Acad. Sci.* 652:253–270.

73. See n. 35.

74. See n. 6 and: Mayer, A. D., Freeman, N. G., & Rosenblatt, J. S. (1979). Ontogeny of maternal behavior in the laboratory rat: Factors underlying changes in responsiveness from 30 to 90 days. *Devel. Psychobiol.* 12:425–439.

75. Mayer, A. D., & Rosenblatt, J. S. (1979). Ontogeny of maternal behavior in the laboratory rat: Early origins in 18–27 day old young. *Devel. Psychobiol.* 12:407–424.

Kinsley, C. H. (1990). Prenatal and postnatal influences on parental behavior in rodents. In *Mammalian parenting* (N. A. Krasnegor & R. S. Bridges, eds.), pp. 348–371. New York: Oxford Univ. Press.

76. Kinsley, C. H., & Bridges, R. S. (1988). Prenatal stress and maternal behavior in intact virgin rats: Response latencies are decreased in males and increased in females. *Horm. Behav.* 22:76–89.

77. Insel, T. R. (1986). Postpartum increases in brain oxytocin binding. *Neuroendocrinol.* 44:515–518.

Insel, T. R., & Shapiro, L. E. (1992). Oxytocin receptor distribution reflects social organization in monogamous and polygamous voles. *Proc. Nat. Acad. Sci.* 89:5981–5985.

Insel, T. R., & Shapiro, L. E. (1992). Oxytocin receptors and maternal behavior. *Ann. N.Y. Acad. Sci.* 652:122–141.

78. Keverne, E. B., & Kendrick, K. M. (1992). Oxytocin facilitation of maternal behavior in sheep. *Ann. N.Y. Acad. Sci.* 652:83–101.

79. Keverne, E. B., & Kendrick, K. M. (1990). Neurochemical changes accompanying parturition and their significance for maternal behavior. In *Mammalian parenting* (N. A. Krasnegor & R. S. Bridges, eds.), pp. 281–304. New York: Oxford Univ. Press.

80. Keverne, E. B., Levy, F., Poindron, P., & Lindsay, D. R. (1983). Vaginal stimulation: An important determinant of maternal bonding in sheep. *Science* 219:81–83.

81. Kendrick, K. M., Keverne, E. B., & Baldwin, B. A. (1987). Intracerebroventricular oxytocin stimulates maternal behaviour in the sheep. *Neuroendocrinol.* 46:56–61.

82. See n. 78, and: Keverne, E. B., & Kendrick, K. (1991). Morphine and corticotrophin releasing factor potentiate maternal acceptance in multiparous ewes after vaginocervical stimulation. *Brain. Res.* 540:55–62.

83. Hupka, R. B. (1981). Cultural determinants of jealousy. *Alternative Lifestyles* 4:310–356.

Zahn-Waxler, C., Cummings, E. M., & Iannotti, R. (eds.) (1986). *Altruism and aggression: Biological and social origins.* New York: Cambridge Univ. Press.

84. Fletcher, D. J. C., & Michener, C. D. (eds.) (1987). *Kin recognition in animals.* London: Wiley.

85. Corter, C. M., & Fleming, A. S. (1990). Maternal responsiveness in humans: Emotional, cognitive, and biological factors. *Advances in the Study of Behavior* 19:83–136.

Brunelli, S. A., Shindledecker, R. D., & Hofer, M. A. (1987). Behavioral responses of juvenile rats (*Rattus norvegicus*) to neonates after infusion of maternal blood plasma. *J. Comp. Psych.* 101:47–59.

86. The mere-exposure effect can increase social attraction. See: Saegert, S., Swap, W., & Zajonc, R. B. (1973). Exposure, context, and interpersonal attraction. *J. Personal. Soc. Psychol.* 25:234–242.

However, this effect reduces sociosexual attraction. For instance, young Israeli children who grew up in a kibbutz generally preferred not to date the people they knew well. See: Shepher, J. (1972). Mate selection among second-generation kibbutz adolescents and adults: Incest avoidance and negative imprinting. *Arch. Sex. Behav.* 1:293–307.

Also, increased exposure to individuals you do not like can increase your dislike of them. See: Swap, W. C. (1977). Interpersonal attraction and repeated exposure to rewarders and punishers. *Person. Soc. Psych. Bull.* 33:248–252.

87. Hill, W. F. (1978). Effects of mere exposure on preferences in nonhuman mammals. *Psych. Bull.* 85: 1177–1198.

88. See n. 87 and: Rozin, P., & Zellner, D. (1985). The role of Pavlovian conditioning in the acquisition of food likes and dislikes. *Ann. N.Y. Acad. Sci.* 443: 189–202.

89. Advertisers often repeat their message to increase the attractiveness of their products. See: Born-stein, R. F. (1989). Exposure and affect: Overview and meta-analysis of research, 1968–1987. *Psych. Bull.* 106: 265–289.

Such effects can also increase interpersonal attraction. See: Moreland, R. L., & Beach, S. R. (1992). Exposure effects in the classroom: The development of affinity among students. *J. Exp. Soc. Psych.* 28:255–276.

90. Morelan, R. L., & Zajonc, R. B. (1982). Exposure effects in personal perception: Familiarity, similarity, and attraction. *J. Exp. Soc. Psychol.* 18:395–415.

Nuttin, J. M., Jr. (1987). Affective consequence of mere ownership: The name letter effect in twelve European languages. *Eur. J. Soc. Psych.* 17:381–402.

91. Cairns, R. B. (1966). Attachment behavior of mammals. *Psych. Rev.* 73:409–426.

92. Zajonc, R. B. (1980). Feeling and thinking: Preferences need no inferences. *Amer. Psychol.* 35: 151–175.

Zajonc, R. B. (1984). On the primacy of affect. *Amer. Psychol.* 39:117–123.

93. We rapidly become habituated to new situations, and a sense of strangeness is replaced with a sense of comfort and familiarity. Essentially nothing is known about the chemistries that mediate this effect. As we will see in the next chapter, it is possible that the ancient mechanisms of place attachment provided a neural impetus for the emergence of social attachments. If so, we should be able to demonstrate that they share certain chemistries. Presently it does appear to be the case that brain opioids, in addition to other brain chemistries, participate in the mediation of both.

Chapter 14

1. For an English summary of this work, see: Bowlby, J. (1980). *Attachment and loss.* Vol. 1, *Attachment.* New York: Basic Books.

2. Hofer, M. A. (1984). Relationships as regulators: A psychobiologic perspective on bereavement. *Psychosom. Med.* 46:183–197.

Hofer, M. A. (1987). Early social relationships: A psychobiologist's view. *Child Devel.* 58:633–647.

Mendoza, S. P., Lyons, D. M., & Saltzman, W. (1991). Sociophysiology of squirrel monkeys. *Amer. J. Primatol.* 23:37–54.

Reite, M., & Capitanio, J. P. (1985). On the nature of social separation and social attachment. In *The psychobiology of attachment and separation* (M. Reite & T. Field, eds.), pp. 223–255. Orlando, Fla.: Academic Press.

3. Panksepp, J., Nelson, E., & Bekkedal, M. (1997). Brain systems for the mediation of social separation-distress and social-reward. *Ann. N. Y. Acad. Sci.* 807: 78–100.

4. Carden, S. E., & Hofer, M. A. (1990). Independence of benzodiazepine and opiate actions in the suppression of isolation distress in rat pups. *Behav. Neurosci.* 104:160–166.

Kalin, N. H., Shelton, S. E., & Barksdale, C. M. (1988). Opiate modulation of separation-induced distress in non-human primates. *Brain Res.* 440:285–292.

Kehoe, P., & Blass, E. M. (1986). Opioid-mediation of separation distress in 10-day-old rats: Reversal of stress with maternal stimuli. *Devel. Psychobiol.* 19: 385–398.

Panksepp, J., Herman, B. H., Conner, R., Bishop, P., & Scott, J. P. (1978). The biology of social attachments: Opiates alleviate separation distress. *Biol. Psychiat.* 13:607–613.

5. Cocteau, J. (1957). *Opium: The diary of a cure.* New York: Grove Press. Quotation on p. 53.

6. Quote from Book 4 of Fitzgerald, R. (trans.). (1963). *Homer's The Odyssey.* Garden City, N.Y.: Anchor Books. Quotation on p. 58.

7. Lewin, L. (1964). *Phantastica narcotic and stimulating drugs* (2d ed.). London: Routledge and Kegan Paul.

8. Panksepp, J. Vilberg, T., Bean, N. B., Coy, D. H., & Kastin, A. J. (1978). Reduction of distress vocalization in chicks by opiate-like peptides. *Brain Res. Bull.* 3:663–667.

9. Panksepp, J. (1981). Brain opioids: A neurochemical substrate for narcotic and social dependence. In *Progress in theory in psychopharmacology* (S. Cooper, ed.), pp. 149–175. London: Academic Press.

10. Childers, S. R., Sexton, T., & Roy, M. B. (1993). Effects of anandamide on cannabinoid receptors in rat brain membranes. *Biochem. Pharmacol.* 47:711–715.

11. See chap. 13, n. 60.

12. Ainsworth, M. D. S., Blehar, M., Waters, E., & Wall, S. (1978). *Patterns of attachment: Strange situation behavior of one year olds.* Hillsdale, N.J.: Lawrence Erlbaum.

Bowlby, J. (1988). *A secure base: Parent-child attachment and healthy human development.* New York: Basic Books.

13. Gerwitz, J. L., & Kurtines, W. M. (1991). *Intersections with attachment.* Hillsdale, N.J.: Lawrence Erlbaum.

14. Pettijohn, T. F. (1979). Attachment and separation distress in the infant guinea pig. *Devel. Psychobiol.* 12:73–81.

15. Hoffman, K. A., Mendoza, S. P., Hennessy, M. B., & Mason, W. A. (1995). Responses of infant titi monkeys, *Callicebus moloch*, to removal of one or both parents: Evidence for paternal attachment. *Devel. Psychobiol.* 28:399–407.

16. For summaries of such issues, see contributions in: Newman, J. D. (ed.) (1988). *The physiological control of mammalian vocalization.* New York: Plenum Press.

17. Pettijohn, T. F. (1977). Reaction of parents to recorded infant guinea pig distress vocalizations. *Behav. Biol.* 21:438–442.

18. Larson, C. R., Ortega, J. D., & DeRosier, A. (1988). Studies on the relation of the midbrain periaqueductal gray, the larynx and vocalization in awake monkeys. In *The physiological control of mammalian* *vocalization* (J. D. Newman, ed.), pp. 43–65. New York: Plenum Press.

Schuller, G., & Radtke-Schuller, S. (1988). Neural control of vocalization in bats at peripheral to midbrain levels. In *The physiological control of mammalian vocalization* (J. D. Newman, ed.), pp. 67–85. New York: Plenum Press.

Buchwald, J. S., Shipley, C., Altafullah, I., Hinman, C., Harrison, J., & Dickerson, L. (1988). The feline isolation call. In *The physiological control of mammalian vocalization* (J. D. Newman, ed.), pp. 119–135. New York: Plenum Press.

19. Keverne, E. B., Martensz, N., & Tuite, B. (1989). ß-Endorphin concentrations in CSF of monkeys are influenced by grooming relationships. *Psychoneuroendocrinol.* 14:155–161.

Montagu, A. (1978). *Touching: The human significance of the skin.* New York: Harper and Row.

20. Although there is no direct evidence that such chemical changes in the brain mediate human feelings of love and devotion, this theoretical proposal is bolstered by a great deal of evidence in animals, such as summarized in nn. 9, 19, and 21.

21. Panksepp, J., Herman, B. H., Vilberg, T., Bishop, P., & De Eskinazi, F. G. (1980). Endogenous opioids and social behavior. *Neurosci. Biobehav. Revs.* 4:473–487.

22. De Lanerolle, N. C., & Lang, F. F. (1988). Functional neural pathways for vocalization in the domestic cat. In *The physiological control of mammalian vocalization* (J. D. Newman, ed.), pp. 21–41. New York: Plenum Press.

Jürgens, U., & Ploog, D. (1988). On the motor coordination of monkey calls. In *The physiological control of mammalian vocalization* (J. D. Newman, ed.), pp. 7–19. New York: Plenum Press.

Lloyd, R. L., & Kling, A. S. (1988). Amygdaloid electrical activity in response to conspecific calls in squirrel monkey (*S. sciureus*): Influence of environmental setting, cortical inputs, and recording site. In *The physiological control of mammalian vocalization* (J. D. Newman, ed.), pp. 137–151. New York: Plenum Press.

Robinson, B. W. (1967). Vocalization evoked from forebrain in *Macaca mulata. Physiol. Behav.* 2:345–354.

23. In primates and birds, CRF increases DVs, but in infant rats it decreases them. See:

Panksepp, J. (1990). A role for affective neuroscience in understanding stress: The case of separation distress circuitry. In *Psychobiology of stress.* NATO ASI Series D: Behavioural and Social Sciences, Vol. 54 (S. Puglisi-Allegra & A. Oliverio, eds.), pp. 41–57. Dordrecht: Kluwer Academic.

Harvey, A. T., & Hennessy, M. B. (1995). Corticotropin-releasing factor modulation of the ultrasonic vocalization rate of isolated rat pups. *Devel. Brain Res.* 87:125–134.

24. For a summary of these unpublished findings of T. Sahley and J. Panksepp, see: Panksepp, J., & Miller, A. (1996). Emotions and the aging brain. In *Handbook of emotion, adult development, and aging* (C. Magai & S. H. McFadden, eds.), pp. 3–26. San Diego: Academic Press.

25. See n. 24 and: Andrew, R. J. (1969). The effects of testosterone on avian vocalizations. In *Bird vocalizations* (R. A. Hinde, ed.), pp. 97–130. Cambridge: Cambridge Univ. Press.

We have also done a great deal of work on testosterone modulation of DVs in young chicks, but the results are not published. One small experiment conducted just for illustrative purposes is shown in Figure 14.5.

26. Rachman, S. (ed.) (1996). *Panic disorder: The facts.* Oxford: Oxford Univ. Press.

27. Herman, B. H., & Panksepp, J. (1981). Ascending endorphin inhibition of distress vocalization. *Science* 211:1060–1062.

Panksepp, J., Normansell, L., Herman, B., Bishop, P., & Crepeau, L. (1988). Neural and neurochemical control of the separation distress call. In *The physiological control of mammalian vocalizations* (J. D. Newman, ed.), pp. 263–299. New York: Plenum Press.

28. Panksepp, J. (1991). Affective neuroscience: A conceptual framework for the neurobiological study of emotions. In *International reviews of emotion research*, vol. 1. (K. Strongman, ed.), pp 59–99. Chichester, U.K.: Wiley.

29. See n. 28 and: Panksepp, J., Siviy, S. M., & Normansell, L. A. (1985). Brain opioids and social emotion. In *The psychobiology of attachment and separation* (M. Reite & T. Fields, eds.), pp 3–49. New York: Academic Press.

30. Normansell, L. (1988). Effects of excitatory amino acids on emotional and sensorimotor behaviors in the domestic chick. Ph.D. diss., Bowling Green State University.

Panksepp, J. (1996). Affective neuroscience: A paradigm to study the animate circuits for human emotions. In *Emotions: Interdisciplinary perspectives* (R. D. Kavanaugh, B. Zimmerberg, & S. Fein, eds.), pp 29–60. Mahwah, N.J.: Lawrence Erlbaum.

31. See nn. 8, 9, 21, 28, 29, 32, and 66.

32. Panksepp, J., Bean, N. J., Bishop, P., Vilberg, T., & Sahley, T. L. (1980). Opioid blockade and social comfort in chicks. *Pharmacol. Biochem. Behav.* 13: 673–683.

33. Hofer, M. A. (1996). Multiple regulators of ultrasonic vocalization in the infant rat. *Psychoneuroendocrinol.* 21:203–217.

Panksepp, J., Newman, J., & Insel, T. (1992). Critical conceptual issues in the analysis of separation-distress systems in the brain. In *International reviews of emotion research*, vol 2 (K. Strongman, ed.), pp. 51–72. Chichester, U.K.: Wiley.

For an analysis of the neurochemical substrates of rodent ultrasonic vocalizations, see:

Hard, E., & Engel, J. (1991). Ontogeny of ultrasonic vocalization in the rat: Influence of neurochemical transmission systems. In *Behavioral biology: Neuroendocrine axis* (T. Archer & S. Hansen, eds.), pp. 37–52. Hillsdale, N.J.: Lawrence Erlbaum.

Miczek, K. A., Tornatzky, W., & Vivian, J. (1991). Ethology and neuropharmacology: Rodent ultrasounds.

In *Animal models in psychopharmacology* (B. Olivier, J. Mos, & J. L. Slangen, eds.), pp. 409–427. Basel: Birkhauser Verlag.

34. Meyerson, B. J., & Linstrom, L. H. (1973). Sexual motivation in the female rat: A methodological study applied to the investigation of estradiol benzoate. *Acta Physiol. Scand.* (suppl 389).

Spruijt, B. M., Meyerson, B. J., & Hoglund, U. (1989). Aging and sociosexual behavior in the male rat. *Behav. Brain Res.* 32:51–61.

Hetta J., & Meyerson B. J. (1978). Sex-specific orientation in the male rat. A methodological study. *Acta Physiol. Scand.* 453 (suppl):5–27.

35. Berger, J. (1978). Group size, foraging, and antipredator ploys: An analysis of bighorn sheep decisions. *Behav. Ecol. Sociobiol.* 4:91–99.

Mooring, M. S., & Hart, B. L. (1992). Animal grouping for protection from parasites: Selfish herd and encounter-dilution effects. *Behaviour* 213:173–193.

Warburton K., & Lazarus J. (1991). Tendency-distance models of social cohesion in animal groups. *J. Theor. Biol.* 150:473–488.

36. Latane, B., & Hothersall, D. (1972). Social attraction in animals. In *New horizons in psychology, II* (P. C. Dodson, ed.). New York: Penguin Books.

For a summary and perspective taking on this work, see: Latane, B. (1987). From student to colleague: Retracing a decade. In *A distinctive approach to psychological research: The influence of Stanley Schachter* (N. E. Gunberg, R. E. Nisbett, J. Rodin, & J. E. Singer, eds.), pp. 66–86. Hillsdale, N.J.: Lawrence Erlbaum.

37. Jonason, K. R., & Enloe, R. J. (1971). Alterations in social behavior following septal and amygdaloid lesions in the rat. *J. Comp. Physiol. Psychol.* 75:286–301.

38. Jonason, K. R., Enloe, L. J., Contrucci, J., & Meyer, P. M. (1973). Effects of simultaneous and successive septal and amygdaloid lesions on social behavior of the rat. *J. Comp. Physiol. Psychol.* 83:54–61.

39. Panksepp, J., Nelson, E., & Siviy, S. M. (1994). Brain opioids and mother-infant social motivation. *Acta Paediatrica* 397(suppl.):40–46.

40. Panksepp, J., Najam, N., & Soares, F. (1980). Morphine reduces social cohesion in rats. *Pharmacol. Biochem. Behav.* 11:131–134.

41. Knowles, P. A., Conner, R. L., & Panksepp, J. (1989). Opiate effects on social behavior of juvenile dogs as a function of social deprivation. *Pharmacol. Biochem. Behav.* 33:533–537.

42. See nn. 5, 19 and: Kurland, A. A. (1978). *Psychiatric aspects of opiate dependence.* West Palm Beach, Fla.: CRC Press.

43. For contrasting findings, see:

Panksepp, J., Nelson, E., & Bekkedal, M. (1997). Brain systems for the mediation of social separation-distress and social-reward. *Ann. N.Y. Acad. Sci.* 807: 78–100.

Witt, D. M., Winslow, J. T., & Insel, T. R. (1992). Enhanced social interactions in rats following chronic, centrally infused oxytocin. *Pharmacol. Biochem. Behav.* 43:855–861.

44. See nn. 19, 41 and: Fabre-Nys, C., Meller, R. E., & Keverne, E. B. (1982). Opiate antagonists stimulate affiliative behavior in monkeys. *Pharmacol. Biochem. Behav.* 16:653–659.

45. Kalin, N. H., Shelton, S. E., & Lynn, D. E. (1995). Opiate systems in mother and infant primates coordinate intimate contact during reunion. *Psychoneuroendocrinol.* 7:735–742.

Schino, G., & Troisi, A. (1992). Opiate receptor blockade in juvenile macaques: Effect on affiliative interactions with their mothers and group companions. *Brain Res.* 576:125–130.

46. Martel, F. L., Nevison, C. M., Rayment, F. D., Simpson, M. J., & Keverne, E. B. (1993). Opioid receptor blockade reduces maternal affect and social grooming in rhesus monkeys. *Psychoneuroendocrinol.* 18:307–321.

Martel, F. L., Nevison, C. M., Simpson, M. J., & Keverne, E. B. (1995). Effects of opioid receptor blockade on the social behavior of rhesus monkeys living in large family groups. *Devel. Psychobiol.* 28:71–84.

47. Gantt, W. H., Newton, J. E., O. Royer, F. L., & Stephens, J. H. (1966). Effect of person. *Cond. Reflex* 1:18–35.

Barnard, K. E., & Brazelton, T. B. (1990). *Touch: The foundation of experience.* Madison, Conn.: International Univ. Press.

Field, T. M. (1993). The therapeutic effect of touch. In *The undaunted psychologists: Adventures in research* (G. Branningan & M. Merrens, eds.), pp. 3–12. New York: McGraw-Hill.

48. See n. 32.

49. See n. 19.

50. Insel, T. R. (1992). Oxytocin: A neuropeptide for affiliation—evidence from behavioral, autoradiographic and comparative studies. *Psychoneuroendocrinol.* 17:3–35.

Insel, T. R., & Shapiro, L. E. (1992). Oxytocin receptor distribution reflects social organization in monogamous and polygamous voles. *Proc. Nat. Acad. Sci.* 89:5981–5985.

Insel, T. R., Wang, Z.-X., & Ferris, C. F. (1994). Patterns of brain vasopressin receptor distribution associated with social organization in microtine rodents. *J. Neurosci.* 14:5381–5392.

Shapiro, L. E., & Insel, T. R. (1989). Ontogeny of oxytocin receptors in rat forebrain: A quantitative study. *Synapse* 4:259–266.

51. Zahn-Waxler, C., Cummings, E. M., & Iannotti, R. (eds.) (1986). *Altruism and aggression.* Cambridge: Cambridge Univ. Press.

52. Nelson, E., Bird, L., Deak, T., Vaningan, M., & Panksepp, J. (1995). Social behavior in the young, vasopressin-deficient Brattleboro rat. *Soc. Neurosci. Abst.* 20:366.

53. For various theoretical views, see nn. 9, 21, and 29.

54. Panksepp, J., Jalowiec, J., De Eskinazi, F. G., & Bishop, P. (1985). Opiates and play dominance in juvenile rats. *Behav. Neurosci.* 99:441–453.

55. Keverne, E. B., Levy, F., Guevara-Guzman, R., & Kendrick, K. M. (1993). Influence of birth and maternal experience on olfactory bulb neurotransmitter release. *Neuroscience* 56:557–665.

Moffat, S. D., Suh, E. J., & Fleming, A. S. (1993). Noradrenergic involvement in the consolidation of maternal experience in postpartum rats. *Physiol. Behav.* 53:805–811.

Sullivan, R. M., Wilson, D. A., & Leon, M. (1989). Norepinephrine and learning-induced plasticity in infant rat olfactory system. *J. Neurosci.* 9:3998–4006.

56. Horn, G. (1985). *Memory, imprinting and the brain: An inquiry into mechanisms.* New York: Clarendon Press.

For a recent *cfos* analysis of imprinting in the chick brain, highlighting activation of the IMHV, see: McCabe, B. J., & Horn, C. (1994). Learning-related changes in Fos-like immunoreactivity in the chick forebrain after imprinting. *Proc. Natl. Acad. Sci.* 91:11417–11421.

57. Nicol. A. U., Brown, M. W., & Horn, G. (1995). Neurophysiological investigations of a recognition memory system for imprinting in the domestic chick. *Eur. J. Neurosci.* 7:766–776.

McCabe, B. J., Davey, J. E., & Horn, G. (1992). Impairment of learning by localized injection of an N-methyl-D-aspartate receptor antagonist into the hyperstriatum ventrale of the domestic chick. *Behav. Neurosci.* 106:947–953.

McCabe, B. J., & Horn, G. (1991). Synaptic transmission and recognition memory: Time course of changes in N-methyl-D-aspartate receptors after imprinting. *Behav. Neurosci.* 105:289–294.

58. Panksepp, J. (1986). The psychobiology of prosocial behaviors: Separation distress, play and altruism. In *Altruism and aggression: Biological and social origins* (C. Zahn-Waxler, E. M. Cummings, & R. Iannotti, eds.), pp. 19–57. Cambridge: Cambridge Univ. Press.

59. Panksepp, J., Siviy, S., Normansell, L., White, K., & Bishop, P. (1982). Effects of ß-chlornaltexamine on separation distress in chicks. *Life Sci.* 31:2387–2390.

60. Panksepp (1995, unpublished data).

61. I have evaluated this possibility in several experiments using central administration of vasotocin, but the results have been ambiguous (Panksepp, 1987–1994, unpublished data). In my estimation, studies with peripheral peptides are not convincing, since such peptides do not adequately cross into the brain.

62. Gittelman, R., & Klein, D. F. (1985). Childhood separation anxiety and adult agoraphobia. In *Anxiety and the anxiety disorders* (A. H. Tuma & J. Mascr, eds.), pp. 389–402. Hillsdale, N.J.: Lawrence Erlbaum.

63. Pettijohn, T. F., Wong, T. W., Ebert, P. D., & Scott, J. P. (1977). Alleviation of separation distress in 3 breeds of young dogs. *Devel. Psychobiol.* 10:373–381.

Davis, K. L., Gurski, J. C., & Scott, J. P. (1977). Interaction of separation distress with fear in infant dogs. *Devel. Psychobiol.* 10:203–212.

64. Hennessy, M. B., Long, S. J., Nigh, C. K., Williams, M. T., & Nolan, D. J. (1995). Effects of peripherally administered corticotropin-releasing factor (CRF) and a CRF antagonist: Does peripheral CRF activity mediate behavior of guinea pig pups during isolation? *Behav. Neurosci.* 109:1137–1145.

65. Opiates are not especially effective in reducing fear-motivated active avoidance behaviors in some studies, but they are quite effective in others. See:

Blanchard, D. C., Weatherspoon, A., Shepherd, J. K., & Rodgers, R. J. (1991). "Paradoxical" effects of morphine on antipredator defense reactions in wild and laboratory rats. *Pharmacol. Biochem. Behav.* 40:819–828.

Rodriquez, R. (1992). Effects of various psychotropic drugs on the performance of avoidance and escape behaviors in rats. *Pharmacol. Biochem. Behav.* 43: 1155–1159.

Smith, J. B. (1985). Effects of single and repeated daily injections of morphine, clonidine, and l-nantradol on avoidance responding of rats. *Psychopharmacol.* 87:425–429.

66. There is great species variability in the efficacy of benzodiazepines in reducing distress vocalizations. Primates, dogs, and domestic chicks exhibit comparatively modest effects, while young rat pups exhibit large effects. See n. 33 and:

Carden S. E., & Hofer, M. A. (1990). The effects of opioid and benzodiazepine antagonists on dam-induced reductions in rat pup isolation distress. *Devel. Psychobiol.* 23:797–808.

Kalin, N. H., Shelton, S. E., & Barksdale, C. M. (1987). Separation distress in infant rhesus monkeys: Effects of diazepam and Ro 15-1788. *Brain Res.* 408: 192–198.

Panksepp, J., Meeker, R., & Bean, N. J. (1980). The neurochemical control of crying. *Pharmacol. Biochem. Behav.* 12:437–443.

Scott, J. P. (1974). Effects of psychotropic drugs on separation distress in dogs. In *Proceedings of IX Congress of the Collegium International Neuropsychopharmacologicum. Excerpta Medica International Congress Series*, no. 359:735–745.

Winslow, J. T., & Insel, T. R. (1991). Endogenous opioids: Do they modulate the rat pup's response to social isolation? *Behav. Neurosci.* 105:253–263.

67. Torgersen, S. (1986). Childhood and family characteristics in panic and generalized anxiety disorders. *Am. J. Psychiat.* 143:630–632.

68. Uhde, T. W., & Tancer, M. (1988). Chemical models of panic: A review and critique. In *Psychopharmacology of anxiety* (P. Tyrer, ed.), pp. 110–131. New York: Oxford Univ. Press.

69. Klein, D. F. (1964). Delineation of two drug-responsive anxiety syndromes. *Psychopharmacol.* 5: 397–408.

70. See fourth article cited in n. 66 and: Suomi, S. J., Seaman, S. F., Lewis, J. K., DeLizio, R. D., & McKinney, Jr., W. T. (1978). Effects of imipramine treatment on separation-induced disorders in rhesus monkeys. *Arch. Gen. Psychiat.* 35:321–329.

71. Klein, D. F. (1981). Anxiety reconceptualized. In *Anxiety: New research and changing concepts* (D. F. Klein & J. Rabkin, eds.), pp. 235–264. New York: Raven Press.

Klein, D. F. (1996). Pharmacological probes in panic disorder. In *Advances in the neurobiology of anxiety disorders* (H. G. M. Westenberg, J. A. den Boer, & D. L. Murphy, eds.). New York: Wiley.

72. See n. 62.

73. See n. 29 and: Nastiti, K., Benton, D., Brain, P. F., & Haug, M. (1991). The effects of 5-HT receptor ligands on ultrasonic calling in mouse pups. *Neurosci. Biobehav. Revs.* 15:483–487.

74. Boyer, W. (1995). Serotonin uptake inhibitors are superior to imipramine and alprazolam in alleviating panic attacks: A meta analysis. *Int. Clin. Psychopharm.* 1:45–49.

75. Klein, D. F. (1993). False suffocation alarms, spontaneous panics, and related conditions. *Arch. Gen. Psychiat.* 50:306–317.

76. Liebowitz, M. R. (1988). Pharmacotherapy of personality disorders. In *Emotions and psychopathology* (M. Clynes & J. Panksepp, eds.), pp. 77–94. New York: Plenum Press.

77. Kramer, P. D. (1993). *Listening to Prozac.* New York: Penguin Books.

78. Mendoza, S. P., Smotherman, W. P., Miner, M. T., Kaplan, J., & Levine, S. (1978). Pituitary-adrenal response to separation in mother and infant squirrel monkeys. *Devel. Psychobiol.* 11:169–175.

For related endocrine issues, see: Sapolsky, R. M. (1993). The physiology of dominance in stable versus unstable social hierarchies. In *Primate social conflict* (W. A. Mason & S. P. Mendoza, eds.), pp. 171–204. Albany: State Univ. of New York Press.

For a review of the potential neurotoxic consequences of stress, see: Sapolsky, R. M. (1996). Stress, glucocorticoids, and damage to the nervous system: The current state of confusion. *Stress* 1:1–19.

79. For a review of such work, see: Panksepp, J., Yates, G., Ikemoto, S., & Nelson, E. (1991). Simple ethological models of depression: Social-isolation induced "despair" in chicks and mice. In *Animal models in psychopharmacology* (B. Olivier, J. Mos, & J. L. Slangen, eds.), pp. 161–181. Basel: Birkhauser Verlag.

80. Harlow, H. F., & Harlow, M. K. (1962). Social deprivation in monkeys. *Sci. Amer.* 207:136–146.

Harlow, H. F. (1971). *Learning to love.* San Francisco: Albion.

Harlow, C. M. (ed.) (1986). *Learning to love: The selected papers of H. F. Harlow.* New York: Praeger.

81. Mason, W. A. (1968). Early social deprivation in nonhuman primates: Implications for human behavior. In *Biology and behavior: Environmental influences* (D. C. Glass, ed.), pp. 70–101. New York: Rockefeller Univ. Press.

Suomi, S. J. (1995). Influence of attachment theory on ethological studies of biobehavioral development in nonhuman primates. In *Attachment theory: Social, developmental, and clinical perspectives* (S. Goldberg, R. Muir, & J. Kerr, eds.), pp. 185–201. Hillsdale, N.J.: Analytic Press.

82. Mason, W. A. (1986). Early socialization. In *Primates, the road to self-sustaining populations* (K. Benirschke, ed.), pp. 321–329. New York: Springer-Verlag.

Suomi, S. J., Harlow, H. F., & McKinney, W. T. (1972). Monkey psychiatrists. *Amer. J. Psychiat.* 128: 41–46.

83. Mason, W. A., & Capitanio, J. P. (1988). Formation and expression of filial attachment in rhesus monkeys raised with living and inanimate mother substitutes. *Devel. Psychobiol.* 21:401–430.

Mason, W. A., & Kenney, W. D. (1974). Redirection of filial attachments in rhesus monkeys: Dogs as mother surrogates. *Science* 183:1209–1211.

84. See n. 79 and: Wilner, P. (1985). *Depression: A psychobiological synthesis.* New York: Wiley.

85. Kraemer, G. W. (1992). A psychobiological theory of attachment. *Behav. Brain Sci.* 15:493–511.

86. Higley, J. D., Suomi, S. J., & Linnoila, M. (1992). A longitudinal study of CSF monoamine metabolite and plasma cortisol concentrations in young rhesus monkeys: Effects of early experience, age, sex, and stress on continuity of individual differences. *Biol. Psychiat.* 32:127–145.

Kraemer, G. W., Ebert, M. H., Schmidt, D. E., & McKinney, W. T. (1989). A longitudinal study of the effects of different rearing environments on cerebrospinal fluid norepinephrine and biogenic amine metabolites in rhesus monkeys. *Neuropsychopharmacol.* 2: 175–189.

87. Hennessy, M. B. (1997). Hypothalamic-pituitary-adrenal responses to brief social separation. *Neurosci. Biobehav. Rev.* 21:11–29.

88. Heilig, M., Koob, G. F., Ekman, R., & Britton, K. T. (1994). Corticotropin-releasing factor and neuropeptide Y: Role in emotional integration. *Trends Neurosci.* 17:80–85.

Valentino, R. J., Foote, S. L., & Page, M. (1993). The locus coeruleus as a site for integrating corticotropin-releasing factor and noradrenergic mediation of stress responses. *Ann. N.Y. Acad. Sci.* 697:173–188.

89. France, R. D., Urban, B., & Krishnan, K. R. (1988). CSF corticotropin-releasing factor–like immunoreactivity in chronic pain patients with or without major depression. *Biol. Psychiat.* 23:86–88.

Nemeroff, C. B. (1984). Elevated concentrations of CSF corticotrophin-releasing factor–like immunoreactivity in depressed patients. *Science* 226:1342–1344.

90. Bisette, G. (1991). Neuropeptides involved in stress and their distribution in the mammalian central nervous system. In *Stress, neuropeptides, and systemic disease* (J. A. McCubbin, P. G. Kaufmann, & C. B. Nemeroff, eds.). San Diego: Academic Press.

Nemeroff, C. B. (1991). Corticotropin-releasing factor. In *Neuropeptides and psychiatric disorders* (C. B. Nemeroff, ed.), pp. 77–91. Washington, D.C.: American Psychiatric Press.

Owens, M. J., & Nemeroff, C. B. (1991). Physiology and pharmacology of corticotrophin-releasing factor. *Pharmacol. Revs.* 43:425–473.

91. Frank, E., Karp, J. F., & Rush, A. J. (1993). Efficacy of treatments for major depression. *Psychopharmacol. Bull.* 29:457–475.

Richelson, E. (1991). Biological basis of depression and therapeutic relevance. *J. Clin. Psychiat.* 52(suppl.): 4–10.

Stewart, J. W., Quitkin, F. M., & Klein, D. F. (1992). The pharmacotherapy of minor depression. *Amer. J. Psychother.* 46:23–36.

92. Barondes, S. H. (1994). Thinking about Prozac. *Science* 263:1102–1103.

Feighner, J. P., & Boyer, W. F. (1991). *Selective serotonin reuptake inhibitors: The clinical use of citalopram, fluoxetine, fluvoxamine, paroxetine and sertraline.* New York: Wiley.

93. Opium, an age-old antidepressant, has never been properly documented according to modern scientific standards, but it was a common treatment of melancholia and many other disorders since its introduction into medicine by Paracelsus in the middle of the 16th century. The following highlights its common use in 19th century medicine: "For the relief of the psychic pains nothing equals opium. . . . It is almost as specific in its action in relieving the mental suffering and depression. . . . As a matter of fact, I have yet to see the first case of opium habit as a result of the use of this drug in melancholia. The physician, however, should dispense the drug himself in these cases, as an added precaution and for the advantage in moral effect." Loomis, A. L., & Thompson, W. G. (eds.) (1898). *A system of practical medicine by American authors.* New York: Lea Brothers. Quotation on p. 779.

94. Also see n. 79.

95. Allman, W. F. (1994). *The stone age present: How evolution has shaped modern life: From sex, violence, and language to emotions, morals, and communities.* New York: Simon and Schuster.

Gazzaniga, M. S. (1985). *The social brain: Discovering the networks of the mind.* New York: Basic Books.

96. Kanner, L. (1943). Autistic disturbance of affective contact. *Nervous Child* 2:217–250. Quotation on p. 250.

97. Baron-Cohen, S., Tager-Flusberg, H., & Cohen, D. J. (eds.) (1993). *Understanding other minds: Perspectives from autism.* Oxford: Oxford Medical.

98. Bauman, M. L., & Kemper, T. L. (eds.) (1994). *The neurobiology of autism.* Baltimore: Johns Hopkins Univ. Press.

Schopler, E., & Mesibov, G. B. (eds.) (1987). *Neurobiological issues in autism.* New York: Plenum Press.

99. Bauman, M. L., & Kemper, T. L. (1995). Neuroanatomical observations of the brain in autism. In *Advaces in biological psychiatry*, vol 1 (J. Panksepp, ed.), pp. 1–26. Greenwich, Conn.: JAI Press.

100. Gillberg, C., & Coleman, M. (1992). *The biology of the autistic syndromes* (2d ed.). Oxford: Mac Keith Press.

101. Bauman, M. L., & Kemper, T. L. (1994). Neuroanatomic observations of the brain in autism. In *The neurobiology of autism* (M. L. Bauman & T. L. Kemper, eds.), pp. 119–145. Baltimore: Johns Hopkins Univ. Press.

102. Margolis, R. L., Chuand, D.-M., & Post, R. M. (1994). Programmed cell death: Implications of neuropsychiatric disorders. *Biol. Psychiat.* 35:946–956.

103. Campbell, M. (1987). Drug treatment of infantile autism: The past decade. In *Psychopharmacology: The third generation of progress* (H. Y. Meltzer, ed.), pp. 1225–1231. New York: Raven Press.

Cook, E. H. (1990). Autism: Review of neurochemical investigations. *Synapse* 6:292–308.

104. See n. 98.

105. Bachevalier, J. (1994). The contribution of medial temporal lobe structures in infantile autism: A neurobehavioral study in primates. In *The neurobiology of autism* (M. L. Bauman & T. L. Kemper, eds.), pp. 146–169. Baltimore: Johns Hopkins Univ. Press.

Panksepp, J., & Sahley, T. (1987). Possible brain opioid involvement in disrupted social intent and language development of autism. In *Neurobiological issues in autism* (E. Schopler & G. Mesibov, eds.), pp. 357–382. New York: Plenum Press.

106. Coleman, M. (1976). *The autistic syndromes.* New York: Elsevier.

107. Zagon, I. S., Gibo, D. M., & McLaughlin, P. J. (1991). Zeta (z), a growth-related opioid receptor in developing rat cerebellum: Identification and characterization. *Brain Res.* 55:28–35.

Zagon, I. S., Zagon, E., & McLaughlin, P. J. (1989). Opioids and the developing organism: A comprehensive bibliography. *Neurosci. Biobehav. Revs.* 13:207–235.

108. Herman, B. H. (1991). Effects of opioid receptor antagonists in the treatment of autism and self-injurious behavior. In *Mental retardations: Developing pharmacotherapies.* Progress in Psychiatry, No. 32 (J. J. Ratsey, ed.), pp. 107–137. Washington, D.C.: American Psychiatric Press.

109. Panksepp, J. (1989). A neurochemical theory of autism. *Trends in Neurosci.* 2:174–177.

Leboyer, M., Bouvard, M. P., Recasens, C., Philippe, A., Guilloud-Bataille, M., Bondoux, D., Tabuteau, F., Dugas, M., Panksepp, J., & Launay, J.-M. (1994). Differences between plasma N- and C-terminally directed ß-endorphin immunoreactivity in infantile autism. *Am. J. Psychiat.* 151:1797–1801.

110. Bouvard, M. P., Leboyer, M., Launay, J.-M., Recasens, C., Plumet, M.-H., Waller-Perotte, D., Tabuteau, F., Bondoux, D., Dugas, M., Lensing, P., & Panksepp, J. (1995). Low-dose naltrexone effects on plasma chemistries and clinical symptoms in autism: A double-blind placebo-controlled study. *Psychiat. Res.* 58:191–201.

Panksepp, J., Lensing, P., Leboyer, M., & Bouvard, M. P. (1991). Naltrexone and other potential new pharmacological treatments of autism. *Brain Dysfunction* 4:281–300.

111. Gillberg, C. (1988). The role of the endogenous opioids in autism and possible relationships to clinical features. In *Aspects of autism: Biological research* (L. Wing, ed.), pp 31–37. Oxford: Alden.

Gillberg, C., Terenius, L., Hagberg, B., Witt-Engerstrom, I., & Eriksson, I. (1990). CSF beta-endorphins in childhood neuropsychiatric disorders. *Brain Devel.* 12:88–92.

Leboyer, M., Bouvard, M. P., Lensing, P., Launay,

J. M., Tabuteau, F., Waller, D., Plumet, M. H., Recasens, C., Kerdelhue, B., Dugas, M., & Panksepp, J. The opioid excess hypothesis of autism: A double-blind study. *Brain Dysfunction* 3:285–298.

112. Jan, J. E., Espezel, H., & Appleton, R. E. (1994). The treatment of sleep disorders with melatonin. *Devel. Med. Child Neurol.* 36:97–107.

113. Bellugi, U., Wang, P. P., & Jernigan, T. L. (1994). Williams syndrome: An unusual neuropsychological profile. In *Atypical cognitive deficits in developmental disorders* (S. H. Broman & J. Grafman, eds.), pp. 23–56. Hillsdale, N.J.: Lawrence Erlbaum.

114. The effects of intranasal administration of vasopressin and oxytocin are modest, and it remains unclear to what extent they get into the main part of the brain. See: Fehm-Wolfsdorf, G., Born, J., Voigt, K.-H. J., & Fehm, H. L. (1984). Human memory and neurohypophyseal hormones: Opposite effects of vasopressin and oxytocin. *Psychoneuroendocrinol.* 9:285–292.

Some molecular congeners of oxytocin have recently been developed that may cross the blood-brain barrier and may lead to better evaluation of such systems in the governance of human social emotions. See: Williams, P. D., et al. (1994). 1-(((7,7-Dimethyl-2(s)-2(S)-amino-4-(methylsulfonyl)butyramido)bicyclo[2.2.1]-hepan (S)-yl)methyl)sulfonyl)-4-(2–methylphenyl)piperazine (L-368,899): An orally bioavailable, non-peptide oxytocin antagonist with potential utility for managing pre-term labor. *J. Med. Chem.* 37:565–571.

115. Panksepp, J. (1989). Altruism, Neurobiology. In *The encyclopedia of neuroscience: Neuroscience year, 1989* (G. Adelman, ed.), pp. 7–8. Boston: Birkhäuser, Boston.

Also see: Hoffman, R. (1981). Is altruism part of human nature? *J. Personal. Soc. Psych.* 40:121–137.

116. Sloboda, J. (1991). Music structure and emotional response: Some empirical findings. *Psychol. Music* 19:110–120.

117. Panksepp, J. (1995). The emotional sources of "chills" induced by music. *Music Percept.* 13:171–207.

118. Goldstein, A. (1980). Thrills in response to music and other stimuli. *Physiol. Psychol.* 3:126–129.

119. For a full discussion of the brain, bodily, and emotional changes produced by music, see:

Hodges, D. A. (ed.) (1995). *Handbook of music psychology*. San Antonio, Tex.: IMR Press.

Maranto, C. (ed.) (1992). *Applications of music in medicine*. Washington, D.C.: National Association for Music Therapy.

Chapter 15

1. Ikemoto, S., & Panksepp, J. (1992). The effects of early social isolation on the motivation for social play in juvenile rats. *Devel. Psychobiol.* 25:261–274.

2. See Figure 1.1 and: Siviy, S. M., & Panksepp, J. (1985). Energy blance and play in juvenile rats. *Physiol. Behav.* 35:435–441.

3. Goodall, J. (1986). *The chimpanzees of Gombe*. Cambridge, Mass.: Harvard Univ. Press. Quotation on pp. 369–370.

4. Panksepp, J. (1993). Rough-and-tumble play: A fundamental brain process. In *Parent-child play: Descriptions and implications* (K. MacDonald, ed.), pp. 147–184. New York: State Univ. of New York Press.

5. The conclusion that males play more than females has permeated the field. See: Meaney, M. J. (1988). The sexual differentiation of social play. *Trends Neurosci.* 11:54–58.

For an overview, also see: Pellis, S. M. (1993). Sex and the evolution of play fighting: A review and model based on the behavior of muroid rodents. *J. Play Theory Res.* 1:55–75.

Unfortunately, no single credible study of gender differences has yet been published where all relevant variables, such as body weight and past social-reinforcement histories, have been fully controlled. For a discussion of such issues, see n. 10. However, there are modest, hormonally caused differences in play styles among males and females (see n 27).

6. Evans, C. S. (1967). Methods of rearing and social interaction in *Macaca nemestrina*. *Anim. Behav.* 15:263–266.

Harlow, H. F., & Harlow, M. K. (1969). Effects of various mother-infant relationships on rhesus monkey behavior. In *Determinants of infant behavior IV* (B. M. Foss, ed.), pp. 15–36. London: Methuen.

7. Chamove, A. S. (1978). Therapy of isolated rhesus: Different partners and social behavior. *Child Devel.* 49:43–50.

Novak, M. A. (1979). Social recovery of monkeys isolated for the first year of life: II. Long-term assessment. *Devel. Psychol.* 15:50–61.

8. Yates, G., Panksepp, J., Ikemoto, S., Nelson, E., & Conner, R. (1991). Social isolation effects on the "behavioral despair" forced swimming test: Effect of age and duration of testing. *Physiol. Behav.* 49:347–353.

9. Panksepp, J., & Beatty, W. W. (1980). Social deprivation and play in rats. *Behav. Neural Biol.* 30: 197–206.

10. Hole, G. J., & Einon, D. F. (1984). Play in rodents. In *Play in animals and humans* (P. K. Smith, ed.), pp. 95–117. New York: Basil Blackwell.

Panksepp, J., Siviy, S., & Normansell, L. (1984). The psychobiology of play: Theoretical and methodological perspectives. *Neurosci. Biobehav. Revs.* 8:465–492.

11. Thor, D. H., & Holloway, W. R., Jr. (1984). Social play in juvenile rats: A decade of methodological and experimental research. *Neurosci. Biobehav. Revs.* 8:455–464.

12. For an overview, see: Aldis, O. (1975). *Play fighting*. New York: Academic Press.

For detailed analysis of play in one species, see: Pellis, S. M. (1981). A description of social play by the Australian magpie *Gymnorhine tibicien* based on Eshkol-Wachman movement notation. *Bird Behav.* 3:61–79.

13. Slade, A., & Wolf, D. P. (eds.) (1994). *Children at play*. New York: Oxford Univ. Press.

14. Humphreys, A. P., & Smith, P. K. (1984).

Rough-and-tumble in preschool and playground. In *Play in animals and humans* (P. K. Smith, ed.), pp. 241–270. Oxford: Blackwell.

Smith, P. K., & Connolly, K. (1972). Patterns of play and social interaction in pre-school children. In *Ethological studies of child behavior* (N. Blurton Jones, ed.), pp. 65–95. Cambridge: Cambridge Univ. Press.

15. Humphreys, A. P., & Einon, D. F. (1981). Play as a reinforcer for maze learning in juvenile rats. *Anim. Behav.* 29:259–270.

16. Weisler, A., & McCall, R. B. (1976). Exploration and play, resume and redirection. *Amer. Psychol.* 31:492–508.

Welker, W. I. (1971). Ontogeny of play and exploratory behaviors: A definition of problems and a search for new conceptual solutions. In *The ontogeny of vertebrate behavior* (H. Moltz, ed.), pp. 171–228. New York: Academic Press.

17. Beatty, W. W., Dodge, A. M., Dodge, L. J., White, K., & Panksepp, J. (1982). Psychomotor stimulants, social deprivation and play in juvenile rats. *Pharmacol. Biochem. Behav.* 16:417–422.

18. Barrett, P., & Bateson, P. (1978). The development of play in cats. *Behaviour* 66:105–120.

Panksepp, J. (1981). The ontogeny of play in rats. *Devel. Psychobiol.* 14:327–332.

Thor, D. H., & Holloway, W. R., Jr. (1984). Developmental analyses of social play behavior in juvenile rats. *Bull. Psychonom. Soc.* 22:587–590.

19. Panksepp, J., Knutson, B., & Pruitt, D. L. (in press). Toward a neuroscience of emotion: The epigenetic foundations of emotional development. In *What develops in emotional development?* (M. F. Mascolo & S. Griffin, eds.), pp. 53–84. New York: Plenum Press.

20. See nn. 10 and 18.

21. See nn. 10 and 22 and: Knutson, B., Panksepp, J., & Pruitt, D. (1996). Effects of fluoxetine on play dominance in juvenile rats. *Aggr. Behav.* 22:241–257.

22. Panksepp, J., Jalowiec, J., De Eskinazi, F. G., & Bishop, P. (1985). Opiates and play dominance in juvenile rats. *Behav. Neurosci.* 99:441–453.

23. Pellis, S. M., & Pellis, V. C. (1987). Play-fighting differs from serious fighting in both target of attack and tactics of fighting in the laboratory rat *Rattus norvegicus. Aggr. Behav.* 18:301–316.

Pellis, S. M., Pellis, V. C., & Dewsbury, D. A. (1989). Different levels of complexity in the play-fighting by muroid rodents appear to result from different levels of intensity of attack and defense. *Aggr. Behav.* 18:297–310.

24. See n. 11.

25. See n. 10.

26. Normansell, L., & Panksepp, J. (1990). Effects of morphine and naloxone on play-rewarded spatial discrimination in juvenile rats. *Devel. Psychobiol.* 23: 75–83.

Pellis, S. M., & McKenna, M. (1995). What do rats find rewarding in play fighting? An analysis using drug-induced non-playful partners. *Behav. Brain Res.* 68: 65–73.

27. A full analysis of acute testosterone effects on play fighting remains to be published, but our unpublished data clearly indicate that testosterone tends to counteract playfulness. The organizational effects of testosterone on subsequent play are also very modest. See: Beatty, W. W., Dodge, A. M., Traylor, K. L., & Meaney, M. J. (1981). Temporal boundary of the sensitive period for hormonal organization of social play in juvenile rats. *Physiol. Behav.* 26:241–243.

However, some have reported larger effects. See:

Meaney, M. J., Stewart, J., & Beatty, W. W. (1985). Sex differences in social play: The socialization of sex roles. *Adv. Study Behav.* 15:1–58.

Pellis, S. M., Pellis, V. C., & Kolb, B. (1992). Neonatal testosterone augmentation increases juvenile play fighting but does not influence the adult dominance relationships of male rats. *Aggr. Behav.* 18:437–447.

However, in all these studies social learning may be a larger factor than any intrinsic effect of testosterone on unconditional play tendencies. Also, females may be more sensitive to distal play gestures, which allow them to anticipate and evade play attacks more successfully. See: Pellis, S. M., Pellis, V. C., & McKenna, M. M. (1994). Feminine dimension in the play fighting of rats (*Rattus norvegicus*) and its defeminization neonatally by androgens. *J. Comp. Psychol.* 108:68–73.

28. At high doses (e.g., 10 mg/kg), fluprazine can reduce play. See: Selseth, K. J., & Keble, E. D. (1988). Fluprazine hydrochloride decreases play behavior but not social grooming in juvenile male rats. *Bull. Psychonom. Soc.* 26:563–564. However, at 4 mg/kg, the same drug increases dorsal contacts, while leaving pinning undiminished; we have found similar effects with other "serenics" such as eltoprazine (Jalowiec, Panksepp, & Nelson, 1989, unpublished data).

29. For a full analysis of laughter, see: Provine, R. R. (1997). Contagious yawning and laughter: Significance for sensory feature detection, motor pattern generation, imitation, and the evolution of social behavior. In *Social learning in animals: The roots of culture* (C. M. Heyes & B. G. Galef, eds.), pp. 179–208. New York: Academic Press.

30. Andrews, R. J. (1963). The origin and evolution of the calls and facial expressions of the primates. *Behaviour* 20:1–109.

Stroufe, L. A., & Waters, E. (1976). The ontogenesis of smiling and laughter: A perspective on the organization of development in infancy. *Psych. Rev.* 83: 173–189.

Van Hooff, J. A. R. A. M. (1972). A comparative approach to the phylogeny of laughter and smiling. In *Non-verbal communication* (R. A. Binde, ed.), pp. 209–246. Cambridge: Cambridge Univ. Press.

31. Ambrose, J. A. (1961). The development of the smiling response in early infancy. In *Determinants of infant behaviour* (B. M. Foss, ed.), pp. 179–201. London: Methuen.

Haith, M., Watson, J., McCall, R., & Zelazo, P. (1972). The meaning of similing and vocalizing in infancy. *Merril-Palmer: Quart. Behav. Devel.* 18:321–365.

Konner, M. (1991). Universals of behavioral development in relation to brain myelination. In *Brain maturation and cognitive development* (K. Gibson & A. Petersen, eds.), pp. 181–224. New York: Aldine de Gruyter.

32. The studies summarized have been submitted for publication: Panksepp, J., & Burgdorf, J. (1997). Laughing rats? Playful tickling arouses high frequency ultrasonic chirping in young rodents. *Nature*. If this work has not been published by the time this text appears, interested readers can request an electronic version of the manuscript from the first author at jpankse@bgnet.bgsu.edu.

A fine summary of laughter in humans and animals is to be found in: Provine, R. R. (1996). Laughter. *Amer. Sci.* 84:38–45.

33. Eibl-Eibesfelt, I. (1989). *Human ethology*. New York: Aldine de Gruyter.

34. For a thorough summary of historical thinking on this issue, see: Chapman, A. J., & Foot, H. C. (1976). Humour and laughter: Theory, research and applications. Chichester, U.K.: Wiley.

35. Poeck, K. (1969). Pathophysiology of emotional disorders associated with brain damage. In *Handbook of clinical neurology*, vol. 3 (P. J. Vinken & G. W. Bruyn, eds.), pp. 343–367. Amsterdam: North Holland.

36. See n. 35 and: Black, D. (1982). Pathological laughter: A review of the literature. *J. Nerv. Ment. Dis.* 170:67–71.

37. Goodall, J. (1986). *The chimpanzees of Gombe*. Cambridge, Mass.: Harvard Univ. Press.

38. It is noteworthy that all of the drugs that are used to treat hyperactive/attention deficit children—namely, amphetamine, methylphenidate, and pemoline—are powerful antiaggressive agents. See: n. 17 and:

Beatty, W. W., Berry, S. L., & Costello, K. B. (1983). Suppression of play fighting by amphetamine: Effects of catecholamine antagonists, agonists and synthesis inhibitors. *Pharmacol. Biochem. Behav.* 20:747–755.

Field, E. G., & Pellis, S. M. (1994). Differential effects of amphetamine on the attack and defense components of play fighting in rats. *Physiol. Behav.* 56:325–330.

Thor, D. H., & Holloway, W. R. (1984). Play soliciting in juvenile male rats: Effects of caffeine, amphetamine, and methylphenidate. *Pharmacol. Biochem. Behav.* 19:725–727.

39. Knutson, B., & Panksepp, J. (1998). Anticipation of play elicits high-frequency ultrasonic vocalizations in young rats. *J. Comp. Psychol.* 112:1–9.

40. Siviy, S., & Panksepp, J. (1987). Sensory modulation of juvenile play in rats. *Devel. Psychobiol.* 20: 39–55.

41. See n. 40 and: Bierley, R. A., Hughes, S. L., & Beatty, W. W. (1986). Blindness and play fighting in juvenile rats. *Physiol. Behav.* 36:199–201.

But vision does have some effect on the specific movements rats exhibit during play. See: Pellis, S. M., McKenna, M. M., Field, E. F., Pellis, V. C., Prusky, G. T., & Whishaw, I. Q. (1996). Uses of vision by rats in play fighting and other close-quarter social interactions. *Physiol. Behav.* 59:905–913.

42. Siviy, S. M., & Panksepp, J. (1987). Juvenile play in the rat: Thalamic and brain stem involvement. *Physiol. Behav.* 41:103–114.

43. Siviy, S. M., & Panksepp, J. (1985). Dorsomedial diencephalic involvement in the juvenile play of rats. *Behav. Neurosci.* 99:1103–1113.

44. Dafny, N., Reyes-Vazquez, C., & Qiao, J. T. (1990). Modification of nociceptively identified neurons in thalamic parafascicularis by chemical stimulation of dorsal raphe with glutamate, morphine, serotonin and focal dorsal raphe electrical stimulation. *Brain Res.* 24:717–723.

Groenewegen, H. J., & Berendse, H. W. (1994). The specificity of the "nonspecific" midline and intralaminar thalamic nuclei. *Trends Neurosci.* 17:52–57.

45. See nn. 35 and 36, as well as the widespread areas of the brain from which gelastic (laughing) epilepsy is found:

Chen, R.-C., & Forster, F. M. (1973). Cursive epilepsy and gelastic epilepsy. *Neurology* 23:1019–1029.

Sterns, F. R. (1972) *Laughing: Physiology, pathophysiology, psychology, pathopsychology and development*. Springfield, Ill.: Charles C. Thomas.

46. Klüver, H., & Bucy, P. C. (1939). Preliminary analysis of the functions of the temporal lobes in monkeys. *Arch. Neurol. Psychiat.* 42:979–1000. Quotation on p. 991.

47. Bard, P., & Mountcastle, V. B. (1948). Some forebrain mechanisms involved in expression of rage with special reference to suppression of angry behavior. *Res. Pubs. Assoc. Nerv. Ment. Dis.* 27:362–404.

Also see: Shreiner, L., & Kling, A. (1953). Behavioral changes following rhinencephalic injury in cat. *J. Neurophysiol.* 16:643–659.

48. Pellis, S. M., Pellis, V. C., & Whishaw, I. Q. (1992). The role of the cortex in play fighting by rats: Developmental and evolutionary implications. *Brain Behav. Evol.* 39:270–284.

49. Panksepp, J., Normansell, L., Cox, J. F., & Siviy, S. M. (1994). Effects of neonatal decortication on the social play of juvenile rats. *Physiol. Behav.* 56:429–443.

50. See n. 49 and: Panksepp (1985, unpublished data).

51. Panksepp, J. (1996). The psychobiology of prosocial behaviors: Separation distress, play, and altruism. In *Altruism and aggression: Biological and social origins* (C. Zahn-Waxler, E. M. Cummings & R. Iannotti, eds.), pp. 19–57. Cambridge: Cambridge Univ. Press.

52. Siviy, S. (in press). Neurobiological substrates of play behavior: Glimpses into the structure and function of mammalian playfulness. In *Animal play: Evolutionary, comparative, and ecological perspectives* (M. Bekoff & J. A. Byers, eds.). New York: Cambridge Univ. Press.

53. See n. 2.

54. See n. 22 and: Vanderschuren, L. J. M. J., Niesink, R. J. M., Spruijt, B. M., & Van Ree, J. M. (1995). Effects of morphine on different aspects of social play in juvenile rats. *Psychopharmacol.* 117:225–231.

Vanderschuren, L. J. M. J., Niesink, R. J. M., Spruijt, B. M., & Van Ree, J. M. (1995). u and k-opioid receptor-mediated opioid effects on social play in juvenile rats. *Eur. J. Pharmacol.* 276:257–266.

55. See n. 10.

56. Panksepp, J., & Bishop, P. (1981). An autoradiographic map of the (^{3}H) diprenorphine binding in rat brain: Effects of social interaction. *Brain Res. Bull.* 7:405–410.

Vanderschuren, L. J. M. J., Stein, E. A., Wiegant, V. M., & Van Ree, J. M. (1995). Social play alters regional brain opioid receptor binding in juvenile rats. *Brain Res.* 680:148–156.

57. Numan, M. (1988). Maternal behavior. In *The physiology of reproduction* (E. Knobil & J. D., Neill, eds.), pp. 1569–1645. New York: Raven Press.

58. Panksepp, J., Normansell, L., Cox, J. F., Crepeau, L. J., & Sacks, D. S. (1987). Psychopharmacology of social play. In *Ethopharmacology of agonistic behaviour in animals and humans* (B. Olivier, J. Mos, & P. F. Brain, eds.), pp. 132–144. Dordrecht: Martinus Nijhoff.

59. See n. 10

60. Siviy, S. M., Fleischhauer, A. E., Kuhlman, S. J., & Atrens, D. M. (1994). Effects of alpha-2 adrenoceptor antagonists on rough-and-tumble play in juvenile rats: Evidence for a site of action independent of non-adrenoceptor imidazoline binding sites. *Psychopharmacol.* 113:493–499.

Siviy, S. M., Line, B. S., & Darcy, E. A. (1995). Effects of MK-801 on rough-and-tumble play in juvenile rats. *Physiol. Behav.* 57:843–847.

61. One of the great paradoxes of psychopharmacology is the enormous variability of receptors for various biogenic amines. Fifteen presently exist for the serotonin system, but no one has yet suggested how a single transmitter such as serotonin, which is largely released by endogenous pacemaker activity in the brain, selectively activates so many receptors. It remains possible that many of these receptors function concurrently to maintain homeostasis in brain serotonin sytems as opposed to normally mediating distinct behaviors. In any event, selective pharmacological modulation of these receptors can produce many distinct behavior effects. For example, see; Bevan, P., Cools, A. R., & Archer, T. (eds.) (1989). *Behavioural pharmacology of 5-HT*. Hillsdale, N.J.: Lawrence Earlbum.

62. Panksepp, J., Crepeau, L., & Clynes, M. (1987). Effects of CRF on separation distress and juvenile play. *Soc. Neurosci. Abstr.* 13:1320.

Panksepp (1990, unpublished data).

63. See n. 12 and:

Fagen, R. (1981). *Animal play behavior*. New York: Oxford Univ. Press.

Smith, P. K. (1982). Does play matter? Functional and evolutionary aspects of animal and human play. *Behav. Brain Sci.* 5:139–184.

64. Crepeau, L. J. (1989). The interactive influences of early handling, prior play exposure, acute stress, and sex on play behavior, exploration and the HPA reactivity in juvenile rats. Ph.D. diss., Bowling Green State University.

65. Panksepp (1989, unpublished data).

66. Einon, F. D., Morgan, J. M., & Kibbler, C. C. (1978). Brief periods of socialization and later behavior in the rat. *Devel. Psychobiol.* 11:213–225.

67. Potegal, M., & Einon, D. (1989). Aggressive behavior in adult rats deprived of playfighting experience as juveniles. *Devel. Psychobiol.* 22:159–172.

68. Adams, N., & Boice, R. (1983). A longitudinal study of dominance in an outdoor colony of domestic rats. *J. Comp. Physiol. Psychol.* 97:24–33.

Adams, N., & Boice, R. (1989). Development of dominance in domestic rats in laboratory and semi-natural environments. *Behav. Proc.* 19:127–142.

Taylor, G. T. (1980). Fighting in juvenile rats and the ontogeny of agonistic behavior. *J. Comp. Physiol. Psychol.* 95:685–693.

69. See n. 4.

70. See n. 13 and:

Christie, J. F., & Johnsen, E. P. (1983). The role of play in social-intellectual development. *Rev. Educ. Res.* 53:93–115.

Saltz, E., & Brodie, J. (1982). Pretend-play training in childhood: A review and critique. *Control Human Devel.* 6:97–113.

Simon, T., & Smith, P. K. (1983). The study of play and problem solving in preschool children: Have experimenter effects been responsible for previous results? *Br. J. Devel. Psych.* 1:289–297.

71. We have been evaluating the consequences of play deprivation for years and have found no clear effects on fairly complex learning tasks such as two-way avoidance and radial maze learning, nor on the task described in n. 66, nor on the onset of sexual behavior in male rats. Presently we are evaluating the consequences of play deprivation on complex social strategies. Human research on play has also questioned the differential benefits of play over simple tutoring. See:

Smith, P. K., Dalgleish, M., & Herzmark, G. (1981). A comparison of the effects of fantasy play tutoring and skills tutoring in nursery classes. *Int. J. Behav. Devel.* 4:421–441.

Smith, P. K., & Sydall, S. (1978). Play and non-play tutoring in pre-school children: Is it play or tutoring which matters? *Br. J. Ed. Psych.* 48:315–325.

72. This idea has been developed in: Panksepp, J. (1986). The anatomy of emotions. In *Emotions: Theory, research and experience*. Vol. 3, *Biological foundations of emotions* (R. Plutchik & H. Kellerman, eds.), pp. 91–121. New York: Academic Press

73. Greenough, W. T., & Juraska, J. M. (eds.) (1986). *Developmental neuropsychobiology*. Orlando, Fla.: Academic Press.

Greenough, W. T., & Black, J. E. (1992). Induction of brain structure by experience: Substrates for cognitive development. In *Behavioral developmental neuroscience*. Vol. 24, *Minnesota symposia on child psychology* (M. Gunnar & C. A. Nelson, eds.), pp. 35–52. Hillsdale, N.J.: Lawrence Erlbaum.

Rosenzweig, M. R., & Bennet, E. L. (1996). Psychobiology of plasticity: Effects of training and experience on brain and behavior. *Behav. Brain Res.* 78: 57–65.

74. Ferchmin, P.A., & Eterovic, V.A. (1986). Forty minutes of experience increases the weight and RNA content of cerebral cortex in periadolescent rats. *Devel. Psychobiol.* 19:1–19.

75. See n. 64, and: Fagen, R. (1992). Play, fun, and communication of well-being. *Play and Culture* 5:40–58.

76. See nn. 69 and 72 for a discussion of such issues.

77. See nn. 16, 70, and 71 for a discussion of such issues.

78. Armstrong, T. (1995). *The myth of the ADD child.* New York: Dutton.

Bradley, C. (1937). The behavior of children receiving Benzedrine. *Am. J. Psychiat.* 94:556–585.

Klein, R. G. (1987). Pharmacology of childhood hyperactivity: An update. In *Psychopharmacology: The third generation of progress* (H. Y. Meltzer, ed.), pp. 1215–1224. New York: Raven Press.

79. See Chapter 8 and:

Kalivas, P. W. (1993). Neurotransmitter regulation of dopamine neurons in the ventral tegmental area. *Brain Res. Revs.* 18:75–113.

Salamone, J. D. (1994). The involvement of nucleus accumbens dopamine in appetitive and aversive motivation. *Behav. Brain Res.* 61:117–135.

80. Cox, J. F. (1986). Catecholamine control of social play: Mechanisms of amphetamine suppression of play. Master's thesis, Bowling Green State University.

81. Pellis, S. M., Casteneda, E., McKenna, M. M., Tan-Nguyen, L. T. L., & Whishaw, I. Q. (1993). The role of the striatum in organizing sequences of play fighting in neonatally dopamine-depleted rats. *Neurosci. Let.* 158:13–15.

Although the play-modifying effects of amine depletion in the preceding report were fairly modest, reflecting mainly an increase in evasions during dorsal contacts, we have performed large lesions of the dorsal striatum in a few pairs of rats, and play has been completely eliminated (Panksepp, 1985, unpublished data). However, these animals are so debilitated in all behavioral realms that the effects cannot be interpreted meaningfully with regard to normal play functions.

82. See n. 4.

83. A potential relationship between attention deficit/hyperactivity disorders (ADHDs) and excessive activity in play circuits is presently supported only by the fact that both are dramatically reduced by administration of psychostimulants. A therapeutic intervention that needs to be urgently evaluated in ADHD children is the provision of extra opportunities to indulge in rough-and-tumble play early each morning to see if such play will alleviate some of the impulsive symptoms later in the day.

84. ADHD children do appear to have diminished frontal lobe inhibition, especially in the right hemisphere. See: Castellanos, F. X., Giedd, J. N., Marsh, W. L., Hamburger, S. D., Vaituzis, A. C., Dickstein, D. P., Sarfatti, S. E., Vauss, Y. C., Snell, J. W., Lange, N., Kaysen, D., Krain, A. L., Ritchie, G. F., Rajapakse, J. C., & Rapoport, J. L. (1996). Quantitative brain magnetic resonance imaging in attention-deficit hyperactivity disorder. *Arch. Gen. Psychiat.* 53:607–616.

85. See nn. 17, 38, and 58.

86. A reduction of playfulness is a common but poorly documented observation. See: Talmadge, J., & Barkley, R. A. (1983). The interactions of hyperactive and normal boys with their fathers and mothers. *J. Abnorm. Child Psychol.* 11:565–580.

87. Chase, T. N., & Friedhoff, A. J. (eds.) (1982). *Gilles de la Tourette syndrome.* New York: Raven Press.

Comings, D. E. (1990). *Tourette syndrome and human behaviour.* Duarte, Calif.: Hope Press.

88. See n. 87 and: Leckman, J. F., Walkup, J. T., Riddle, M. A., Towbin, K. E., & Cohen, D. J. (1987). Tic disorders. In *Psychopharmacology: The third generation of progress* (H. Y. Meltzer, ed.), pp. 1239–1246. New York: Raven Press.

89. See nn.17, 38, and 58.

90. Wing, L. (1985). *Autistic children: A guide for parents and professionals.* New York: Brunner/Mazel.

91. Cousins, N. (1979). *Anatomy of an illness as perceived by the patient: Reflections on healing and regeneration.* New York: Norton.

92. Bolk, L. (1926). *Das Problem de Menschwerdung.* Jena: Gustav Fisher.

Gould, S. J. (1977). *Ontogeny and phylogeny.* Cambridge, Mass.: Belknap Press of Harvard Univ. Press.

93. Insel, T. R. (1993). Oxytocin and the neuroendocrine basis of affiliation. In *Hormonally induced changes in mind and brain* (J. Schulkin, ed.), pp. 225–251. San Diego: Academic Press.

However, in this context, it should be emphasized that recent work with oxytocin knockout mice indicates that oxytocin gene expression is not absolutely essential for maternal behavior, but such animals are less social and more aggressive. See: Young, L. J., Wang, Z., Nishimori, K., Guo, Q., Matzuk, M., & Insel, T. R. (1996). Maternal behavior and brain oxytocin receptors unaffected in oxytocin knockout mice. *Abstr. Soc. Neurosci.* 22:2070.

94. See nn. 10 and 58.

95. Knoll, J. (1992). (-) Deprenyl-mediation: A strategy to modulate the age-related decline of the striatal dopaminergic system. *J. Am. Geriatr. Soc.* 40: 839–847.

96. Knoll, J. (1988). Extension of lifespan of rats by long-term (-)deprenyl treatment. *Mt. Sinai J. Med.* 55:67–74.

97. The Parkinson Study Group (1989). Effect of deprenyl on the progression of disability in early Parkinson's disease. *N. Eng. J. Med.* 321:1364–1371.

98. Ward, W., Morgensthalen, J., & Fowkes, S. W. (1993). *Smart Drugs II: The next generation.* Menlo Park, Calif.: Health Freedom.

99. Knoll, J. (1988). The striatal dopamine dependency of lifespan in male rats: Longevity study with (-) deprenyl. *Mech. Aging and Devel.* 46:237–262.

Chapter 16

1. The difference between the "easy" and "hard" questions of consciousness is related to the "specific contents" versus the "underlying processes" of consciousness. Many interesting views concerning the nature of consciousness are to be found in: Gray, J. A. (1995). The contents of consciousness: A neuropsychological conjecture. *Behav. Brain Sci.* 18:659–722.

The literature on consciousness has grown enormously in the past decade. A comprehensive view of consciousness is to be found in: Baars, B. J. (1988). *A cognitive theory of consciousness.* New York: Cambridge Univ. Press.

Excellent general discussions concerning the nature of consciousness can be found in the following:

Farthing, G. W. (1993). *The psychology of consciousness.* Englewood Cliff, N. J. Prentice Hall.

Davies, M., & Humphreys, G. W. (eds). (1993). *Consciousness*, Oxford: Blackwell.

Many other recent contributions offer more specific viewpoints, including the following:

Dennett, D. C. (1996). *Kinds of minds: toward an understanding of consciousnes.* New York: Basic Books.

Edelman, G. M. (1992). *Bright air, brilliant fire: On the matter of the mind.* New York: Basic Books.

Also see nn. 19, 25, and 33.

2. With the use of the Wada test, in which the right hemisphere is selectively anesthetized, it has been found that humans shift from expressing deeper primary-process emotions to more superficial social emotions. See: Ross, E. D., Homan, R. W., & Buck, R. (1994). Differential hemispheric lateralization of primary and social emotions. *Neuropsychiat. Neuropsych. Behav. Neurol.* 7:1–19.

3. One of the starting premises of cognitive psychology was the scientifically problematic nature of emotionality. See: Norman, D. A. (1980). Twelve issues for cognitive science. *Cog. sci.* 4:1–32.

4. For some thoughts on the fragmentation of psychology, see chap. 1, n. 8, as well as:

Bower, G. H. (1993). The fragmentation of psychology? *Am. Psychol.* 48:905–907.

Koch, S. (1993). "Psychology" on "the psychological studies"? *Am. Psychol.* 48: 902–904.

5. The varieties of brain stimulation–induced affective experiences in humans are summarized in chap. 1, n. 20.

6. The extent to which we have conscious access to the causes of our behavior has been critically analyzed by many, most prominently by: Nisbett, R. E., & Wilson, T. D. (1977). Telling more than we can know: Verbal reports on mental processes. *Psych. Rev.* 84: 231–259.

However, the documented failures of introspective insight typically come from the analysis of cognitive processes. It remains unclear whether such arguments apply to feelings that arise from the arousal of the basic emotions. Also, it is now important to consider such issues from neural systems perspectives, such as those described in n. 2 and in: Farah, M. J., O'Reilly, R. C., & Vecera, S. P. (1993). Dissociated overt and covert recognition as an emergent property of a lesioned neural network. *Psych. Rev.* 100:571–588.

7. For a recent discussion of issues related to the mental abilities of animals, see: Griffin, D. R. (1992). *Animal minds.* Chicago: Univ. of Chicago Press.

8. For a thorough discussion of the rejections of universals in "human nature" and their gradual acceptance in the social sciences, see: Brown, D. E. (1991). *Human universals.* New York: McGraw-Hill.

9. Fridlund, A. J. (1994). *Human facial expression: An evolutionary view.* San Diego: Academic Press.

However, now critical evidence is also coming directly from an analysis of the genetic issues. See: Hamer, D., & Copeland, P. (1994). *The science of desires: The search for the gay gene and the biology of behavior.* New York: Simon and Schuster.

10. It is, of course, regrettable that the higher psychological concepts will never completely overlap with neural issues, but new ways of using concepts can facilitate progress in specifying critical linkages. The capitalization of key concepts employed in this text may help remind us that all linkages are provisional and shall remain open, no doubt forever, to refinement.

11. The new brain-imaging procedures have a deceptive appeal for the uninitiated. Not only do the traditional pseudocolor images often reflect remarkably small brain changes, but they surely yield many false-negatives: The techniques probably fail to highlight areas that are critical for certain psychological processes because of massive overlap of opposing systems or other biophysical properties of certain brain areas.

12. At the present time, most behavioral neuroscientists remain unwilling to grant intangible conscious processes such as perceptual awareness and internally felt experience to their animal subjects. However, this is commonly done less on the basis of reasoned arguments than habitual assertions that anthropomorphism is bad and the conviction that such internal processes will never be "seen" or "weighed" with sufficient accuracy to be useful scientifically. In addition, the continuing neglect of consciousness (at least at the neuro-empirical level, if not the conceptual one) is partly due to the fact that many investigators of animal brain functions are not primarily interested in how their findings may relate to human issues. Many are simply and justifiably interested in animal behaviors and brain functions for their own sake. However, for others who believe that much of the importance of animal brain research lies in its ability to deeply clarify the human condition, the neglect of consciousness by neuroscientists often seems to be an irrational and uncourageous choice. Of course, it remains much easier to talk about such matters than to do illuminating experiments on them. Most agree that the highest levels of human perceptual consciousness are closely linked to sensory analyzers of the cortex, while intentionality and conscious planning are closely linked to frontal lobe functions. Humans clearly have more frontal lobe tissue than other creatures, which allows our consciousness to be expanded especially far in space and time. However, affective consciousness surely has deeper evolutionary roots in ancestral subcortical processes that we can systematically analyze through animal brain research.

13. To highlight the abundant new levels of intellectual activity in this field, there is now an Association for the Scientific Study of Consciousness (ASSC), which organizes physical and electronic meetings on the topic and supports the publication of several journals (for web site, see: http://www.phil.vt.edu/ASSC/).

14. Even though most students of psychology are familiar with the dubious history of phrenological thought, it should be remembered that the founders of the field established a new level of precision in studying the brain. As Samuel Solly indicated in the preface to the first "modern" textbook of neuroanatomy, "Every honest and erudite anatomist must acknowledge that we are indebted mainly to Gall and Spurzheim for the improvements which have been made in our mode of studying the brain." Solly, S. (1847). *The human brain: Its structure, physiology and disease*, (2d ed.). London: Longman, Brown, Green, and Longmans. Quotation on pp. x-xi.

15. For a discussion of sexual cannibalism in mantises, see: Prete, F. R., Lum H., & Grossman, S. P. (1992). Non-predatory ingestive behaviors of the praying mantids *Tenodera aridifolia sinesnis* (*Sauss.*) and *Sphodromantis lineola* (*Burr.*). *Brain Behav. Evol.*, 329: 124–132.

16. For some perspectives on the consequences of Cartesian dualism in the neurosciences, see: Harrington, A. (ed.) (1992). *So human a brain: Knowledge and values in the neurosciences.* Boston: Birhäuser.

During the past decade, there has been an increasingly vigorous debate over the existence of animal consciousness. The foremost proponent of animal consciousness simply from a behavioral perspective, with few neuroscience underpinnings, has been Donald Griffin (see n. 7). Several other popular books have also advocated the reality of animal emotion. For example see: Thomas, E. M. (1993). *The hidden life of dogs.* Boston: Houghton Mifflin.

17. For an intriguing and novel view on this traditional dilemma, see:

Heyes, C., & Dickinson, A. (1993). The intentionality of animal action. In *Consciousness* (M. Davies & G. W. Humphreys, eds.), pp. 105–120. Oxford: Blackwell.

Barresi, J., & Moore, C. (1996). Intentional relations and social understanding. *Behav. Brain Sci.* 19:107–154.

18. The potentially endless cascade of "awareness of awarenesses" has been humorously depicted by R. A. Gardner and B. T. Gardner in their review of Parker, S. T., Michell, R. W., & Boccia, M. L. (eds.) (1994). *Self-awareness in animals and humans: Developmental perspectives.* New York. Cambridge Univ. Press (which appeared in *Contemporary Psychology* 41[1996]:682–684): "A while back a distinguished Russian colleague visited our chimpanzee laboratory in Reno and asked us if Washoe had in her mind an image of our image of the sign language she addressed to us . . . and pointed out that we must then have in our minds an image of Washoe's image of our image of her signs. Moreover, the fact that he understood us meant that he had in his mind an image of our image of Washoe's image of our image, and the fact that we understood him meant that we had an image of his image of our image of Washoe's image of our image of Washoe's signs." Enough said about "multiple observers"?

19. A recent treatise on consciousness as focused largely on our ability to see has been provided by Nobel laureate Francis Crick. see: Crick, F. (1994). *The astonishing hypothesis: The scientific search for the soul.* New York: Scribner.

If I had to select a single form of sensory deprivation that would most compromise the normal overall coherence of human consciousness, it probably would be somatosensory or vestibular. We are probably deeply dependent on touch for our emotional and perceptual equilibrium, as highlighted by some sensory deprivation experiments that were done before the present era where such types of experiments might be deemed unethical. See: Heron, W., Doane, B.K., & Scott, T. H. (1956). Visual disturbances after prolonged perceptual isolation. *Canad. J. Psychol.* 10:13–18.

However, many of these effects may have been due to demand characteristics. See: Orne, M. T., & Scheibe, K. E. (1964). The contribution of nondeprivation factors in the production of sensory deprivation effects: The psychology of the "panic button." *J. Abnorm. Soc. Psych.* 68:3–12.

Indeed, now it is known that restriction of sensory input can have various therapeutic effects. See: Suedfeld, P. (1980). *Restricted environmental stimulation: Research and clinical applications.* New York: Wiley.

20. For a summary of such studies, see: Nelkin, N. (1993). The connection between intentionality and consciousness. In *The psychology of consciousness* (G. W. Farthing, ed.), pp. 224–239. Englewood Cliffs, N.J.: Prentice Hall.

21. Bauer, R. M., & Verfaellie, M. (1988). Electrodermal discrimination of familiar but not unfamiliar faces. *Brain Cogn.* 8:240–252.

Damasio, A. R. (1990). Category-related recognition defects as a clue to the neural substrates of knowledge. *Trends Neurosci.* 13:95–98.

Damasio, A. R., Tranel, D., & Damasio, H. (1990). Face agnosia and the neural substrates of memory. *Ann. Rev. Neurosci.* 13:89–109.

22. Sano, K., Mayanagi, Y., Sekino, H., Ogashiwa, M., & Ishijima, B. (1970). Results of stimulation and destruction of the posterior hypothalamus in man. *J. Neurosurg.* 33:689–707.

23. Le Doux, J. E. (1985). Brain, mind, and language. In *Brain and mind* (D. A. Oakley, ed.), pp. 197–216. London: Methuen.

Zaidel, D. W. (1993). View of the world from a split-brain perspective. In *Neurological boundaries of reality* (E. M. R. Critchley, ed.). London: Farrand Press.

24. Lambert, A. J. (1991). Interhemispheric interaction in the split-brain. *Neuropsychologia*. 29:941–948.

Pashler, H., Luck, S. J., Hillyard, S. A., Manguin, G. R., O'Brien, S., & Gazzaniga, M. S. (1994). Sequential operation of disconnected cerebral hemispheres in split-brain patients. *NeuroReport* 5:2381–2384.

25. Baars, B. J. (1996). *In the theater of consciousness: The workspace of the mind*. Oxford: Oxford Univ. Press.

26. The likelihood is high that the distinct functions of the two hemispheres are derived more by epigenetic, learning influences than by any dramatic genetically prescribed differential functions. This is suggested by the ability of one hemisphere to assume the functions of the other when damage occurs early in life. For instance, children whose left/speaking hemispheres have been surgically removed to control epilepsy rarely exhibit the dramatic language deficits that are common after similar damage in adults. see: Vargha-Khadem, F., & Polkey, C. E. (1992). A review of cognitive outcome after hemidecortication in humans. *Adv. Exp. Med. Biol.* 325:137–151.

The literature on hemispheric specialization of functions is massive, but the types of issues that are relevant for the present discussion are succinctly summarized in: Davidson, R. J., & Hugdahl, K. (1995). *Brain asymmetry*. Cambridge, Mass.: MIT Press.

27. See n. 2.

28. Tucker, D., & Williamson, P. A. (1984). Asymmetric neural control systems in human self-regulation. *Psych. Rev.* 91:185–215.

29. See chap. 5, nn. 48 and 49. In this context, it must be pointed out that similar types of damage cannot be done in older animals that have come to rely more upon their cortical functions. Indeed, humans are so dependent on cortical functions that their deficit following restricted cortical damage is routinely much more severe than is evident in most "lower" animals. For instance, damage to the motor cortex can lead to total contralateral paralysis, while similar damage in a rat is almost undetectable, with only fine motor skills being affected. See: Whishaw, I. Q., & Kolb, B. (1984). Behavioral and anatomical studies of rats with complete or partial decortication in infancy: Functional sparing, crowding or loss and cerebral growth or shrinkage. In *Recovery from brain damage* (R. Almli & S. Finger, eds.). New York: Academic Press.

For a full analysis of such higher issues, see: Kolb, B., & Tees, C. (eds.) (1990). *The cerebral cortex of the rat*. Cambridge, Mass.: MIT Press.

30. A basic attribute of the primal SELF that must be emphasized is the epigenetic emergence of hierarchical controls in the developing system. Although the lower levels may be essential for the normal development of the higher levels, once those levels have matured in the brain, they have some autonomy. However, without support from the lower levels, the functions of the higher levels might gradually degrade. A parallel is observed in human sexual behavior, where removal of some lower levels, such as the gonads, leads only gradually to a deterioration of sexual interest and competence. Also, it should be noted that in humans, some of the lower levels have special inputs from higher areas, which may provide unique types of emotional controls in the human brain. See: Porges, S. W., Doussard-Roosevelt, J. A., & Maity, A. K. (1994). Vagal tone and the physiological regulation of emotion. In *Emotion regulation: Behavioral and biological considerations*. Monograph of the Society for Research in Child Development, vol. 59 (serial no. 240) (N. A. Fox, ed.), pp. 167–186.

For a more behavioristic analysis of "self"-related issues, see: Rachlin, H. (1995). Self-control: Beyond commitment. *Behav. Brain Sci.* 18:109–159.

31. Many fascinating issues concerning phantom limbs are summarized in: Melzack, R. (1989). Phantom limbs, the self and the brain. The D. O. Hebb Memorial Lecture. *Canad. J. Psychol.* 30:1–16.

Related sensory agnosias are summarized in: Ramachandran, V. S. (1994). Phantom limbs, neglect syndromes, repressed memories, and Freudian psychology. *Int. Rev. Neurobiol.* 37:291–333.

32. For one of the most recent variants of the thalamic reticular theory of consciousness, see: Newman, J. (1995). Review: Thalamic contributions to attention and consciousness. *Conscious. Cogn.* 4:172–193.

Also see the various commentaries on this theory. in this issue of *Consciousness and Cognition*, every issue of which is rich in thought-provoking articles on the nature of consciousness.

33. Dennett, D. C. (1991). *Consciousness explained*. Boston: Little, Brown.

34. According to the present argument (i.e., that a neural entity such as "the SELF" does exist in the brain), the bottom-line statement probably should be "I am, therefore I am." In any event, we probably should not persist in chastising Descartes for giving primacy to "I think, therefore I am." In *The Passions of the Soul*, Descartes did accept the primacy of emotions in experience, but perhaps for political reasons (to avoid religious persecution, to which Galileo suffered) he drew a strict dualistic line between bodily processes (which included emotions) and mind/soul processes (which included thoughts). To quote from p. 344 of the source cited in chap. 2, n. 43: "In Holland, Descartes worked at his system, and by 1634 he had completed a scientific work called *Le Monde*. When he heard, however, of the condemnation of Galileo for teaching the Copernican system, as did *Le Monde*, he immediately had the book suppressed. This incident is important in Descartes's life, for it reveals that spirit of caution and conciliation toward authority which was very marked in him. . . . The suppression also affected the subsequent course of his publications, which were from then on strategically designed to recommend his less orthodox views in an oblique fashion."

35. It should be remembered that the primate homolog of Wernicke's area is also devoted to elaborating cross-modal associations, which presumably are the basis for language. Also, it is generally believed that presemantic vocal signs, such as the many types of natural vocal calls of mammals, emerge from subcortical reaches of the brain that are very distinct from the language cortex. However, the two processes may be coordinated in motivational areas such as the anterior-cingulate cortex which seems to provide the psychic energy for people to communicate linguistically (see Appendix B). In this context, it is noteworthy that to a substantial extent human speech may still serve primitive affective functions such as social grooming at a distance, where "what matters is not what you say, but how you say it," as expanded upon in: Dunbar, R. I. M. (1993). Coevolution of neocortical size, group size and language in humans. *Behav. Brain Sci.* 16:681–735.

For a full comparative view of communication, see: Hauser, M. D. (1996). *The evolution of communication*. Cambridge, Mass.: MIT Press.

36. One of the great achievements in this realm is the demonstration that the environmentally induced neural patterns from waking states can be detected during sleep. See chap. 7, n. 15.

37. Bekoff, M., & Jamieson, D. (eds.) (1995). *Reading in animal cognition*. Cambridge, Mass.: MIT Press.

38. George, M. S., Ketter, T. A., Kimbrell, T. A., Speer, A. M., Steedman, J. M., & Post, R. M. (1996). What functional imaging has revealed about the brain basis of mood and emotion. *Advances in Biological Psychiatry*, vol. 2 (J. Panksepp, ed.), pp. 63–113. Greenwich, Conn.: JAI Press.

39. Kelso J. A. (1995). *Dynamic patterns*. Cambridge, Mass.: MIT Press.

Turbes, C. C. (1993). Brain self-organization dynamics. *Biomed. Sci. Instrum.* 29:135–146.

40. For an example of how this is achieved at a fairly low level of the neuroaxis, see: Kalesnykas, R. P., & Sparks, D. L. (1996). The primate superior colliculus and the control of saccadic eye movements. *Neuroscientist* 2:284–292.

41. Strehler, B. L. (1991). Where is the self? A neuroanatomical theory of consciousness. *Synapse* 7:44–91.

42. It is likely that several coordinated functions of the brain stem are necessary for establishing a network for the basic SELF, but I will limit the present discussion to a simplified outline of the relevant issues. The issue of whether these low areas of the brain stem can elaborate any form of conscious experience is debatable, but the relevant experiments—namely, those in very young organisms—remain to be done. I would suggest that during early development these systems lie at the heart of conscious experience and that only gradually during development do these lower functions become so automatized that they no longer are the focus of active attention. Attention may become more entranced by the flow of information through the thalamic-neocortical axis that comes to constitute the contents of consciousness. Still, I would hypothesize that the lower, primary-process substrates of consciousness remain as an essential neural scaffolding for the higher levels of consciousness to be elaborated.

43. The entertaining notion of a Cartesian theater is discussed by Dennett (see n. 33). Many eschew the concept of a central agency within consciousness. For one prominent example of such a view, see: Minsky, M. (1987). *Society of mind*. New York: Simon and Schuster.

44. The fact that functions are rerepresented within the brain is well established, and there is a great deal of data indicating that the higher brain areas can respecialize readily. For instance, when the visual cortex is damaged early in life, the visual system will project to nearby cortex that is still intact, even though these cortical areas would normally be used for the processing of other sensory modalities. See: Frost, D. O., & Metin, C. (1985). Induction of functional retinal projections to the somatosensory system. *Nature* 517:162–164.

For a broad-ranging discussion of such issues, see: Sporns, O., & Tononi, G. (1994). *Selectionism and the brain*. Special issue of *International Review of Neurobiology*, vol. 37. San Diego: Academic Press.

45. There are powerful interconnections between the mesencephalic areas implicated in the generation of the primal SELF and the frontal cortex. See: Sesack, S. R., Deutsch, A. Y., Roth, R. H., & Bunney, B. (1989). Topographic organization of the efferent projections of the medial prefrontal cortex in the rat: An anterograde tract tracing study with *Phaeolus vulgaris* leucoagglutinin. *J. Comp. Neurol.* 190:213–242.

46. Brudzynski, S. M., Wu, M., & Mogenson, G. J. (1993). Decreases in rat locomotor activity as a result of changes in synaptic transmission to neurons within the mesencephalic locomotor region. *Can. J. Physiol. Pharmacol.* 71:394–406.

Mogenson, G. J., & Yang, C. R., (1991). The contribution of basal forebrain to limbic-motor integration and the mediation of motivation to action. *Adv. Exp. Med. Biol.* 295:267–290.

It is a neuroanatomical fact that all of the basic emotional and motivational systems are represented within PAG tissue. This remarkable confluence of information clearly speaks of the importance of this tissue in the integration of all types of affective information.

47. Sparks, D. L. (1988). Neural cartography: Sensory and motor maps in the superior colliculus. *Brain Behav. Evol.* 31:49–56.

48. See chap. 4, n. 2, and. Eslinger, P. J., Grattan, L. M., Damasio, H., & Damasio, A. R. (1992). Developmental consequences of childhood frontal lobe damage. *Arch. Neurol* 49:764–769.

Goyer, P. F., Andreason, P. J., Semple, W.E., Clayton, A. H., King, A. C., & Compton-Toth, B. (1994). Positron-emission tomography and personality disorders. *Neuropsychopharmacol.* 10: 21–28.

49. For a practical overview of brain rhythms and how they can be harnessed to improve life, see: Abarbanel, A. (1995). Gates, states, rhythms, and resonances: The scientific basis of neurofeedback training. *J. Neurotherapy* 1:15–38.

50. Bailey, P., & Davis, E. W. (1942). Effects of lesions of the periaqueductal gray matter in the cat. *Proc. Soc. Exp. Biol. Med.* 351:305–306.

Bailey, P., & Davis, E. W. (1943). Effects of lesions of the periaqueductal gray matter on the *Macaca mulatta*. *J. Neuropath. Exp. Neurol.* 3:69–72.

51. See n. 50. For an overview of PAG functions,

see: Depaulis, A., & Bandler, R. (eds.) (1991). *The midbrain periaqueductal gray matter: Functional, anatomical, and neurochemical organization*. New York: Plenum Press.

52. See n. 45 and chap. 4, n. 2, as well as: Mantyh, P. W. (1982). Forebrain projections to the periaqueductal gray in the monkey, with observations in the cat and rat. *J. Comp. Neurol.* 206:146–158.

53. See n. 51 and: Bandler, R., & Shipley, M. T. (1994). Columnar organization in the midbrain periaqueductal gray: Modules for emotional expression. *Trends Neurosci.* 17:379–389.

Newman, J. D. (ed.) (1988). *The physiological control of mammalian vocalization*. New York: Plenum Press.

54. Behbehani, M. M. (1995). Functional characteristics of the midbrain periaqueductal gray. *Prog. Neurobiol.* 46:575–605.

Borszcz, G. S. (1995). Increases in vocalization and motor reflex thresholds are influenced by the site of morphine microinjection: Comparisons following administration into the periaqueductal gray, ventral medulla, and spinal subarachnoid space. *Behav. Neurosci.* 109:502–522.

Hsieh, J. C., Stahle-Backdahl, M., Hagermark, O., Stone-Elander, S., Rosenquist, G., & Ingvar, M. (1996). Traumatic nociceptive pain activates the hypothalamus and the periaqueductal gray: A positron emission tomography study. *Pain* 64: 303–314.

55. Eleftheriou, B. E. (ed.) (1972). *The neurobiology of the amygdala*. New York: Plenum Press.

Kalivas, P. W. (ed.). (1992). *Limbic motor circuits and neuropsychiatry*. Boca Raton, Fla.: CRC Press.

Rhawn, J. (1996). *Neuropsychiatry, neuropsychology, and clinical neuroscience: Emotion, evolution, cognition, language, memory, brain damage, and abnormal behavior*, (2d ed,). Baltimore: Williams and Wilkins.

56. Carpenter, W. T., Jr., Buchanan, R. W., & Kirkpatrick, B. (1995). New diagnostic issues in schizophrenic disorders. *Clin. Neurosci.* 3:57–63.

Kirkpatrick, B., Buchanan, R.W., Breier, A., & Carpenter, W. T., Jr. (1994). Depressive symptoms and the deficit syndrome of schizophrenia. *J. Nerv. Ment. Dis.* 182: 452–455.

57. A distinct signal may be obtained only if we learn how to orient our recording electrodes properly among the relevant neuronal ensembles. Obviously, this type of research cannot be done in humans, since it would entail local tissue recordings in real time. Because of the concentrated overlap of many systems within the central midbrain (see n. 53), functional changes there may be hard to resolve using the modern brain-imaging technologies that are so effectively resolving telencephalic functions where the neuronal canopy is especially widely distributed. Accordingly, animal brain research may be essential for the electrophysiological identification of the "signatures" of the primal SELF, but if that can be achieved, we may be able to measure emotional changes in animals relatively directly by monitoring specific types of brain activity.

In this context, it is important to mention that the closest human researchers have gotten to monitoring the mechanisms of consciousness in the brain is through the recording of 40–Hz EEG signals that may reflect information processing in the brain that may have conscious attributes. See:

Jefferys, J. G. R., Traub, R. D., & Whittington, M. A. (1996). Neuronal networks for induced "40 Hz" rhythms. *Trends Neurosci.* 19:202–208.

Plourde, G., & Villemure, C. (1996). Comparison of the effects of enflurane/N20 on the 40–Hz auditory steady-state response versus the auditory middle-latency response. *Anesth. Analg.* 82:75–83.

58. As emphasized throughout this text, glutamate is integrally involved in all functions of the brain, from the top down. See:

Conti, F., & Hicks, T. P. (eds.) (1996). *Excitatory amino acids and the cerebral cortex*. Cambridge, Mass.: MIT Press.

Scheibel, A. B. (1980). Anatomical and physiological substrates of arousal: A view from the bridge. In *The reticular formation revisited* (J. A. Hobson & M. A. B. Brazier, eds.), pp. 55–66. New York: Raven Press.

59. See nn. 25 and 32 and:

Newman, J. (1995). Reticular-thalamic activation of the cortex generates conscious contents. *Behav. Brain Sci.* 18:691–692.

Newman, J., Baars, B. J., & Cho, S.-B. (1997). A neurocognitive model for attention and consciousness. In *Two sciences of mind* (S. O'Nuallain, ed.). Philadelphia: John Benjamins of North America.

60. From the perspective that the SELF-process becomes rerepresented within the brain during development, it is noteworthy that ascending serotonin and norepinephrine systems are situated in the medial parts of the midbrain and pons, and are among the most ancient and widespread of neural systems of the brain, providing possible trophic influences on brain development. Also, pharmacological facilitation of serotonin in adult humans can modify their affective personality structures, making folks more socially confident and less aggressive. Modifications of brain dopamine can have other personality effects. See:

Cloninger, C. R., Svrakic, D. M., & Przybeck, T. R. (1993). A psychobiological model of temperament and character. *Arch. Gen. Psychiat.* 50:975–990.

Cloninger, C. R. (1994). The genetic structure of personality and learning: A phylogenetic model. *Clinical Genet.* 46 124–137.

61. Domino, E. F., & Luby, E. D. (1973). Abnormal mental states induced by phencyclidine as a model of schizophrenia, In *Psychopathology and psychopharmacology* (J. O. Cole, A. M. Freeman, & A. J. Friedhof, eds.), pp. 37–50. Baltimore: Johns Hopkins Univ. Press.

Lahti, A.C., Koffel, B., La Porte, D., & Tamminga, C. A. (1995). Subanesthetic doses of ketamine stimulate psychosis in schizophrenia. *Neuropsychopharmacol.* 13:9–19.

62. The mechanism by which the various anesthetics melt everyday consciousness remains unknown. A large number of brain changes are induced by the various anesthetics. Some will say that this type of manipulation is no more interesting for the understanding of consciousness than hitting someone over the head with a hammer. That is a foolish criticism if we simply consider the kinetic energy of the hammer needed to impair consciousness and the kinetic energy of the molecules of barbiturate anesthetics needed to do the same.

I have done some preliminary studies along these lines, comparing intracerebral injections of pentobarbital into central mesencephalic sites and central telencephalic sites. Both have produced some anesthesia (as measured by motor incoordination), but the caudal injections have been more potent.

63. See nn. 2 and 71. If this line of research can be verified, and if it is in fact correct to assume that the anesthetic administered via the carotid arteries does not compromise subcortical abilities, these types of experiments would suggest that certain affective abilities are highly dependent on higher cerebral functions. This would not be inconsistent with the present thesis, since it is accepted that many of the higher social feelings such as guilt, shame, embarrassment, and pride, although constituted of lower emotional systems, could not exist without the higher brain functions that make subtle social appraisals.

64. See chap. 9, nn. 82–85, for facial measures of taste pleasure, and n. 54 for effects of pain on the brain. Other interesting aspects of pain can be found in:

Eismann, C. H., Jorgensen, W. K., Merrit, D. J., Rice, M. J., Cribb, B. W., Webb, P. D., & Zalucki, M. P. (1984). Do insects feel pain? A biological view. *Experientia* 40:164–167.

Fisichelli, V. R., & Karelitz, S. (1963). The cry latencies of normal infants and those with brain damage. *J. Pediatrics* 62:724–734.

65. Neary, D. (1995). Neuropsychological aspects of frontotemporal degeneration. *Ann. N.Y. Acad. Sci.* 769:15–22.

Valenstein, E. S. (1986). *Great and desperate cures: The rise and decline of psychosurgery and other radical treatments for mental illness.* New York: Basic Books.

66. See chap. 8, n. 18, and: Cummings, J. L. (1995). Anatomic and behavioral aspects of frontal-subcortical circuits *Ann. N.Y. Acad. Sci.* 769:1–13.

67. Baer, L., Rauch, S. L., Ballantine, H. T., Jr., Martuza, R., Cosgrove, R., Cassem, E., Girionas, I., Manzo, P. A., Dimino, C., & Jenike, M. A. (1995). Cingulotomy for intractable obsessive-compulsive disorder. Prospective long-term follow-up of 18 patients. *Arch. Gen. Psychiat.* 52:384–392.

Devinsky, O., Morrell, M. J., & Vogt, B. A. (1995). Contributions of anterior cingulate cortex to behaviour. *Brain* 118:279–306.

Drevets, W. C., Price, J. L., Simpson, J. R., Jr., Todd, R. D., Rich, T., Vannier, M., & Raichle, M. E. (1997). Subgenual prefrontal cortex abnormalities in mood disorders. *Nature* 386:824–827.

Jenike, M. A., Baer, L., Ballantine, T, Martuza, R. L., Tynes, S., & Giriunas I. (1991). Cingulotomy for refractory obsessive-compulsive disorder. A long-term followup of 33 patients. *Arch. Gen. Psychiat.* 48:548–555.

Mayberg, H. S., et al. (1997). Cingulate function in depression: A potential predictor of treatment responses. *NeuroReport* 8:1057–1061.

Vogt, B. A., & Gabriel, M. (eds.) (1993). *Neurobiology of cingulate cortex and limbic thalamus: A comprehensive handbook.* Boston: Birkhäuser.

The many reasons for akinetic mutism are fully discussed in: Ore, G. D. (ed.). *The Apallic syndrome.* Berlin: Springer-Verlag.

68. The flow of information between amygdala and cortex is generally believed to be more heavily in the amygdalopedal direction (i.e., from cortex). Here it is worth noting that human and other primate brains appear to have much stronger amygdalofugal inputs to cortex than do the brains of other mammals that have been studied intensively. See: Burwell, R. D., Witter, M. P., & Amaral, D. G. (1995). Perirhinal and postrhinal cortices of the rat: A review of the neuroanatomical literature and comparison with findings from the monkey brain. *Hippocampus* 5:390–408.

This may indicate that affective processes may have stronger influences on cognitive processes in primates than is the case in other animals.

69. Jacobson, R. (1986). Disorders of facial recognition, social behaviour and affect after combined bilateral amygdalotomy and subcaudate tractotomy: A clinical and experimental study. *Psych. Med.* 16:439–450.

Kling, A. S., Tachiki, K., & Lloyd, R. (1993). Neurochemical correlates of the Klüver-Bucy syndrome by in vivo microdialysis in monkey. *Behav. Brain Res.* 56:161–170.

70. The classic studies of amygdalectomized animals indicated their inability to relate socially. See: Kling, A. (1972). Effects of amygdalectomy on social-affective behavior in non-human primates. In *The neurobiology of the amygdala.* (B. E. Eleftheriou, ed.), pp. 536–551. New York: Plenum Press.

Subsequent studies have indicated how responsive neurons are within the amygdala to various social and emotional stimuli. See:

Brothers, L., Ring, B., & Kling, A. (1990). Response of neurons in the macaque amygdala to complex social stimuli. *Behav. Brain Res.* 41:199–213.

Nishijo, H., Ono, T., & Nishino, H. (1988). Single neuron responses in amygdala of alert monkey during complex sensory stimulation with affective significance. *J. Neurosci.* 8:3570–3583.

71. For a complete update of relevant issues, see: Davidson, R. J., Hugspeth, K. (eds.) (1995). *Brain asymmetry.* Cambridge, Mass.: MIT Press.

The original studies of Richard Davidson's group (summarized in the preceding book and in chap. 5, nn. 72–74), largely conducted in women, have now been replicated in men. See: Jacobs, G. D., & Snyder, D. (1996). Frontal brain asymmetry predicts affective style in men. *Behav. Neurosci.* 110:3–6.

72. Dawson, G., Panagiotides, H., Klinger, L. G., & Hill, D. (1992). The role of frontal lobe functioning in the development of infant self-regulatory behavior. *Brain and Cog.* 20:152–175.

73. See chap. 5, nn. 42 and 78. Also, in our unpublished work evaluating EEG changes to happy and sad music segments, happiness causes more EEG synchronization (disarousal), while sadness produces EEG desynchronization (arousal). See: Panksepp, J., Lensing, P., Klimesch, W., Schimke, H., & Vaningan, M. (1993). Event-related desynchronization (ERD) analysis of rhythmic brain functions in normal and autistic people. *Soc. Neurosci. Abst.* 19:1885.

74. Indeed, neuropeptides such as CRF, which promote anxiety and separation distress, promote cortical arousal. See: Page, M. E., Berridge, C. W., Foote, S. L., & Valentino, R. J. (1994). Corticotropin-releasing factor in the locus coeruleus mediates EEG activation associated with hypotensive stress. *Neurosci. Let.* 164: 81–84.

75. Gainotti, G., & Caltagirone, C. (eds.) (1989). *Emotions and the dual brain.* Berlin: Springer-Verlag.

It is too simplistic to treat the whole right hemisphere in these terms. For instance, there is evidence that the right parietal areas may also help sustain positive affect. See: Robinson, R. G., Kubos, K. L., Starr, L. B., Rao, K., & Price, T. R. (1984). Mood disorders in stroke patients: Importance of location of lesion. *Brain* 107: 81–93.

76. Gainotti, G. (1972). Emotional behavior and hemispheric side of the brain. *Cortex* 8:41–55.

77. For a summary of effects, see chap. 10, n. 101, and: Conca, A., Koppi, S., Konig, P., Swoboda, E., & Krecke, N. (1996). Transcranial magnetic stimulation: A novel antidepressive strategy? *Neuropsychobiol.* 34:204–207.

78. Ross, E. D. (1981). The aprosodias: Functional-anatomic organization of the affective components of language in the right hemisphere. *Arch. Neurol.* 38: 561–569.

79. Liotti, M., & Tucker, D. M. (1994). Emotion in asymmetric corticolimbic networks. In *Human brain laterality* (R. J. Davidson & K. Hugdahl, eds.), pp. 389–424. New York: Oxford Univ. Press.

Tucker, D. M., Luu, P., & Pribram, K. H. (1995). Social and emotional self-regulation. *Ann. N.Y. Acad. Sci.* 769:213–239.

80. Although there are some animal data indicating lateralization of emotional functions (Denenberg, V. H. [1981]. Hemispheric laterality in animals and the effects of early experience. *Behav. Brain Sci.* 4:1–49), I have spent a great deal of effort looking for cerebral lateralization of basic emotions in animals, with little success, as summarized elsewhere. See: Panksepp, J. (1989). The psychobiology of emotions: The animal side of human feelings. In *Emotions and the dual brain* (G. Gainotti & C. Caltagirone, eds.), pp. 31–55. Berlin: Springer-Verlag.

Briefly, after preparing various groups having total unilateral decortication of the right and left hemispheres, I was not able to observe any systematic differences in the sexual courting vocalizations of adult male guinea pigs, the distress vocalizations of young domestic chicks, or the rough-and-tumble play of juvenile rats. For this reason, I strongly suspect that the lateralization effects described by others are largely the consequence of learning effects rather than intrinsic emotional specializations of the two hemispheres.

Indeed, such types of brain damage have only modest effects in humans, as long as the damage occurred quite early in childhood: See n. 26.

81. See chap. 3, n. 15.

82. The evolutionary view of higher human functions has been beautifully summarized by: Wright, R. (1994). *The moral animal.* New York: Pantheon.

83. See chap. 4, n. 21.

84. See chap. 2, n. 5, as well as the debate between Parrott and Schulkin and Le Doux in: Watts, F. N. (1993). Special issue: Neuropsychological perspectives on emotion. *Cognition and Emotion* 7: 43–69.

85. For current controversies in the facial analysis of emotions, see the controversy between Russell, Ekman, and Izard (chap. 3, n. 14), as well as n. 9.

For a discussion of the laterality of facial expression, see:

Borod, J. C., & Koff, E. (1984). Asymmetries in affective facial expression: Behavior and anatomy. In *The psychobiology of affective development* (N. Fox & R. Davidson, eds.), pp. 293–324. Hillsdale, N.J.: Lawrence Erlbaum.

Etcoff, N. (1986). The neuropsychology of emotional expression. In *Advances in clinical neuropsychology*, vol. 2 (G. Goldstein & R. E. Tarter, eds.). New York: Plenum Press.

Fridlund, A. J. (1988). What can asymmetry and laterality in facial EMG tell us about the face and brain? *Int. J. Neurosci.* 39:53–69.

86. Even when we are not being challenged by strong needs, desires, and other feelings, our higher mental apparatus still tends to be guided by the welling up of mood-congruent memories. There is an abundance of data in the recent cognitive literature for mood-congruent memory effects. If one induces negative moods in a variety of ways, people tend to retrieve negative memories, while positive moods coax people to dwell on positive memories. See:

Bower, G. H. (1987). Commentary on mood and memory. *Behav. Res. Ther.* 6:23–35.

Bullington, J. C. (1990). Mood congruent memory: A replication of symmetrical effects for both positive and negative moods. *J. Soc. Behav. Person.* 5(special issue): 123–134.

Similar effects can be achieved by modifying mood with drugs. For instance, the broad-spectrum antipsychotic haloperidol tends to make people dysphoric and much less likely to come up with positive memories when cued with a variety of concepts. See: Kumari, V., Hemsley, D. R., Cotter, P. A., Checkley, S. A., Gray, J. A. (1997). Haloperidol-induced mood and retrieval of happy and unhappy memories. *Cog. Emot.* In press.

Mood-congruent memory retrieval can also be evoked by music. See: Parrott, W. G., & Sabini, J. (1990). Mood and memory under natural conditions: Evidence for mood incongruent recall. *J. Person. Soc. Psych.* 59: 321–336.

87. Various empirical contributions allow us to forecast the impressive riches that such work will provide. Consider one example: Investigators have recently identified brain areas that exhibit long-term plastic changes as a function of previous maternal experience. See: Fleming, A. S., & Korsmit, M. (1996). Plasticity in the maternal circuit: Effects of maternal experience on Fos-Lir in hypothalamic, limbic, and cortical structures in the postpartum rat. *Behav. Neurosci.* 110:567–582.

Not surprisingly, the largest changes were among the brain circuits discussed in Chapter 13, but many other higher areas were also involved, including parietal and prefrontal cortical zones.

It is intriguing to note that some hormonal effects on neuronal plasticity occur only if animals are conscious. See: Quinones-Jenab, V., Zhang, C., Jenab, S., Brown, H. E., & Pfaff, D. W. (1996). Anesthesia during hormone administration abolishes the estrogen induction of preproenkephalin mRNA in ventromedial hypothalamus of female rats. *Mol. Brain Res.* 35:297–303.

88. This famous quote by William James (James, W. [1890/1961]. *The principles of psychology: The briefer course.* New York: Harper and Row. Quotation on pp. 16–17) is being supported by modern research on the development of sensitization within underlying brain craving systems as a function of psychostimulant abuse (see "Afterthought," Chapter 6). These brain systems are also modulated by stress in similar ways. See: Chrousos, G. P., McCartly, R., Pacak, K., Cizza, G., Sternberg, E., Gold, P. W., & Kvetnansky, R. (eds.) (1995). *Stress: Basic mechanisms and clinical implications.* Special issue of *Ann N. Y. Acad. Sci.*, Vol. 771, New York: New York Academy of Sciences.

89. Naturalistic fallacies are attempts to derive "should" statements from "is" statements. Obviously, biological facts do not yield any unambiguous moral imperatives for the construction of social systems or even personal conduct. However, not taking the available facts into consideration in discussing such issues is tantamount to not thinking clearly about the issues.

90. Much of this last "Afterthought" is adapted from my published comments on a theoretical paper that attempted to synthesize our understanding of basic emotional systems with classical views concerning political systems (i.e., Miller, T. C. [1993]. The duality of human nature. *Politics and Life Sci.* 12:221–241).

My response was: Panksepp, J. (1994). The role of brain emotional systems in the construction of social systems. *Politics and Life Sci.* 13:116–119.

For an extensive analysis of emotion-culture interactions, see:

Mesquite, B., & Frijda, N. H. (1992). Cultural variations in emotions: A review. *Psych. Bull.* 112:179–204.

Scherer, K. R., Walbott, H. G., & Summerfield, A. S. (1986). *Experiencing emotion: A cross-cultural study.* Cambridge: Cambridge Univ. Press.

91. For reviews of sensitization, see chap. 8, nn. 5 and 99.

92. The functions of play are diverse and probably include promoting the growth and solidification of neural circuits, perhaps via the genetic activation of various neurotrophins. Although this idea remains to be empirically tested, it has recently been demonstrated that touch can activate the genetic expression of one neurotrophin. See: A Rocamora, N., Welker, E., Pascual, M., & Soriano E. (1996). Upregulation of BDNF mRNA expression in barrel cortex of adult mice after sensory stimulation. *J. Neurosci.* 16:4411–4419.

93. It is hard to imagine how such a proposition could ever be empirically evaluated. Obviously, the expression of emotional and motivational urges will be critically dependent on the environments in which they occur.

94. This phrase originally comes from the title of an etching from a pessimistic series by Francisco Goya (1746–1828), Spain's first great modern artist.

95. There are many evolutionary stories that need to be empirically evaluated, but we can never experimentally determine "why" something happened in evolution. For instance, we will never really know why all human societies practice religion. Presumably, the human brain contains functions that promote worship, reverence, and the feeling of belonging, but it may be impossible to unambiguously identify how those functions emerged in brain evolution. For a discussion of some possibilities, see: Burkert, W. (1996). *Creation of the sacred: Tracks of biology in early religions.* Cambridge, Mass.: Harvard Univ. Press.

In addition to the half dozen possibilities outlined by Burkert, we should also consider the possibility that religious urges arise partly from our brain mechanisms for social bonding (see Chapters 12 and 13), as well as our tendency to interpret correlated events in nature as reflective of causal processes (see Chapter 8).

96. For an excellent discussion of the sources of criminal behavior, see:

Marsh, F. H., & Katz, J. (eds.) (1985). *Biology, crime and ethics: A study of biological explanations for criminal behavior.* Cincinnati, Ohio: Anderson.

Raine, A. (1993). *The psychopathology of crime: Criminal behavior as a clinical disorder.* San Diego: Academic Press.

97. Mealey, L. (1995). The sociobiology of sociopathy: An integrated evolutionary model. *Behav. Brain Sci.* 18:523–599.

98. For a discussion of this issue, see our commentary to Mealey (n. 97), which includes our views on the matter. See: Panksepp, J., Knutson, B., & Bird, L. (1995). On the brain and personality substrates of psychopathy. *Behav. Brain Sci.* 18:568–570.

99. For a discussion of tit-for-tat strategies not working in certain social environments, see: Wright, R. (1994). *The moral animal.* New York: Pantheon.

For a discussion of "cosmetic psychopharmacology," see: Kramer, P. D. (1993). *Listening to Prozac.* New York: Viking.

100. For a discussion of such issues, see: Goleman, D. (1995). *Emotional intelligence.* New York: Bantam Books.

The viewpoint of this text has been that to scientifically understand the basic emotions of the mammalian brain as evolved neurobiological entities, we will have to build from the ground up. See: Ekman, P. (1992). An argument for basic emotions. *Cog. Emot.* 6:169–200.

Because of space limitations, I have not endeavored to thoroughly cover the neuropsychological and neuropsychiatric aspects of emotions; for some in-depth discussion of those issues, see: Heilman, K. M., & Satz, P. (eds.) (1983). *Neuropsychology of human emotion.* New York: Guilford Press.

Also see third book cited in n. 55.

Fortunately, some of the higher emotional functions of humans are finally being probed in neurologically credible ways. See: Davidson, R. J. (1993). Cerebral asymmetry and emotion: Conceptual and methodological conundrums. *Cog. Emot.* 7:115–138.

We can be confident that the higher cerebral dynamics that are affected by emotions will follow specifiable mental laws that as often as not may be manifested in behavior. See: Frijda, N. H. (1988). The laws of emotion. *Am. Psychol.* 43:349–358.

If we continue to pursue a systematic course of inquiry, explicating first the evolutionary foundations and then more recent developments, we will eventually be able to understand the full complexity of human emotions that has just barely started to be scientifically described. See: Scherer, K. R. (1993). Neuroscience projections to current debates in emotion psychology. *Cog. Emot.* 7:1–41.

Appendix A

1. Leakey, R. E. (1977). *Origins: The emergence and evolution of our species and its possible future.* New York: Dutton, Inc.

Leakey, R. E. & Lewin, R. (1979). *People of the lake: Man, his origins, nature, and future.* London: Collins.

Wilcock, C. (1974). *Africa's Rift Valley.* Amsterdam: Time-Life.

2. Ardrey, R. (1961). *African genesis.* New York: Atheneum. Quotations on p. 11.

3. Futuyma, D. J. (1983). *Science on trial: The case for evolution,* New York: Pantheon.

Johanson, D. C., & Edey, M. A. (1981). *Lucy: The beginnings of humankind.* New York: Simon and Schuster.

Leakey, M. (1984). *Disclosing the past.* Garden City, N.Y.: Doubleday.

Lewin, R. (1987). *Bones of contention: Controversies in the search for human origins.* New York: Simon and Schuster.

Shapiro, R. (1986). *Origins: A skeptic's guide to the creation of life on earth.* New York: Bantam Books.

4. Sarich, V., & Wilson, A. (1967). An immunological timescale for hominid evolution. *Science* 158: 1200–1203.

Gribbin, J., & Cherfas, J. (1982). *The monkey puzzle: Reshaping the evolutionary tree.* New York: McGraw-Hill.

5. Alvarez, W., Claes, P., & Kieffer, S. W. (1995). Emplacement of cretaceous-tertiary boundary shocked quartz from Chicxulub crater. *Science* 269:930–935.

Alvarez, W., & Asaro, F. (1992). *The extinction of the dinosaurs.* Cambridge: Cambridge Univ. Press.

6. See n. 4, but also: Benveniste, R. E., & Todaro, G. J. (1976). Evolution of type C viral genes: evidence for an Asian origin of man. *Nature* 261:101–107.

7. As quoted in Gribbin & Cherfas (1982), n. 4.

8. Strum, S. (1987). *Almost human: A journey into the world of baboons.* New York: Random House.

9. De Waal, F. (1982). *Chimpanzee politics,* New York: Harper and Row.

Goodall, J. (1986). *The chimpanzees of Gombe: Patterns of behavior.* Cambridge, Mass.: Harvard Univ. Press.

10. Finlay, B. L., & Darlington, R. B. (1995). Linked regularities in the development and evolution of mammalian brain. *Science* 268:1578–1584.

Jerison, H. J. (1991). *Brain size and the evolution of the mind.* New York: American Museum of Natural History.

Passingham, R. E. (1985). Rates of brain development in mammals including man. *Brain Behav. Evol.* 26:167–175.

11. Deacon, T. W. (1990). Rethinking mammalian brain evolution. *Amer. Zool.* 30:629–705.

12. The "mitochondrial Eve" hypothesis was proposed by: Cann, R. L., Stoneking, M., & Wilson, A. C. (1987). Mitochondrial DNA and human evolution. *Nature* 325:31–36.

The criticisms and discussions of this idea can be found in: Willis, C. (1993). *The runaway brain: The evolution of human uniqueness.* New York: HarperCollins.

13. See n. 2.

14. Lewin, R. (1988). *In the age of mankind.* Washington, D.C.: Smithsonian Books.

Ruspoli, M. (1987). *The cave of Lascaux: The final photographs.* New York: Abrams.

15. Tattersall, I., Delson, E., & Couvering, J. V. (eds.) (1988). *Encyclopedia of human evolution and prehistory.* New York: Garland.

16. Vander Wall, S. B. (1990). *Food hoarding in animals.* Chicago: Univ. of Chicago Press.

17. Axelrod, R. (1984). *The evolution of cooperation,* New York: Basic Books.

18. See n. 17 and: Axelrod, R. (1984). The laws of life, *The Sciences* 27: 44–51.

Trivers, R. L. *Social evolution.* Menlo Park, Calif.: Benjamin/Cummings.

19. The level of integration between brain areas may be changing as a function of cerebral evolution. One reasonable way for corticocognitive evolution to proceed is via the active inhibition of more instinctual subcortical impulses. It is possible that evolution might actually promote the disconnection of certain brain functions from others. For instance, along certain paths of cerebral evolution, perhaps in emerging branches of the human species, there may be an increasing disconnection of cognitive from emotional processes. This may be the path of autism, in its various forms.

There is also a special neurodevelopmental path, called *Williams syndrome*, where emotional processes are more integrally linked to impoverished intellectual skills, except for the spoken word. See: Bellugi, U., Wang, P. P., & Jernigan, T. L. (1994). Williams syndrome: An unusual neuropsychological profile. In *Atypical cognitive deficits in developmental disorders* (S. H. Broman & J. Grafman, eds.), pp. 23–56. Hillsdale, N.J.: Lawrence Erlbaum.

It has recently been determined that this syndrome arises from a microdeletion of a segment of chromosome 7 that codes for the elastin protein, as well as a brain enzyme (i.e., LIM-kinasel) of unknown function. See:

Lowery, M. C., Morris, D. A., Ewart, A., Brothman, L. J., Zhu, X. L., Leonard, C. O., Carey, J. C., Keating, M., & Brothman, A. R. (1995). Strong correlation of elastin deletions, detected by FISH, with Williams syndrome: Evaluation of 235 patients. *Amer. J. Human Gen.* 57:49–53

Frangiskakis, J. M., et al. (1996). *LIM-kinasel* hemizygosity implicated in impaired visospatial constructive cognition. *Cell* 86: 59–69.

20. Since one of the core symptoms of autism is social aloneness, it is possible that the brain areas that mediate cognitive processes are substantially disconnected from those processes that mediate affect, leading to deficits of joint attention and a diminution of social learning. See: Sigman, M. (1994). What are the core deficits in autism? In *Atypical cognitive deficits in developmental disorders* (S.H. Broman & J. Grafman, eds.), pp. 139–157. Hillsdale, N.J.: Lawrence Erlbaum.

The cerebral patterns that have been observed in autism—where hippocampal neurons are extremely numerous and small—suggest the possibility of such a neuroevolutionary process. See:

Raymond, G. V., Bauman, M. L., & Kemper, T. L. (1996). Hippocampus in autism: A Golgi analysis. *Acta Neuropathological* 91:117–119.

Bauman, M. L. (1996). Brief report: Neuroanatomic observations of the brain in pervasive developmental disorders. *J. Autism Devel. Dis.* 26:199–203.

Courchesne, E., et al. (1994). A new finding: Impairment in shifting attention in autistic and cerebellar patients. In *Atypical cognitive deficits in developmental disorders* (S. H. Broman & J. Grafman, eds.), pp. 101–137. Hillsdale, N.J.: Lawrence Erlbaum.

21. Harris, G. J., & Hoehn-Saric, R. (1995). Functional neuroimaging in biological psychiatry. In *Advances in biological psychiatry,* vol. 1. (J. Panksepp, ed.), pp. 113–160. Greenwich, Conn.: JAI Press.

22. Courchesne, E., Townsend, J., & Saitoh, O. (1994). The brain in infantile autism: Posterior fossa structures are abnormal. *Neurology* 44:214–223.

Courchesne, E., Saitoh, O., Yeung-Courchesne, R., Press, G. A., Lincoln, A. J., Haas, R. H., & Schreibman, L. (1994). Abnormality of cerebellar vermian lobules VI and VII in patients with infantile autism: Identification of hypoplastic and hyperplastic subgroups with MR imaging. *Amer. J. Roentgenology* 162:123–130.

Kemper, T. L., & Bauman, M. L. (1993). The contribution of neuropathologic studies to the understanding of autism. *Neuro. Clin.* 11:175–187.

Appendix B

1. For an overview of information theory, see: Campbell, J. (1982). *Grammatical man: Information, entropy, language and life.* New York: Simon and Schuster.

The issue of metaphors in science and language has been discussed in a provocative way in the following:

Lakoff, G., & Johnson, M. (1980). *Metaphors we live by.* Chicago: Univ. of Chicago Press.

Lakoff, G. (1987). *Women, fire, and dangerous things: What categories reveal about the mind.* Chicago: Univ. of Chicago Press.

2. Caplan, D. (1987). *Neurolinguistics and linguistic aphasiology.* New York: Cambridge Univ. Press.

Kranegor, N. A., Rumbaugh, D. M., Schiefelbusch, R. L., & Studdert-Kennedy, M. (eds.) (1991). *Biological and behavioral determinants of language development.* Hillsdale, N.J.: Lawrence Erlbaum.

Ojemann, G. A. (1991). Cortical organization of language. *J. Neurosci.* 11:2281–2287.

3. See chap. 4, n. 4.

4. The brains of autistic children, especially boys, are larger than normal. See: Piven. J., & Andreasen, N. (1996). Regional brain enlargement in autism: A magnetic resonance imaging study. *J. Amer. Acad. Child Adolesc. Psychiat.* 35:530–536.

However, unlike normal children, the left (or speech) hemisphere is not larger than the right hemisphere, even though this lack of asymmetry does not appear to correlate with speech deficits. See: Tsai, L. Y., Jacoby, C. G., Stewart, M. A., & Beisler, J. M. (1982). Unfavorable left-right asymmetries of the brain and autism: A question of methodology. *Br. J. Psychiat.* 140:312–319.

Also, autistic children tend to exhibit reduced EEG power in brain areas that mediate language. See: Dawson, G., Klinger, L. G., Panagiotides, H., Lewy, A., & Castelloe, P. (1995). Subgroups of autistic children based on social behavior display distinct patterns of brain activity. *J. Abn. Child. Psych.* 23:569–583.

5. Corina, D. P., Vaid, J., & Bellugi, U. (1992). The linguistic basis of left hemisphere specialization. *Science* 255:1258–1260.

6. Shaywitz, B. A., Shaywitz, S. E., Pugh, K. R., Constable, R. T., Skudlarski, P., Fulbright, R. K., Bronen, R. A., Fletcher, J. M., Shankeweiler, D. P., Katz, L., & Gore, J. C. (1995). Sex differences in the functional organization of the brain for language. *Nature* 373:607–609.

Schultz, R. T., Cho, N. K., Staib, L. H., Kier, L. E., Fletcher, J. M., Shaywitz, S. E., Shankweiler, D. P., Katz, L., Gore, J. C., Duncan, J. S. (1994). Brain morphology in normal and dyslexic children: The influence of sex and age. *Ann. Neurol.* 35:732–742.

7. For reviews of brain plasticity, see: chap. 2, n. 59, and chap. 15, n. 73.

In the language realm, it seems that there is a relationship between educational level and the complexity of neuronal organization in speech-processing cortex. See: Jacobs, B., Schall, M., & Scheibel, A. B. (1993). A quantitative dendritic analysis of Wernicke's area in humans: II. Gender, hemispheric, and environmental factors. *J. Comp. Neurol.* 327: 97–111.

In general, the more complex the linguistic usage, the more brain tissue has to be recruited, including more circuits of the right hemisphere. See: Just, M. A., Carpenter, P. A., Keller, T. A., Eddy, W. F., & Thulborn, K. R. (1996). Brain activation modulated by sentence comprehension. *Science* 274:114–116.

8. For a recent overview of plasticity in the visual system, see: Katz, L. C., & Schatz, C. J. (1996). Synaptic activity and the construction of cortical circuits. *Science*, 274:1133–1138.

Plasticity probably is evident in the brain for every human endeavor. For instance, musical training seems to facilitate different areas of the brain working together. See: Johnson, J. K., Petsche, H., Richter, P., von Stein, A., & Filz, O. (1996). The effects of coherence estimates of EEG at rest on differences between subjects with and without musical training; In *MusicMedicine*, vol. 2 (R. R. Pratt & R. Spintge, eds.), pp. 65–84. Saint Louis, Mo.: MMB Music.

9. Bellugi, U., & Hickok, G. (1995). Clues to the neurobiology of language. In *Neuroscience, memory, and language: Decade of the brain*, vol. 1 (R. D. Broadwell, ed.), pp. 87–107. Washington, D.C.: U.S. Government Printing Office.

Haglund, M. M., Ojemann, G. A., Lettich, E., & Bellugi, U. (1993). Dissociation of cortical and single unit activity in spoken and signed languages. *Brain Lang.* 44:19–27.

10. Deacon, T. W. (1989). The neural circuitry underlying primate calls and human language. *Human Evol.* 4:367–401.

Poizner, H., Klima, E. S., & Bellugi, U. (1990). *What the hands reveal about the brain.* Cambridge, Mass.: MIT Press.

For a summary of brain lateralization issues, see:

Corballis, M. (1991). *The lopsided ape.* New York: Oxford Univ. Press.

Zeidel, D. W. (ed.) (1994). *Neuropsychology.* San Diego: Academic Press.

11. Sebeok, T. A., & Rosenthal, R. (ed.). *The Clever Hans phenomenon: Communication with horses, whales, apes, and people.* Special issue of *Ann. N.Y. Acad. Sci.*, vol. 364. New York: New York Academy of Sciences.

The controversy of facilitated communication in the treatment of autism is summarized in: Jacobson, J. W., Mulick, J. A., & Schwartz, A. A. (1995). A history of facilitated communication: Science, pseudoscience, and antiscience science working group on facilitated communication. *Amer. Psychol.* 50:750–765.

Some still report positive evidence for facilitated communication. See: Cardinal, D. N., Hanson, D., & Wakeham, J. (1996). Investigation of authorship in facilitated communication. *Mental Ret.* 34:231–242.

12. This term was coined by Nietzsche in the quotation "We have to cease to think if we refuse to do it in the prison-house of language for we cannot reach further than the doubt which asks whether the limit we see is really a limit." This quote was also the lead epigraph in a renowned book on literary criticism by: Jameson, F. (1972). *The prison-house of language.* Princeton, N.J.: Princeton Univ. Press.

A key question is to what extent language reflects the intrinsic cognitive channels of the brain and to what extent it reflects the ability of the human brain to arbitrarily generate symbolic structures and meaning. Since Chomsky's work, the pendulum has been swinging, at least in certain intellectual circles, from the latter toward an acclamation of the former. See: Chomsky, N. (1975). *Reflections on language.* New York: Random House.

For an overview of modern linguistic theory, see: Pinker, S. (1994). *The language instinct: How the mind creates language.* New York: HarperCollins.

Appendix C

1. For a summary of this interpretation of the actions of Descartes, see chap. 16, n. 34.

2. For overviews of such approaches, see: Gazzaniga, M. S. (ed.) (1995). *The cognitive neurosciences.* Cambridge, Mass.: MIT Press.

3. Campbell, J. (1982). *Grammatical man: Information, entropy, language, and life.* New York: Simon and Schuster.

4. See the references to Chapter 16 and all issues of the journal *Consciousness and Cognition.*

5. Penfield, W. (1975). *The mystery of the mind: A critical study of consciousness and the human brain.* Princeton, N.J.: Princeton Univ. Press. Quotation on pp. 56, 79, 80, 81 (emphasis in original).

6. Sperry, R. W. (1969). A modified concept of consciousness. *Psych. Rev.* 76: 532–536.

Sperry, R. W. (1970). An objective approach to subjective experience: Further explanation of a hypothesis. *Psychol. Rev.* 77:585–590.

Sperry, R. (1982). Bridging science and values: A unifying view of mind and brain. In *Mind and brain: The many-faceted problem* (J. Eccles, ed.), pp. 255–269. Washington, D.C.: Paragon House. Quotation on p. 258.

7. For a full description of Sperry's social views, see: Sperry, R. (1992). *Science and moral priority: Merging mind, brain, and human values.* New York: Columbia Univ. Press.

Also see:

Sperry, R. W. (1993). Psychology's mentalist paradigm and the religion/science tension. In *Brain, culture, and the human spirit: Essays from an emergent evolutionary perspective* (J. B. Ashbrook, ed.), pp. 109–128. Lanham, Md.: Univ. Press of America.

Sperry, R. W. (1984). Consciousness, personal identity and the divided brain. *Neuropsychologia* 22:661–673.

Sperry, R. W. (1986). The new mentalist paradigm and ultimate concern. *Persp. Biol. Med.* 29:413–422.

Sperry, Roger W. (1995). The riddle of consciousness and the changing scientific worldview. *J. Humanistic Psych.* 35:7–33.

8. Quotation from third book in n. 6, p. 261.

9. Eccles, J. C. (1989). *Evolution of the brain: Creation of the self.* London: Routledge.

Eccles, J. C. (1992). *The human psyche.* London: Routledge.

Eccles, J. C. (1994). *Evidence of purpose: Scientists discover the creator* (J. M. Templeton, ed.). New York: Continuum.

Eccles, J. C. (1994). *How the self controls its brain.* Berlin: Springer-Verlag.

10. Quotation from third book in n. 6, pp. 366-367.

11. This section of Eccles's book provides a critical review of all the major modern theories of consciousness, including those put forward by Crick, Dennett, Penrose, and Sperry. It is a remarkable document.

12. This creative view of how an immaterial mind may control matter was published in one of the most prestigious scientific journals in the world. See: Beck, F., & Eccles, J.C. (1992). Quantum aspects of brain activity and the role of consciousness. *Proc. Nat. Acad. Sci.,* 89:11357–11361.

13. Quotation from fourth book in n. 9, p. 180.

14. The study of neurochemical modulation of mood in normal individuals is in its infancy. For instance, recent work indicates that increased serotonin activity increases social affiliation perhaps by reducing negative affect: Knutson, B., Wolkowitz, O. W., Cole, S. W., Chan, T., Moore, E. A., Johnson, R. C., Terpstra. J., Turner, R. A.. & Reus, V. I. (1998). Serotonergic intervention selectively alters aspects of personality and social behavior in normal humans. *American Journal of Psychiatry* 155:373–379.

15. LeDoux, J. (1996). *The emotional brain.* New York: Simon and Schuster. Quotation on p. 302.

16. See chap. 15, n. 49.

Although I have tried earnestly to update relevant literature citations in the notes, work in this area is moving at a rapid pace. There would be much to incorporate from the year and a half since this manuscript was submitted to the publisher. Rather than attempt the impossible, I would like to symbolically select the one paper that I have found to be most impressive from this time period. It is a paper analyzing the cerebral consequences of social stress by Kollack-Walker, S., Watson, S. J., & Akil, H. (1997) Social stress in hamsters: Defeat activates specific neurocircuits within the brain. *J. Neurosci.* 15:8842–8855.

I select this paper partially because I have been contemplating the possible existence of a basic "DOMINANCE" system for some time, and this work provides the best evidence to date (using *cFos* in situ hybridization) concerning how such a process might be elaborated in the mammalian brain. This paper carefully analyzed genetic arousal of neural systems in dominant and submissive animals after half an hour of social confrontation/aggression using a resident-intruder paradigm in pairs of males who did not know each other well. It helps highlight for us not only the powerful effect of social submission (and FEAR) on the brain, but how much less the emotional systems of the dominant animals are aroused. The largest increase in arousal seen in the victors was in the supraoptic nucleus of the hypothalamus, where vasopressin systems are concentrated.

This paper again helps highlight for us the widespread consequences of emotional arousal within the brain (also see, chap. 11, n. 97). To some extent, such widespread effects may seem inconsistent with the existence of fairly discrete emotional systems in the brain, but such findings are, in fact, very compatible with the present thesis. The basic anatomical fact about emotional systems is that they have remarkably widespread consequences in the brain (Figure 3.3), and they also interact with many general modulatory systems (Figures 3.6, 6.5, and 6.6) of the brain. It must obviously be the case that emotions have diverse effects on the brain—for the mental consequences of emotional arousal in humans affect essentially all other brain and bodily functions. It will be a most interesting chapter of future research when we begin to dissect, anatomically and functionally, those subcomponents within the brain that lead to the final integrated psychobehavioral response.

Author Index

Subject Index

9 780195 178050